Springer Texts in Statistics

Series Editors:
G. Casella
S. Fienberg
I. Olkin

Springer Texts in Statistics

(continued after index)

Nicholas T. Longford

Studying Human Populations

An Advanced Course in Statistics

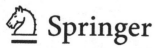 Springer

N.T. Longford
SNTL Statistics Research and Consulting, Reading
England

ISBN : 978-1-4419-3156-6   e-ISBN : 978-0-387-73251-0

To Shenki Xhadni and his sponsors

Preface

This monograph is for postgraduate students of statistics, statistical analysts, and other professionals who are interested in the design and analysis of studies in which responses are elicited from human subjects. Emphasis is placed on dealing with data that arise in imperfectly conducted studies. The reasons for imperfection include a sampling plan that cannot be implemented, measurement or elicitation of information by imperfect instruments, poor motivation of the subjects and their unwillingness to cooperate, and a multitude of other unavoidable shortcomings in relation to textbook-like settings that would be easy to analyse.

The subject of statistics is defined as making decisions in the presence of uncertainty. The context of a population and one or several variables defined for each member of this population is presented, and complete information is at first defined as having established the values of these variables for every member of the population. Making decisions with such complete information is regarded as a task outside the remit of statistics and is assumed to be a resolved problem or a problem for another profession. The raison d'être for statistics is that the available resources (time, manpower, expertise, funding, respondents' goodwill, and the like) are not sufficient for collecting the complete information.

With insufficient resources, we may establish the values of the variables for only some of the members of the population, and we may establish them imprecisely using imperfect instruments. Estimation is defined as forming a summary of the collected incomplete information (the data) with the purpose of getting as close as possible to the complete-information quantity of interest (the target). The quality of such a process (efficiency of the estimator) is described in frequentist terms by the mean squared error (MSE), defined by replications of the data-generating and estimation processes. Study design is defined generally as doing the best that can be done with the available resources. 'Doing the best' entails designing a study, implementing it (collecting the data), and estimating the target with the smallest possible MSE.

This scheme can be adapted for other forms of inference (such as confidence intervals and hypothesis tests) and measures of quality different from MSE.

The text assumes that the reader is familiar with the basics of statistics: the frequentist perspective; the definition of discrete and continuous distributions, including conditional and multivariate distributions; the concepts of independence, density, and distribution function; the common classes of distributions (normal and distributions derived from it, uniform, beta, gamma, binomial, and Poisson); sampling design and measurement process; the elementary statistical calculus (evaluating expectations and variances and fitting ordinary regression); and hypothesis testing and confidence intervals for some simple settings. This material is condensely presented in the Appendix, intended both for revision before reading Chapter 1 and for reference throughout the study. The exercises at the end of the Appendix are a suitable material for an entrance or revision exam.

Chapter 1 follows the standard curriculum of the analysis of variance and ordinary regression but parts company with the established solutions by adhering to the goals of efficient estimation and unbiased assessment of the efficiency. Chapter 2 introduces maximum likelihood as a general method of estimation, presents the basic results (without proofs), and discusses model selection and model uncertainty, issues broached in the previous chapter.

With limited resources, we can record the values of the relevant variables for only some members of the population and may have to do so imprecisely. These two forms of incompleteness lead to two general topics: survey sampling (Chapter 3) and measurement processes (Chapter 6). Between them, Chapter 4 introduces the Bayesian perspective as an alternative to the frequentist one, although it can be argued that there are three perspectives—model-based, design-based, and Bayesian, introduced in the respective Chapters 2, 3, and 4.

Chapter 5 returns to the frequentist perspective to discuss data incompleteness as a ubiquitous problem in implementing a design for studying a human population and introduces methods for dealing with missing data, data that we intended to collect but failed to. Complete information is defined here as the result of a perfectly implemented study design, a dataset that would be relatively easy to analyse. EM algorithm and multiple imputation are presented as two generic methods for dealing with incompleteness. Some other applications of these methods are outlined. In Chapter 6, imperfect measurement is presented as one of them.

Chapter 7 discusses experiments and observational studies and highlights the importance of the treatment-assignment process. Chapter 8 deals with clinical trials and presents them as a model example of experiments, emphasising the key role of their design, in the context of high ethical costs. Here, as well as in some earlier chapters, hypothesis testing is discussed, with the criticism that it fails to integrate information about the consequences (severity) of the two kinds of error that may be committed. Model selection criteria are subjected to similar criticism.

Chapters 9 and 10 discuss methods for multilevel and generalised linear models, respectively, as two indispensable elements of a statistician's analytical (computational) armoury. Chapter 11 deals with longitudinal and time-series analysis, treating them as applications of the methods presented in the previous two chapters.

Chapter 12 concludes with meta-analysis, a method for summarising the results of studies with a common or similar inferential agenda. The multivariate version of meta-analysis is discussed and connected to the problem of estimating one or several of a large number of interrelated quantities.

The chapters are designed so that they can be read or studied in order, with logical stopping points after Chapters 6, 8, and 10, which are followed by increasingly demanding material. They are intended as both a textbook for a semester, with some of the last few chapters optional, and a reference, with chapters as self-contained units. Chapters 1–8 can be covered in an academic quarter.

Several themes straddle the chapters. First among them is the view of nonstandard problems as involving missing data. That is, the problem at hand would be (more) tractable if some additional information were available. With the EM algorithm and multiple imputation, this is a natural approach to expanding the horizon of problems that we can deal with. Second is the pursuit of efficiency (small MSE) and of honesty (unbiased estimation of MSE) in estimation. Combining estimators (synthesis) is presented as an alternative to model selection, and their properties are compared in several settings, starting with the analysis of variance (ANOVA) in Chapter 1. Third is that we should be concerned with analysis of information, not merely analysis of one dataset at a time, and that study design is much more important than analysis. There is no reprieve for the deficiencies in the study design, whereas a reanalysis is a relatively inexpensive affair. The value of computing, for simulations in particular, and graphics, for effective data exploration and to summarise the results, is emphasised as a companion and, in some instances, an alternative, to (mathematical) analytical effort.

Background in elementary calculus and linear algebra is assumed, and experience in some statistical software, such as R [151] or S-plus [191], at an introductory level at least, is essential. In the spirit of object orientation, I tried to avoid subscripting whenever possible by defining suitable vectors and matrices. At a slower pace, the text could be combined with a course in R or other software for statistical analysis and graphics. Although all the computing and graphics was prepared in R, the text has very few references to R, and all the examples in the text, including simulations, can be reproduced with other software. The code used for the analyses and illustrations, mostly in the form of R functions, and the datasets for the exercises can be downloaded from www.sntl.co.uk/BookA.

Each chapter has a few references for further reading and more detailed study (for example, the monographs [168] for Chapter 3, [110] for Chapter 5, [113] for Chapter 9, [132] for Chapter 10, [37] for Chapter 11, and [72] for Chapter 12) and 16–26 exercises, some directly connected to the text of the chapter and to its examples in particular. They range in difficulty and complexity from those for solving within a few minutes to open-ended problems suitable for projects for individual or small groups of students.

I have thought hard about the notation, whether to design rules that could be used consistently throughout the book or to adhere to the conventions that are consistent within narrow subject areas represented by the chapters but not across them. For example, capital letters are used for population quantities and lowercase for sample quantities in survey sampling, whereas in linear models capital letters are used for matrices and lowercase for vectors. I have settled for the prevailing conventions, with a few exceptions. As is common, I use the same notation for a random variable (estimator, dataset) and its realisation (estimate, realised dataset), but preface the latter by the term 'value of' whenever the two might be confused. In a few instances I simply ran out of suitable symbols or wanted to stick to established conventions and had to reuse some symbols. For example, β is used for both regression parameters and the power of a selection (or a test) in Chapter 2.

I could not avoid a few forward references in the text. None of them requires a detailed study of the section referred to, and when the section is reached later, the introduction made earlier is useful because the topic is not completely new. To smooth the text, I have set aside some mathematical niceties in favour of terms that are commonly used, but strictly speaking are not correct. Thus, by continuous distribution I mean throughout absolutely continuous distribution, and every one-to-one continuous function is assumed to be monotone.

I want to thank University Pompeu Fabra (UPF), Barcelona, Spain, and other institutions for opportunities to use draft chapters of this book in my lectures. I wrote and revised most of the manuscript in 2006 at UPF. I have benefited from attending the annual Applied Statistics Weeks organised by UPF and from eye-opening lectures by Don Rubin in particular. Support for this work by grants from the Spanish Ministry of Education and Science is acknowledged. Comments and encouragement from Anna Cuxart, Albert Satorra, and Frederic Udina, my colleagues at UPF, are acknowledged.

I had a fair number of false starts and postponed deadlines, and I want to commend Springer-Verlag for its near-asymptotic patience.

Reading, England   *Nick Longford*
September 2007

Contents

ANOVA and Ordinary Regression

In this chapter, we address the standard task of learning about a process when it is observed incompletely, by means of a finite number of its realisations. We study two simple settings, analysis of variance (ANOVA) and simple regression, with the standard assumptions of normality and equal residual variance. We are interested in efficient estimation of a priori specified population quantities.

1.1 Analysis of Variance

Analysis of variance is a historical term for the setting with $K > 1$ contexts (groups) within which the studied process generates observations as random samples from normal distributions with a common variance σ_W^2 but (possibly) distinct means μ_k, $k = 1, \ldots, K$. The observations are denoted by y_{jk}, $j = 1, \ldots, n_k$, where n_k are the sample sizes within the contexts. The overall sample size is $n = n_1 + \cdots + n_K$. For simplicity, we assume that $n_1, \ldots, n_K$ are fixed (constant across replications). The setting with $n_1 = \ldots = n_K$ is referred to as *balanced*.

This description of ANOVA corresponds to the model

$$(y_{11}, y_{21}, \ldots, y_{n_1 1}, y_{12}, \ldots, y_{n_K K})^\top \sim \mathcal{N}_n \left\{ \begin{pmatrix} \mu_1 \mathbf{1}_{n_1} \\ \mu_2 \mathbf{1}_{n_2} \\ \vdots \\ \mu_K \mathbf{1}_{n_K} \end{pmatrix}, \sigma_W^2 \mathbf{I}_n \right\}. \quad (1.1)$$

The symbols $\mathbf{1}$, $\mathbf{I}$, and $\mathbf{0}$ are used for the vector of unities, the identity matrix, and the matrix of zeros; their dimensions are given in their subscripts but are omitted when they are obvious from the context. Although accurate, this description is most inelegant and uninstructive, because it does not readily convey our assumptions or beliefs about the studied process. A more instructive description is by one or several *model equations*, algebraic expressions that state how the observations (outcomes) are assumed to be related to the contexts. For the class of distributions in (1.1), one such description is

$$y_{jk} = \mu_k + \varepsilon_{jk},$$ (1.2)

where the n terms ε_{jk} are a random sample from $\mathcal{N}(0, \sigma_{\mathrm{W}}^2)$. This description is much neater and easy to interpret as follows: in context k, observations are dispersed around their context-specific mean μ_k, with independent deviations that are normally distributed with variance σ_{W}^2. Note that the small print following equation (1.2) is essential to complete the description.

We can regard the entire set of n_k observations as a single multivariate observation, $\mathbf{y}_k = (y_{1k}, \dots, y_{n_k k})^\top$, and write

$$\mathbf{y}_k = \mu_k \mathbf{1}_{n_k} + \boldsymbol{\varepsilon}_k,$$ (1.3)

where the vectors $\boldsymbol{\varepsilon}_k \sim \mathcal{N}_{n_k}\left(\mathbf{0}, \sigma_{\mathrm{W}}^2 \mathbf{I}\right)$, $k = 1, \dots, K$, are mutually independent. Such matrix notation focuses much better on the relevant without omitting any detail. For completeness, we define the vector of all observations $\mathbf{y} = (\mathbf{y}_1^\top, \dots, \mathbf{y}_K^\top)^\top$, obtained by vertical stacking of the vectors $\mathbf{y}_1, \dots, \mathbf{y}_K$.

Suppose the task is to estimate one of the means, say μ_1. An obvious solution is the sample mean of the observations made in context 1, $\hat{\mu}_1 = (y_{11} + \cdots + y_{n_1 1})/n_1 = n_1^{-1} \mathbf{y}_1^\top \mathbf{1}$. As $\hat{\mu}_1 \sim \mathcal{N}(\mu_1, \sigma_{\mathrm{W}}^2/n_1)$, $\hat{\mu}_1$ is unbiased. More information, in the form of greater sample size n_1 in context 1, is rewarded by smaller sampling variance. However, $\hat{\mu}_1$ ignores all the remaining $n - n_1$ observations.

If the within-context distributions were identical, $\mu_1 = \dots = \mu_K = \mu$, the context would be irrelevant and $\mu_1 = \mu$ would be estimated much more efficiently by $\hat{\mu} = n^{-1} \mathbf{y}^\top \mathbf{1}$. Like $\hat{\mu}_1$, $\hat{\mu}$ would also be unbiased, but its variance, σ_{W}^2/n, would be much smaller than $\mathrm{var}(\hat{\mu}_1) = \sigma_{\mathrm{W}}^2/n_1$, unless n_1 is a substantial fraction of n. In the long established approach, the hypothesis that the context is irrelevant is tested, and if this (null-)hypothesis of equal means, $\mu_1 = \dots = \mu_K$, is rejected, μ_1 is estimated by $\hat{\mu}_1$. Otherwise, having failed to find evidence against the hypothesis, μ_1 is estimated by $\hat{\mu}$. Hypothesis testing is discussed in greater detail in Chapter 2; here we use it merely as a means of choosing between two models.

This approach is flawed because failure to reject the null-hypothesis is confused with confirming it. Failure to reject should be interpreted as 'do not know whether ...', as a state of ignorance. Not only hypothesis testing, but any other approach that commits us to either the assumption that $\mu_1 = \dots = \mu_K = \mu$ or its alternative ('not all means are equal') is also deficient unless the choice made is unfailingly correct; that is, hypothetical replications of the process generating the observations $\mathbf{y}$ would also yield the same decision, and this decision would be correct. In one perspective, the decision is obvious. Since the equality of the means, $\mu_1 = \dots = \mu_K$, is an extremely special case, we can safely bet that the means differ, especially when we have no prior information why they should not, at least by a little bit.

Another deficiency of the commitment to a model can be illustrated by the following comparison. Consider two scenarios, both with the same overall sample size $n = 100$. In the first, the sample size of context 1 is $n_1 = 2$ and in the other $n_1 = 80$. In the first scenario, the two observations of context 1 tell us very little about μ_1; $\text{var}(\hat{\mu}_1) = \frac{1}{2}\sigma_W^2$ is large, yet there may be a lot of information in the $n - n_1 = 98$ observations from the other contexts that could contribute to estimating μ_1. If the means μ_k are equal, $\hat{\mu}$ is very efficient, since $\text{var}(\hat{\mu}) = \sigma_W^2/100$ is 50 times smaller than $\text{var}(\hat{\mu}_1)$. In the second scenario, $\text{var}(\hat{\mu}_1) = \sigma_W^2/80$ is much smaller, and there is no urgency to improve on $\hat{\mu}_1$, since the best that we might achieve is that the mean squared error (MSE) would be equal to $\sigma_W^2/100$, a reduction by a mere 20%. Thus, our eagerness to estimate μ_1 by $\hat{\mu}$ should be informed by the sample size n_1. However, the hypothesis test treats all the sample sizes $n_1, \ldots, n_K$ symmetrically and implies the same decision regarding estimation of each mean μ_k, irrespective of its sample size.

When we nonetheless make, with uncertainty, a decision as to whether or not the context is irrelevant, we estimate μ_1 by neither $\hat{\mu}_1$ nor $\hat{\mu}$, but by

$$\hat{\mu}_1^\dagger = (1 - \mathcal{I})\,\hat{\mu}_1 + \mathcal{I}\hat{\mu},$$

where $\mathcal{I}$ indicates failure to reject the null-hypothesis; $\mathcal{I} = 0$ if we reject it, and $\mathcal{I} = 1$ otherwise. The distribution of this estimator is neither $\mathcal{N}(\mu_1, \sigma_W^2/n_1)$ nor $\mathcal{N}(\mu_1, \sigma_W^2/n)$; in fact, it is not normal, not even symmetric, except in some esoteric settings. Certainly, $\hat{\mu}_1^\dagger$ is biased, and its variance or MSE are equal to neither σ_W^2/n_1 nor σ_W^2/n.

In the established approach, the within-group (population) variance σ_W^2 is estimated, and the sampling variance of $\hat{\mu}_1^\dagger$ is estimated by $\hat{s}_1^2 = \hat{\sigma}_W^2/n_1$ or $\hat{s}^2 = \hat{\sigma}_W^2/n$, depending on the decision made as a result of hypothesis testing. This estimator of the sampling variance is

$$\hat{s}_1^{2\,\dagger} = (1 - \mathcal{I})\,\hat{s}_1^2 + \mathcal{I}\hat{s}^2$$

and is a very inefficient and biased estimator of MSE $\left(\hat{\mu}_1^\dagger\,;\,\mu_1\right)$ or of var $\left(\hat{\mu}_1^\dagger\right)$. It underestimates the MSE, often severely so. Details are postponed until Chapter 2.

The cause of all the problems described in this example is *model uncertainty*; if we knew which model applies we could estimate μ_1 more efficiently. By ignoring model uncertainty, we conclude with an inferential statement that generates an impression of relative certainty that is not justified. By the a priori made assumption, the more general model applies, but we were hoping to do better by reducing the range of plausible distributions or by narrowing the associated parameter space.

1.1.1 Synthetic Estimation

The solution to the problem of estimating μ_1 in an ANOVA setting rests not in committing ourselves to one of the estimators, $\hat{\mu}_1$ or $\hat{\mu}$, depending on a fallible criterion, however well it may be devised. Instead, we explore how the relative strengths of the two estimators can be exploited more fully.

We consider the combinations

$$\tilde{\mu}_1 = (1 - b_1)\,\hat{\mu}_1 + b_1\hat{\mu}, \tag{1.4}$$

with a constant b_1 that is specific to estimating μ_1, more completely denoted as b_{μ_1}. We select this coefficient to further our aim of efficient estimation of μ_1. For estimating the mean for a different context or for estimating another quantity, we may choose a different coefficient. The MSE of $\tilde{\mu}_1$ is

$$\mathrm{MSE}(\tilde{\mu}_1;\,\mu_1) = \mathrm{var}(\tilde{\mu}_1) + \{\mathrm{B}(\tilde{\mu}_1;\,\mu_1)\}^2$$

$$= (1 - b_1)^2\frac{\sigma_{\mathrm{W}}^2}{n_1} + b^2\frac{\sigma_{\mathrm{W}}^2}{n} + 2b_1(1 - b_1)\,\mathrm{cov}(\hat{\mu}_1,\hat{\mu}) + b_1^2(\mu - \mu_1)^2;$$

$\mathrm{B}(\hat{\eta},\eta)$ denotes the bias of $\hat{\eta}$ as an estimator of the target η. Further,

$$\mathrm{cov}(\hat{\mu}_1,\hat{\mu}) = \frac{n_1}{n}\,\mathrm{var}(\hat{\mu}_1) = \frac{\sigma_{\mathrm{W}}^2}{n},$$

derived from the fact that $\hat{\mu} = (n_1\hat{\mu}_1 + \cdots + n_K\hat{\mu}_K)/n$ is a sum of mutually independent contributions from the contexts. Therefore

$$\mathrm{MSE}(\tilde{\mu}_1;\,\mu_1) = b_1^2\left\{g_1\sigma_{\mathrm{W}}^2 + (\mu_1 - \mu)^2\right\} - 2b_1g_1\sigma_{\mathrm{W}}^2 + \frac{\sigma_{\mathrm{W}}^2}{n_1}, \tag{1.5}$$

where $g_1 = 1/n_1 - 1/n$. This is a quadratic function of b_1, with a positive quadratic coefficient, so it has a unique minimum, attained for

$$b_1^* = \frac{g_1\sigma_{\mathrm{W}}^2}{g_1\sigma_{\mathrm{W}}^2 + (\mu_1 - \mu)^2}. \tag{1.6}$$

The MSE of $\tilde{\mu}_1$ with this coefficient is

$$\mathrm{MSE}\left\{\tilde{\mu}_1(b_1^*);\,\mu_1\right\} = \frac{\sigma_{\mathrm{W}}^2}{n_1} - \frac{\left(g_1\sigma_{\mathrm{W}}^2\right)^2}{g_1\sigma_{\mathrm{W}}^2 + (\mu_1 - \mu)^2}. \tag{1.7}$$

We have added the argument b_1^* to the estimator $\tilde{\mu}_1$ to distinguish it from $\tilde{\mu}_1(b)$ based on some other (suboptimal) coefficient b.

At first, this development seems to lead us nowhere because we can set the coefficient b_1 in (1.4) to its optimal value only when we know the target μ_1 itself, or at least its deviation from μ. However, suppose prior information about the contexts allows us to assume that the absolute deviation $|\mu_1 - \mu|$

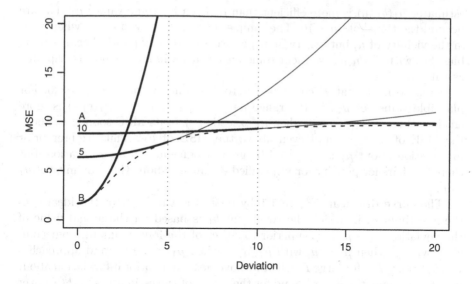

Fig. 1.1. The MSEs of the estimators of μ_1 as functions of the deviation $\mu_1 - \mu$. The estimators are $\hat{\mu}_1$, marked as A; $\hat{\mu}$, marked as B; and $\tilde{\mu}_1(b_{1,r})$ for $\Gamma = 10$ and $\Gamma = 5$, marked as 10 and 5, respectively. The MSE of the ideal synthetic estimator is drawn by dashes. Based on the setting $\sigma_W^2 = 100$, $n_1 = 10$, and $n = 60$.

does not exceed a certain threshold Γ. We will use $\tilde{\mu}_1$ with the coefficient b_1 that is optimal when $\mu_1 = \mu \pm \Gamma$ and then assess the loss of efficiency arising from the fact that μ_1 is closer to μ.

Denote by $b_{1,\Gamma}$ the coefficient b_1 that would be optimal if $|\mu_1 - \mu| = \Gamma$; it is obtained by substituting Γ^2 for $(\mu_1 - \mu)^2$ in (1.6). For this coefficient, the identity in (1.5) yields

$$\mathrm{MSE}\{\tilde{\mu}_1(b_{1,\Gamma}); \mu_1\} = \left(\frac{g_1\sigma_W^2}{g_1\sigma_W^2 + \Gamma^2}\right)^2 \{g_1\sigma_W^2 + (\mu_1 - \mu)^2\} - \frac{2\left(g_1\sigma_W^2\right)^2}{g_1\sigma_W^2 + \Gamma^2} + \frac{\sigma_W^2}{n_1}.$$
(1.8)

This is an increasing linear function of the squared distance $(\mu_1 - \mu)^2$. For the largest plausible distance, when $|\mu_1 - \mu| = \Gamma$, the MSE reaches its maximum, and yet, among the combinations in (1.4), $\tilde{\mu}_1(b_{1,\Gamma})$ is efficient for μ_1.

Figure 1.1 gives an illustration for the following setting: $\sigma_W^2 = 100$, $n_1 = 10$, $n = 60$, and $\Gamma = 10$. As the MSE of $\tilde{\mu}_1(b_{1,\Gamma})$ depends on μ_1 only through its (absolute) deviation from μ, it suffices to explore its MSE for $\mu_1 > \mu$. As a reference, we use the two originally considered estimators, $\hat{\mu}_1$ and $\hat{\mu}$; their MSEs are marked in the diagram by the respective symbols 'A' and 'B'. The former is unbiased and its sampling variance is constant, equal to $\sigma_W^2/n_1 = 10$. Unbiasedness offers little comfort when the variance is so large, exceeding $\mathrm{MSE}\{\tilde{\mu}_1(b_{1,10})\}$, marked as '10', for any plausible value of μ_1. The estimator $\tilde{\mu}_1(b_{1,10})$ is more efficient than $\hat{\mu}_1$ even for some values μ_1 that are beyond the threshold $\mu + 10$. The sample mean $\hat{\mu}$ is very efficient when μ_1 is in the vicinity of μ, but otherwise it performs extremely poorly because of its bias. So, with $\tilde{\mu}_1(b_{1,10})$ we incur some bias, but its impact is not as crippling as with $\hat{\mu}$.

Suppose next that Γ could be set to a smaller value, say, $\Gamma' = 5$. For plausible values of μ_1, in the range $\mu - 5 \leq \mu_1 \leq \mu + 5$, $\tilde{\mu}_1(b_{1,5})$ is more efficient than $\tilde{\mu}_1(b_{1,10})$, but when μ_1 exceeds $\mu + 5$, its MSE soon rises above the MSE of $\tilde{\mu}_1(b_{1,10})$ and even above the MSE of $\hat{\mu}_1$. Thus, tighter prior information about μ_1 is rewarded by greater efficiency in its estimation, but there is a harsher penalty for unjustified optimism about the proximity of μ_1 to μ.

The curve drawn in Figure 1.1 by dashes is the MSE of the ideal synthetic estimator, in which the coefficient b_1 is based on the actual value of the deviation $\mu_1 - \mu$. It is superior to either of the four estimators but coincides with $\hat{\mu}$ when $\mu_1 = \mu$, with $\tilde{\mu}_1(b_{1,\Gamma})$ when $\mu_1 = \mu \pm \Gamma$, and approaches $\mathrm{var}(\hat{\mu}_1) = \sigma_{\mathrm{W}}^2/n_1$ for large Γ, when we have next to no prior information about μ_1. It represents the lower bound for the MSEs of the estimators $\tilde{\mu}_1(b_{1,\Gamma})$ over all values of Γ. It is also the lower bound for the MSEs of all the synthetic estimators $\tilde{\mu}_1(\hat{b}_1)$, because with uncertainty about b_1 we could not possibly estimate μ_1 more efficiently than when the value of b_1 is known.

Our final point of criticism of model selection is that, in a flawed perspective that ignores model uncertainty, it aims to match the better of the alternative estimators $\hat{\mu}_1$ and $\hat{\mu}$. With the synthetic estimator $\tilde{\mu}_1$, we set our sights higher, aiming to outperform both estimators. Admittedly, we fail to achieve this goal, but we fail in scenarios in which improvement is least necessary (small distance of μ_1 from μ) and rule out disasters that may be brought on by selecting an inappropriate model.

Estimated Coefficient

The optimal coefficient b_1^* depends on σ_{W}^2 and, more disconcertingly, on the target μ_1 itself. So, when we are not willing to commit ourselves to a threshold Γ, we face a circular problem. If we knew μ_1, we could set b_1 to estimate μ_1 efficiently. We are less concerned with the uncertainty about σ_{W}^2, because all n observations contribute to its estimation. In contrast, only n_1 observations from group 1 provide direct information for estimating μ_1.

A remedy is to estimate the coefficient b_1^*, and the obvious estimator replaces the unknown parameters σ_{W}^2, μ, and μ_1 by their estimates,

$$\hat{b}_1^* = \frac{g_1}{g_1 + \dfrac{(\hat{\mu}_1 - \hat{\mu})^2}{\hat{\sigma}_{\mathrm{W}}^2}} . \tag{1.9}$$

(Such an estimator is called *naive*.) We could have estimated $(\mu_1 - \mu)^2$ by zero, assuming the null-hypothesis, but this would not be rational as it is the smallest possible value of a square. That would be a poor response to our uncertainty about the deviation $|\mu_1 - \mu|$. Another alternative might be to correct $(\hat{\mu}_1 - \hat{\mu})^2$ for its bias in estimating $(\mu_1 - \mu)^2$. We have

$$\mathrm{E}\left\{(\hat{\mu}_1 - \hat{\mu})^2\right\} = (\mu_1 - \mu)^2 + \mathrm{var}\,(\hat{\mu}_1 - \hat{\mu})$$
$$= (\mu_1 - \mu)^2 + g_1 \sigma_{\mathrm{W}}^2 .$$

Hence, $(\hat{\mu}_1 - \hat{\mu})^2 - g_1 \hat{\sigma}_{\mathrm{W}}^2$ is unbiased for $(\mu_1 - \mu)^2$, so long as $\hat{\sigma}_{\mathrm{W}}^2$ is unbiased for σ_{W}^2. The resulting estimator of b_1^* is $\hat{b}_1^* = g_1/(\hat{\mu}_1 - \hat{\mu})^2$. Whereas $0 < b_1^* \leq 1$, $\hat{b}_1^*$ can attain values greater than 1.0. Then $\tilde{\mu}_1(\hat{b}_1^*) = (1 - \hat{b}_1^*)\hat{\mu}_1 + \hat{b}_1^* \hat{\mu}$ would accord negative weight to $\hat{\mu}_1$, contradicting common sense. Bias adjustment does not seem to improve estimation of μ_1. In any case, even when σ_{W}^2 is estimated by $\hat{\sigma}_{\mathrm{W}}^2$ without bias, the reciprocal, $1/\sigma_{\mathrm{W}}^2$ is estimated by $1/\hat{\sigma}_{\mathrm{W}}^2$ with bias, although the bias is small when $\mathrm{var}\,(\hat{\sigma}_{\mathrm{W}}^2)$ is small. A more fruitful avenue to improving the synthetic estimator $\tilde{\mu}_1$ is by reducing the impact of the uncertainty about $(\mu_1 - \mu)^2$ and estimating b_1^* by

$$\hat{b}_1^* = \frac{g_1}{g_1 + r \dfrac{(\hat{\mu}_1 - \hat{\mu})^2}{\hat{\sigma}_{\mathrm{W}}^2}} ,$$

with a positive factor $r < 1$.

Yet another approach replaces $(\mu_1 - \mu)^2$ in (1.9) with the variance of the context-level means, $\sigma_{\mathrm{B}}^2 = \frac{1}{K} \sum_k (\mu_k - \bar{\mu})^2$, where $\bar{\mu} = (\mu_1 + \cdots + \mu_K)/K$ is the mean of the context-level means. When this variance is not known, an estimate is used instead. The rationale for this approach is that the *context-level* variance σ_{B}^2 may in some settings be known or an intelligent guess of its value can be made. Observations from all contexts k with $n_k > 1$ contribute to any reasonable estimator of σ_{B}^2, so σ_{B}^2 can be estimated with greater precision than $(\mu_1 - \mu)^2$. In effect, we replace $(\mu_1 - \mu)^2$ or its estimate with (an estimate of) the average of $(\mu_k - \mu)^2$ over the contexts k. It is preferable to err on the side of positive bias in estimating σ_{B}^2. By overstating σ_{B}^2 we reduce the coefficient b_1, and therefore assign more weight to $\hat{\mu}_1$ in $\tilde{\mu}_1$, weighing more in favour of unbiased estimation over variance reduction.

1.2 Ordinary Regression

Regression is defined as the conditional expectation $\mathrm{E}(Y \mid X = x)$ of a variable Y, regarded as a function of the value of another variable (covariate) X in the condition. The value x of covariate X can be regarded as a *stimulus* that results in a particular distribution of the outcomes Y. This description motivates the general model that assumes that the values of the covariate X are set, by the analyst's *design* (intent), to $x_1, \ldots, x_n$, and the resulting values of the *outcome variable* Y are observed; these outcomes are denoted as $y_1, \ldots, y_n$.

The outcomes are subject to uncertainty (variation in hypothetical replications). A general model for this setting is

$$(y_j \mid x_j) \sim \mathcal{D}\left\{f(x_j); g(x_j)\right\},\qquad(1.10)$$

independently, where $\mathcal{D}$ denotes a class of distributions specified by expectation $f(x)$ and variance $g(x)$. Important features of this model are that the outcomes are independent (autonomous) and the impact of the stimulus X is isolated to the associated observation; the stimulus set for observation j exerts no influence on $y_{j'}$ for any $j' \neq j$. The model in (1.10) can be generalised by including further arguments in $\mathcal{D}$, all of them dependent only on x_j, by defining more complex stimuli that combine several variables, and by allowing some form of dependence among the outcomes.

All this is an agenda for later. Here we focus on a substantial simplification of the model in (1.10), which is nevertheless of central importance in statistics. First, we assume that the variance is constant; that is, $g(x_j) = \sigma^2$ for every j. This property is called *homoscedasticity*. Next, we assume that f is a linear function; $f(x_j) = \beta_0 + \beta_1 x_j$. And finally, we assume that the distribution $\mathcal{D}$ is normal.

Thus, the model we consider is

$$y_j \sim \mathcal{N}(\beta_0 + \beta_1 x_j, \sigma^2),\qquad(1.11)$$

independently. This is equivalent to the model equation

$$y_j = \beta_0 + \beta_1 x_j + \varepsilon_j,$$

where ε_j, $j = 1, \ldots, n$, are a random sample from $\mathcal{N}(0, \sigma^2)$. The following matrix notation is very useful: let $\mathbf{x} = (x_1, \ldots, x_n)^\top$, $\mathbf{y} = (y_1, \ldots, y_n)^\top$, and $\boldsymbol{\beta} = (\beta_0, \beta_1)^\top$. Further, we define $\mathbf{X}$ as the $n \times 2$ matrix composed of the columns $\mathbf{1}_n$ and $\mathbf{x}$. Now

$$\mathbf{y} = \mathbf{X}\boldsymbol{\beta} + \boldsymbol{\varepsilon}$$

and $\boldsymbol{\varepsilon} \sim \mathcal{N}_n(\mathbf{0}, \sigma^2\mathbf{I})$. The linear function $\beta_0 + \beta_1 x$ is called the regression (function or line) and σ^2 is referred to as the *residual variance*. The parameters β_0 and β_1 are called the *intercept* and *slope*, respectively, and collectively they are referred to as the *regression parameters*. The model with linear regression and the assumptions of normality and homoscedasticity is called the *ordinary regression* model.

It is straightforward to generate an example by simulation. Such an example is presented in the left-hand panel of Figure 1.2, generated by setting the values of X on the grid of points 1.0, 1.1, ..., 2.9, 3.0 and repeating each value three times. More difficult is the task of locating the regression line when all we have are the vectors $\mathbf{x}$ and $\mathbf{y}$. This problem is presented in the right-hand panel.

A well-motivated approach is to estimate the regression (or *fit a regression*) by a line from which the points have the smallest possible total of their distances. There are several analytical advantages when this proposal is altered

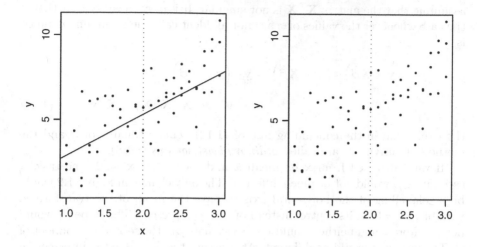

Fig. 1.2. Data $(\mathbf{x}, \mathbf{y})$ generated according to the regression model $y = \beta_0 + \beta_1 x + \varepsilon$, with $\beta_0 = 0.5$, $\beta_1 = 2.4$, and $\varepsilon \sim \mathcal{N}(0, 3)$. The right-hand panel is a copy of the left-hand panel with the regression line removed.

to minimising the total of the squared distances and measuring the distances vertically. That is, we minimise the sum of squares

$$(\mathbf{y} - \mathbf{X}\boldsymbol{\beta})^\top (\mathbf{y} - \mathbf{X}\boldsymbol{\beta}) = \sum_{j=1}^{n} (y_j - \beta_0 - \beta_1 x_j)^2.$$

We prefer to work with the expression on the left-hand side because it is easier to generalise, it relegates the indexing to the small print and is typographically more convenient. We find the minimum of this expression either by completing the square,

$$(\mathbf{y} - \mathbf{X}\boldsymbol{\beta})^\top (\mathbf{y} - \mathbf{X}\boldsymbol{\beta})$$
$$= \left\{ \boldsymbol{\beta} - (\mathbf{X}^\top \mathbf{X})^{-1} \mathbf{X}^\top \mathbf{y} \right\}^\top \mathbf{X}^\top \mathbf{X} \left\{ \boldsymbol{\beta} - (\mathbf{X}^\top \mathbf{X})^{-1} \mathbf{X}^\top \mathbf{y} \right\}$$
$$+ \mathbf{y}^\top \mathbf{y} - \mathbf{y}^\top \mathbf{X} (\mathbf{X}^\top \mathbf{X})^{-1} \mathbf{X}^\top \mathbf{y}, \tag{1.12}$$

or, more elegantly, by matrix differentiation,

$$-\frac{1}{2} \frac{\partial}{\partial \boldsymbol{\beta}} \left\{ (\mathbf{y} - \mathbf{X}\boldsymbol{\beta})^\top (\mathbf{y} - \mathbf{X}\boldsymbol{\beta}) \right\} = \mathbf{X}^\top (\mathbf{y} - \mathbf{X}\boldsymbol{\beta}).$$

Either way we obtain the unique solution

$$\hat{\boldsymbol{\beta}} = (\mathbf{X}^\top \mathbf{X})^{-1} \mathbf{X}^\top \mathbf{y}, \tag{1.13}$$

assuming that the matrix $\mathbf{X}^\top\mathbf{X}$ is not singular. It is easy to verify that that is the case whenever the values of x are not all identical. The minimum attained is

$$\left(\mathbf{y} - \mathbf{X}\hat{\beta}\right)^\top \left(\mathbf{y} - \mathbf{X}\hat{\beta}\right) = \mathbf{y}^\top \left(\mathbf{y} - \mathbf{X}\hat{\beta}\right)$$
$$= \mathbf{y}^\top\mathbf{y} - \mathbf{y}^\top\mathbf{X}\left(\mathbf{X}^\top\mathbf{X}\right)^{-1}\mathbf{X}^\top\mathbf{y}, \qquad (1.14)$$

the expression in the concluding line of (1.12). This estimator of β and the method of deriving it are called *ordinary least squares* (OLS).

If we subtracted from $\mathbf{x}$ its mean $\bar{x}$ and used $\mathbf{x}^\circ = \mathbf{x} - \bar{x}\mathbf{1}$, the task of estimating β would not be much different. The only change in Figure 1.2 would be a relabelling of the horizontal axis to have the mean of the transformed variable, $\bar{x}^\circ = 0$, in its centre, instead of $\bar{x} = 2$ at present. The slope $\hat{\beta}_1$ would not be altered, and neither would be its estimate $\hat{\beta}_1$, the second component of $\hat{\beta}$. The intercept would be different. At present, it is $\beta_0 = 0.5$, the intersection of the regression line with the vertical axis. With $\mathbf{x}^\circ$, it would be equal to its value at $x = 2$, that is, $0.5 + 2 \times 2.4 = 5.3$.

One advantage of using $\mathbf{x}^\circ$ is that $\mathbf{x}^{\circ\top}\mathbf{1} = 0$, and so the corresponding matrix or crossproducts $\mathbf{X}^{\circ\top}\mathbf{X}^\circ$, required in (1.13), is diagonal:

$$\mathbf{X}^{\circ\top}\mathbf{X}^\circ = \begin{pmatrix} n & 0 \\ 0 & \mathbf{x}^{\circ\top}\mathbf{x}^\circ \end{pmatrix}.$$

Hence $\hat{\beta}_0^\circ = \bar{y}$ and $\hat{\beta}_1 = \mathbf{x}^{\circ\top}\mathbf{y}/(\mathbf{x}^{\circ\top}\mathbf{x}^\circ)$. The circle $^\circ$ in the superscript of β_0 and $\hat{\beta}_0$ indicates the association with $\mathbf{x}^\circ$. Apart from obtaining the estimates without having to invert any matrix, these expressions help us to establish a connection with the regression as defined originally. The estimator of the slope is

$$\hat{\beta}_1 = \frac{(\mathbf{x} - \bar{x}\mathbf{1})^\top(\mathbf{y} - \bar{y}\mathbf{1})}{n} \frac{n}{(\mathbf{x} - \bar{x}\mathbf{1})^\top(\mathbf{x} - \bar{x}\mathbf{1})}$$
$$= \frac{\widehat{\mathrm{cov}}(X,Y)}{\widehat{\mathrm{var}}(X)},$$

where the wide circumflex $^\frown$ indicates naive estimation.

The population version of the regression is defined as $\mathrm{E}(Y \mid X = x)$. When (X, Y) have the bivariate normal distribution,

$$\mathrm{E}(Y \mid X = x) = \mathrm{E}(Y) + \frac{\mathrm{cov}(X,Y)}{\mathrm{var}(X)}\{X - \mathrm{E}(X)\},$$

so the regression is linear, with slope $\beta_1 = \mathrm{cov}(X,Y)/\mathrm{var}(X)$ and intercept $\beta_0 = \mathrm{E}(Y) - \beta_1\mathrm{E}(X)$. Thus, the two meanings of the term 'regression', as a population and a sample quantity, are in agreement.

The conditional variance,

$$\text{var}(Y \mid X = x) = \text{var}(Y) - \frac{\{\text{cov}(X, Y)\}^2}{\text{var}(X)},$$

coincides with the residual variance $\sigma^2 = \text{var}(\varepsilon)$, and the minimum derived in (1.14) is closely related to it; it is a naive estimator of the n-multiple of $\text{var}(Y \mid X = x)$:

$$\hat{\sigma}_\dagger^2 = \frac{1}{n} \mathbf{e}^\top \mathbf{e}, \tag{1.15}$$

where $\mathbf{e} = \mathbf{y} - \mathbf{X}\hat{\beta}$ is the vector of *residuals*. These should not be confused with the model deviations $\varepsilon = \mathbf{y} - \mathbf{X}\beta$ but can be regarded as their estimates in a peculiar form of replications in which $\hat{\beta}$ varies according to its sampling distribution but the same ε_j is realised every time for the target observation j.

The regression parameter estimator $\hat{\beta}$ is unbiased:

$$\text{E}\left(\hat{\beta}\right) = \left(\mathbf{X}^\top \mathbf{X}\right)^{-1} \mathbf{X}^\top \text{E}(\mathbf{y}) = \beta,$$

since $\text{E}(\mathbf{y}) = \mathbf{X}\beta$, and its variance (and MSE) matrix is

$$\text{var}\left(\hat{\beta}\right) = \left(\mathbf{X}^\top \mathbf{X}\right)^{-1} \mathbf{X}^\top \sigma^2 \mathbf{I}_n \mathbf{X} \left(\mathbf{X}^\top \mathbf{X}\right)^{-1} = \sigma^2 \left(\mathbf{X}^\top \mathbf{X}\right)^{-1};$$

it can be estimated without bias by substituting for σ^2 an unbiased estimator $\hat{\sigma}^2$ of σ^2.

Estimating the Residual Variance

The estimator $\hat{\sigma}_\dagger^2$ defined in (1.15) is biased for σ^2. To show it, denote $\mathbf{P}_X = \mathbf{X} \left(\mathbf{X}^\top \mathbf{X}\right)^{-1} \mathbf{X}^\top$ and $\mathbf{Q}_X = \mathbf{I} - \mathbf{P}_X$; $\mathbf{P}_X$ is called the *projection matrix*. It is *idempotent*; that is, $\mathbf{P}_X^2 = \mathbf{P}_X$. The matrix $\mathbf{Q}_X$ is also idempotent. Further, $\mathbf{Q}_X$ is orthogonal to $\mathbf{X}$,

$$\mathbf{Q}_X \mathbf{X} = \mathbf{0}.$$

More generally, $\mathbf{Q}_X$ is orthogonal to any matrix that is premultiplied by $\mathbf{X}$; we say that it is orthogonal to the regression space (spanned by $\mathbf{X}$). All the eigenvalues of $\mathbf{P}_X$ and $\mathbf{Q}_X$ are either equal to zero or unity. This is obvious when we realise that the eigenvalues of $\mathbf{P}_X$ and $\mathbf{P}_X^2$ have to coincide, so they have to be the squares of themselves. With this background, we are ready for the following sequence of identities:

$$\text{E}\left(\hat{\sigma}_\dagger^2\right) = \frac{1}{n} \text{E}\left(\mathbf{y}^\top \mathbf{Q}_X \mathbf{y}\right)$$

$$= \frac{1}{n} \text{tr}\left\{\mathbf{Q}_X \text{E}\left(\mathbf{y}\mathbf{y}^\top\right)\right\}$$

$$= \frac{1}{n} \sigma^2 \text{tr}(\mathbf{Q}_X) + \text{tr}\left(\mathbf{Q}_X \mathbf{X}\beta\beta^\top \mathbf{X}^\top\right),$$

using first the identity $\text{tr}(\mathbf{AB}) = \text{tr}(\mathbf{BA})$ for any conformable matrices $\mathbf{A}$ and $\mathbf{B}$, then the commutative property of the expectation and linear operations, $\text{E}\{\text{tr}(\mathbf{CU})\} = \mathbf{C}\,\text{tr}\{\text{E}(\mathbf{U})\}$ for any random matrix $\mathbf{U}$ and a conformable matrix of constants $\mathbf{C}$, followed by the identity $\text{E}(\mathbf{yy}^\top) = \text{var}(\mathbf{y}) + \text{E}(\mathbf{y})\{\text{E}(\mathbf{y})\}^\top$. The second term in the concluding expression vanishes because $\mathbf{Q_X X} = \mathbf{0}$, and

$$\text{tr}(\mathbf{I} - \mathbf{P_X}) = n - \text{tr}(\mathbf{I}_2) = n - 2\,.$$

Hence $\text{E}(\hat{\sigma}_{\dagger}^2) = \sigma^2(n-2)/n$, and an unbiased estimator of σ^2 is obtained by reducing the denominator in $\hat{\sigma}_{\dagger}^2$ from n to $n-2$:

$$\hat{\sigma}^2 = \frac{1}{n-2}\,\mathbf{e}^\top\mathbf{e}\,. \tag{1.16}$$

This is the estimator of choice by the vast majority of analysts. However, the appropriateness of this choice depends on how $\hat{\sigma}^2$ is going to be used. Often it appears in the denominator of a ratio of independent unbiased estimators, $\hat{\sigma}_A^2/\hat{\sigma}^2$, of two unrelated variances σ_A^2 and σ^2. This ratio is biased for the ratio of the targets, σ_A^2/σ^2, because

$$\text{E}\left(\frac{\hat{\sigma}_A^2}{\hat{\sigma}^2}\right) = \text{E}\left(\sigma_A^2\right)\text{E}\left(\frac{1}{\hat{\sigma}^2}\right)$$

and $\text{E}(1/\hat{\sigma}^2) \neq 1/\sigma^2$. The property of no bias is lost by the nonlinear transformation. We postpone efficient estimation of σ^2 and $1/\sigma^2$ to Section 2.3. The '2' in $n-2$ is referred to as the two *degrees of freedom* lost due to not knowing the values of β_0 and β_1. If one of the regression parameters, say β_1, were known, σ^2 would be estimated without bias by (1.16), with $\mathbf{e} = \mathbf{y} - \hat{\beta}_0 - \beta_1\mathbf{x}$, but with the divisor $n-1$. If both β_0 and β_1 were known, $\mathbf{e}$ would be equal to $\boldsymbol{\varepsilon}$, and $\boldsymbol{\varepsilon}^\top\boldsymbol{\varepsilon}/n$ would estimate σ^2 without bias.

1.2.1 Prediction

A frequent task associated with ordinary regression is to estimate the value of the outcome y in response to a specific stimulus x^*. In the usual setting that motivates this problem, the process generating the values of y is triggered by the values $x_1, \ldots, x_n$, at each turn independently from the previous outcomes y, conditionally on the values of x. We would like to anticipate the value of y that would be observed when the process is set off next time, with the value $x_{n+1} = x^*$. Hence the commonly used term *prediction* for this problem, although it is equivalent to estimating the linear combination $\mathbf{x}^*\boldsymbol{\beta}$ of the regression parameters for $\mathbf{x}^* = (1, x^*)$.

It may seem that the problem is solved because $\hat{y} = \mathbf{x}^*\hat{\boldsymbol{\beta}}$ is a suitable *predictor* of the outcome in response to x^*. It is unbiased, as $\text{E}(\hat{y}) = \mathbf{x}^*\boldsymbol{\beta}$, and its variance is

$$\mathrm{var}(\hat{y}) = \sigma^2 \mathbf{x}^* \left(\mathbf{X}^\top \mathbf{X}\right)^{-1} \mathbf{x}^{*\top}$$

$$= \frac{\sigma^2}{n} + \frac{\sigma^2}{S_\mathrm{x}} (x^* - \bar{x})^2 , \tag{1.17}$$

where $S_\mathrm{x} = \sum_{j=1}^{n}(x_j - \bar{x})^2$ is the corrected sum of squares of the stimuli applied thus far. For the identity in (1.17) we used the centred parameterisation (from x to $x^\circ = x - \bar{x}$), for which $\mathbf{X}^{\circ\top}\mathbf{X}^\circ$ is diagonal. Note that in addition to the sampling (or prediction) variance in (1.17) the anticipated outcome y is associated with the residual variance σ^2, which is inherent to the studied process. The sampling variance can be reduced by increasing n and S_x, but σ^2 is a source of uncertainty that cannot be affected, because prior to applying the stimulus x^* we have no information about the next deviation ε^*.

The predictor $\hat{y} = \mathbf{x}\hat{\boldsymbol{\beta}}$ can be improved. If the slope β_1 were equal to zero, the sample mean of the outcomes, $\bar{y}$, would be more efficient, because its bias would be $\mathrm{B}(\bar{y}; x^*\boldsymbol{\beta}) = 0$ and $\mathrm{var}(\bar{y}) = \sigma^2/n$. The difficulty is that we cannot establish whether $\beta_1 = 0$. In any case, the bias incurred by using $\bar{y}$ when β_1 is not zero, but not very large in absolute value, may be more than compensated by the variance reduction, equal to $\sigma^2(x^* - \bar{x})^2/S_\mathrm{x}$; see (1.17).

To find the more efficient of the predictors $\bar{y}$ and $\hat{y}$ of $\mathbf{x}^*\boldsymbol{\beta}$, we compare the two estimators, assuming the linear regression model in (1.11). We have

$$\mathrm{MSE}\,(\bar{y}; x^*\boldsymbol{\beta}) = \frac{\sigma^2}{n} + \beta_1^2(x^* - \bar{x})^2 ,$$

so (1.17) implies that $\bar{y}$ is more efficient than $\hat{y}$ when $\beta_1^2 < \sigma^2/S_\mathrm{x}$. Thus, we might choose $\bar{y}$ when $\hat{\beta}_1^2 < \hat{\sigma}^2/S_\mathrm{x}$, although it would be more appropriate to estimate β_1^2 without bias and compare $\hat{\beta}_1^2 - \mathrm{var}(\hat{\beta}_1)$ with $\hat{\sigma}^2/S_\mathrm{x}$ instead of $\hat{\beta}_1^2$ with $\hat{\sigma}^2/S_\mathrm{x}$.

A more ambitious approach searches for the combination of $\bar{y}$ and $\hat{y}$ that has the smallest MSE. We consider the combinations

$$\tilde{y}(b) = (1 - b)\hat{y} + b\bar{y} , \tag{1.18}$$

evaluate their MSE as a function of b, and choose the coefficient b^* for which $\mathrm{MSE}\,\{\tilde{y}(b); \mathbf{x}^*\boldsymbol{\beta}\}$ attains its minimum. This coefficient will turn out to depend on the model parameters β_1 and σ^2, so we will have to resort to its estimation and consider the associated loss in efficiency.

The sought MSE is

$$\mathrm{MSE}\,\{\tilde{y}(b); \mathbf{x}^*\boldsymbol{\beta}\} = (1-b)^2\sigma^2\left\{\frac{1}{n} + \frac{(x^* - \bar{x})^2}{S_\mathrm{x}}\right\} + b^2\left\{\frac{\sigma^2}{n} + \beta_1^2(x^* - \bar{x})^2\right\}$$

$$+ 2b(1-b)\frac{\sigma^2}{n}$$

$$= b^2(x^* - \bar{x})^2\left(\frac{\sigma^2}{S_\mathrm{x}} + \beta_1^2\right) - 2b(x^* - \bar{x})^2\frac{\sigma^2}{S_\mathrm{x}}$$

$$+\sigma^2 \left\{ \frac{1}{n} + \frac{(x^* - \bar{x})^2}{S_x} \right\}. \tag{1.19}$$

This is a quadratic function of b, with a positive quadratic coefficient, so it has a unique minimum, attained for

$$b^* = \frac{\sigma^2/S_x}{\sigma^2/S_x + \beta_1^2} = \frac{1}{1 + S_x \omega}, \tag{1.20}$$

where $\omega = \beta_1^2/\sigma^2$ is the relative squared slope. If ω were known, $\mathbf{x}^*\boldsymbol{\beta}$ would be predicted with MSE

$$\text{MSE}\{\tilde{y}(b^*); \mathbf{x}^*\boldsymbol{\beta}\} = \frac{\sigma^2}{n} + \frac{\beta_1^2(x^* - \bar{x})^2}{1 + S_x \omega}.$$

This is smaller than both $\text{var}(\hat{y})$ and $\text{MSE}(\bar{y}; \mathbf{x}^*\boldsymbol{\beta})$, because these two quantities correspond to the choices $b = 0$ and $b = 1$ in (1.18), and they were rejected in favour of a compromise, $b^* \in (0, 1)$, given by (1.20).

It remains to address the uncertainty about ω. One solution, parallel to the development illustrated by Figure 1.1 for ANOVA, is to identify an upper bound for ω, denoted by Ω, and explore how the estimator (or predictor) $\tilde{y}(b_\Omega^*)$, which is optimal when $\omega = \Omega$, performs when in fact $\omega < \Omega$. For a fixed coefficient b and variance σ^2, $\text{MSE}\{\tilde{y}(b); \mathbf{x}^*\boldsymbol{\beta}\}$ is an increasing function of σ^2:

$$\text{MSE}\{\tilde{y}(b); \mathbf{x}^*\boldsymbol{\beta}\} = \frac{\sigma^2}{S_x}(x^* - \bar{x})^2 \left\{ b^2(1 + S_x \omega) - 2b \right\} + \sigma^2 \left\{ \frac{1}{n} + \frac{(x^* - \bar{x})^2}{S_x} \right\}; \tag{1.21}$$

see (1.19). Thus, for any fixed σ^2, we minimise the MSE for the plausible scenario that is least favourable for predicting $\mathbf{x}^*\boldsymbol{\beta}$. Therefore the estimator $\tilde{y}(b_\Omega^*)$ is more efficient than $\hat{y}$ for any pair of plausible values of σ^2 and β_1 and is more efficient than $\bar{y}$ from a certain value of β_1^2 on. The loss of efficiency due to not knowing ω is

$$\text{MSE}\{\tilde{y}(b_\Omega); \mathbf{x}^*\boldsymbol{\beta}\} - \text{MSE}\{\tilde{y}(b^*); \mathbf{x}^*\boldsymbol{\beta}\}$$

$$= \sigma^2 \frac{(x^* - \bar{x})^2}{S_x} \left\{ \frac{1 + S_x \omega}{(1 + S_x \Omega)^2} - \frac{2}{1 + S_x \Omega} + \frac{1}{1 + S_x \omega} \right\}$$

$$= \sigma^2 (x^* - \bar{x})^2 \frac{S_x}{1 + S_x \omega} \frac{(\Omega - \omega)^2}{(1 + S_x \Omega)^2}.$$

This is an increasing function of Ω for any $\omega < \Omega$. Therefore, specifying a smaller Ω is advantageous, so long as it is still an upper bound for ω. By reducing Ω, the squared coefficient b^2 increases, and with it the curvature of the MSE in (1.21) as a function of $\sigma^2 \omega = \beta_1^2$. As a consequence, false confidence in the small size of Ω is punished more harshly the smaller the value of Ω. Note the close parallels with our conclusions in Section 1.2.1.

In Section 2.3, we describe a general theory of which these two cases are particular applications.

Suppose we use for combining $\hat{y}$ and $\bar{y}$ a value $\omega^\dagger$ that differs from the population quantity ω. We explore how large an error $|\omega^\dagger - \omega|$ can be committed before the synthetic estimator $\tilde{y}$ is no longer more efficient than both $\hat{y}$ and $\bar{y}$. By comparing (1.17) and (1.21), we conclude that $\tilde{y}$ based on $\omega^\dagger$ is more efficient than $\hat{y}$ so long as

$$\frac{\sigma^2}{S_x}(x^* - \bar{x})^2 \left\{ \frac{1 + S_x\omega}{(1 + S_x\omega^\dagger)^2} - \frac{2}{1 + S_x\omega^\dagger} \right\} < 0\,;$$

that is,

$$\omega < 2\omega^\dagger + \frac{1}{S_x}\,.$$

By similar operations, we conclude that $\tilde{y}$ is more efficient than $\bar{y}$ so long as

$$\sigma^2(x^* - \bar{x})^2 \left\{ \frac{1 + S_x\omega}{(1 + S_x\omega^\dagger)^2} - \frac{2}{1 + S_x\omega^\dagger} + 1 \right\} - \beta_1^2 S_x(x^* - \bar{x})^2 < 0\,,$$

which reduces first to

$$S_x\left(\omega + S_x\omega^{\dagger2}\right) < S_x\omega\left(1 + S_x\omega^\dagger\right)^2$$

and then to the condition

$$\omega > \frac{\omega^\dagger}{2 + S_x\omega^\dagger}\,.$$

The two conditions,

$$\frac{\omega^\dagger}{2 + S_x\omega^\dagger} < \omega < 2\omega^\dagger + \frac{1}{S_x}\,, \tag{1.22}$$

are not very restrictive. Even if we err by setting $\omega^\dagger$ to one-half or double of ω, $\tilde{y}$ remains more efficient than both $\hat{y}$ and $\bar{y}$. Further, as we always choose a positive $\omega^\dagger$, the right-hand condition is redundant when $S_x\omega < 1$.

In practice, ω is not known, so we have to estimate it and use the coefficient $\hat{b} = 1/(1 + S_x\hat{\omega})$ or another estimator of b. Efficient estimation of b is difficult because b is a nonlinear function of the model parameters β_1 and σ^2. Although β_1 is estimated by $\hat{\beta}_1$ without bias, $\hat{\beta}_1^2$ is biased for β_1^2;

$$\mathrm{E}\left(\hat{\beta}_1^2\right) = \beta_1^2 + \frac{\sigma^2}{S_x}\,.$$

Hence, $\hat{\beta}_1^2 - \hat{\sigma}^2/S_x$ is unbiased for β_1^2. By substituting this estimator in b, we obtain

$$\hat{b} = \frac{\hat{\sigma}^2}{\hat{\beta}_1^2 S_x}\,.$$

For estimating b this is not satisfactory because, unlike b, $\hat{b}$ may attain values in excess of 1.0. Dividing by $\hat{\beta}_1^2$, which may attain arbitrarily small positive values, is problematic even when β_1 is estimated by $\hat{\beta}_1$ efficiently. An obvious improvement may be achieved by adding a positive constant to the denominator in $\hat{b}$; if we add unity we obtain the naive estimator of b. Similarly, even though $\hat{\sigma}^2$ is unbiased and independent of $\hat{\beta}_1$, its reciprocal $1/\hat{\sigma}^2$ is biased for $1/\sigma^2$. However, even if we corrected for the bias of $1/\hat{\sigma}^2$, this would be in vain as b is a distinctly nonlinear function of both σ^2 and $1/\sigma^2$.

Although efficient estimation of b is an open problem, we can explore how 'tampering' with the naive estimator $\hat{b}$ affects the predictor $\tilde{y}(\hat{b})$. Of particular interest is avoiding very poor performance of $\tilde{y}$. By choosing $b = 0$, and therefore $\tilde{y}(0) = \hat{y}$, we act conservatively and obtain an unbiased predictor. In contrast, choosing $b = 1$ might seem to be reckless because, without any prior information, there is no limit on the bias, and therefore not on the MSE of $\tilde{y}(1) = \bar{y}$ either. This suggests that, since MSE $\{\tilde{y}(b); \mathbf{x}^*\boldsymbol{\beta}\}$ is a smooth function of b, we are on safer ground when we use an estimator $\hat{b}$ that underestimates b. Some efficiency may be lost in the process, but we protect our inference about $\mathbf{x}^*\boldsymbol{\beta}$ against very poor performance in some settings that are plausible.

An obvious way to underestimate b or to reduce $E(\hat{b}) - b$, which may be positive, is to use $r\hat{b}$ with a positive factor $r < 1$. It is difficult to recommend a factor r universally, or even for a specific setting, because it should ideally be informed by the clients' preferences, willingness to take risks, and prior information. Playing out some scenarios by simulations may be informative, without taxing the analyst's theoretical prowess.

1.3 Model Diagnostics

Models are our intermediaries between data and inferences. We specify one or several models that capture what we know about the studied process and attempt to narrow down the range of plausible distributions that govern this process.

A model is associated with its *fit*, our data-based estimator of the model parameters, such as $\hat{\boldsymbol{\beta}}$ for $\boldsymbol{\beta}$ in (1.13) and $\hat{\sigma}^2$ for σ^2 in (1.16). Having fitted a model, it is advisable to assess whether the model is appropriate—whether there are any signs that some of the assumptions made, such as linearity and normality in ordinary regression, are violated. Such procedures are referred to as *model diagnostics*.

In the ordinary regression model, most assumptions focus on the deviations $\boldsymbol{\varepsilon}$. If we ignore the uncertainty about the regression parameters $\boldsymbol{\beta}$, the deviations $\boldsymbol{\varepsilon}$ coincide with the residuals $\mathbf{e}$. Thus, we may explore whether the residuals $\mathbf{e}$ have the appearance of a random sample from a centred normal distribution, bearing in mind the licence taken by equating $\boldsymbol{\varepsilon}$ to $\mathbf{e}$.

Checking the assumption that $E(\varepsilon) = 0$ requires no scrutiny because $e^\top 1 = 0$ by construction, as $e^\top X = 0$ and 1 is a column of X. A histogram of e is likely to be useful only for large samples, when the shape of the empirical distribution of e can reasonably be expected to resemble its underlying distribution. For example, substantial asymmetry of e is a telltale sign of a departure from normality.

Outliers can be regarded similarly. A component of e (or of any other vector) is called an outlier if it stands out among the other components, for instance, by being far away from the vast majority of them. A small group of values may also be outliers, if they are far away from the remaining values, even though they may be close to one another. The obvious question arises: when is a group small enough to be declared as a set of outliers? There is no clinical answer. However, both situations, when a group of values is an outlier and when it represents another population or process, indicate a violation of the assumptions. It may result from using an inappropriate variable x or from its inappropriate definition, or from the model being too simple a description of the studied process. But it may be that one or a few observational units behave exceptionally. Models have no intrinsic right to be valid.

The residuals can be regarded as random variables; their joint distribution can be derived from the identity

$$e = y - X\hat{\beta}$$

$$= Q_X y = Q_X \varepsilon.$$

Thus, each residual e_j is normally distributed, and jointly they have the multivariate normal distribution $\mathcal{N}_n(0, \sigma^2 Q_X)$. The variance matrix of this distribution is singular because its rank is $n - 2$; Q_X has the unit eigenvalue with multiplicity $n - 2$ and the zero eigenvalue with multiplicity 2. Further, each diagonal element of Q_X, equal to $\mathrm{var}(e_j)/\sigma^2$, is smaller than or equal to unity. However, the variances $\mathrm{var}(e_j)$, $j = 1, \ldots, n$, are not necessarily equal to one another. The residuals e_j can be standardised, adjusted to have identical distributions, by the transformation $e_j^\dagger = e_j/\sqrt{(Q_X)_{jj}}$. The jth diagonal element of Q_X is

$$(Q_X)_{jj} = 1 - \frac{1}{n} - \frac{(x_j - \bar{x})^2}{S_x}.$$

It is exceptionally small only when x_j is in a much greater distance from the mean $\bar{x}$ than the remaining stimuli $x_{j'}$, $j' \neq j$. In fact, when $n > 2$, the only configuration of the stimuli x_j that results in one diagonal entry of Q_X vanishing is that $n - 1$ values of x_j coincide and the remaining one differs.

One or a few values x_j distant from the remainder raise the following problem. As the linear regression fit minimises the sum of squares of the residuals, it is averse to large residuals. For a distant (outlying) stimulus x_j, a small change in $\hat{\beta}_1$, interpretable as a rotation of the regression line around $\hat{\beta}_0 + \hat{\beta}_1\bar{x}$, results in a much greater change of the residual e_j than for the

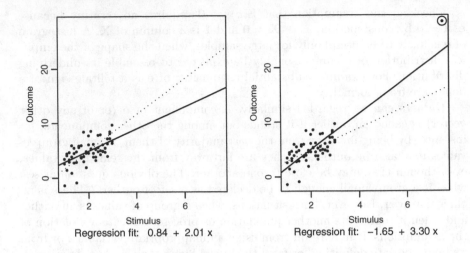

Fig. 1.3. Example of high leverage in linear regression. The same set of observations (x_j, y_j) are plotted in the two panels, with a high-leverage observation added in the right-hand panel (encircled).

other observations. Therefore, the model fit will come close to matching the outcome y_j, and so the corresponding residual e_j has a small variance.

Figure 1.3 gives an illustration. The two panels contain the plot of the same 63 pairs of values (x_j, y_j), but another pair (x_{64}, y_{64}) is added in the right-hand panel. The solid line in either panel is the fit to the respective 63 and 64 displayed observations, and the dotted line indicates the other fit. The substantial change in the regression (see the subtitles) is brought about by the single observation No. 64 (marked by a circle). This observation is said to have *high leverage*. High leverage is connected to the small value of the corresponding diagonal entry of $\mathbf{Q_X}$. Observations with high leverage are best avoided because with them the inference is strongly influenced by a single (or a few) observation. Note that high leverage is a property of the stimuli (values of x) and is related to the outcome solely through x.

For outlying stimuli, the standardisation of e_j to $e_j^\dagger$ amounts to a substantial inflation, to compensate for the propensity of the fit to match the outcomes. Both e_j and $e_j^\dagger$ are problematic as representations (estimates) of the deviation ε_j, even more so than their counterparts for the remaining observations. In any case, ε_j are mutually independent, whereas e_j are not.

A useful device for diagnosing nonlinearity of the regression $\mathrm{E}(Y \mid X = x)$ is to plot the residuals against the values of x. Any pattern of the residuals indicates a departure from linearity. It is meaningful to consider departures from independence only when there are credible alternatives, such as dependence due to the order of the observations, especially when the order (sequencing) relates to time. Patterns in the plot of the order number against the residuals may indicate dependence, although we have to take into account the influence of the values of the stimuli. This is particularly difficult when the stimuli are administered in the ascending or descending order of its values. The study design should attend to this problem by mixing up the order of the values of x_j, so that they do not follow any obvious pattern.

Departures from homoscedasticity, that is, from equal residual variance, can be brought on by recording the value of the outcome on an inappropriate scale. For example, the dependence of the residual variance on the stimulus can be greatly reduced by a particular transformation of x or y or both. To see this, suppose the linear model in (1.10) is appropriate. Then

$$\mathrm{E}\left\{\exp(y_j)\,|\,\mathbf{x}_j\right\} = \exp\left(\mathbf{x}_j\boldsymbol{\beta} + \frac{\sigma^2}{2}\right),$$

$$\mathrm{var}\left\{\exp(y_j)\,|\,\mathbf{x}_j\right\} = \exp\left(2\mathbf{x}_j\boldsymbol{\beta} + \sigma^2\right)\left\{\exp(\sigma^2) - 1\right\}. \tag{1.23}$$

This suggests that *heteroscedasticity* (the negation of homoscedasticity) goes hand in hand with nonlinearity. That is the case when the underlying mechanism, with x and y recorded on suitable scales, relates y to x linearly. Of course, this need not be the case; a transformation may arrange one assumption to be palatable at the expense of another. More general models are the way to resolve this problem.

By way of a summary of model diagnostics, concerns about the validity of the assumptions, Figure 1.4 gives examples of departures from normality, linearity, homoscedasticity, and independence. The panels in the left-hand column plot the outcomes and stimuli, and the panels in the right-hand column contain the graphs of residuals suitable for assessing the type of departure concerned.

1.3.1 Simulation-Based Diagnostics

The examples in Figure 1.4 were constructed deliberately to be clear cut. In practice, we may come across plots of residuals for which it is much more difficult to conclude whether they indicate a failure of a particular model assumption. In some instances, what appears to be an obvious pattern of the residuals may in fact arise purely by chance; that is, it would not be present in the analysis of a replication of the study. It may also arise as a consequence of the configuration of the values of x, and so it would be present in replications. A random sample from a normal distribution is not always 'normal' in an exemplary way. This calls for caution and a balance in the eagerness to identify patterns in the residuals $\mathbf{e}$ that contradict the assumptions about $\boldsymbol{\varepsilon}$. The more detailed an inspection of the data we conduct, the more likely we are to discover an aberrant pattern, but at the same time, an aberrant pattern is more likely to appear even when the corresponding assumption is satisfied. There is no ready formula for the balance of thoroughness and sound judgment of what indicates a genuine model violation.

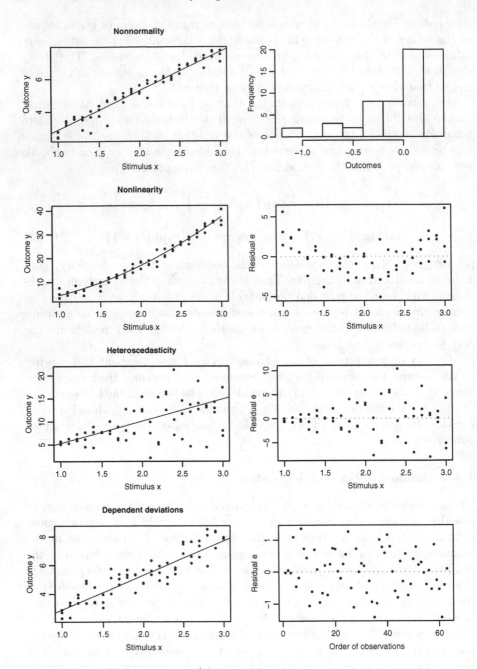

Fig. 1.4. Examples of departures from the assumptions of the linear model and diagnostic plots.

An alternative approach to model diagnostics is based on simulations. The analyst defines a *feature*; this may be a statistic, table, graph, or any other object and the process for generating it. The feature is evaluated on the observed data; the result is called the *realised feature*. Next, outcomes are generated by simulation from the fitted model and the feature is evaluated for each replication, generating several *simulated* (replicate) features. The realised and simulated features are shuffled, so that the location of the realised feature is not known. If the realised feature stands out among all the features, for instance, if another analyst identifies it as outlying, the model should be rejected as unsuitable (not fitting well).

A feature may comprise several elements. For example, a graph may comprise several panels, and an array (table or matrix) of several sub-arrays or individual entries. A feature may comprise elements of different kinds, such as a graph and a matrix (e.g., the matrix may be displayed in the graph). If each element can be regarded as a feature on its own, the collection of the elements is called a *multifeature*. The purpose of a multifeature is to avoid the natural human inclination to be more likely to spot something unusual when several sets of objects are inspected. It is practical to generate 19 (49 or 99) replicate features, so that false identification of a feature is associated with probability 0.05 (0.02 or 0.01).

How should a feature be defined? Matching its choice to our concerns (a priori suspicions) is the principal difficulty, but it is shared to a large extent with the established methods discussed earlier. A residual plot can be regarded as a feature, so no innovation is required. However, *any* other object is suitable, and it is up to the analyst's ingenuity to match the concern about the studied process and the model applied with a suitable feature. For example, if symmetry of the distribution of the deviations is a concern, a suitable feature is

$$s = (\mathbf{e}_U + \mathbf{e}_D)^\top (\mathbf{e}_U + \mathbf{e}_D),$$

where $\mathbf{e}_U$ and $\mathbf{e}_D$ are the permutations of the residuals $\mathbf{e}$ in ascending and descending order, respectively. We note in passing that the *symmetry plot* is defined as the scatterplot of $\mathbf{e}_U$ and $-\mathbf{e}_D$, although it suffices to plot these values for only half the units.

The rationale for using s as a feature is that $s = 0$ corresponds to perfect symmetry; otherwise s is positive. A greater value of s corresponds to greater asymmetry, although the residual variance σ^2 also exerts an impact on the distribution of s. Randomness in the model used for simulation causes the replicate values of s to be positive, but the distribution of these values indicates how large they tend to be when the distribution is in fact symmetric.

A disadvantage of this simulation approach is that the evidence, in the form of 20 (50 or 100) replicates, is awkward to present in a publication that has to be concise and contained in a few pages. However, good practice should be granted primacy over good appearance. Of course, a single-number feature does not suffer from this drawback. Even 100 features (99 simulated and 1

```
0. | 001111111111111111122222222222222222222223333333333333333333444444
0. | 55555555555555666666688899
1. | 4
1. | 5
2. | 0
2. |
3. | 0
```

Fig. 1.5. Stem-and-leaf plot of the realised (highlighted) and 99 replicate values of the statistic s as a diagnostic feature.

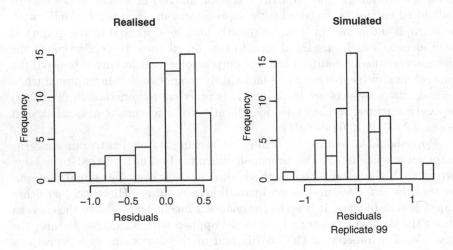

Fig. 1.6. The realised and a simulated (replicate) set of residuals summarised by the stem-and-leaf plot of the feature s in Figure 1.5.

realised) can be compactly presented in a stem-and-leaf plot, with the realised feature highlighted. If it is at the extreme, among the highest or lowest of the values, it is appropriate to reject the model.

Figure 1.5 displays the stem-and-leaf plot of the one realised and 99 replicate values of the statistic s for an example of non-normality similar to that displayed in the top panels of Figure 1.4. The realised value, equal to 3.01, is highlighted. Being by far the largest, it leaves little doubt that symmetry, and hence normality, is not a suitable assumption for the model deviations. Figure 1.6 displays the histograms of the realised set of residuals and one set of replicate residuals. It is much more difficult to make a diagnostic assessment based only on these two histograms. The histogram itself could be adopted as a feature, but the statistic s is much more practical for that purpose.

Finally, we discuss what action to take when we identify a contradiction of the data with the model. The generic answer is to review the model, for example, by replacing the inappropriate assumption with an alternative or a more general one. Thus, the analyst has to have in store models, methods for fitting and interpreting them, and diagnostic procedures for them. This does not resolve everything, however, because every diagnostic procedure is a process that leaves a trace, however subtle, on the distribution of the estimators, and of sample quantities in general.

By way of an example, suppose a particular model A is fitted and a diagnostic procedure applied, the outcome of which is to either approve the model or fit a more general model B based on which the target θ would be estimated. Suppose the models are associated with estimators $\hat{\theta}_A$ and $\hat{\theta}_B$. Then the estimator of θ is neither $\hat{\theta}_A$ nor $\hat{\theta}_B$, but their mixture

$$\hat{\theta}_{AB} = \mathcal{I}\hat{\theta}_A + (1 - \mathcal{I})\hat{\theta}_B,$$

where $\mathcal{I}$ is the indicator of adopting model A after the diagnostic procedure. If the decision based on the diagnostic procedure is subject to uncertainty, $\hat{\theta}_{AB}$ need not be efficient, even if both $\hat{\theta}_A$ and $\hat{\theta}_B$ are efficient when the corresponding model, A or B, is appropriate. In brief, our inferences are not as efficient when we are uncertain about the model assumptions (and have to check them), as when we are certain (and rightly skip some or all diagnostic procedures). This should not be regarded as an invitation to skip diagnostics, because the penalty for unjustified confidence is unpredictable. But the diagnostics does not come free, even if we can conduct it effortlessly and competently. Intelligence, in the form of prior information about the behaviour of the studied processes, is irreplaceable.

It is important to bear in mind that diagnostic procedures can find a contradiction with the assumptions of a model but cannot confirm the model. Failure to find a contradiction is more appropriately interpreted as ignorance—not knowing whether the model is appropriate or not. However, a well-conducted search, using features targeted for the particularly suspect points in the model-building exercise, can be pragmatically regarded as giving some comfort that the model is appropriate, or that the outcomes are not in any glaring contradiction with the model assumptions.

1.4 Toward Causal Inference

The methods discussed thus far deal with *observable* (visible) properties of the outcomes—properties or features that can be constructed from the outcomes. Some assumptions of the linear model cannot be confirmed by inspecting the data because departures from them leave no trace in the outcomes. Foremost among them are that the stimuli are defined up front, prior to observing the outcomes, and that no influences other than the subject's stimulus are at play.

The ultimate understanding of a process is attained when we can influence (*manipulate*) the outcomes by the stimuli directly, without intermediation of any other variables. In such a case, we say that the stimulus is a *cause* of the response. Suppose the response is related to the stimulus by the linear model $y = \beta_0 + \beta_1 x + \varepsilon$. If x is a cause of y, then for every unit j a change of x by Δ, to $x + \Delta$, brings about the change, called the *effect* of the response, from y to $y + \beta_1\Delta$. The effect usually depends on Δ but may also be specific to the unit and the value of x. When we can engage a unit in the study only once, we cannot apply both stimuli x and $x + \Delta$ (on separate occasions) but may nevertheless speculate what the response would be to the stimulus that was not applied.

Regression is often used when x cannot be manipulated because x is an inherent attribute or characteristic of the unit. This does not amount to an abuse of the regression, so long as we do not interpret the results as inferences about causes and effects. The most common example of this is estimation of the 'sex effect' and 'age effect', the difference between men and women, or young and old, with respect to a particular outcome variable, such as intelligence, a physical attribute, health, attitude, or the like. The term *effect* would be meaningful in either of these contexts only if we had a straightforward means of altering subjects' sexes or ages in isolation, without any impact on the subjects in any other way. This is clearly an absurdity, for the time being at least, and so are the associated 'effects'—it is more accurate to refer to them as (average) differences. We revisit this issue in Chapter 7.

1.5 Designing Regression Studies

Linear regression can be applied to any dataset in which one variable is identified as the stimulus and one as the outcome. However, interpretation of the results is much easier for a designed study, in which the values of the stimuli are set by the analyst. So, when design is feasible and can be afforded, how should the sample size, the values of x, and other details be chosen, and how should the study be conducted?

The first consideration should be given to the desired inferences—the substantive questions (purposes) that have generated the impulse to conduct the study. Usually there is a collection of questions, and so some compromise of the purposes is necessary. Suppose a population quantity, such as $\mathbf{x}^*\boldsymbol{\beta}$, should be estimated with a particular precision. Equation (1.17) indicates that $\mathrm{var}(\mathbf{x}^*\hat{\boldsymbol{\beta}})$ is a decreasing function of the sample size n and the corrected sum of squares S_x, so these two quantities should be sufficiently large; we require a sufficiently large sample without neglecting the dispersion of the covariate X. Sample size contributes to an increase of S_x, as does increased dispersion of the values of X.

The squared deviation $(x - \bar{x})^2$ is a factor in $\mathrm{MSE}(\bar{y}; \mathbf{x}\boldsymbol{\beta})$, $\mathrm{var}(\mathbf{x}^*\hat{\boldsymbol{\beta}})$, and the associated synthetic estimator [see (1.21)] so the optimal choice of $\bar{x}$ is the stimulus for which we wish to make a prediction. Prediction is usually desired for a range of values of X; then $\bar{x}$ should be chosen near the middle of this range, taking into account the relative importance of the inferences for the various values of X.

The association of the outcome with the stimulus X need not be linear, but when restricted to a narrow range of the values of X it may be indistinguishable from linearity. Therefore, we should resist applying a very wide range of values of X, unless the shape of the (nonlinear) association is of interest, we know that the regression is linear, or we want to establish whether linearity applies for a wide range of values of X. Observations with high leverage should be avoided—esoteric or uneven distributions of the values of X often make the subsequent inferences problematic.

The term *interpolation* is used for approximating the value of a smooth function f at a point x based on points x_1 and x_2 such that $x_1 < x < x_2$. *Extrapolation* is the complement of interpolation; it refers to approximating the value of f at x based on points x_1 and x_2 such that $x \notin (x_1, x_2)$. This term is borrowed for prediction; extrapolation refers to predicting the outcome y for a stimulus x^* that lies outside the range of values x_j used in the study. Such extrapolation should be avoided for two reasons. First, MSE of the prediction, using $\hat{y}$ or $\tilde{y}$, is an increasing (linear) function of $(x^* - \bar{x})^2$; this is really an argument against predicting a large distance from the average stimulus $\bar{x}$. Second, the regression of y on x may be (approximately) linear and homoscedastic for a narrow range of stimuli, but in a wider range the departure from linearity or homoscedasticity may be substantial. Prediction in a long distance from $\bar{x}$ is then problematic. Extrapolation can be avoided, in principle, by anticipating at the planning stage the range of values of x for which prediction will be sought. By setting the stimuli in a wider range, we increase the summary S_x and reduce the variance of the prediction, so long as we do not stretch the assumption of linearity too far. An alternative is to conduct two or several studies that cover the entire range of x in which inferences might be sought and base each prediction on the study for which it amounts to interpolation. Nonlinear regression and other generalisations, discussed in Chapter 10, offer other analytically more challenging alternatives.

Some of the model assumptions call for particular arrangements in the conduct of the study. Independence of the deviations is ensured when the incidents of outcome (data) generation for the subjects do not interfere with one another. If the values of Y are realised in a sequence, a realisation should not be affected in any way by the previous realisations. Any conscious action by the personnel conducting the study, or a mechanism that acts outside our control, that excludes responses based on their values y, is highly problematic. If we have an opportunity to discard observations that we do not like, our agenda, for instance, to distort the inference, can be very successful, especially when the residual variance σ^2 is relatively large. Ideally, all such action should be ruled out; when it cannot be, it should be documented in detail, with the reasons for exclusion. Its impact, in replications, can in principle be explored by simulations.

1.6 Observational Studies and Experiments

We conclude this chapter with a discussion of types of studies. In observational studies, values of variables are recorded without any intention to influence them by imposition, incentives, or any other means. By analysing such studies we can compare subpopulations (strata) defined by the values of the covariates—we can learn about the existing aspects of the studied population.

The purpose of experiments is to make inferences about effects, in the sense of causal analysis. The variable that represents a cause is called the *treatment*. Unfortunately, the values of such a variable are also called treatments; to distinguish between them, we shall use the terms *treatment variable* and *treatment* for the variable and value (type), respectively. Further, an effect refers to a comparison (*contrast*), so it has to be qualified by the two treatments that are being compared. Thus, we are interested in the effect of treatment B over A on the outcome—the change in the outcome that is attributable to the change of the treatment from A to B. In the ideal setting, the treatments are set by design, in such a manner that the treatment variable is not associated with and exercises no influence on any of the other (incidental) variables. As a consequence, any differences observed among the groups of subjects defined by the treatment applied can be attributed to the sampling variation and systematic differences among the treatments. The sampling variation is limited by the sample size (design), enabling us to make inferences about the systematic differences that can be interpreted as average effects.

For simplicity, we focus on a simple experimental design used for comparing two values of a treatment variable, A and B. The subjects (experimental units) administered a treatment form the *treatment group* named after the treatment. If administration of both treatments is equally expensive, symmetry suggests that the same number of subjects should be assigned to each treatment. The model for this setting is

$$y_{jk} = \mu_k + \varepsilon_{jk}, \qquad (1.24)$$

where k is the treatment (A or B) and $j = 1, \ldots, n_1 = n_2 = \frac{1}{2}n$ identifies the subject within each treatment group. The distribution of ε_{jk} is immaterial for the discussion, although we assume that it does not depend on the treatment group, has a finite variance σ^2, and the distinct deviations ε_{jk} are uncorrelated. To be able to attach a meaning to μ_k, we assume that $E(\varepsilon_{jk} \mid k) = 0$ within each treatment k.

With the normality assumptions for ε, the model represented by (1.24) is ANOVA with two categories, A and B. At the same time, it is a special case of the linear regression model, with intercept μ_A and slope $\Delta\mu = \mu_B - \mu_A$, and the covariate which indicates whether treatment B is applied ($x = 0$ for A and $x = 1$ for B).

The target of estimation is the treatment difference $\Delta\mu$. It is estimated naively by $\Delta\hat{\mu} = \hat{\mu}_B - \hat{\mu}_A$, where $\hat{\mu}_k$, $k = $ A or B, is the sample mean of the outcomes in group k. The estimator $\Delta\hat{\mu}$ is unbiased, and its variance is $\mathrm{var}(\Delta\hat{\mu}) = 2\sigma^2/n$. Setting the sample size n involves balancing the outlay on the study against the precision of the inferences. The outlay on the study can usually be approximated as a linear function of n, $C + 2Dn$, with its absolute term C equal to the costs that are not affected by the sample size, and unit cost D associated with each subject. If we could construct a function that expresses the (monetary) gain in terms of precision, as $G\left(n; \sigma^2\right)$, finding the optimal sample size would be relatively easy, for instance, by maximising the difference $G\left(n; \sigma^2\right) - C - 2Dn$.

Several factors make such optimisation difficult. First, the variance σ^2 is usually not known, although the study designer may have some idea of its value. Next, summarising the costs by monetary values is often nontrivial. When human subjects are involved, especially when they are patients who suffer from a particular condition (for which the treatments are intended), ethical 'costs' are involved, and these are difficult to convert to monetary values. Further, the gains achieved as a result of the study depend not only on the precision but also on the difference $\Delta\mu$, which itself may not represent fully the benefits derived from the tested (new) treatment. In a commercial setting, the gains may be strongly influenced by actions of competitors and are therefore subject to considerable uncertainty. And finally, one study is often only part of a sequence of studies that may lead to a (nearly) definite conclusion about a treatment. Therefore, the study design cannot be considered in isolation from its convoluted context.

An important element of the study design is ensuring that the difference $\Delta\mu$ can be regarded as the effect of the treatment and interpreted as the hypothetical difference between the mean outcomes in the two treatment groups that comprise perfectly matched pairs of subjects. In this hypothetical setting, a pair of clones is available for each of n subjects. One clone is assigned to treatment A and the other to treatment B. This ensures that the comparison of the two treatment groups is of like with like. Instead of this unrealistic scenario, the $2n$ subjects are assigned to the treatment groups at random, paying no respect for any of the subjects' attributes. This process (and principle) is referred to as *randomisation*. Randomisation does not arrange the two groups to be identical in any respect, but in a large number of replications the groups would be nearly identical *on average*.

Randomisation is problematic in very small experiments because chance may bring about substantial differences among the subjects prior to the experiment. However, any form of deliberate allocation, based on the values of relevant recorded variables threatens to introduce differences between the treatment groups due to variables that were not recorded—variables that are relevant but have not been recognised as such. In any case, small experiments with subjects that have substantial a priori differences on relevant variables are problematic, because the analysis cannot disentangle the contributions of the a priori differences and the differences due to the administered treatments to the estimator $\Delta\hat{\mu}$.

1.6.1 Human Subjects

When humans are involved, as subjects, informants or administrators of the treatments, it is necessary to ensure that their conduct is not influenced by any prejudice (or valid information) they may have about the treatments. In *clinical trials*, in which medical treatments and procedures are compared, this is enforced by making the treatments anonymous. For example, when the treatments are drugs, alternative formulations are prepared so that they are indistinguishable by sight, taste, or smell (e.g., by pills having identical coating). This principle is referred to as *blinding*. *Double-blinding* is an established practice in clinical trials in which neither the subject (patient) nor the administrator (nurse) is informed about the identity of the treatment. A treatment may be compared with 'no action'. To disguise the latter, the principle of blinding calls for administering the same procedure as for the *active treatment*, but with the active ingredient removed, with neither the administrator nor subject informed about it or being able to notice it when the treatment is administered. Such a treatment is called *placebo*. Having a placebo treatment group protects the study from an uneven influence (in the everyday care and interaction and the like) exercised by the staff who administer the treatments. The identities of the treatments are disclosed for the sole purpose of the analysis at the conclusion of the trial.

The model in (1.24) assumes that the treatment difference (or effect) $\Delta\mu$ applies to every member of the relevant population. That is, *if* a member of the population could be subjected to both treatments A and B, independently and without any influence (interference) of the other treatment, the difference of the responses would be $\Delta\mu$ or would differ from it by small values that can be attributed to the measurement process and the inexplicable everyday influences. Alternatively, if the pair of treatments A and B could be applied in such a manner in replications, the average treatment difference would be the same value $\Delta\mu$ for every subject. In practice, not even one pair of treatments can be applied in this way when the (healing) effect of a treatment cannot be wiped out instantly. The hypothetical difference between the outcomes of two such administrations is therefore called a *counterfactual* effect.

The assumption of independent deviations ε_{jk} can be interpreted as no interference among the subjects. For a given treatment, the outcome for one subject is not affected in any way by the outcome for another subject. When subjects do not communicate with one another, this is a reasonable assumption, although some correlation might still be introduced by the staff administering the treatments and caring for the subjects.

The assumption of universal $\Delta\mu$, applicable to every member of the population, is often problematic, because it assumes that we have identified the scale for measuring the responses that is linear. If a scale has this property its nonlinear transformation does not, unless there are no differences in the outcome variable among the members. Thus, the treatment effect $\Delta\mu$ may be constant on one scale and variable on another. Furthermore, the treatment effect may be variable on *any* scale, for instance, when one treatment is more beneficial to one subpopulation, the other treatment to another, and the treatments are equally (or indistinguishably) beneficial to the remainder of the population. Variable treatment effect is also referred to as *treatment heterogeneity*.

Clinical trials, and any other experiments on human subjects, cannot select subjects by any sampling design because the ethical standards dictate that participants have to give *informed consent*—they have to be informed about the nature and substance of the trial, the risks involved, and the role of the subjects in the trial, including that none of their statutory rights would be affected in any way if they refused to participate or agreed but subsequently withdrew from participation at some stage. Also, a sampling frame of the population of sufferers from a particular condition usually cannot be compiled. In any case, the target population of the study are the *future* sufferers, some of whom are yet to contract the condition. Admittedly, we can reasonably assume that current sufferers are a population very similar to the sufferers in the future. In brief, a clinical trial is both an experiment and a survey, but the aspects associated with good survey design cannot be implemented. Yet, under treatment heterogeneity they are not innocuous.

As inclusion in the study cannot be controlled by a sampling design, the participating subjects may be a poor representation of the relevant population. When the treatment effect is variable, the representation of the subject-specific treatment effects may be distorted in the sample. This problem is not alleviated by randomisation. As an example, suppose treatment B is superior to treatment A for 50% of the population, inferior for 20%, and is about the same for 30%. The recruitment process may conspire to select mainly subjects for whom treatment B is inferior, likely to lead to the inappropriate conclusion that B is inferior to A. However, estimating the distribution of treatment effects requires unrealistically large samples that in practice cannot be afforded, and identifying subpopulations for whom a treatment is (uniformly) beneficial is a problem that has to rely on the expertise of the medical profession.

1.6.2 Observational Studies and Estimation of Effects

Experimental design is essential, although not always sufficient, for making inferences about effects. Drawbacks of experiments include their relatively high expense, difficulties with their conduct on large samples and, over long periods of time, adherence to their protocols and maintenance of the realistic nature of the study in the setting in which control is imposed. Observational studies have fewer restrictions in their protocols, can usually afford substantially greater sample sizes, and can be conducted over longer periods of time. But they yield much less credible inferences or require a host of assumptions and prior information to support such inferences.

In an observational study, a sample of subjects from the relevant population is interviewed or observed. For contrast with experiments, we consider a study in which the treatment applied, A or B, to a subject is recorded together with the response to the treatment. As no control was exercised over the treatment applied in the past, the treatments could not have been randomised; subjects or their representatives *selected* their treatments and exercised their free will, sometimes with minimum supervision, in adhering to the details of the treatment. Of course, they were aware of which treatment was applied and were informed about alternatives. Lack of randomisation and blinding are serious barriers to unbiased estimation of the (average) treatment effect. The bias cannot be reduced by increasing the sample size of the study. With large sample size it becomes the dominant contributor to the MSE of the estimator of the treatment effect, even when the estimator is unbiased for the treatment difference, the difference between the means of the outcomes within the treatment groups.

Any arrangements to combat the problems of subjects having selected themselves into treatment groups can at best be regarded as a limitation of the damage caused by the lack of experimental control. One approach finds a match for each subject in one treatment group with a subject in the other treatment group. Two such subjects have the same values on a set of *matching variables*. These variables have to be selected with care; if too many variables are selected a lot of subjects will end up being neither matched nor used as matches, and the comparisons, using the matched pairs, will be based on too small a fraction of the sample. Instead of an exact match on a variable, a modicum of deviation may be allowed; this is relevant especially for variables that are continuous or have many categories. To make the matching process easier, some categories may be aggregated. Variables not identified as relevant or not recorded represent a threat to the success of the inferences based on matched (sub-)samples. An analytically more challenging approach defines a score for each subject and the subjects are matched on this score, possibly after some coarsening. Another approach defines or estimates adjustments due to the process of subjects being selected or self-selecting themselves to the treatments. Further details are given in Chapters 5 and 7.

Observational studies of responses to treatments can be classified as *retrospective* and *prospective*. In retrospective studies subjects are asked to recall their treatment regime for the studied condition in the past. Prospective studies recruit from a population of healthy subjects or a population susceptible to the studied condition, and incidences of the condition are recorded as and when they occur. Prospective studies are usually conducted over very long periods of time (years); otherwise too few subjects contract the condition and comparisons involving them would have very large sampling variation.

Prospective studies require very large sample sizes, but their protocols are less demanding. They are suitable for treatments that are administered over long periods of time, such as altered diet, physical exercise, primary health care, and education, which could not be assigned by randomisation. For example, a study may recruit middle-aged women, ask them about their diet, extent of daily exercise, occupation, housing conditions, and the like, and collect over the next decade or so information about breast cancer cases, either from the subjects directly or from a maintained register of cases.

Suggested Reading

The material for this chapter is adapted from several journal articles by the author, including [120] and [121]. Useful references to linear algebra in the context of ANOVA and linear regression, which is indispensable for this and most of the later chapters, are [70], [153], [176], and [178].

Problems and Exercises

1.1. Generate data according to the ANOVA model in (1.3) with $K = 2$ groups, within-group sample sizes $n_1 = n_2 = 10$, population means $\mu_1 = 0$ and $\mu_2 = 1.25$, and common within-group variance $\sigma_W^2 = 0.25$. Apply the within-group mean ($\hat{\mu}_1$), the sample mean ($\hat{\mu}$), and the selected-model-based estimator which uses $\hat{\mu}_1$ if the hypothesis of equal means, $\mu_1 = \mu_2$, is rejected and uses $\hat{\mu}$ otherwise. Repeat this exercise 1000 times, storing the values of the three estimates, and estimate the MSEs of these estimators. Check that $\mathrm{MSE}(\hat{\mu}_1; \mu_1) = \sigma^2/n_1$ and that $\mathrm{MSE}(\hat{\mu}; \mu_1) = \sigma^2/n + \frac{1}{4}(\mu_1 - \mu_2)^2$.
Hint: The hypothesis of equal means is rejected when

$$\frac{|\hat{\mu}_1 - \hat{\mu}_2|}{\hat{\sigma}} \sqrt{\frac{1}{n_1} + \frac{1}{n_2}}$$

($\hat{\sigma}^2$ is the pooled estimator of the within-group variance) exceeds the 97.5th percentile of the t-distribution with $n_1 + n_2 - 2$ degrees of freedom. In this exercise, this percentile is equal to 2.101.

1.2. Repeat the simulations in Exercise 1.1 for a range of values of μ_2, including $\mu_2 = \mu_1$, while keeping all the other settings intact. Compare the efficiencies of the estimators for the different values of μ_2. Can you anticipate the results for different values of μ_1 and σ^2?

1.3. In the simulations in the previous two exercises, evaluate also the estimator of the sampling variance: $\hat{\sigma}^2/n_1$ when $\hat{\mu}_1$ is used and $\hat{\sigma}^2/(n_1 + n_2)$ when $\hat{\mu}$ is used. Compare the empirical means of these estimators with the MSEs (or variances) of the simulated values of the estimates of μ_1.

1.4. Implement the synthetic estimator $\tilde{\mu}_1$ given by (1.4) with the coefficient b_1 estimated by (1.6). Simulate values of $\tilde{\mu}_1$ using one of the settings in the previous exercises and compare the alternative estimators of μ_1. Compare $MSE(\tilde{\mu}_1 ; \mu_1)$ with the MSE of the estimator $\tilde{\mu}_1(b^*)$ based on the ideal coefficient b_1^*.

1.5. Suppose that for the setting of the previous exercises, the absolute difference $|\mu_1 - \mu_2|$ is unlikely to exceed 1.0. Derive the MSE of the estimator that is efficient when $|\mu_1 - \mu_2| = 1.0$ and compare it with the MSE of $\tilde{\mu}_1(\hat{b}^*)$. How would you describe the value of the information that $|\mu_1 - \mu_2| \leq 1.0$? Describe the additional rewards (MSE reduction) when we know that $|\mu_1 - \mu_2| < 0.5$. Suppose we have inappropriately assumed that $|\mu_1 - \mu_2| < 0.5$ and applied the estimator $\tilde{\mu}_1(b_{1,0.5})$. The threshold of $\Gamma = 1$ would have been more appropriate than $\Gamma = 0.5$. Find the deviation $\Delta\mu_1(0.5, 1) = |\mu_1 - \mu|$ for which $\tilde{\mu}_1(b_{1,0.5})$ and $\tilde{\mu}_1(b_{1,1})$ have identical MSEs. Show that this deviation is in the range $\left(0.5, \sqrt{0.625}\right)$ or, in general, in the range

$$\left(\Gamma_1, \sqrt{\frac{\Gamma_1^2 + \Gamma_2^2}{2}}\right).$$

Interpret the value $\Delta\mu_1(\Gamma_1, \Gamma_2)$ as *forgiveness* of the synthetic estimator (with respect to an optimistic threshold Γ_1 and a conservative threshold Γ_2).

1.6. For the setting of the previous exercises, compare the synthetic estimators of μ_1 based on $r\hat{b}_1^*$ for $r = 0.5, 0.6, \ldots, 1.0, 1.1$ and make a recommendation as to which value of r to use for estimating μ_1.

1.7. For the linear regression model with two continuous covariates and their interaction,

$$y_j = \beta_0 + \beta_1 x_j^{(1)} + \beta_2 x_j^{(2)} + \beta_{12} x_j^{(1)} x_j^{(2)} + \varepsilon_j,$$

with the assumptions of normality and homoscedasticity, express in terms of β_1, β_2, and β_{12} the regression parameters when $u_j^{(2)} = 3x_j^{(2)} - 7$ is used instead of $x_j^{(2)}$. Similarly, describe the changes when the outcome Y is replaced with $y_j' = 7y_j + 4$ and when both y_j' and u_j are used.

1.8. Suppose the linear regression model has a continuous and categorical covariate (K categories), together with their interaction. Write down the model formula with the first category as reference, so that there are $K - 1$ regression parameters for the differences between categories 2, 3, $\ldots$, K and category 1, and $K - 1$ regression parameters for the differences in the within-category slopes. Describe the changes in the model formula when category K is used as the reference.

1.9. Generalise the problem in Exercises 1.7 and 1.8 as follows. Suppose we have regression $E(\mathbf{y} \mid \mathbf{X}) = \mathbf{X}\boldsymbol{\beta}$. Express the regression of $b + c\mathbf{y}$ on $\mathbf{XA}$ for scalars (constants) b and $c \neq 0$ and a nonsingular matrix $\mathbf{A}$. Construct the matrix $\mathbf{A}$ for the example in Exercise 1.7. Discuss what would happen if matrix $\mathbf{A}$ were singular. What would happen if the vector of outcomes $\mathbf{y}$ were replaced by $\mathbf{y} + \mathbf{Xd}$ for a (column) vector $\mathbf{d}$ of suitable length?

1.10. Draw 20 independent random samples, each of size 50, from the standard normal distribution $\mathcal{N}(0, 1)$, and assess each sample separately whether it has the features of the normal distribution: unimodality (consider carefully its definition for a finite sample), symmetry and 'thin' tails. Should you reject any of the samples based on this inspection?

1.11. Write a programme for fitting linear regression by ordinary least squares for the setting with a single continuous covariate X. Generate a set of 50 values $\mathbf{x}$ of a covariate by drawing them from the standard (continuous) uniform distribution. Repeat Exercise 1.10 and use the samples to define 20 sets of outcomes according to the linear regression model with X, using the the the same set of values $\mathbf{x}$ and intercept $\beta_0 = 2$ and slope $\beta_1 = 0.27$. Fit the regression to each dataset and calculate the 20 sets of residuals $\mathbf{e}$. Inspect each vector $\mathbf{e}$ and note any unusual features. Should the model be revised in any way in cases in which you have noticed something that might be interpreted as a contradiction with the assumptions of normality and homoscedasticity of ε?

1.12. Find realistic examples of studies in which the values of one or several covariates X are set by design, but the outcomes y are subject to interference. For example, the (human) subjects may discuss their participation in the study or the outcomes may be recorded in time order and the values already recorded can be inspected; the subjects may find it desirable to have or not to have exceptional outcomes.

1.13. The χ^2 distribution with $M > 0$ degrees of freedom is defined as the distribution of the sum of squares of a set of m independent variables, each with the standard normal distribution:

$$X^2 = Y_1^2 + \cdots + Y_2^2 + \cdots + Y_M^2, \qquad (1.25)$$

where Y_m, $m = 1, \ldots, M$, are independent and $Y_m \sim \mathcal{N}(0, 1)$. We write $X^2 \sim \chi_M^2$. Derive the expectation and variance of the χ_M^2 distribution. The noncentral χ^2 distribution with M degrees of freedom and a noncentrality parameter $\xi \geq 0$ is defined similarly to (1.25), except that

$$Y_1 \sim \mathcal{N}\left(\sqrt{\xi}, 1\right) ;$$

the other variables, $Y_2, \ldots, Y_M$, have standard normal distributions and all the Ys are mutually independent. We use the notation $\chi_{M,\xi}^2$. Derive the expectation and variance of $\chi_{M,\xi}^2$.

1.14. A variable X is said to have a scaled χ^2 distribution if for a constant $c > 0$, X/c has a χ^2 distribution; c is referred to as the *scale* of the distribution. Show that the estimator of σ^2 in ordinary regression model with a single continuous covariate has the scaled χ^2 distribution with scale $\sigma^2/(n-2)$ and $n-2$ degrees of freedom.

Hint: Express the vector of residuals $\mathbf{y} - \mathbf{X}\hat{\boldsymbol{\beta}}$ in terms of the projection matrix $\mathbf{P_X} = \mathbf{X}\left(\mathbf{X}^\top \mathbf{X}\right)^{-1}\mathbf{X}$.

1.15. Derive the expectation and variance of the estimator $\hat{\sigma}^2$ in the setting of the previous exercise. Find the efficient estimator of σ^2 among the estimators $d\hat{\sigma}^2$ for $d > 0$.

1.16. The χ^2_M distribution has the density

$$f(x) = \Gamma\left(\tfrac{1}{2}M\right) x^{\frac{M}{2}-1} \exp\left(-\tfrac{1}{2}x\right).$$

(Γ is the Gamma function, defined as $\Gamma(a) = \int_0^{+\infty} x^{a-1}e^{-x}\,dx$.) The reciprocal χ^2_M is defined as the distribution of $1/X$ for a variable X distributed according to χ^2_M. Derive the density of the reciprocal χ^2_M. Derive the bias and variance of the estimator $1/\hat{\sigma}^2$ for the reciprocal of the residual variance σ^2 in ordinary regression. Find among the estimators $d/\hat{\sigma}^2$, with a positive constant d, the one that has no bias and the one that has minimum MSE.

Hint: Let $F(x) = P(X < x)$ for $x > 0$ be the distribution function of χ^2_M. Then $G(x) = 1 - F(1/x)$ is the distribution function of the reciprocal χ^2_M. The corresponding density is obtained by differentiating G.

1.17. Plot the MSE in (1.19) as a function of b for a setting ($\mathbf{X}$, σ^2, and $\bar{x}$) of your choice and check that its minimum is attained for $b^* = 1/(1 + S_x \omega)$. Check the conclusions related to the inequalities in (1.22).

1.18. Derive the synthetic estimator $\tilde{y}$ for the prediction problem in Section 1.2.1 with the criterion $\text{var}(\tilde{y}) + \rho B^2(\tilde{y}; \mathbf{x}^*\boldsymbol{\beta})$ instead of MSE (ρ is a positive constant). Check that the solution agrees with the text when $\rho = 1$. Discuss the solutions for $\rho = 0$ and $\rho \to +\infty$.

1.19. Discuss the difference between an observation that is an outlier and one that is associated with high leverage. Is being an outlier a population or a sample (replication-specific) quantity? What about a unit (subject) with high leverage? What, if anything, can be done about outliers and high-leverage units when designing a study?

1.20. Reproduce Figure 1.3 for a dataset of your choice or one generated on the computer, and add to it an observation with high leverage, unless the dataset already has one. Illustrate how the regression slope changes as the outcome for this subject is altered. Find among the subjects one for which the residual $e_j = y_j - \mathbf{x}\hat{\boldsymbol{\beta}}$ is altered only slightly and one for which e_j is changed much more. Discuss the problems arising from having a high-leverage observation when the regression is in fact not linear.

1.21. Prove the identities in (1.23). Derive the corresponding identities for the square transformation, $E\left(y_j^2 \mid \mathbf{x}_j\right)$ and $\mathrm{var}\left(y_j^2 \mid \mathbf{x}_j\right)$, when $y_j \sim \mathcal{N}(\mathbf{x}_j\beta, \sigma^2)$.

1.22. Generate a random sample of size 50 from the standard uniform distribution. Denote it by $\mathbf{U}$. Evaluate $\mathbf{y} = \mathbf{U}^{1.1}$ (elementwise). Suppose you do not know how Y was generated but have information that it may be a random sample from the standard uniform distribution. Define a suitable feature and apply simulation-based diagnostics to assess whether $\mathbf{y}$ is such a random sample.
Hint: By raising the random sample $\mathbf{U}$ to a power, the symmetry of the underlying distribution is spoilt and the expectation of the distribution is reduced from $\frac{1}{2}$.

1.23. Repeat the previous exercise with a range of powers of $\mathbf{U}$, including 1.0, and assess the effectiveness of your method. Suppose the median of the distribution underlying $\mathbf{y}$ is estimated as 0.5 if it is concluded that the sample is from $\mathcal{U}(0,1)$, and as the sample median otherwise. Discuss the properties of this estimator and devise some improvements on it.

1.24. Inflation can be described as the effect of time on the price of a product. Apply this definition to the house prices in a region given that there is a great variety of houses, only some are sold in any given period of time, and the sale price depends on a variety of factors, such as the professionals involved (estate agent, solicitor, etc.), the bargaining positions of the seller and buyer, and the details of the sales contract. The dataset in file EX1a.dat on www.sntl.co.uk/BookA/Data contains an example. Explore how it can be presented graphically.

1.25. Discuss the difficulties in estimating the average effect of a method of teaching. The teachers participating in a study would be instructed about the novel teaching style and encouraged to apply it in their classes. Discuss whether (and how) the principles of experimental design can be applied. Consider the 'novelty factor': as a novelty, the teaching style is attractive and brings about better outcomes, but over time the novelty wears off and it is no longer effective.

1.26. Consider the design of a study in which ordinary regression of the outcome Y is to be fitted to the stimulus X, the value of which can be set at the designer's will. Discuss the advantages of the values of the stimuli set in a wide range (interpolation possible for a wide range of values of X) and in a narrow range (the assumptions of the linear regression are more palatable). Apply your conclusions to a study in which the effect of an active compound on the time it takes for an open wound of a particular kind to heal is to be estimated.

Maximum Likelihood Estimation

Maximum likelihood is a very general method for estimation of model parameters. It has good properties in large samples and when a valid model is used. Therefore it has to be accompanied by a method that addresses model uncertainty. In this chapter, we give details of the method of maximum likelihood and compare two approaches to dealing with model uncertainty—selecting a model and combining estimators based on the alternative models.

2.1 Likelihood

The *likelihood* is defined as the joint density or probability of the outcomes, with the roles of the values of the outcomes $\mathbf{y}$ and the values of the parameters θ interchanged. Thus, let $f(\mathbf{y}; \theta)$ be a class of joint densities with the parameter vector θ in a set (parameter space) Θ. For each $\theta \in \Theta$, $f(\mathbf{y}; \theta)$ is a joint density of a continuous distribution. It will be expedient to use the same notation for joint probabilities of discrete distributions; for them, $f(\mathbf{y}; \theta) = \mathrm{P}(\mathbf{Y} = \mathbf{y}; \theta)$, where $\mathbf{Y}$ is the random vector of the outcomes. The likelihood is defined, after recording the values $\mathbf{y}$ of the vector $\mathbf{Y}$, as the function

$$L(\theta; \mathbf{y}) = f(\mathbf{y}; \theta), \tag{2.1}$$

with $\theta \in \Theta$ as its argument. This definition reflects the task at hand. Having observed, and therefore fixed, $\mathbf{Y}$ at $\mathbf{y}$, we consider all possible values of θ, intending to estimate the value that underlies the observed process, delineate a plausible range of values of θ, or make an inference about θ that is formulated in some other way. When we planned the study, we considered the configurations of values of $\mathbf{y}$ that might arise and how likely they are to arise if the studied process is governed by a particular joint density f; that is, we temporarily fixed θ and explored the plausible outcomes $\mathbf{y}$. After observing $\mathbf{y}$, we now want to identify values of θ that are compatible with the vector of outcomes $\mathbf{y}$, pursuing the unattainable ideal of identifying the value of θ that governs the process of generating $\mathbf{Y}$.

The maximum likelihood estimator of θ for the model given by the joint densities or probabilities $f(\mathbf{y}; \theta)$, with $\theta \in \Theta$, is defined as the value of θ at which the corresponding likelihood $L(\theta; \mathbf{y})$ attains its maximum:

$$\hat{\theta}_{\mathrm{ML}} = \arg\max_{\theta} L(\theta; \mathbf{y}).$$

This definition is not complete because there is no guarantee that such a maximum exists or, when it does exist, it is unique. However, in many settings this definition turns out to be very useful and constructive, yielding an estimator with good properties.

The principal theoretical results about the efficiency of the maximum likelihood estimators relate to *asymptotic* settings, corresponding, roughly speaking, to large sample sizes or increasing amounts of information. A ubiquitous caveat associated with all the results is that the model has to be valid; it has to contain the distribution according to which the outcomes are generated. Another important assumption is that the likelihood L is a smooth function of the parameter vector θ, usually interpreted as L being twice differentiable with all its second-order partial differentials continuous and bounded. Further, the distributions are distinct; if two distributions in the class coincide, then so do the values of their parameter vectors θ. In most practical settings, these conditions are satisfied, as a small change in the values of the parameters θ corresponds to small changes in the likelihood L. Further, the parameter vector θ must be in the interior of the parameter space Θ. Notable cases in which this condition is not satisfied include a zero variance and constraints, such as $\theta_1 \geq \theta_2$, when the data-generating process satisfies the identity $\theta_1 = \theta_2$.

Suppose the outcomes $\mathbf{y}$ are conditionally independent given the values of the other (observed) variables, a matrix $\mathbf{X}$, so that the model for them can be expressed as

$$f(\mathbf{y}; \mathbf{X}, \theta) = \prod_{j=1}^{n} f(y_j; \mathbf{x}_j; \theta)$$

($\mathbf{x}_j$ is the jth row of $\mathbf{X}$). The corresponding likelihood is

$$L(\theta; \mathbf{y}, \mathbf{X}) = \prod_{j=1}^{n} f(y_j; \mathbf{x}_j; \theta). \tag{2.2}$$

A standard approach to maximising this likelihood searches for values of $\hat{\theta}$ for which the partial derivatives of L vanish. Instead of L it is more convenient to work with its logarithm, called the *log-likelihood*,

$$l(\theta; \mathbf{y}, \mathbf{X}) = \log\{L(\theta; \mathbf{y}, \mathbf{X})\},$$

because the product in the likelihood L converts to a summation in l,

$$l(\theta; \mathbf{y}, \mathbf{X}) = \sum_{j=1}^{n} \log\{f(y_j; \mathbf{x}_j; \theta)\}.$$

This simplifies the differentiation;

$$\frac{\partial l}{\partial \boldsymbol{\theta}} = \sum_{j=1}^{n} \frac{\partial f}{\partial \boldsymbol{\theta}}(y_j\,;\mathbf{x}_j\,;\bullet)$$

for the likelihood in (2.2). The black disc indicates the argument over which the differentiation is carried out.

The vector of the first-order partial differentials of the log-likelihood is called the *score* vector; we denote it by $\mathbf{s}(\boldsymbol{\theta})$, with further arguments (as in l) if it is necessary to avoid any ambiguity. Thus, the maximum likelihood estimator should be sought among the roots of the score vector, solutions of the equation $\mathbf{s}(\boldsymbol{\theta}) = \mathbf{0}$, where the score vector is not defined, and on the boundary of the parameter space $\boldsymbol{\Theta}$. The matrix of the negative second-order partial differentials, defined as the matrix with elements

$$-\frac{\partial l^2}{\partial \theta_k\, \partial \theta_h}$$

as functions of $\boldsymbol{\theta}$ and $\mathbf{y}$, is called the *observed information matrix*. The expectation of the observed information matrix, with elements

$$-\mathrm{E}\left(\frac{\partial l^2}{\partial \theta_k\, \partial \theta_h}\right)$$

as functions of $\boldsymbol{\theta}$, is called the *expected information matrix*. It is denoted by $\mathcal{I}(\boldsymbol{\theta},\boldsymbol{\theta})$. The argument $\boldsymbol{\theta}$ appears twice, so that we can use the notation also for submatrices of $\mathcal{I}$. For example, the vector $\boldsymbol{\theta}$ may be split into a subvector $\boldsymbol{\theta}_1$ of parameters of interest and subvector $\boldsymbol{\theta}_2$ of nuisance parameters; $\boldsymbol{\theta} = \left(\boldsymbol{\theta}_1^{\top},\boldsymbol{\theta}_2^{\top}\right)^{\top}$. Then the complete notation for the square submatrix of $\mathcal{I}$ that corresponds to $\boldsymbol{\theta}_1$ is $\mathcal{I}\left(\boldsymbol{\theta}_1,\boldsymbol{\theta}_1\,;\,\boldsymbol{\theta}_1,\boldsymbol{\theta}_2\right)$, emphasising that the submatrix depends on the entire parameter vector.

Example 1. Ordinary Regression. Suppose the vector of outcomes $\mathbf{y}$ is generated according to the ordinary regression model

$$\mathbf{y} = \mathbf{X}\boldsymbol{\beta}+\boldsymbol{\varepsilon}\,,$$

where $\mathbf{X}$ is a matrix of covariates, with $\mathbf{1}$ as its first column, and the deviations $\boldsymbol{\varepsilon}$ are distributed according to $\mathcal{N}(\mathbf{0},\sigma^2\mathbf{I})$ for a positive σ^2. We derive the maximum likelihood estimators of $\boldsymbol{\beta}$ and σ^2. We assume that $\mathbf{X}$ is of full rank p, the number of its columns, and $p < n$, so that the $p \times p$ matrix $\mathbf{X}^{\top}\mathbf{X}$ is nonsingular. The log-likelihood for this model is

$$l(\boldsymbol{\beta},\sigma^2;\,\mathbf{y},\mathbf{X}) = -\frac{1}{2}\left\{n\log(2\pi\sigma^2)+\frac{1}{\sigma^2}\mathbf{e}^{\top}\mathbf{e}\right\}\,, \qquad (2.3)$$

where $\mathbf{e} = \mathbf{y}-\mathbf{X}\boldsymbol{\beta}$. This vector $\mathbf{e}$ differs from $\boldsymbol{\varepsilon}$; $\mathbf{e}$ is a function of $\boldsymbol{\beta}$, whereas $\boldsymbol{\varepsilon}$ is the value of $\mathbf{e}$ for the population ('true') value of $\boldsymbol{\beta}$. The log-likelihood in

(2.3) is a quadratic function of β, involved in $\mathbf{e}$, so its extremes are easy to find. As $\partial \mathbf{e}/\partial \beta = -\mathbf{X}$, we have

$$\frac{\partial l}{\partial \beta} = \frac{1}{\sigma^2}\mathbf{X}^\top \mathbf{e},$$

and this score vector has the unique root

$$\hat{\beta} = \left(\mathbf{X}^\top \mathbf{X}\right)^{-1}\mathbf{X}^\top \mathbf{y},$$

irrespective of the value of σ^2. (The inverse is well defined because $\mathbf{X}$ has full column rank.) This coincides with the ordinary least squares estimator derived in Section 1.2.

The observed information matrix for β is obtained by differentiating the score vector $\partial l/\partial \beta$, yielding

$$-\frac{\partial l^2}{\partial \beta\,\partial \beta^\top} = \frac{1}{\sigma^2}\mathbf{X}^\top \mathbf{X}.$$

Being constant (not depending on $\mathbf{y}$), it is also equal to the expected information matrix. Its inverse, assuming that $\mathbf{X}^\top \mathbf{X}$ is nonsingular, is the sampling variance matrix of $\hat{\beta}$. The two related results, that the maximum likelihood estimator is efficient and that the inverse of its information matrix is equal to the sampling variance matrix, hold more generally, but, unlike for ordinary regression, they do only approximately and with some qualifications. These are discussed in Section 2.1.2.

The maximum likelihood estimator of σ^2 is obtained by finding the root of the score function for σ^2:

$$-\frac{n}{2\sigma^2} + \frac{1}{2\sigma^4}\mathbf{e}^\top \mathbf{e} = 0,$$

that is,

$$\hat{\sigma}^2 = \frac{1}{n}\hat{\mathbf{e}}^\top \hat{\mathbf{e}} = \frac{1}{n}\left(\mathbf{y}^\top \mathbf{y} - \mathbf{y}^\top \mathbf{X}\hat{\beta}\right),$$

where $\hat{\mathbf{e}} = \mathbf{y} - \mathbf{X}\hat{\beta}$ is the vector of residuals. This estimator differs from its ordinary least squares counterpart by its denominator (n instead of $n-p$). It is biased; $\mathrm{E}(\hat{\sigma}^2/\sigma^2) = (n-p)/n$. This might appear as a deficiency of the maximum likelihood, although the bias of $\hat{\sigma}^2$ is small for large n.

2.1.1 Consistency

Consistency is a property of an estimator that it would recover the value of the target if it were based on many observations. To formalise this, we represent the idea of many observations by a sequence of sets of observations and models for them, with sample sizes increasing beyond all bounds. The sets, as well as observations within each set, are mutually independent. Each set is associated with a different model, but the models share the same vector of model parameters. The simplest, yet still quite general, setting has the same density (or probability) conditional on some covariates $\mathbf{x}$ with observation-specific values, $f(\mathbf{y}; \boldsymbol{\theta}, \mathbf{x})$.

To avoid contorted verbal expressions, we refer to the sequence of (univariate) estimators $\hat{\theta}_n$ based on the nth set of observations $\mathbf{y}_n$ as a single estimator. Consistency of such an estimator $\hat{\theta}$ of a target θ is defined as convergence of $\hat{\theta}_n$ to the target θ as $n \rightarrow +\infty$. For distributions, there are several definitions of convergence, and each corresponds to a different definition of consistency. In practice, these differences are not important, and we can focus on weak convergence, defined as convergence of the distribution functions of $\hat{\theta}_n$ to the degenerate distribution with all its mass (a single jump) at θ.

An important result about maximum likelihood estimators is that under some regularity conditions they are consistent. The regularity conditions include smoothness of the likelihood, its distinctness for each vector of model parameters and finite dimensionality of the parameter space, independent of the sample size. This result has extensions in several directions. First, univariate outcomes can be replaced by multivariate ones. Next, some correlation among the observations can be allowed, so long as it is distant from ± 1. And finally, the parameter space may be expanding with the sample size, but its dimension has to grow at a rate much slower than n.

Consistency of the maximum likelihood estimator is a key condition for deriving other properties of maximum likelihood estimators that are of practical importance.

2.1.2 Asymptotic Efficiency and Normality

Asymptotic efficiency and asymptotic normality are key properties of maximum likelihood estimators. The qualifier *asymptotic* refers to properties in the limit as the sample size increases above all bounds. Asymptotic efficiency supports the everyday application of maximum likelihood estimators, and asymptotic normality enables us to make a convenient reference to a familiar distribution.

For a set of many conditionally independent outcomes (large sample size n), given covariates and a finite-dimensional set of parameters $\boldsymbol{\theta}$, the maximum likelihood estimator is approximately unbiased, and its distribution is well approximated by the normal distribution with sampling variance matrix equal to the inverse of the expected information matrix. This result is referred to as *asymptotic normality*. Further, the maximum likelihood estimator is *asymptotically efficient* and, asymptotically, the sampling variance of the estimator is equal to the corresponding diagonal element of the inverse of the expected information matrix. That is, for large n, there are no estimators substantially more efficient than the maximum likelihood estimator. This result is the main underpinning of maximum likelihood estimation. In the next section, we construct estimators that are more efficient than maximum likelihood, but not substantially so for large sample sizes.

The *Cramér–Rao inequality* is a powerful result that relates to all unbiased estimators. It gives a lower bound for the variance of an unbiased estimator. Let $l(\theta; \mathbf{y})$ be a log-likelihood and $s(\theta; \mathbf{y})$ and $\mathcal{I}(\theta)$ the corresponding score function and expected information. Suppose l satisfies the regularity conditions listed earlier. Then any unbiased estimator $\hat{\theta}$ of θ satisfies the inequality

$$\mathrm{var}\left(\hat{\theta}\right) \geq \frac{1}{\mathcal{I}(\theta)};\tag{2.4}$$

that is, there are no unbiased estimators that are more efficient than the maximum likelihood estimator.

A more general result related to (2.4) states that, under the same regularity conditions, any estimator $\hat{\theta}$ of θ, with bias $\mathrm{B}(\hat{\theta}; \theta)$, satisfies the inequality

$$\mathrm{var}\left(\hat{\theta}\right) \geq \frac{\left\{1 + \mathrm{B}'(\hat{\theta}; \theta)\right\}^2}{\mathcal{I}(\theta)}.\tag{2.5}$$

Hence, there may be biased estimators with smaller MSE than any unbiased estimator. This may at first appear as a contradiction, because any estimator $\hat{\theta}$ might be improved by removing its bias. However, the bias itself has to be estimated, and so its removal may be accompanied by a variance inflation. The inequality in (2.5) suggests that efficient biased estimators should be sought among those with bias $\mathrm{B}(\hat{\theta}; \theta)$ that is a decreasing function of θ. Some shrinkage estimators have this property, so it makes sense to search for improvement on maximum likelihood estimators among them; see Example 4.

The Cramér–Rao inequality (2.4) justifies our focus on maximum likelihood only for large samples, when unbiasedness is essential for efficiency. There is no clinical formula that would arbitrate whether a given sample size in a particular setting is large enough for a specified purpose. Also, small-sample behaviour of the maximum likelihood estimator may differ from what the asymptotic expression would suggest. A further difficulty is that all the results associated with maximum likelihood estimation are subject to the caveat of working with the appropriate model. Sufficiently large samples can come close to confirming that a particular model is appropriate, but model uncertainty has to be reckoned with in small or moderate samples. The aim of achieving the lower bound in (2.4) may either be too optimistic or not particularly attractive because too complex a model has to be specified. In any case, equality in (2.4) and (2.5) is attained only when the estimator $\hat{\theta}$ is a linear function of the score $\partial l / \partial \theta$.

Asymptotic normality and efficiency of the maximum likelihood estimator confer the central role on the normal distribution in statistics. The proof of asymptotic normality relies on the weak law of large numbers, which confers a similar role on the normal distribution in probability theory. We are rather fortunate that the normal distribution is relatively easy to handle, it has a comprehensive generalisation to many dimensions that is closed with respect to addition, taking margins and conditioning.

The results of asymptotic normality and efficiency have been extended to settings other than those of independent and conditionally identically distributed outcomes, such as for correlated observations and observations that do not have identical distributions, even after conditioning on the values of the covariates in regression or similar quantities. Features common to these extensions are that none of the observations and groups of observations that have finite sizes make an unbounded (disproportionately large) contribution to the expected information. A complication in formulating the assumptions is that asymptotics requires a much more careful definition than for independent observations. For example, for the random-effects ANOVA, the number of clusters should diverge to infinity, but the fraction n_k/n of the sample size of each cluster k and the overall sample size (the representation of cluster k) should converge to zero in such a way that even $n_k/\sqrt{n}$ converges.

The assumptions necessary for these results are that the log-likelihood is smooth, with all its second-order partial differentials continuous, the expected information matrix exists, the value of the parameter vector is in the interior of the parameter space, and the distributions constituting the model are distinct and contain the data-generating ('true') distribution. Further, all the eigenvalues of the expected information matrix diverge to $+\infty$ as $n \to \infty$. These are the regularity conditions referred to earlier.

In brief, maximum likelihood has no competitor for large samples. The theoretical results provide no formula for establishing what constitutes a large enough sample in any particular setting. Often only trial and error with simulations can provide an indication for how close we are to asymptotics. For some simple models, such as ordinary regression, maximum likelihood estimators coincide with established estimators or are very close to them. Together with its universality, this gives maximum likelihood a strong appeal and justifies its role as the workhorse of statistical analysis. With small or moderate sample sizes, maximum likelihood is applied as a default when there is no obvious alternative. In evaluating maximum likelihood estimators we may have to call on (iterative) numerical methods for maximisation of real functions.

In Chapter 1, we came across examples in which $\hat{\theta}$ was an unbiased and efficient estimator of a parameter θ, yet a monotone nonlinear transformation $g(\hat{\theta})$ was neither unbiased nor efficient for $g(\theta)$. Maximum likelihood has the converse property. If $\hat{\theta}$ is the maximum likelihood estimator of θ, then $g(\hat{\theta})$ is the maximum likelihood estimator of $g(\theta)$ for any monotone (one-to-one) transformation g. This may at first appear to be a very convenient property. However, it implies that not all maximum likelihood estimators are efficient. A maximum likelihood estimator $\hat{\theta}$ is efficient only *asymptotically* (assuming that the regularity conditions apply). As the sample size diverges, the sampling variance of $\hat{\theta}$ diminishes; only when it vanishes can the operations of estimation and (nonlinear) monotone transformation be interchanged.

Under regularity conditions, the bias of a maximum likelihood estimator converges to zero. We say that such estimators are asymptotically unbiased. Together with the sampling variance converging to zero (as $n \to \infty$), this is equivalent to consistency, with the appropriate definition of convergence (convergence in expectation). Consistency is a valuable property in connection with large samples but is not particularly relevant otherwise, when the sampling variance is the dominating contributor to the mean squared error (MSE).

2.2 Sufficient Statistics

The log-likelihood function $l(\boldsymbol{\theta}; \mathbf{y})$ sometimes depends on the outcomes $\mathbf{y}$ only through one or a few summaries of $\mathbf{y}$; $l(\boldsymbol{\theta}; \mathbf{y}) = l\{\boldsymbol{\theta}; \mathbf{u}(\mathbf{y})\}$. To evaluate such a likelihood, we do not have to provide the n-dimensional data vector $\mathbf{y}$; it suffices to provide the summaries $\mathbf{u}(\mathbf{y})$. A set of summaries that enables the evaluation of the log-likelihood is called a *set of sufficient statistics*. When there is such a set of statistics the score vector depends on $\mathbf{y}$ also only through them: $\mathbf{s}(\boldsymbol{\theta}; \mathbf{y}) = \mathbf{s}\{\boldsymbol{\theta}; \mathbf{u}(\mathbf{y})\}$. As the main use of the likelihood is for its maximisation with respect to the vector of its parameters $\boldsymbol{\theta}$, we do not have to be concerned with its factors that do not involve $\boldsymbol{\theta}$, even if they involve $\mathbf{y}$. A set of sufficient statistics can be motivated as a condensed version of the data that is complete; any additional statistic (data summary) would be redundant for maximum likelihood estimation.

A set of sufficient statistics is qualified by the model (a class of distributions) and the vector of its parameters. Formally, it is defined as follows. A set of statistics $\mathbf{u}$ is sufficient for a parameter vector $\boldsymbol{\theta}$ in a model if the conditional distribution of $\mathbf{y}$ given the value of $\mathbf{u} = \mathbf{u}(\mathbf{y})$, $(\mathbf{y} \mid \mathbf{u})$, does not depend on $\boldsymbol{\theta}$. This conditional distribution may depend on model parameters that are not included in $\boldsymbol{\theta}$. Also, it need not depend on $\boldsymbol{\theta}$ in a particular model, but may depend on it in a more general model.

Checking that a vector $\mathbf{u}$ is sufficient by applying this definition directly is often tedious because it entails derivation of the (joint) density of $\mathbf{u}$. A much more practical equivalent definition refers to the form of the likelihood. A random vector $\mathbf{u}$ is sufficient for a parameter vector $\boldsymbol{\theta}$ in a model if and only if the log-likelihood can be expressed as

$$l(\boldsymbol{\theta}; \mathbf{y}) = l_1\{\boldsymbol{\theta}; \mathbf{u}(\mathbf{y})\} + l_2(\mathbf{y}). \tag{2.6}$$

This equivalence is known as the *factorisation theorem*, referring to the factors $\exp(l_1)$ and $\exp(l_2)$ of the likelihood $\exp(l)$. Note that maximising the likelihood is equivalent to maximising the 'essential' factor $l_1(\boldsymbol{\theta}, \mathbf{u})$ and is related to the problem of finding the roots of $\mathbf{s}(\boldsymbol{\theta}) = \partial l_1(\boldsymbol{\theta}, \mathbf{u})/\partial \boldsymbol{\theta}$.

For example, $\mathbf{X}^\top \mathbf{y}$ is a set of sufficient statistics for β in the ordinary regression, and when supplemented with $\mathbf{y}^\top \mathbf{y}$ it is sufficient also for σ^2. This is obvious from the expression

$$l = -\frac{1}{2}\log(2\pi) - \frac{n}{2}\log(\sigma^2) - \frac{1}{2\sigma^2}\beta^\top \mathbf{X}^\top \mathbf{X}\beta + \frac{1}{\sigma^2}\mathbf{y}^\top \mathbf{X}\beta - \frac{1}{2\sigma^2}\mathbf{y}^\top \mathbf{y};$$

the first three terms on the right-hand side do not depend on $\mathbf{y}$, and the last term does not involve β but does involve σ^2. A set of sufficient statistics $\mathbf{u}(\mathbf{y})$ is not unique because sufficiency is retained, for instance, when the components of $\mathbf{u}(\mathbf{y})$ are subjected to strictly monotone transformations or when further summaries are added to $\mathbf{u}(\mathbf{y})$. In particular, $\mathbf{y}$ itself is a set of sufficient statistics.

A set of sufficient statistics $\mathbf{u}$ that has m components is said to be *minimal* if for every transformation f from $\mathcal{R}^m$ to $\mathcal{R}^{m'}$, $m' < m$, $f(\mathbf{u})$ is not sufficient. That is, a set of sufficient statistics is minimal if all of its reductions to fewer statistics are not sufficient. For example, if we drop one of the components of a set of minimal sufficient statistics or replace a pair of them by their total, the result is not a set of sufficient statistics. In ordinary regression with $\mathbf{X}$ of full column rank, $\mathbf{y}$ as a set of statistics is not minimal sufficient because $(\mathbf{X}\ \mathbf{y})^\top \mathbf{y}$ is a reduction of $\mathbf{y}$ to fewer dimensions. A set of sufficient statistics $\mathbf{u}(\mathbf{y})$ is said to be *linear* if l_1 in the factorisation (2.6) is a linear function of $\mathbf{u}$.

The importance of sufficient statistics is that they reduce the range of data summaries that have to be considered for any inference about the model parameters. Thus, immediately after data collection we can reduce the outcomes $\mathbf{y}$ to the statistics $\mathbf{u}(\mathbf{y})$ without discarding any relevant information. This is particularly valuable when $\mathbf{u}$ has only a small number of components, and their number does not depend on the sample size n. In iterative procedures for maximising the likelihood, we do not have to work with the entire vector $\mathbf{y}$ in each iteration if we evaluate a vector of sufficient statistics before the first iteration. We can consider similar summaries for $(\mathbf{X}\ \mathbf{y})$, formally by regarding the covariates $\mathbf{X}$ also as outcomes. With such summaries, we could conduct the analysis without requiring any access to $\mathbf{X}$ or $\mathbf{y}$. For example, the ordinary least squares requires the summaries in $(\mathbf{X}\ \mathbf{y})^\top(\mathbf{X}\ \mathbf{y})$.

A theoretical result supporting our focus on sufficient statistics is the *Rao–Blackwell theorem*. It states that any estimator $\hat{\theta}$ of a model parameter θ is at least as efficient as the conditional expectation $\mathrm{E}(\hat{\theta}\,|\,\mathbf{u})$ where $\mathbf{u}$ is a set of sufficient statistics. Thus, any estimator of θ can be associated with an estimator that is at least as efficient and depends on $\mathbf{y}$ only through $\mathbf{u}$.

Example 2. Exponential Distributions. The class of exponential distributions is given by the densities

$$f(x;\theta) = \theta \exp(-\theta x)$$

for argument $x > 0$ and parameter $\theta > 0$. We derive the maximum likelihood estimator of θ based on a random sample $\mathbf{x}$ of size n from an exponential distribution. The log-likelihood is equal to

$$l(\theta; \mathbf{x}) = n \log(\theta) - \theta x_+ ,$$

where $x_+ = \mathbf{x}^\top \mathbf{1}$ is the sample total. Thus, x_+ is a linear sufficient statistic. Of course, it is minimal. The score for θ is equal to

$$l'(\theta; \mathbf{x}) = \frac{n}{\theta} - x_+ ,$$

so the maximum likelihood estimator is $\hat\theta = 1/\bar{x}$, the reciprocal of the sample mean.

The sample total x_+ has the gamma distribution with parameters θ and n:

$$f_n(u) = \frac{\theta^n x^{n-1}}{\Gamma(n)} \exp(-\theta x) .$$

This can be proved by induction. For $n = 1$ the result is obvious. Assuming the result for a given n, the density of the total of $n + 1$ random values is

$$\int_0^x \frac{\theta^n y^{n-1}}{\Gamma(n)} \exp(-\theta y) \, \theta \exp\{-\theta(x - y)\} \mathrm{d}y = \frac{1}{n} \frac{\theta^{n+1}}{\Gamma(n)} \exp(-\theta x) \left[y^n\right]_0^x ,$$

from which the result follows immediately.

The expectation of the reciprocal total $1/x_+$, assuming that $n > 1$, is

$$\mathrm{E}\left(\frac{1}{X_+}\right) = \int_0^{+\infty} \frac{\theta^n x^{n-2}}{\Gamma(n)} \exp(-\theta x) \, \mathrm{d}x$$

$$= \frac{\theta}{n-1} \int_0^{+\infty} \frac{\theta^{n-1} x^{n-2}}{\Gamma(n-1)} \exp(-\theta x) \, \mathrm{d}x = \frac{\theta}{n-1} ,$$

after realising that the latter integrand is the density of a gamma distribution. By similar steps, we obtain the identity

$$\mathrm{E}\left(\frac{1}{X_+^2}\right) = \frac{\theta^2}{(n-2)(n-1)} ,$$

so long as $n > 2$. Hence the maximum likelihood estimator $\hat\theta = n/X_+$ has the expectation $\{1 + 1/(n-1)\}\theta$, that is, bias $\theta/(n-1)$, and MSE

$$\mathrm{MSE}\left(\frac{n}{X_+}; \theta\right) = \frac{n^2\theta^2}{(n-2)(n-1)^2} + \frac{\theta^2}{(n-1)^2}$$

$$= \frac{(n+2)\theta^2}{(n-2)(n-1)} . \tag{2.7}$$

The estimator n/X_+ is biased; the bias can be eliminated by replacing the numerator n with $n - 1$. This is more efficient than the maximum likelihood estimator, as

$$\text{var}\left(\frac{n-1}{X_+}\right) = \frac{\theta^2}{n-2};$$

compare with (2.7). In this example, we eliminated the bias and at the same time reduced the MSE. More precisely, we simultaneously reduced the (squared) bias and the variance. In some cases such a 'correction for bias' is counterproductive—it is accompanied by variance inflation that results in a net increase of MSE. Note, however, that the bias of n/X_+ converges to zero as $n \to \infty$, as does the gain in efficiency of $(n-1)/X_+$ over n/X_+. Asymptotically, n/X_+ is unbiased and efficient.

Next we consider maximum likelihood estimation of the expectation $1/\theta$. The estimator is the sample mean $\bar{X}$. Its expectation and variance are $1/\theta$ and $1/(n\theta^2)$, respectively, derived immediately from the expectation and variance of a random draw. We explore the estimators $c\bar{X}$ for positive constants c. Their biases are $(1-c)/\theta$ and MSEs

$$\frac{c^2}{n\theta^2} + \frac{(1-c)^2}{\theta^2} = \frac{c^2}{\theta^2}\left(1+\frac{1}{n}\right) - 2\frac{c}{\theta^2} + \frac{1}{\theta^2}.$$

This quadratic function of c attains its minimum at

$$c^* = \frac{n}{n+1}.$$

The corresponding estimator, $n\bar{X}/(n+1)$, is biased,

$$\text{B}\left\{\frac{n}{n+1}\bar{X}; \frac{1}{\theta}\right\} = \frac{1}{(n+1)\theta},$$

but its MSE,

$$\text{MSE}\left(\frac{n}{n+1}\bar{X}; \frac{1}{\theta}\right) = \frac{1}{(n+1)\theta^2},$$

is smaller than for the maximum likelihood estimator $\bar{X}$. Asymptotically, as $n \to \infty$, the gain vanishes. But in practice we work (almost) exclusively with finite samples.

Example 3. Continuous Uniform Distributions. Let $x_1, x_2, \ldots, x_n$ be a random sample from the continuous uniform distribution on $(0, \theta)$, with an unknown positive parameter θ. We derive the maximum likelihood estimator of θ, and show that it is not efficient, not even asymptotically. Denote by $x_{\max}$ the largest outcome x_j, $j = 1, \ldots, n$, and by $X_{\max}$ its random-variable counterpart. The joint density of the outcomes is

$$f(\mathbf{x}; \theta) = \frac{1}{\theta^n} I\left(x_{\max} < \theta\right),$$

where I is the indicator function, equal to unity when its argument is true and to zero when it is false. This density is positive when θ is greater than or equal to all x_j, that is, when $\theta \geq x_{\max}$. The log-likelihood for $\mathbf{x}$ is defined only when $\theta > x_{\max}$. Then

$$L(\theta; \mathbf{x}) = -n\log(\theta);$$

$x_{\max}$ is a linear minimal sufficient statistic. The log-likelihood is a decreasing function for all $\theta > x_{\max}$. Therefore, its maximum is at $\hat{\theta} = x_{\max}$. Note that the likelihood is not continuous at this point.

The distribution of this estimator is derived as the probability that no outcome x_j exceeds x:

$$P\left(X_{\max} \leq x\right) = \prod_{j=1}^{n} P(X_j < x) = \frac{x^n}{\theta^n}.$$

The corresponding density is

$$f(x) = \frac{nx^{n-1}}{\theta^n}.$$

The expectation and variance of this distribution are

$$E\left(X_{\max}\right) = n \int_0^\theta \frac{x^n}{\theta^n}\, \mathrm{d}x = \frac{n}{n+1}\, \theta,$$

$$\operatorname{var}\left(X_{\max}\right) = n \int_0^\theta \frac{x^{n+1}}{\theta^n}\mathrm{d}x - \left\{E\left(X_{\max}\right)\right\}^2$$

$$= \theta^2 \left\{ \frac{n}{n+2} - \frac{n^2}{(n+1)^2} \right\} = \frac{n\theta^2}{(n+1)^2(n+2)}.$$

Therefore,

$$\operatorname{MSE}\left(X_{\max}; \theta\right) = \frac{n\theta^2}{(n+1)^2(n+2)} + \frac{\theta^2}{(n+1)^2} = \frac{2\theta^2}{(n+1)(n+2)}.$$

We can eliminate the bias of $X_{\max}$ by multiplying the estimator by $1 + 1/n$. The sampling variance of the resulting estimator is

$$\operatorname{var}\left(\frac{n+1}{n} X_{\max} \right) = \frac{\theta^2}{n(n+2)}.$$

For large n, this is only about half of the MSE of the maximum likelihood estimator $X_{\max}$. In this example, the maximum likelihood theory breaks down because the likelihood is not smooth in the neighbourhood of θ.

2.3 Synthetic Estimation

In this section, we describe a generalisation of the synthetic estimator defined in Sections 1.1.1 and 1.2.1. We contrast it with model selection, selecting one of the candidate models.

Suppose there are $M + 1$ candidate models for a particular study; the models are indexed by integers $0, 1, \ldots, M$. Let $\hat{\theta}_m$ be the estimator derived under the assumption that model m is valid. Further, suppose $\hat{\theta}_0$ is unbiased, irrespective of which model is valid, and the estimators $\hat{\theta}_m$ are not linearly dependent, so that a combination $b_0 \hat{\theta}_0 + b_1 \hat{\theta}_1 + \cdots + b_M \hat{\theta}_M$ has zero variance only when all the coefficients b_m vanish.

A setting for which the general result that is derived next is intended in particular is that model 0 is a general model and all the other models are its submodels. In this setting, we say that model 0 is a *supermodel* or an *envelope* of models $1, \ldots, M$; model 0 contains their union. Model 0 is assumed to be valid at the outset, prior to data inspection. Denote by $\hat{\boldsymbol{\theta}}$ the vector of estimators $\hat{\theta}_m$, $m = 1, \ldots, M$, by $\mathbf{V}$ its variance matrix, by $\mathbf{B}$ the vector of its biases in estimating $\theta \mathbf{1}$ and by $\mathbf{C}$ the vector of the covariances of $\hat{\boldsymbol{\theta}}$ with $\hat{\theta}_0$:

$$\hat{\boldsymbol{\theta}} = \left(\hat{\theta}_1, \ldots, \hat{\theta}_M \right)^{\mathsf{T}},$$

$$\mathbf{V} = \mathrm{var} \left(\hat{\boldsymbol{\theta}} \right),$$

$$\mathbf{C} = \mathrm{cov} \left(\hat{\boldsymbol{\theta}}, \hat{\theta}_0 \right),$$

$$\mathbf{B} = \mathrm{E} \left(\hat{\boldsymbol{\theta}} \right) - \boldsymbol{\theta}. \tag{2.8}$$

These (co-)variances and biases are evaluated assuming model 0. Note that $\hat{\theta}_0$ is not involved in $\hat{\boldsymbol{\theta}}$, $\mathbf{V}$, or $\mathbf{B}$. Let $V_0 = \mathrm{var}(\hat{\theta}_0)$.

The ideal composition of the estimators $\hat{\theta}_m$, $m = 0, 1, \ldots, M$, is defined as their convex combination with the smallest MSE. We show later that this combination is

$$\tilde{\theta}^* = \left(1 - \mathbf{b}^{*\mathsf{T}} \mathbf{1} \right) \hat{\theta}_0 + \mathbf{b}^{*\mathsf{T}} \hat{\boldsymbol{\theta}}, \tag{2.9}$$

where $\mathbf{b}^* = \mathbf{Q}^{-1} \mathbf{P}$, with

$$\mathbf{Q} = \mathrm{E} \left\{ \left(\hat{\boldsymbol{\theta}} - \hat{\theta}_0 \mathbf{1} \right) \left(\hat{\boldsymbol{\theta}} - \hat{\theta}_0 \mathbf{1} \right)^{\mathsf{T}} \right\},$$

$$\mathbf{P} = \mathrm{cov} \left(\hat{\theta}_0 \mathbf{1} - \hat{\boldsymbol{\theta}}, \hat{\theta}_0 \right).$$

The matrix $\mathbf{Q}$ is positive definite.

To prove this assertion, we consider the composition

$$\tilde{\theta} = \left(1 - \mathbf{b}^{\mathsf{T}} \mathbf{1} \right) \hat{\theta}_0 + \mathbf{b}^{\mathsf{T}} \hat{\boldsymbol{\theta}}$$

for arbitrary $M \times 1$ vector $\mathbf{b}$. Its MSE in estimating θ is

$$\mathrm{MSE} \left(\tilde{\theta}; \theta \right) = \left(1 - \mathbf{b}^{\mathsf{T}} \mathbf{1} \right)^2 V_0 + \mathbf{b}^{\mathsf{T}} \mathbf{V} \mathbf{b} + 2 \left(1 - \mathbf{b}^{\mathsf{T}} \mathbf{1} \right) \mathbf{b}^{\mathsf{T}} \mathbf{C} + \mathbf{b}^{\mathsf{T}} \mathbf{B} \mathbf{B}^{\mathsf{T}} \mathbf{b}.$$

This is a quadratic function of $\mathbf{b}$, with its matrix-quadratic term equal to

$$V_0 \mathbf{1}\mathbf{1}^\top + \mathbf{V} - \mathbf{1}\mathbf{C}^\top - \mathbf{C}\mathbf{1}^\top + \mathbf{B}\mathbf{B}^\top = \mathbf{Q},$$

and so it is positive definite. Therefore $\mathrm{MSE}(\tilde{\theta}; \theta)$ has a unique minimum, and it can be found as the root of the vector of first-order partial differentials. Elementary matrix operations yield the identity

$$\frac{1}{2} \frac{\partial \mathrm{MSE}\left(\tilde{\theta}; \theta\right)}{\partial \mathbf{b}} = \left(V_0 \mathbf{1}\mathbf{1}^\top + \mathbf{V} - \mathbf{1}\mathbf{C}^\top - \mathbf{C}\mathbf{1}^\top + \mathbf{B}\mathbf{B}^\top\right)\mathbf{b} + \mathbf{C} - V_0 \mathbf{1}$$

$$= \mathbf{Q}\mathbf{b} - \mathbf{P}.$$

Hence the ideal synthetic estimator has the vector of coefficients $\mathbf{b}^* = \mathbf{Q}^{-1}\mathbf{P}$. Its MSE is

$$\mathrm{MSE}\left(\tilde{\theta}^*; \theta\right) = V_0 - \mathbf{P}^\top \mathbf{Q}^{-1}\mathbf{P}. \tag{2.10}$$

If the matrix $\mathbf{Q}$ and vector $\mathbf{P}$ were known, $\tilde{\theta}^*$ would be more efficient than any of the estimators $\hat{\theta}_m$, because the latter correspond to particular choices of $\mathbf{b}$, equal to $\mathbf{0}_M$ for $m = 0$ and to the unit vectors which comprise $M - 1$ zeros except for unity in location m for $m = 1, \ldots, M$. The MSE in (2.10) could be attained only if the matrices $\mathbf{Q}$ and $\mathbf{P}$ were known. In practice, the vector $\mathbf{b}^*$ is estimated, eroding some of the advantage of the composition $\tilde{\theta} = \tilde{\theta}(\mathbf{b}^*)$ over any one of the estimators $\hat{\theta}_m$. The composition $\tilde{\theta}$ can be defined for any collection of estimators $\hat{\theta}_m$; neither of them has to be maximum likelihood, although $\hat{\theta}_0$ has to be unbiased, or its bias should be very small. In the context of maximum likelihood or other estimators that are connected with a model, we refer to $\hat{\theta}_m$, $m = 0, 1, \ldots, M$, as *single-model-based* and, because they contribute to $\tilde{\theta}^*$, as its *constituent* estimators. Note that these estimators may have good properties when the model they are derived for is valid. However, derivation of the synthetic estimator is based on their properties (joint distribution) when only the a priori specified (designated) model 0 is valid.

Example 4. Variance Estimation. We explore estimation of the variance of a random sample from a centred normal distribution $\mathcal{N}(0, \sigma^2)$. The mean square of the observations,

$$S = \frac{1}{n}\left(X_1^2 + \cdots + X_n^2\right),$$

is an obvious candidate. Its distribution is related to the χ^2 distribution with n degrees of freedom. This distribution is defined by the sum of squares of a sequence of n independent variables, each with standard normal distribution; see Exercise 1.13. From the properties of $\mathcal{N}(0, 1)$, it is easy to derive that $\mathrm{E}\left(\chi_n^2\right) = n$ and $\mathrm{var}\left(\chi_n^2\right) = 2n$. The number of generating variables (degrees of freedom), n, is indicated by the subscript.

We have

$$\frac{n}{\sigma^2}S \sim \chi_n^2,$$

confirming that S is unbiased for σ^2; further, $\mathrm{var}(S) = 2\sigma^4/n$. As a much less credible alternative, consider the constant zero. Its bias is σ^2 and MSE is σ^4. For $n = 1$, zero is more efficient than S, and for $n = 2$ their MSEs coincide. For greater n, S is more efficient. The synthesis of S and zero corresponds to an estimator cS with suitably chosen $c > 0$. For $c < 1$, this can be interpreted as a *shrinkage*, pulling the 'original' unbiased estimator closer to zero. The minimum of the MSE,

$$\mathrm{MSE}\left(cS; \sigma^2\right) = \left\{(1 - c)^2 + \frac{2c^2}{n}\right\}\sigma^4,$$

is attained for $c^* = n/(n + 2)$, when the MSE is $2\sigma^4/(n + 2)$. Thus, a small bias, $\mathrm{E}(c^*S) - \sigma^2 = 2\sigma^2/(n+2)$, is accompanied by a $(1+2/n)$-fold reduction of the MSE. This is modest for large n, but far from trivial for small n.

We come across χ^2 distributions frequently in variance estimation. For example, the ordinary least squares estimator of the residual variance in linear regression, $\hat{\sigma}^2 = \mathbf{e}^{\top}\mathbf{e}/(n - p)$, has a scaled χ^2 distribution; $(n - p)\hat{\sigma}^2/\sigma^2 \sim \chi^2_{n-p}$. Standard textbooks emphasise unbiased estimation; for small sample sizes we can do a bit better.

2.4 Model Selection

An alternative to synthetic estimation commits us to one of the single-model-based estimators, the selection of which is also based on the data. The importance of such a selection arises from the caveat of the maximum likelihood estimator (in addition to asymptotics)—when the model is valid the estimator is (asymptotically) efficient. Other model-based estimators are subject to similar caveats. Note that the theory does not state that the estimator is not efficient when the model is not valid.

We could protect our inferences against the lack of validity by defining very general models. Although they still cannot ensure validity, they do no harm to the chances of attaining this goal; if a narrower model is valid, then so is its generalisation. If we are committed to basing our inferences on a single model we have a strong incentive to select a narrower model because estimation is in general more efficient in a smaller parameter space, so long as it contains the parameter vector that governs the studied process. However, as we make our model narrower, we may drop the data-generating distribution, ending up with an invalid model.

A procedure for narrowing the model on which we base our inferences is called *model selection*. Model selection entails uncertainty; a different model may be selected in a replication. A typical model selection procedure arbitrates between two models, A and B, where B is a submodel of A. A statistic $t(\mathbf{y})$ is defined, together with a *critical value* t^*. If the realised value of $t(\mathbf{y})$ falls below t^*, model B is adopted; otherwise model A is adopted. Following the selection (adoption) of either model, further model selection procedures may be applied. A collection of such procedures is called *multistage*. Instead of a critical value, a *critical region*, denoted by $\mathcal{C}$, may be specified. This may be an interval, such as (t_L^*, t_U^*) or its complement, with respective lower and upper limits t_L^* and t_U^*, but in principle any division of the support of the statistic $t(\mathbf{y})$ can be declared a critical region.

There is no straightforward recipe for choosing the statistic $t(\mathbf{y})$, but there are several well-founded criteria for assessing them. In many settings, model A is defined by a parameter space Θ and model B by its subspace, such as $\Theta_B = (\boldsymbol{\theta}; \theta_1 = 0)$, constraining the first component of $\boldsymbol{\theta}$ to a specific value. This setting is made much more general by allowing transformations of $\boldsymbol{\theta}$ or by imposing a constraint on a subvector of $\boldsymbol{\theta}$; $\Theta_B = \{\boldsymbol{\theta}; g(\boldsymbol{\theta}) = \mathbf{0}\}$. The constraint function g is usually linear.

For the constraint $\theta_1 = 0$, we may use an estimator $\hat{\theta}_1$ of θ_1; the critical region for θ_1 comprises values of $\hat{\theta}_1$ that are distant from the 'special' value 0. The choice of the critical region can be guided by the desire to minimise the probability of making an erroneous choice. In one view, model A is always a correct choice because we assume it to be valid. However, when model B is also valid, we would regard the choice of A as an error, because we would forego some gains in efficiency by not using the narrower model. Therefore, we choose the critical region so that the probability of (inappropriately) selecting A when B is valid does not exceed a small value, such as $\alpha = 0.05$. Note that this probability is conditional or, more accurately, hypothetical, because it refers to the setting of model B, which need not be valid. The critical region is usually set to one or both tails of the hypothetical distribution of $t(\mathbf{y})$; t_L^* and t_U^* are set so that

$$\mathrm{P}\left\{t(\mathbf{y}) \notin (t_L^*; t_U^*) \,|\, \mathrm{B}\right\} \leq \alpha, \tag{2.11}$$

or equal to α when it can be arranged. Special cases of practical importance are $t_L^* = -t_U^*$ (symmetric critical region), and $t_L^* = -\infty$ or $t_U^* = +\infty$ (one-sided critical regions). Another choice includes in the critical region the part of the support of $t(\mathbf{y})$ that has the smallest density; that is, a constant c is sought for which

$$\mathrm{P}\left[f\{t(\mathbf{y})\} < c \,|\, \mathrm{B}\right] \leq \alpha,$$

where f is the density of $t(\mathbf{y})$. When the density f is symmetric and increasing to the left and decreasing to the right of its single mode at zero, this criterion coincides with that in (2.11) with $t_L^* = -t_U^*$. Values of $\hat{\theta}_1$ may fall in the critical region even when $\theta_1 \neq 0$, but the probability of this event, when $\theta_1 = 0$, is small, so such cases can be regarded as exceptional.

A critical region is difficult to choose when the probability in (2.11) depends on $\boldsymbol{\theta}$ or, more accurately, on $\boldsymbol{\theta}_{-1}$, the subvector of $\boldsymbol{\theta}$ with the constrained component θ_1 removed. It may be opportunistic to simplify our task by choosing a statistic $t(\mathbf{y})$ that depends only on $\hat{\theta}_1$. However, this goal should be subordinated to the principal purpose, appropriate model selection, or selection that results in an efficient estimator.

When choosing A or B, two kinds of error may be committed. One, described by (2.11), is a failure to narrow down to model B. The other is the inappropriate choice of B when B is not valid. The probability of such an error usually depends on θ, and almost always on θ_1. For example, it is close to $1 - \alpha$ when θ_1 is close to zero and the likelihood corresponding to model A is smooth. The probability of appropriately selecting model A,

$$P\left\{t(\mathbf{y}) \in \mathcal{C}\right\},$$

as a function of θ, is called the *power* of the selection; it is denoted by β. (Note the potential conflict with the notation for regression parameters.)

The ideal choice of t and t^* for a given probability α is such that it has the highest possible power. As power is a function, procedures for model selection can be compared only partially. Some procedures may be more 'powerful' in certain regions of the parameter space Θ and less powerful elsewhere. A procedure is called unbiased if its power exceeds α for all θ associated with the complement of B in A (denoted by B \ A) and is smaller than or equal to α for any θ when model B is valid. One procedure is said to be uniformly more powerful than another if it has a greater power (is more powerful) for any value of the parameter vector θ in B \ A.

Example 5. ANOVA. Suppose outcomes y_{jk}, $j = 1, \ldots, n_k$, $k = 1, 2$, with $n_1 = 5$ and $n_2 = 50$, are generated according to the ANOVA model introduced in Section 1.1. We discuss estimation of the mean μ_1 for group $k = 1$. We consider the general model (A) in which the two groups have unrelated means μ_1 and μ_2 and its submodel (B) defined by the constraint $\mu_1 = \mu_2$. In both models we assume that the two groups have the same within-group variance σ_W^2, assumed to be known.

We base the model choice on the difference of the sample means $\Delta\hat{\mu} = \bar{y}_1 - \bar{y}_2$, an unbiased estimator of the population difference $\Delta\mu = \mu_1 - \mu_2$. If $|\Delta\hat{\mu}|$ is large we choose model A. If model B is valid, $\Delta\hat{\mu}$ is distributed according to $\mathcal{N}(0, g\sigma_W^2)$, where $g = 1/n_1 + 1/n_2$. We set the critical region to $(-t^*, t^*)$, where t^* is the $(1 - \frac{1}{2}\alpha)$-quantile of $\mathcal{N}(0, g\sigma_W^2)$; that is,

$$t^* = \sigma_W \sqrt{g}\, \Phi^{-1}\left(1 - \tfrac{1}{2}\alpha\right),$$

where Φ is the distribution function of $\mathcal{N}(0, 1)$. Thus, we choose A, and with it $\hat{\mu}_1 = \bar{y}_1$ if $|\Delta\hat{\mu}| > t^*$, and B and $\hat{\mu}_1 = \bar{y} = (n_1\bar{y}_1 + n_2\bar{y}_2)/n$ otherwise.

The power of this selection procedure is

$$P(|\Delta\hat{\mu}| > t^*; \Delta\mu) = \Phi\left(\frac{-t^* - \Delta\mu}{\sigma_W\sqrt{g}}\right) + 1 - \Phi\left(\frac{t^* - \Delta\mu}{\sigma_W\sqrt{g}}\right),$$

calculating the probabilities separately for negative and positive values of $\Delta\hat{\mu}$, distributed according to $\mathcal{N}(\Delta\mu, g\sigma_W^2)$.

The model selection procedure defined by $\Delta\hat{\mu}$ and t^* is unbiased. This can be proved by differentiating the power function with respect to the difference $\Delta\mu$:

$$\frac{\partial P(|\Delta\hat{\mu}| > t^*; \Delta\mu)}{\partial\Delta\mu} = \frac{1}{\sigma_W\sqrt{g}}\left\{-\phi\left(\frac{-t^* - \Delta\mu}{\sigma_W\sqrt{g}}\right) + \phi\left(\frac{t^* - \Delta\mu}{\sigma_W\sqrt{g}}\right)\right\}.$$

As the density $\phi(x)$ of $\mathcal{N}(0,1)$ is symmetric and monotone for negative and positive values of x, the differential vanishes only when $\Delta\mu = 0$. So the power, as a function of $\Delta\mu$, attains its extreme at $\Delta\mu = 0$, and it is easy to check that this extreme is a minimum. Therefore, when $\Delta\mu \neq 0$, the power exceeds α.

Two model selection procedures are said to be *equivalent* if they yield the same decision (A or B) for every possible outcome **y**. In particular, a procedure based on statistic t and critical value t^* is equivalent to the procedure based on $u(t)$ and $u(t^*)$ for any increasing function u.

2.4.1 Hypothesis Testing

The model selection procedure described in the previous section is also referred to as *hypothesis testing*. In its terminology, model B corresponds to the *null-hypothesis* and model A to the *alternative* hypothesis. We assume that the null-hypothesis is valid and abandon it in favour of the alternative only if the outcomes present sufficient evidence against B. That is, the null-hypothesis is regarded as the status quo and is overturned only when successfully challenged.

To test a particular hypothesis, a *test statistic* t is defined, together with its critical region, just like for model selection. When the realised value of the test statistic, $t(\mathbf{y})$, falls in the critical region, we regard it as evidence against the null-hypothesis. When $t(\mathbf{y})$ is outside the critical region, we adhere to the status quo, although the logically appropriate conclusion is that 'we do not know' whether the null-hypothesis is valid—we adhere to the null-hypothesis by default, not as a result of any evidence that confirms it. After adopting the null-hypothesis as an assumption, we have found no statistical contradiction with it—we have merely *failed to reject it*.

Instead of defining a test statistic $t(\mathbf{y})$ it suffices to split the outcome space, the set of all possible outcomes **y**, into two subsets and designate one of them the critical region. Although this is a more general definition of a hypothesis test, it is of little practical use. Similarly, any subset of the parameter space Θ can be declared as the null-hypothesis and its complement as the alternative. However, many practical settings can be expressed in the narrower format of the null-hypothesis being a subspace of the parameter space, defined by constraining one or several components of $\boldsymbol{\theta}$ to default (special) values.

One notable exception arises when the null-hypothesis has the form $\theta_1 > \theta_1^*$ or a similar inequality for one or several components of $\boldsymbol{\theta}$. Such a hypothesis is called *one-sided*. For instance, in Example 5, adapted for hypothesis testing, we could replace the null-hypothesis defined by $\mu_1 = \mu_2$ with $\mu_1 < \mu_2$. We can use the same test statistic, $\Delta\hat{\mu}$, but a more suitable critical region is an interval $(t^*, +\infty)$, so that the hypothesis would be rejected for large (positive) values of $\Delta\hat{\mu}$. We choose the limit t^* as

$$t^* = \sigma_W \sqrt{g}\, \Phi^{-1}(1 - \alpha),$$

so that the probability of rejecting the null-hypothesis under the borderline assumption $\mu_1 = \mu_2$ is equal to α. It is easy to check that when $\mu_1 < \mu_2$, the probability of rejecting the null-hypothesis is smaller than α and that the power exceeds α whenever the alternative is valid. Thus, the hypothesis test based on $\Delta\hat{\mu}$ and t^* is unbiased.

2.4.2 Inference Following Model Selection

Having selected a model, A or B, we may apply further selection procedures, each time pitting the previous 'winner' against a new challenger model. At the end of such a string of selections we come to the concluding part of inference, a statement about a quantity of interest θ. We might regard the 'winning' model as valid and formulate all inferences assuming so. The profound drawback of this approach is that we ignore *model uncertainty*. In each model selection step, we may have been led astray by an inappropriate selection, not by our (the analyst's) fault, but by the inherent nature of each model selection step that it does not yield the 'correct' answer with certainty. This is easy to confirm by simulations, replicating the process of generating data and model selection.

Figure 2.1 provides an illustration based on the setting of Example 5, with $\mu_1 = 1$, $\mu_2 = 0$, $\sigma_W^2 = 1$, $n_1 = 5$, and $n_2 = 50$. The left-hand panel, containing the plot of a simple random sample of 100 pairs of simulated values of the within-group sample means $\hat{\mu}_1$ and $\hat{\mu}_2$, shows that the hypothesis of equal means is rejected mostly when $\hat{\mu}_1$ is greater than μ_1. This should come as no surprise, because $\hat{\mu}_2$ has a small sampling variance $(1/50)$, and so the outcome of the hypothesis test depends mainly on the value of $\hat{\mu}_1$.

In the right-hand plot, the empirical distribution of the estimator $\hat{\mu}_1^{\dagger}$ that is based on the selected model is drawn. The distribution is distinctly bimodal, with the two mounds corresponding to rejection of the null-hypothesis (using $\hat{\mu}_1$, the shaded part of the histogram) and estimating μ_1 by $\hat{\mu}$. The solid vertical line indicates the target $(\mu_1 = 1)$ and the vertical dashes the expectation $E(\hat{\mu}_1^{\dagger})$. The MSEs of the estimators we considered are: $\text{var}(\hat{\mu}_1) = \sqrt{1/5} = 0.45$, $\text{MSE}(\hat{\mu}; \mu_1) = \sqrt{1/55 + (50/55)^2} = 0.92$, and $\text{MSE}(\hat{\mu}_1^{\dagger}; \mu_1) = 0.46$, the last established by simulations. Note that the two mounds in the right-hand panel deviate from the normal distribution; they are *conditional* distributions of the form $(Y \,|\, I)$ where Y is normally distributed and I is a dichotomous variable correlated with Y. Thus, we set out with two normally distributed estimators,

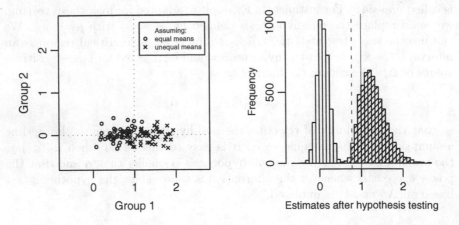

Fig. 2.1. Estimates based on hypothesis testing; the setting of Example 5 ($\mu_1 = 1$, $\mu_2 = 0$, $n_1 = 5$, $n_2 = 50$, and $\sigma^2 = 1$). In the left-hand panel, a random sample of simulated estimates of $\hat{\mu}_1$ and $\hat{\mu}_2$ is plotted; the right-hand panel is the histogram of the estimates of μ_1 after testing the hypothesis that $\mu_1 = \mu_2$; the values obtained after rejecting the null-hypothesis are represented by shading.

$\hat{\mu}_1$ and $\hat{\mu}$, attempting to use the better of them. In this task we have almost succeeded (0.46 vs. 0.45), but we ended up with an estimator that is biased and distinctly not normally distributed.

In the 10 000 replications that are summarised in Figure 2.1, the null-hypothesis was rejected in 5720 instances. If model uncertainty is ignored in these cases the standard error of $\sqrt{1/5} = 0.45$ would be reported, with a reference to $\mathcal{N}(0, 1/5)$, whereas in the remaining 4280 instances, $\sqrt{1/50} = 0.14$ would be reported. Thus the standard error would be substantially underestimated.

In summary, the process of model selection has a nontrivial impact not only on which model is selected and with what probability, but also on the distribution of the estimator, on the quality of the inference made, and on the assessment of this quality. We can rephrase this problem in the language of hypothesis testing as follows. Whichever test we apply, we cannot proceed by pretending that the outcome of the hypothesis test was known in advance of data inspection. We cannot ignore the uncertainty of the steps taken prior to the concluding act of applying the estimator that corresponds to the selected model.

The problem illustrated in Figure 2.1 cannot be resolved by applying a different test (different test statistic or different critical region). It does not appear for all configurations of means μ_1 and μ_2 and sample sizes n_1 and n_2, because in some settings the 'correct' decision is made by hypothesis testing with high probability. However, without knowing the values of μ_1 and μ_2, we are exposed to the risk of poor performance of the two-stage estimator. (The two stages are model selection and evaluation of the estimator associated with the selected model.)

A more complete overview of the problem is given in the next section where two other model-selection criteria are introduced.

2.5 Model Selection Criteria Related to Likelihood

This section describes some common model selection criteria. They are all related to likelihood and to one test statistic in particular, the *likelihood ratio*. Throughout, we consider the setting with a general model A, assumed to be valid, with a p-dimensional parameter space Θ, and its submodel B defined by constraining the parameter vector θ to a $(p - r)$-dimensional subspace of Θ, by means of a constraint (to zero) on each of r components of θ.

Let l_A and l_B be the maxima of the log-likelihood under the respective models A and B. That is, $l_A = l(\hat{\theta}_A ; \mathbf{y})$ and $l_B = l(\hat{\theta}_B ; \mathbf{y})$, where $\hat{\theta}_A$ and $\hat{\theta}_B$ are the maximum likelihood estimators under the respective models A and B. The likelihood ratio statistic is defined as $\Delta l = 2(l_A - l_B)$. Its practical importance is that the asymptotic sampling distribution of Δl is χ^2 with r degrees of freedom. This motivates the likelihood ratio test, which selects the general model A when Δl exceeds the 95th percentile of the χ_r^2 distribution. This test can be used for model selection, selecting the submodel B when Δl falls short of the 95th percentile of the χ_r^2 distribution. Under the regularity conditions, the likelihood ratio test based on Δl is asymptotically most powerful; that is, as the sample size increases, any other test of the same hypothesis is at best only slightly more powerful.

The test and the model selection procedure can be interpreted as follows. We strive for *model adequacy*, to obtain as high a (log-)likelihood as possible, while pursuing *model parsimony*, to use models with as few parameters (dimensions of the parameter space) as possible. Therefore, we select the more general model A only when it yields a much higher likelihood than the submodel B does. The likelihood ratio requires fitting both models A and B; this is a drawback only for some very complex models and large-scale datasets, because usually both estimation procedures require the same software.

The score test of the hypothesis $\theta_1 = 0$ is defined as

$$ s = \frac{\hat{\theta}_1}{\sqrt{\mathcal{I}(\theta_1)}}, $$

where $\mathcal{I}$ is the diagonal element of the information matrix that corresponds to parameter θ_1 and is evaluated at the default value $\theta_1 = 0$. Its asymptotic (large-sample) distribution, assuming model B, is standard normal. The general model is adopted when the value of $|s|$ is large, $|s| > \Phi^{-1}(1 - \alpha/2)$, so s^2 is an alternative form of the test statistic and its distribution under model B is χ_1^2, approximately, in large samples. The score test can be regarded as comparing a model and its submodel defined by the constraint $\theta_1 = 0$. It requires fitting only the general model.

The *Akaike information criterion* (AIC) is an adjustment of the likelihood ratio test statistic. It is based on the statistic $2(l_A - l_B + r)$; it selects the submodel B when its value falls short of the 95th percentile of the χ_r^2 distribution. It corrects some of the deficiencies of the likelihood ratio criterion (for model selection) but is subject to uncertainty, just like any other procedure.

The *Bayesian information criterion* (BIC) adjusts the likelihood ratio statistic by $2r \log(n)$, where n is the sample size, so it is more likely to prefer the submodel B in all but very small datasets.

We revisit Example 5 with the ANOVA setting with two groups. The likelihood ratio test is equivalent to the test conducted in ANOVA. This is shown by elementary operations:

$$l_A - l_B = -\frac{1}{2\sigma_W^2} \sum_{k=1}^{2} \sum_{j=1}^{n_k} \left(y_{jk} - \hat{\mu}_k\right)^2 + \frac{1}{2\sigma_W^2} \sum_{k=1}^{2} \sum_{j=1}^{n_k} \left(y_{jk} - \hat{\mu}\right)^2$$

$$= \frac{1}{2\sigma_W^2} \sum_{k=1}^{2} n_k \left(\hat{\mu}_k - \hat{\mu}\right)^2$$

$$= \frac{n_1 n_2}{n\sigma_W^2} \left(\hat{\mu}_1 - \hat{\mu}_2\right)^2.$$

This statistic is an increasing function of $\Delta\hat{\mu} = |\hat{\mu}_1 - \hat{\mu}_2|$.

Figure 2.2 summarises the selected-model-based estimators for the range of differences $\Delta\mu \in (0,3)$. In panel A, each curve represents the bias $B(\hat{\mu}_1 ; \mu_1)$ as a function of $\mu_2 - \mu_1$. Each curve is based on empirical evaluation (50 000 replicates) for the 31 points $0.0, 0.1, \ldots, 3.0$. The biases and MSEs are plotted in the respective panels A and B for the probabilities α equal to 0.005, 0.01, 0.025, and 0.05. The MSEs in panel B and the powers of selection in panel C are constructed similarly. For the synthetic estimator, no model selection takes place, so the power of selection is not defined. In panel C, the synthetic estimator is represented by the empirical mean of the shrinkage coefficient.

As MSE is our criterion for efficiency, panel B is key. The MSEs of the model-based estimators are constant for model A, equal to 0.2, and quadratic for model B, equal to $0.02 + \Delta\mu^2$. The estimator $\hat{\mu}_B = \hat{\mu}$ based on B is inefficient for all but very small differences $\Delta\mu$. The estimators based on model selection criteria (LR, AIC and BIC) are also efficient for small values of $\Delta\mu$ but are very inefficient for a wide range of values of $\Delta\mu$. For large values of $\Delta\mu$ they are almost as efficient as estimator $\hat{\mu}_A$.

Except for estimator $\hat{\mu}_A = \hat{\mu}_1$, the synthetic estimator has by far the smallest maximum MSE over the range $(0,3)$. It is not uniformly more efficient than the selected-model-based estimators, but it does not have their glaring weaknesses. It is least efficient when $\Delta\mu$ is small—when the estimation problem is, in a way, the easiest. Similarly, for large $\Delta\mu$, when the data should

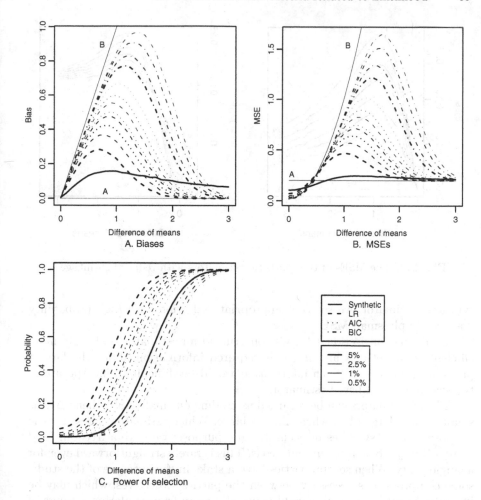

Fig. 2.2. The biases, MSEs, and powers of selection using likelihood ratio (LR), AIC and BIC, and synthesis, using a range of probabilities α, with the ANOVA setting of Example 5: $n_1 = 5$, $n_2 = 50$, $\mu_1 = 0$, $\sigma^2 = 1$, and μ_2 in the range $(0,3)$. For synthesis, the power of selection in panel C is replaced by the mean of the shrinkage coefficient. A and B in panel B denote the MSEs of the estimators based on the respective models A and B.

strongly indicate that $\Delta\mu$ is positive, the synthetic estimator is not the most efficient, but the MSEs of the competing estimators differ little. Thus, the main strength of the synthetic estimator is that it does not have any weaknesses; for no values of $\Delta\mu$ is its performance very poor. Panel A indicates that the bias is a substantial contributor to the MSE for the selected-model-based estimators. Panel C shows that the power of selection is related to the MSE. Using the mean shrinkage coefficient as a substitute for the power for the

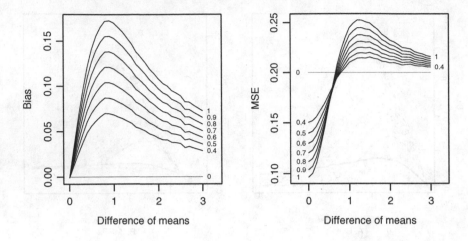

Fig. 2.3. The MSEs of the synthetic estimators with reduced shrinkage.

synthetic estimator, we see that appropriate selection with high probability does not imply small MSE.

Recall that in Section 1.1.1 we constructed an estimator uniformly more efficient than both $\hat{\mu}_1$ and $\hat{\mu}$ but it required information about the largest plausible value of $\Delta\mu$. Such information would be difficult to incorporate in the selected-model-based estimators.

All the estimators can be regarded as trading off small MSE when $|\Delta\mu|$ is small against large MSE when $|\Delta\mu|$ is large. Which estimator is best for the purpose? The answer lies in declaring *our* purpose; we have a freedom (and responsibility) to do it to suit our needs. This is rarely straightforward even for a single party. When several parties have a stake in the outcome of the study, some compromise is necessary between the parties' objectives, which may be in mutual conflict. But we should never shy away from exploring a range of purposes and then settle on an estimator that represents their compromise. Such an exploration should not look at the possible results (estimates) but at properties of estimators, MSEs as functions of parameters and design settings.

The synthetic estimator is attractive if we wish to minimise the maximum of $\text{MSE}(\hat{\mu}; \mu_1)$, which we interpret as having no weaknesses. However, by this criterion the sample mean estimator $\hat{\mu}_1$ is superior, negating all our efforts to improve on it. We can explore some variations of the synthetic estimator, by reducing its shrinkage coefficient. As a result, the estimator is improved for large values of $\Delta\mu$, at the price or reduced efficiency for small values of $\Delta\mu$. Figure 2.3 presents the results graphically, using the estimators $\tilde{\mu}_1(b)$ with the shrinkage coefficients $b = rg_1/(g_1 + \hat{\gamma}^2)$, for $r = 0.4, 0.5, \ldots, 1.0$.

The diagram shows that as we reduce the coefficient b we also reduce the bias uniformly and trade off efficiency at small values of $\Delta\mu$ for improvement at large values of $\Delta\mu$. (The breakpoint at which all the plotted functions intersect is around $\Delta = 0.7$.) At the extreme, for $r = 0$, we match the even performance of $\hat{\mu}_1$.

This extended example should in no way be interpreted as evidence of superiority of the synthetic estimator over selected-model-based estimators. Instead, the example outlines how alternative estimators can be explored and what entails the decision to choose one of them. First, the search is rarely complete and definite, because we can rarely identify an estimator that is uniformly more efficient than all its competitors. Second, we have to weigh carefully the advantages and drawbacks of the alternative estimators and, possibly, supplement our criteria with what we regard as 'good' estimation. And finally, the search may indicate how prior information, additional to the analysed dataset, can make the search more effective. For example, if in Example 5 we knew that $|\Delta| < 0.5$ we would zoom in our attention on the appropriate part of panel B in Figure 2.2.

Nevertheless, some general comments can be made about the two classes of estimators, synthetic and selected-model-based. By model selection, we aim to match the most efficient of the competing estimators. This 'ambition' is not achieved because the selection is imperfect. Synthesis aims higher, to outperform each of the constituent estimators. It fails to achieve this goal because the ideal shrinkage coefficient can only be estimated.

For two constituent estimators (models), both classes of estimators have the form

$$\tilde{\theta} = \left(1 - \hat{B}_\theta\right)\hat{\theta}_1 + \hat{B}_\theta\,\hat{\theta}_2. \tag{2.12}$$

With model selection, $\hat{B}_\theta$ 'estimates' the model to be used ($\hat{B}_\theta$ is a binary variable, with possible values 0 and 1), whereas with synthesis it estimates the ideal combination of the constituent estimators. The description by (2.12) has an obvious extension to more than two constituent estimators for synthesis:

$$\tilde{\theta} = \sum_{m=0}^{M} \hat{B}_{\theta,m}\,\hat{\theta}_m,$$

with the constraint that $\hat{B}_{\theta,0} + \hat{B}_{\theta,1} + \cdots + \hat{B}_{\theta,M} = 1$. Model selection entails the additional constraint that $(\hat{B}_{\theta,0}, \hat{B}_{\theta,1}, \ldots, \hat{B}_{\theta,M})$ is multinomial—it contains M zeros and one unity.

Although model selection usually proceeds by choices within pairs, leading to multistage selection, it is equivalent to a single-stage selection from among several models. Synthesis can also be conducted in stages, for example, first by combining estimators A and B, then by combining their synthesis with C, and so on. At first, this might seem not to be useful because the constituent estimators could be combined directly. However, synthesis of many estimators is problematic because the matrix $\mathbf{Q}_\theta^{-1}$ may be estimated inefficiently even when $\mathbf{Q}_\theta$ is estimated efficiently, especially when $\mathbf{Q}_\theta$ or $\hat{\mathbf{Q}}_\theta$ is close to singularity. In such a case, some estimators (models) can be discarded from the synthetic estimator because they can themselves almost be combined from the other constituent estimators.

As the number of observations increases and the parameter space is unaltered, the probability of selecting the appropriate model increases and the shrinkage coefficients converge to a unit vector $(0, \ldots, 0, 1, 0, \ldots, 0)$ or the zero vector $\mathbf{0}$, so that synthesis is based on a single model. Thus, asymptotically, model selection is not an issue. As the sampling variance of every estimator converges to zero, our attention should focus on eliminating the bias, and this is best done by applying the most complex model. Asymptotically, we do not have to pursue model parsimony, because one or a few redundant parameters (degrees of freedom used unnecessarily) inflate the sampling variance only slightly when we have degrees of freedom in abundance. Asymptotically, maximum likelihood has no competitors, so long as the regularity conditions are satisfied, and model adequacy should be the only concern. In practice, asymptotics is usually far away and, if we are committed to working with a single model, parsimony is highly relevant. Synthesis frees us up from this constraint but does not offer a uniformly more efficient solution.

Suggested Reading

The classical text [27] contains a comprehensive treatment of the likelihood theory, including proofs of all the key properties of maximum likelihood estimators. For a more recent monograph on likelihood, see [143]. The original references to the two information criteria, AIC and BIC, are [3] and [175], respectively. Maximum likelihood estimators for many models are evaluated using methods for numerical optimisation. Useful references to such methods are [35, 58], and [94]. A more recent monograph [98] is addressed specifically to statisticians.

Problems and Exercises

2.1. Write down the likelihood for a random sample of size n from the binary distribution with unknown probability p. How does it differ from the likelihood for a single draw from the binomial distribution $\mathcal{B}(n, p)$ with known sample size n and unknown probability p? Find a linear sufficient statistic for p. Derive the maximum likelihood estimator of p. Check that its sampling variance agrees with the reciprocal of the expected information and explain why this agreement is not maintained for the parameter $v = p(1 - p)$.

2.2. Generate random samples from a binomial distribution of your choice and verify empirically the properties of the maximum likelihood estimator $\hat{p}$ of the proportion p. Experiment with estimators of the form $c\hat{p}$ for a range of values of c near unity. Show that if p were known the minimum MSE would be attained for $c = p/\{p + (1 - p)/n\}$.

2.3. Suppose the probability $p > 0$ is known but the sample size n in a random sample from a binary distribution is not. Derive the likelihood for this setting with parameter n. How does this likelihood differ from the likelihood(s) in Exercise 2.2? Compare the maximum likelihood estimator of n with $\hat{n} = k/p$, where k is the number of positive outcomes.

2.4. Consider the following experiment comprising binary outcomes (success and failure). We keep generating outcomes independently from a binary distribution with probability $p > 0$ and stop when we reach a given positive number M of successes. Derive the likelihood for p and the maximum likelihood estimator. Explain why you would expect it to have a positive bias, especially for small M. Check your conclusion by simulations.

2.5. Derive the results in Example 1 without the aid of matrix algebra and matrix differentiation.

2.6. The *beta distributions* are defined by the densities

$$f(y; a, b) = \frac{\Gamma(a + b)}{\Gamma(a)\Gamma(b)} y^{a-1}(1 - y)^{b-1}$$

for positive constants (parameters) a and b; their support is the interval $(0, 1)$. (Note that the uniform distribution corresponds to $a = b = 1$.) Find a set of sufficient statistics for a and b. Suppose we know that a and b are integers. How would you go about maximising the likelihood? Derive the expectation and variance of the beta distribution and use them to derive a moment-matching estimator.

Hint: A *moment-matching estimator* is defined as a solution of an equation, or of a set of equations, that matches sample moments (expectation, variance, and the like) to the population moments expressed as functions of parameters. This method is called the *method of moments*.

2.7. The beta distributions with $b = 1$ are called *power distributions*. Show that they can be derived as powers of the continuous uniform distribution. Derive the Cramér–Rao inequality for the power distributions. Compare it with the sampling variance of the moment-matching estimator based on the expectation and variance. Explain why the moment-matching estimator is not efficient.

Hint: Look at the sufficient statistic for a.

2.8. Show that the χ^2 distributions are a subset of the gamma distributions. Hint: Show this first for χ_1^2 distribution and then proceed by induction. Using the densities of the gamma distributions, check that the expectation and variance of χ_n^2 are n and $2n$, respectively. Check these results using the definition of χ_n^2 by construction from a random sample from $\mathcal{N}(0, 1)$; see Exercise 1.13. Derive the expectation and variance of the reciprocal of χ^2, that is, of a variable X such that $1/X \sim \chi_n^2$.
Hint: Relate the integrals $\int y^{-k} f(y) dy$, $k = 1, 2$ to the densities of some χ^2 distributions.

2.9. Either using Exercise 1.14 or independently, prove that the (unbiased) estimator of the population variance σ^2, $\hat{\sigma}^2 = (\mathbf{y} - \bar{y})^{\top}(\mathbf{y} - \bar{y})/(n-1)$, based on a random sample $\mathbf{y}$ of size n from $\mathcal{N}(\mu, \sigma^2)$ has χ^2 distribution with $n-1$ degrees of freedom. Compare the efficiencies of the estimators with denominators n (the maximum likelihood estimator), $n-1$, and $n+1$. Find the denominator that yields the efficient estimator. Extend this result to estimating the residual variance in ordinary regression.

2.10. Estimate the reciprocal of the variance σ^2 in the setting of the previous example. Find an estimator more efficient than $1/\hat{\sigma}^2$.
Hint: Use the results of Exercise 2.8.

2.11. Suppose $\hat{\boldsymbol{\beta}}_1$ and $\hat{\boldsymbol{\beta}}_2$ are the ordinary least squares estimators with respective models 1 and 2. Models 1 and 2 may be invalid. Let $\hat{\beta}_{\mathsf{x}}$, $\hat{\beta}_{\mathsf{x}1}$, and $\hat{\beta}_{\mathsf{x}2}$ be the slopes on a covariate included in both models. Show that $\operatorname{cov}(\hat{\beta}_{\mathsf{x}1}, \hat{\beta}_{\mathsf{x}2}) = \operatorname{var}(\hat{\beta}_{\mathsf{x}2})$. Generalise this result to a sequence of K nested models and describe the pattern of the variance matrix of the K estimators of the coefficient with respect to the same covariate.

2.12. Let $(v_1, \ldots, v_K)$ be a decreasing sequence of positive numbers and $\mathbf{V}$ the matrix defined by its elements $V_{kh} = v_{\max(k,h)}$. Find the determinant and inverse of $\mathbf{V}$.
Hint: Proceed by induction. Find in the literature on matrices formulae for the determinant and inverse of a partitioned matrix $\begin{pmatrix} \mathbf{A} & \mathbf{B} \\ \mathbf{B}^{\top} & \mathbf{C} \end{pmatrix}$; in our case, $\mathbf{B} = v_K \mathbf{1}_{K-1}$ and $\mathbf{C} = v_K$.

2.13. Compile a programme for simulating the selected-model-based and synthetic estimators of the expectation for a group in the setting of ANOVA with several (say, eight) groups of ten observations each. Set the differences among the groups in such a way that the target group has in one case an extreme expectation, in another case is close to the mean of the expectations, and in another has about the average deviation from the mean of the within-group expectations. Describe the results of the simulations and present them in a diagram.

2.14. The *F-distribution* with n_1 and n_2 degrees of freedom is defined as the ratio of two scaled independent χ^2-distributed variables with n_1 and n_2 degrees of freedom in the numerator and denominator, respectively:

$$X = \frac{X_1}{X_2}\frac{n_2}{n_1}$$

where $X_1 \sim \chi^2_{n_1}$ and $X_2 \sim \chi^2_{n_2}$. Derive the expectation and variance of these distributions.

2.15. Consider the ordinary regression model

$$y_j = \beta_0 + \beta_1 x_{1j} + \beta_2 x_{2j} + \varepsilon_j$$

for two covariates, X_1 and X_2, with $\varepsilon \sim \mathcal{N}(0, \sigma^2)$, independently. Derive the likelihood ratio test statistic for the hypothesis that $\beta_2 = 0$.
Hint: Replace the variable X_2 with $X_2^* = X_2 - b_1 X_1 - b_0$ with b_1 and b_0 set so that X_2 is orthogonal to both X_1 and the intercept **1**.
Show that the test is equivalent to rejecting the hypothesis for large values of $\hat{\beta}_2^* / \sqrt{\widehat{\text{var}}\left(\hat{\beta}_2^*\right)}$, where $\hat{\beta}_2^*$ is the least squares estimator of the slope on X_2.

2.16. Compare (analytically) the estimators $(1 + 1/n) \max_j X_j$ and $2\bar{X}$ for the parameter θ of the uniform distribution on $(0, \theta)$. Do you think the estimator $\min_j X_j + \max_j X_j$ is more efficient than either of these? Check your view by simulations.

Explore the analogous problem with the uniform distribution replaced by the distribution that is formed as the mean of a random sample of size K from $\mathcal{U}(0, \theta)$. Show that this distribution is beta. Check by simulations that this distribution converges to the normal as $K \to \infty$. Presumably, as K increases, twice the sample mean becomes a relatively more efficient estimator of θ than $(1 + 1/n) \max_j X_j$. Can you confirm this? For which K are the two estimators about equally efficient? (You may consider all positive numbers for K, not only integers.)

2.17. The *Poisson distributions* are defined by the probabilities

$$P(Y = k) = \frac{e^{-\lambda} \lambda^k}{k!}$$

for $k = 0, 1, \ldots$ and parameter $\lambda > 0$. Show that $E(Y) = \text{var}(Y) = \lambda$ and that the sum of two independent variables, each with a Poisson distribution, also has a Poisson distribution. For a simple random sample from a Poisson distribution, find the maximum likelihood estimator of λ and its sampling variance. Explain why and verify by simulations that λ is estimated more efficiently as the sample mean than as the sample variance.

2.18. A local authority conducted an experiment in which all men below the age of 21 were encouraged to be at home by 11 pm every night during the months April to October 2004. To evaluate its success, they compared the numbers of reported public-order offences that involved young men in this period of 30 weeks with the same period in 2003 (dataset `EX2a.dat` on `www.sntl.co.uk/BookA/Data`). Test by the likelihood ratio the hypothesis that the average weekly numbers of offences are the same in the two years, assuming that each sequence of 30 outcomes is a random sample from a Poisson distribution. Assess how valuable it is to know that both samples are from Poisson distributions. Check and discuss how realistic such an assumption is. Discuss the problems with interpreting the result of the test given that it is not possible to implement all the principles of experimental design.

Hint: Generate many pairs of random samples from the Poisson distributions with the same means as the two years have in the data, calculate their variances as features, and plot the pairs of these variances, together with the realised pair of the within-year means which, according to the adopted model, are unbiased estimators of the variances.

2.19. *Permutation test.* As an alternative to the solution in the previous exercise consider the following. Generate a *permutation dataset* by assigning the two observations for a week to the years 2003 and 2004 at random, with these assignments being independent across the weeks. Evaluate the difference of the within-year sample means. Replicate this process many times and compare the (realised) version of this difference with the distribution of its permutation counterparts. Reject the null-hypothesis of equal means if the realised difference is in the tail of the distribution of simulated (permutation) differences. Discuss the relevance of the assumptions of the Poisson distributions and of independence among the weeks for this test.

3

Sampling Methods

This chapter deals with estimation of population quantities in surveys with a known sampling design, specified (controlled) by the designer of the survey. Sampling theory treats the values of variables as constants, and chance decides whether or not they are observed for any given member of the population. By sampling design, we set the joint probabilities associated with these observations. In Sections 3.7 and 3.7.1, pursuing efficient estimation of population quantities, we bring into play regression and related models, making use of the experience with them in the infinite population setting of Chapters 1 and 2.

3.1 Preliminaries

With unlimited resources and ready access to them, a population could be studied by enumeration—by collecting the values of the relevant variables from each member of the population. A more economic alternative is to collect such information only from a subset of the members of the population. These (selected) members are referred to as *subjects*, and collectively as a *sample*. The sampling process, by which a sample is drawn, is governed by a sampling design S defined as the function that assigns to each subset **s** of the studied population $\mathcal{P}$ a probability, $P(\mathbf{s})$, that **s** would form the sample. In practice, only one such sample is realised, by a single application of the sampling process, but inferential statements refer to distributions over samples drawn by infinitely many replications of the sampling process.

Let I be the indicator of selection of a member into the sample: $I(i) = 1$ if member i is included and $I(i) = 0$ otherwise. For each member i, $I(i)$ is a binary random variable with expectation $p_i = \mathrm{E}\{I(i)\}$ equal to the probability of including member i in the sample. The variance of $I(i)$ is $p_i(1 - p_i)$. The probability p_i can be derived solely from the sampling design, by adding up the probabilities of all the subsets of the population that contain member i:

$$p_i = \sum_{\mathbf{s}\in\exp(\mathcal{P});\, i\in\mathbf{s}} P(\mathbf{s}).$$

This is an impractical prescription for evaluating p_i in all but some very small populations and simple designs. In most cases, p_i is derived much more easily from a mechanistic description of the sampling design (the sampling *mechanism*) and various considerations of symmetry. For example, in simple random sampling without replacement and fixed sample size n, $p_i = n/N$. This follows from elementary combinatorics, but also by solving the equation $E\left(\sum_i I_i\right) = \sum_i p_i = n$ for identical probabilities $p_i \equiv p$.

For simplicity, we consider the setting with a single variable X and estimation of its population mean $\mu = \sum_i X_i/N$. The sample mean $\hat{\mu}^\dagger = \sum_j x_j/n$, the naive estimator of μ, can be expressed in terms of the population values as

$$\hat{\mu}^\dagger = \frac{\sum_{i=1}^{N} I(i)\, X_i}{\sum_{i=1}^{N} I(i)}.$$

Evaluating the mean and variance of this estimator is difficult when the denominator is random. This problem is sometimes sidestepped by conditioning on the realised sample size n. If the variation of n is to be ignored, then the size equal to the rounded expectation of the denominator, $\left[\sum_i p_i\right]$, might seem to be the obvious choice for n. The conditional variance of $\hat{\mu}^\dagger$ given n is usually a steeply decreasing function of n, especially for small n.

Of course, the conditioning on the sample size is redundant when n is fixed, when only subsets of size n have positive probabilities of forming the sample. Then

$$E\left(\hat{\mu}^\dagger\right) = \frac{1}{n}\sum_{i=1}^{N} p_i X_i,$$

$$\operatorname{var}\left(\hat{\mu}^\dagger\right) = \frac{1}{n^2}\sum_{i=1}^{N} p_i(1-p_i)X_i^2 + \frac{2}{n^2}\sum_{i=1}^{N}\sum_{i'=i+1}^{N}(p_{ii'}-p_i p_{i'})X_i X_{i'}$$

$$= \frac{1}{n^2}\sum_{i=1}^{N}\sum_{i'=1}^{N} p_{ii'} X_i X_{i'} - \left(\frac{1}{n}\sum_{i=1}^{N} p_i X_i\right)^2, \tag{3.1}$$

where $p_{ii'}$ is the probability of including both members i and i' in the sample; we refer to it as the *pairwise inclusion probability* and set $p_{ii} = p_i$. The result for the variance uses the identity

$$\operatorname{cov}\{I(i), I(i')\} = p_{ii'} - p_i p_{i'},$$

derived by equating the expectation of an indicator to the probability of it being positive. The first double summation in (3.1) would vanish if $p_{ii'} = p_i p_{i'}$, that is, if the events of including pairs of distinct members in the sample were independent. However, independence and fixed sample size are not compatible because, with independence, the variance of the sample size $n = I_1 + \cdots + I_N$,

$$\text{var}(n) = \sum_{i=1}^{N} p_i(1 - p_i),$$

is positive. An important implication of the expression for $\text{var}(\hat{\mu}^\dagger)$ in (3.1) is that the inclusion probabilities p_i are not sufficient for deriving the properties of the sample mean (or of other statistics), because they depend also on the pairwise inclusion probabilities $p_{ii'}$.

The estimator $\hat{\mu}^\dagger$ is biased when the probabilities p_i are correlated with the values of X. The expression for its bias,

$$B(\hat{\mu}^\dagger) = \frac{1}{n} \sum_{i=1}^{N} \left\{ p_i - \frac{\text{E}(n)}{N} \right\} X_i,$$

highlights the advantage of equiprobability sampling, when all inclusion probabilities p_i are equal. For such a sampling design, with n fixed, $\hat{\mu}^\dagger$ is unbiased. In practice, this is a very weak argument in favour of such designs—control over the survey costs is usually a more important consideration. In any case, efficiency (small MSE) overrides unbiasedness as a desirable property of an estimator and we are at liberty to define other estimators of μ.

Among sampling designs, we consider only those for which each inclusion probability p_i is positive. Such designs are called *proper*. Improper designs can be regarded as excluding the subpopulation of members with $p_i = 0$ from the study. An improper design becomes proper by reducing the target population to the members with $p_i > 0$. But the definition of a population should in general not be influenced by the sampling design. In proper designs, the reciprocals of the probabilities, $w_i = 1/p_i$, are called the *sampling weights*.

3.2 Horvitz–Thompson Estimator

Equation (3.1) for $\text{E}(\hat{\mu}^\dagger)$ suggests that μ can be estimated without bias by

$$\hat{\mu} = \frac{1}{N} \sum_{i=1}^{N} I(i) \, w_i X_i, \tag{3.2}$$

as $\text{E}\{I(i)w_i\} = 1$ for each member i. This estimator, or its version for estimating the population total $N\mu$, which does not involve the divisor N, is called the *Horvitz–Thompson* (HT) estimator. When the population size N is not known its estimate has to be substituted in (3.2). Its nonlinear involvement in the estimator raises no substantial problems when N is estimated with high precision. We assume first that N is known. The estimator in (3.2) involves a summation of only n terms, those for the subjects (selected members):

$$\hat{\mu} = \frac{1}{N} \sum_{j=1}^{n} \frac{x_j}{q_j},$$

where q and x are the sample versions of the respective variables p and X. Note that X_i is related to x_j for $j = i \leq n$ only through being the values of the same variable X. The ordering of the subjects is not related to the ordering of the members in any way; p_i and q_j are related similarly.

The sampling variance of the HT estimator is

$$\text{var}\,(\hat{\mu}) = \frac{1}{N^2} \sum_{i=1}^{N} \sum_{i'=1}^{N} \left(\frac{p_{ii'}}{p_i\, p_{i'}} - 1 \right) X_i X_{i'}. \tag{3.3}$$

This identity does not have the form of an average squared deviation from the mean, which might be easier to motivate. However, it will turn out to be useful for a straightforward definition of its estimator. The expression

$$\text{var}\,(\hat{\mu}) = \frac{1}{N^2} \sum_{i=1}^{N} \sum_{i'=1}^{N} \frac{p_{ii'}}{p_i\, p_{i'}} X_i X_{i'} - \mu^2,$$

equivalent to (3.3), is closer in form to some common expressions for the sampling variance.

When all the pairwise probabilities of inclusion are positive, we can apply the HT estimator to the N^2 values of products $X_i X_{i'}$, which have probabilities of being observed equal to $p_{ii'}$. These products are defined in the population of all pairs $i, i' \in \mathcal{P}$, denoted by $\mathcal{P} \times \mathcal{P}$. Denote by $I^{(2)}(i, i') = I(i)\, I(i')$ the indicator of presence in the sample of both members i and i'. Then the HT estimator of var($\hat{\mu}$) is

$$\widehat{\text{var}}(\hat{\mu}) = \frac{1}{N^2} \sum_{i=1}^{N} \sum_{i=1}^{N} \frac{1}{p_{ii'}} \left(\frac{p_{ii'}}{p_i p_{i'}} - 1 \right) I^{(2)}(i, i')\, X_i X_{i'}$$

$$= \frac{1}{N^2} \sum_{j=1}^{n} \sum_{j'=1}^{n} \left(\frac{1}{q_j\, q_{j'}} - \frac{1}{q_{jj'}} \right) x_j x_{j'}, \tag{3.4}$$

defined with reference to the population $\mathcal{P} \times \mathcal{P}$. This variance estimator requires a design for proper sampling from $\mathcal{P} \times \mathcal{P}$. In Section 3.2.2, we explore systematic sampling designs in which most pairs (i, i') cannot appear in a sample together. In brief, a systematic sampling design is defined by a *random start* a and *step length* b, and it includes in the sample all the members with indices $i = a + kb$. The integer b is set by design, and a is drawn from the discrete uniform distribution on $(1, 2, \ldots, b)$. Of course, $p_{ii'} = 0$ unless $i - i'$ is divisible by b.

The singularity in (3.4) for the systematic sampling designs can be motivated as follows. A single sample s provides next to no information about the values of the other possible samples. On the one hand, the values of X may be in a regimented order, constant within the sets of $b \doteq N/n$ members that are represented in the sample by a single subject; on the other hand, the values may be dispersed much more than they are in any possible sample. This diagnosis exposes a weakness of the estimator in (3.4): it allows no input of information about the association of the values of X for neighbouring members and, more generally, members i and i' in a distance $| i - i' |$ shorter than the step length b. However, unlike model-based estimators discussed in Chapters 1 and 2, which could be incorrect because the adopted model may be invalid, the variance estimator in (3.4) is 'correct' (unbiased) *if* the probabilities p_i and $p_{ii'}$, set by design, are correctly specified. In practice, such correctness is not attained because of numerous imperfections and compromises in the conduct of the survey, foremost among them nonresponse and imperfect sampling frame.

The obvious strength of the HT estimator is its universality; it can be applied to any proper sampling design and any variable X. Some of its drawbacks can be exposed on some admittedly esoteric examples. Suppose X is a constant variable, equal to μ for every member. Then its HT estimator $\hat{\mu}$ has a positive variance for a variety of designs. For illustration, consider any sampling design with unequal probabilities p_i and sample size $n = 1$. The estimator is $\hat{\mu} = \mu/(Nq_1)$ and its sampling variance is

$$\mathrm{var}\,(\hat{\mu}) = \frac{\mu^2}{N^2} \left(\sum_{i=1}^{N} \frac{1}{p_i} - 1 \right). \tag{3.5}$$

This summation is nonnegative, because it can be related to the difference between the harmonic and arithmetic averages of the probabilities. The variance vanishes only when the p_i are constant, equal to $1/N$. When the p_i are constant but the sample size n is variable, $\hat{\mu}$ is constant conditionally on the value of n, but not without such conditioning.

A further deficiency of the HT estimator relates to the division by some very small probabilities q_j. The corresponding subjects exercise strong influence over the value of $\hat{\mu}$, and the problem is further exacerbated in the estimator $\widehat{\mathrm{var}}(\hat{\mu})$, in which $1/(q_j q_{j'})$ and $1/q_{jj'}$ are involved. These problems show how important it is to incorporate our intelligence about X in the sampling and estimation processes. We address these issues in Sections 3.7.1 and 3.7.2.

For designs with fixed sample size there is an alternative expression for the variance of the HT estimator, namely

$$\text{var}\,(\hat{\mu}) \;=\; -\frac{1}{2N^2}\sum_{i=1}^{N}\sum_{i'=1}^{N}(p_{ii'}-p_i p_{i'})\left(\frac{X_i}{p_i}-\frac{X_{i'}}{p_{i'}}\right)^2. \qquad (3.6)$$

To show that it is equivalent to (3.3), expand the square and collect the terms involving the squares X_i^2:

$$-\frac{1}{N^2}\sum_{i=1}^{N}\frac{X_i^2}{p_i^2}\sum_{i'=1}^{N}(p_{ii'}-p_i p_i').$$

This summation vanishes because fixed sample size implies the identity $\sum_{i'=1}^{N}(p_{ii'}-p_i p_{i'})=0$ for any fixed i. The remainder of (3.6) coincides with the right-hand side of (3.3). The expression in (3.6) suggests that $\text{var}(\hat{\mu})$ is small in sampling designs in which $p_\bullet$ as a variable defined in $\mathcal{P}$ is close to being proportional to X. We develop this theme in Section 3.7.2, after introducing some commonly used sampling designs.

3.2.1 Simple Random Sampling

The HT estimator simplifies considerably for equiprobability sampling designs and for simple random sampling (SRS) designs in particular. For the SRS design with fixed sample size n and without replacement, $p_i = n/N$ and $p_{ii'} = n(n-1)/\{N(N-1)\}$. The latter identity is obtained from elementary combinatorics or by solving the equation $\text{var}\{\sum_i I(i)\}=0$ when $p^{(2)}=p_{ii'}$ for every pair $i \neq i'$, and $p_i = p$ for every member i. In general, fixed sample size n is equivalent to the identity

$$\sum_{i=1}^{N}\sum_{i'\neq i}p_{ii'} = n^2-n.$$

To prove this, recall that fixed sample size n implies that $\sum_i p_i = n$. Further,

$$\text{var}\left\{\sum_{i=1}^{N}I(i)\right\} = \sum_{i=1}^{N}p_i(1-p_i)+\sum_{i=1}^{N}\sum_{i'\neq i}(p_{ii'}-p_i p_{i'})$$

$$= n-n^2+\sum_{i=1}^{N}\sum_{i'\neq i}p_{ii'},$$

and this vanishes if and only if the $N(N-1)$ pairwise probabilities of inclusion of two distinct members add up to $n(n-1)$. When all these probabilities coincide, $p^{(2)}=n(n-1)/\{N(N-1)\}$, as claimed earlier.

For SRS with replacement and fixed sample size, the HT estimator of the population mean μ is equal to the sample mean, and its sampling variance is equal to

$$\text{var}\,(\hat{\mu}) = \frac{1}{N^2}\frac{N-n}{n}\left\{\sum_{i=1}^{N}X_i^2 - \frac{1}{N-1}\sum_{i=1}^{N}\sum_{i'\neq i}X_i\,X_{i'}\right\}$$

$$= \left(\frac{1}{n}-\frac{1}{N}\right)\frac{1}{N-1}\sum_{i=1}^{N}(X_i-\mu)^2. \tag{3.7}$$

This expression is a product of the population variance σ^2, with the finite-sample divisor $N-1$, and the scalar $1/n - 1/N$ that can be written as f/n, where $f = 1 - n/N$. The factor f is referred to as the finite-population correction; it would be equal to unity if the population size were infinite. The variance in (3.7) is estimated by its sample version.

Sampling designs with replacement are of little practical relevance, especially in surveys of human populations and their organisations (families, schools, businesses, and the like), because multiple inclusion of a subject in the sample would amount to multiple representation of the subject's record in the dataset. Most populations studied by surveys are large and the sample fractions n/N are small, so that in a sampling design with replacement the probability of multiple inclusion is very small. In such a setting, for every sampling design with replacement there is a very similar sampling design without replacement.

With independent draws of subjects into the sample, $p_{ii'} = p_i\,p_{i'}$ for $i \neq i'$, so the formula for var$(\hat{\mu})$ is simplified. Suppose each member of a population is included in the sample with a common probability p and the events of inclusion are independent. Then the population mean of X is estimated by $\hat{\mu} = \bar{x}/(pN)$, where $\bar{x}$ is the sample mean. The sampling variance of this estimator is

$$\text{var}(\hat{\mu}) = \frac{1-p}{pN^2}\sum_{i=1}^{N}X_i^2.$$

Let $Y = a + bX$ for some constants a and $b \neq 0$. The population mean of this variable is $\mu_Y = a + b\mu$, and its HT estimator is $\hat{\mu}_Y = a + b\hat{\mu}$. However, the sampling variance of $\hat{\mu}_Y$,

$$\text{var}\,(\hat{\mu}_Y) = \frac{1-p}{pN^2}\sum_{i=1}^{N}(a+bX_i)^2,$$

differs from $b^2\text{var}(\hat{\mu})$. In contrast, when the sample size is fixed, we have the equality var$(\hat{\mu}_Y) = b^2\text{var}(\hat{\mu})$; see (3.7).

3.2.2 Systematic Sampling Designs

To derive an estimator of var$(\hat{\mu})$, we require, instead of properness of the sampling design, a stricter condition, that of properness of the sampling design with the joint probabilities of inclusion $p_{ii'}$ in the population $\mathcal{P}\times\mathcal{P}$. *Systematic*

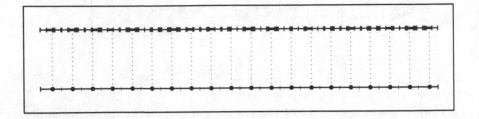

Fig. 3.1. Illustration of a general systematic sampling design. The segment at the top represents the 130 members of a fictional population and the segment at the bottom the sample selection points separated by the (constant) step length. The vertical dots connect the selected points to the corresponding subject, whose segments are highlighted.

sampling designs are a practical example of designs with $p_{ii'} = 0$ for some pairs (i, i'). For drawing a sample of size n, assuming for simplicity that $b = N/n$ is an integer, an integer a is selected at random from the sequence $1, 2, \ldots, b$, and the members $a + bh$, $h = 0, 1, \ldots, n - 1$, are selected into the sample. Thus, two members can be selected into the sample only if the distance of their positions in the sampling frame is a multiple of b. For any other pair of members i and i', $p_{ii'} = 0$.

Systematic sampling designs and their various generalisations can be described geometrically. We represent each member by a segment of unit length and join the segments into a single segment of length N. We choose the *step length b* and draw a *random start a* from the (continuous) uniform distribution on $(0, b)$. The sample comprises all subjects whose segments contain the points in distances $a + b(j - 1)$, $j = 1, \ldots, n$, from the origin. The unit-length segments can be joined to form a circle (or N-hedron); then $b = 2\pi/n$ and a can be replaced by an angle. With such a scheme, the sampling can go round the circle several times and may draw some elements repeatedly. Next, the members' segments may have unequal lengths, x_i, enabling sampling with probabilities proportional to these lengths. An illustration is given in Figure 3.1. With such a sampling design, a member represented by a segment longer than b may be selected more than once. If we insist on sampling without replacement we retain only one selection. As an alternative, the lengths x_i may be truncated at b. The members for whom we set $x_i = b$ are selected into the sample with certainty and the remainder of the sample is drawn from among the other members.

Systematic sampling designs are easy to implement, but there are no obvious estimators of the sampling variance of $\hat{\mu}$. The number of distinct samples that can be drawn is very limited (often equal to an integer close to b) and, without some additional information, one (realised) sample contains no information about the other possible samples because they do not overlap. This can in principle be remedied by supplementing the systematic sample with subjects drawn at random from the other possible samples; these subjects may be in preset or randomly set distances from the subjects in the original sample.

3.2.3 Some Other Sampling Designs

Next we introduce two classes of sampling designs. In the first, each member i is associated with probability p_i, and the events of inclusion are mutually independent for all the members. Thus, the (variable) sample size has expectation $E(n) = p_1 + \cdots + p_N$ and variance $E(n) = p_1(1-p_1) + \cdots + p_N(1-p_N)$. Independence of the inclusions implies that $p_{ii'} = p_i p_{i'}$ whenever $i \neq i'$, and so the variance of the HT estimator reduces to

$$\text{var}(\hat{\mu}) = \frac{1}{N^2} \sum_{i=1}^{N} \frac{1 - p_i}{p_i} X_i^2$$

and is estimated without bias by

$$\widehat{\text{var}}(\hat{\mu}) = \frac{1}{N^2} \sum_{j=1}^{n} \frac{1 - q_j}{q_j^2} x_j^2 .$$

The variable sample size has an undesirable impact on the estimation of the population mean, especially when $E(n)$ is not very large, because sample sizes much smaller than $E(n)$ cannot be ruled out. The HT estimator can be improved by 'correcting' it for the population size:

$$\hat{\mu}^* = \frac{1}{\hat{N}} \sum_{j=1}^{n} \frac{x_j}{q_j},$$

where $\hat{N} = 1/q_1 + \cdots + 1/q_n$ can be interpreted and, when N is not known, used as the HT estimator of the population size N. The estimator $\hat{\mu}^*$ is a weighted mean, using the sampling weights. The variance of $\hat{\mu}^*$ is, approximately,

$$\text{var}(\hat{\mu}^*) \doteq \frac{1}{N^2(N-1)} \sum_{i=1}^{N} \frac{N(1 - p_i) - 1}{p_i} (X_i - \mu)^2. \tag{3.8}$$

The method for deriving this approximation is presented in greater generality in Section 3.7.

The next general sampling design is with replacement and has a fixed sample size. Suppose each member is associated with a probability $r_i > 0$, and $r_1 + \cdots + r_N = 1$. The sampling mechanism comprises n replicates of drawing (with replacement) one member from the population, with the probabilities r_i. The HT estimator is a sum of n independent contributions, each being a random draw from the distribution given by the values $X_1/r_1, \ldots, X_N/r_N$. Let V be the variance of these values. Then the variance of the HT estimator is V/n. The population variance V can be estimated by its sample version.

The expressions for the (approximate) sampling variances of the estimators $\hat{\mu}$ in these two general schemes indicate that μ could be estimated with high precision if the probabilities p_i in one scheme and r_i in the other were proportional to X_i. Of course, the values X_i are not known. However, if the values of another (observed or constructed) variable Z, known to be highly correlated with X, are available, then the probabilities p_i (or r_i) could be set proportional to their values. This motivates the sampling designs in which the selection probabilities are proportional to a variable that has positive values. These designs are said to be with probability proportional to size.

3.3 Stratification

Stratification is a general device for converting the unwieldy task of conducting a survey in a large population to conducting several smaller surveys in a set of subpopulations that form a division (partition) of the studied population. The subpopulations are called *strata* and the sampling designs in the strata are independent. The strata are often geographical (regions), taking advantage of information available about the regions and of the management structures that the survey organisation in charge may have in place.

When inferences are required about the strata, stratification enables the designers to control the precision of the estimators of the within-stratum population quantities because the sampling plan specifies, in effect, a separate design for each stratum. When the strata (regions) are relatively homogeneous in comparison with the domain (country) as a whole, estimation within each stratum is relatively precise. Estimation of the corresponding national quantities then has a potential to be more efficient than with designs that do not use stratification.

Stratification should be used sparingly. Each stratum can be associated with a degree of freedom lost, so stratification that is too detailed or in which the strata are not any more homogeneous than the entire population is ineffective, resulting in an estimator that is not efficient. In this respect, an analogy can be drawn with model-based estimation. The ideal stratification is based on a few strata that have substantially different subpopulation means, or distributions, of the target variable. Thus, stratification promotes smoother organisation of a survey, and with it cost-effectiveness, and has a potential to increase efficiency.

Stratification does not generate any analytical difficulties beyond those of estimation for each stratum separately. Let $\hat{\mu}_h$ be unbiased estimators of within-stratum population means μ_h, $h = 1, \ldots, H$, of a variable X, and N_h the within-stratum population sizes. Then the (national) population mean μ is estimated without bias by

$$\hat{\mu} = \frac{1}{N} \sum_{h=1}^{H} N_h \hat{\mu}_h$$

and, as μ_h are independent, its sampling variance is

$$\text{var}\,(\hat{\mu}) = \frac{1}{N^2} \sum_{h=1}^{H} N_h^2 \,\text{var}\,(\hat{\mu}_h) \,.$$

This variance is estimated by the same linear combination of the estimators of the within-stratum variances $\text{var}(\hat{\mu}_h)$. Of course, difficulties arise when the within-stratum population sizes N_h are not known, but this problem is encountered also at the planning stage, when setting the sampling design.

3.4 Clustering

Most target populations are structured, and grouping into clusters in several layers, such as of individuals in families within postal sectors, communities, and districts, is a common structure. We consider first a population with only one layer of K clusters. Just like the strata in the previous section, such clusters form a division of the domain. In a simple (single-stage) *clustered sampling design*, a sample of clusters is drawn by a sampling design, and each member of a selected cluster is included in the sample. Subjects within a cluster often provide similar responses, so the data collected from them contain some (near) duplication. On the one hand, this may appear to be wasteful; on the other hand, most of the effort and expenditure associated with the data collection are spent on arranging and realising the interview—travel costs and time of the interviewer, sometimes requiring additional calls. Thus, collecting information from all members of a selected cluster may represent a relatively small expenditure in addition to collecting information from some or only one of them. Other factors may favour including the entire cluster in the survey. For example, in educational surveys, data collection in the form of a test may become part of the curriculum, so it is practical to administer it to entire clusters (schools or classrooms). Administering it selectively may also be disruptive and encourage some subjects to refuse cooperation, preferring alternative activities.

Multistage clustered design is applied when a sample of clusters at the most aggregate level H (the *primary sampling units*) is selected (the first stage), and then samples at the lower level of aggregation, $H - 1$ (*secondary sampling units*), are selected only from the clusters selected in the first stage, and so on, until in stage H, in which individuals (*elementary-level sampling units*) are selected from the clusters at level 2 that were selected to the sample in stage $H - 1$. The sampling designs in the various stages are independent and may include enumeration within the clusters selected in the previous stage, and the within-cluster sampling designs at each level are also independent.

Fixed overall sample size is possible to arrange only by imposing fixed sample sizes within all clusters in all the stages. This is rarely feasible, especially when the clusters at the various levels have unequal population sizes.

Another important consideration is that a sampling frame for the entire population may not be available or is too costly and time-consuming to compile. In multistage clustered sampling, it suffices to compile sampling frames within the selected clusters and only for the level of selection in the stage concerned. For example, in a clustered design with students within schools and schools within districts of a country, lists of schools need to be compiled only for the selected districts, and lists of students only in the selected schools.

3.4.1 Two-Stage Clustered Sampling

A two-stage clustered sampling design is described easiest of all by the sampling design at the first stage, in which clusters play the role of members and subjects, and by the *conditional sampling designs*, one for each cluster, given that the cluster is selected in the first stage. We use the superscripts I and II to indicate the sampling stage. For stage II we have to indicate both the cluster and its members. Thus, $p_{ii'\,|\,k}^{II}$ stands for the pairwise conditional (second-stage) probability of inclusion of members i and i' in cluster k, given that the cluster was selected in stage I. Other notation is defined by analogy.

The unconditional probabilities, required for the HT estimator $\hat{\mu}$, are the products of the first-stage selection probabilities of the clusters and the conditional probabilities of selection in stage II:

$$p_i = p_k^I \, p_{i\,|\,k}^{II} \, .$$

The notation is incomplete, because it does not indicate that member i belongs to cluster k. We omit this to avoid a clutter of subscripts. For pairwise inclusion probabilities, required for the sampling variance of $\hat{\mu}$ and its estimator, different identities apply for two members from the same cluster and from different clusters.

Although the general identity (3.3) applies also for the two-stage design, it is instructive to express the sampling variance of $\hat{\mu}$ in terms of the cluster-level and within-cluster design probabilities and variances:

$$\text{var}\,(\hat{\mu}) \; = \; \text{var}_I\,(\hat{\mu} \,|\, \{\mu_k\}) + \frac{1}{N^2} \sum_{k=1}^{N^I} N_k^2 \text{var}_{II}\,(\hat{\mu}_k) \, , \qquad (3.9)$$

where the first variance (var_I) is for the estimator of $\hat{\mu}$ in the hypothetical setting of the cluster-level means μ_k observed in the selected clusters directly (with precision) and the second variance (var_{II}) is for estimating the cluster-level means. The decomposition in (3.9) can be extended to multistage clustered sampling designs by substituting for var_{II} the variances that add up the contributions from the stages after the first. Also, the identity (3.9) can be 'composed' from the conditional variances, and so no new analytical development is required when the sampling design is changed at one of the stages. However, we emphasise that independence of the stages as well as of the within-cluster designs is an important assumption of the formula.

To prove (3.9), we make use of the identity

$$\text{var}\,(\hat{\mu}) = \text{var}_\text{I}\,\{E_\text{II}\,(\hat{\mu})\,|\,I\} + E_\text{I}\,\{\text{var}_\text{II}\,(\hat{\mu}\,|\,I)\}\,, \qquad (3.10)$$

where the subscripts I and II indicate, respectively, replications over the first stage of sampling and over the second stage conditionally on the first. Given the first stage (conditionally on the clusters in the sample),

$$E_\text{II}\,(\hat{\mu}\,|\,I) = \sum_{k \in s^\text{I}} \mu_k\,/p_k^\text{I}\,, \qquad (3.11)$$

because the means μ_k within the selected clusters k are estimated without bias. The right-hand side of (3.11) has the form of the HT estimator with μ_k as the observations, so it would be unbiased for μ if the means μ_k involved were observed. Therefore, the first-stage variance of (3.10) is equal to the first term on the right-hand side of (3.9). Each sampled cluster contributes (additively) to the estimator $\hat{\mu}$ by $N_k\hat{\mu}_k$, and the sampling variance of this contribution is $N_k^2\text{var}_\text{II}\,(\hat{\mu}_k)$ The first-stage expectation of their total is

$$\sum_{k=1}^{N^\text{I}} N_k^2\text{var}_\text{II}\,(\hat{\mu}_k)\,.$$

This concludes the proof of (3.9).

The sampling variance given by (3.9) is estimated without bias by

$$\widehat{\text{var}}\,(\hat{\mu}) = \widehat{\text{var}}_\text{I}\,(\hat{\mu}\,|\,\{\mu_k\}) + \frac{1}{N^2}\sum_{k \in s^\text{I}} \frac{N_k^2}{p_k^\text{I}}\,\widehat{\text{var}}_\text{II}\,(\hat{\mu}_k)\,, \qquad (3.12)$$

where

$$\widehat{\text{var}}_\text{I}\,(\hat{\mu}\,|\,\{\mu_k\}) = \sum_{k \in s^\text{I}}\sum_{k' \in s^\text{I}}\left(\frac{1}{p_k^\text{I}\,p_{k'}^\text{I}} - \frac{1}{p_{kk'}^\text{I}}\right)\hat{\mu}_k\,\hat{\mu}_{k'} - \sum_{k \in s^\text{I}}\frac{1}{p_k^\text{I}}\left(\frac{1}{p_k^\text{I}} - 1\right)\widehat{\text{var}}(\hat{\mu}_k)\,.$$

In fact, both contributions are unbiased for their counterparts in (3.9).

Design Effect

The term *design effect* is used for the ratio of the sampling variances of two unbiased estimators of the same population quantity with two different sampling designs. The two estimators have similar or identical forms, so that the design effect can be regarded as a comparison of the designs. A level playing field is ensured by comparing two designs with the same (fixed or expected) sample size. The sampling design in the denominator is the standard or reference, against which the nonstandard design in the numerator is compared. The most commonly adopted reference design is SRS without replacement. The design effect has its 'financial' equivalent, in which two designs that require the same (or comparable) outlay of resources are compared.

Most large-scale surveys are used for a multitude of inferences, and each of them is associated with a design effect. These design effects may vary, and one sampling design need not have all the design effects greater (or smaller) than another design. This complicates the choice among the alternative designs. Priorities among the planned inferences have to be taken into account to resolve this problem.

3.5 Planned and Realised Sampling Designs

Most large-scale surveys plan to have a set sample size. Stratification is commonly employed to ensure that certain subpopulations, usually defined by the geography or administrative division of the domain, also have planned sample sizes. The statistical rationale for this is to secure sufficient information for inferences about each subpopulation. Interviewers require training and instruction and may be renumerated by a fixed amount, so not engaging them fully is wasteful. The survey management may therefore want to match the contracted interviewers with agreed workloads. This can also be arranged, or promoted, by stratification.

Despite careful planning, the conduct of a survey involves a lot of improvisation because most human subjects are disinterested and often reluctant, unwilling, or unavailable for an interview. The generally adopted standards rule out any coercion and any rewards for cooperation other than nominal. In longitudinal surveys, one rejection is often interpreted as intention not to cooperate in the future. Nonresponse raises profound difficulties because it alters the sampling process as described by the probabilities $P(\mathbf{s})$, $\mathbf{s} \in \exp(\mathcal{P})$, or by p_i and $p_{ii'}$. Chapter 5 deals with this topic in greater detail and generality.

As nonresponse entails a great deal of uncertainty about the size and representativeness of the sample, it reduces the importance and relevance of planning to have a fixed sample size, and it is more constructive to insist on a sample size that has a small variance. Arranging fixed sample sizes within strata may also be unrealistic, but measures to reduce their (within-stratum) variation are important, especially when inferences are required for some or all the strata.

An equiprobability sampling design is the natural choice for surveying a population when no information other than a sampling frame is available about it or if we do not wish to use any such information. Sampling designs can be classified as those that apply one or several equiprobability designs and those that apply designs with sampling probabilities dependent on one or several variables. An example of the former, apart from SRS design, is the stratified sampling design with a distinct SRS design in each stratum and clustered sampling design with an equiprobability design in each selected cluster. A simple example of a design with probabilities dependent on a variable is a clustered design in which the first-stage probabilities depend on a variable, such as urbanity of the cluster.

To plan and implement a sampling design with unequal probabilities, the variable(s) on which these probabilities are based have to be set first, and this is practical only in populations that have been well researched in the past and for which the values of the relevant variables are available and, preferably, included in the sampling frame. Administrative registers may be suitable sources of such information, even when they are constructed and maintained for an unrelated purpose.

In multistage clustered sampling designs, the collection of the information about the clusters can be postponed until their selection, sparing such work in the clusters that are not selected. In principle, the 'conditional' sampling design given the selection of the cluster could be set at that stage. However, in a national survey this would involve instructing several administrators who are in charge of the data collection processes in the clusters. Such procedures are regarded by management as fragile and prone to imperfect (inconsistent) implementation, so it is preferable to control the later-stage designs centrally.

Sampling with probability proportional to the size of the stratum ensures that more populous strata have a richer representation in the sample. Such a strategy is effective for estimating quantities associated with the entire population but may be inefficient for inferences about the strata. The targets for the most populous strata will then be estimated with abundant precision. In contrast, greater sample sizes could have been used in the most sparsely populated strata without increasing the expenditure substantially. Thus, altering the sample sizes in favour of the less populous strata may be advantageous. However, the sampling costs per subject, pro-rated to strata and other aggregate sampling units, may differ, making this problem of sample allocation difficult not only to solve but even to formulate. Section 3.6 addresses some of these problems but, by necessity, in settings that are much simpler, both to formulate and to deal with, than those encountered in practice.

3.5.1 Adjusting and Trimming the Weights

A well-established method for compensating for nonresponse adjusts the original sampling weights $w_j = 1/q_j$ so that their summaries would agree with certain known population summaries. As a simple example, suppose the studied population is known to contain $P = 52\%$ women, but the HT estimate based on the realised sample is only $p = 45\%$. The sampling weights are adjusted for every woman by the factor P/p and for every man by $(1-P)/(1-p)$, so that the sample total of the weights remains unchanged. Such a weight adjustment can be regarded as a *poststratification*—introducing a new layer of stratification to force the within-stratum totals of 'sampling' weights to agree with the corresponding subpopulation sizes. All inferences are then drawn with the adjusted weights as if they were the original ones.

Generalisations to several categories are obvious in principle. When the population composition is available for several categorical variables that are recorded also in the survey, various iterative weight adjustment schemes have to be applied. They adjust for one set of subpopulation percentages at a time and cycle through these sets for other variables until the changes in the weights since the previous cycle become very small. These schemes are referred to as *raking*.

The adjusted weights engender a superficial respectability because some cosmetic features of the sample agree with their population versions. Such an adjustment is 'too good', because even if the planned sampling design were implemented perfectly, with a perfect sampling frame, such an agreement would not be achieved. Estimation with the weights adjusted by raking may lead to underestimation of the sampling variances (unjustified optimism or dishonesty), because the weights adjusted by a random process are regarded as the original weights—the uncertainty involved in the adjustment is ignored. In practice, this problem is often ignored, claiming that the uncertainty entailed is only minute. The adjustment of the sampling weights is difficult to follow up by a corresponding adjustment of the pairwise sampling weights, the reciprocals of the pairwise inclusion probabilities.

Large sampling weights or large values of $w_j x_j$ make disproportionately large contributions to the sampling variance of $\hat{\mu}$. Recognising that, with or without various adjustments, the weights are approximations to the reciprocals of the probabilities of inclusion, analysts adjust them further by trimming them. A threshold W is set and each weight w_j that exceeds W is reduced to W. If w_j were the original weights in a survey with perfectly implemented sampling design, such trimming would make the HT estimator biased. However, empirical evidence, supported by theoretical considerations, suggests that this is well worth doing as the sampling variance of $\hat{\mu}$ is reduced substantially at the price of a slight bias.

Smoother trimming schemes may be more effective. One such scheme is motivated by shrinkage. Let $\bar{w}$ be the (sample) mean of the sampling weights w_j. Then the weights w_j are replaced by

$$\tilde{w}_j = (1 - b)w_j + b\bar{w} \tag{3.13}$$

for a small positive constant b. This constant may be specific to each stratum or to each category of some other division of the population and may be set so as to reduce the dispersion of the adjusted weights $\tilde{w}_j$ to a desired level. If σ_{w}^2 is the variance of the original weights w_j, then the variance of the adjusted weights is $(1 - b)^2 \sigma_{\mathrm{w}}^2$. Weights are often more naturally compared on a multiplicative scale, especially when interpreted as numbers of members of the population they effectively represent. This motivates a more radical way of trimming the weights in which the shrinkage in (3.13) is applied to the logarithms of the weights.

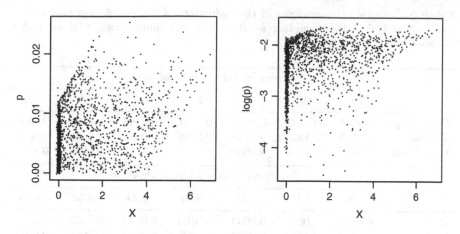

Fig. 3.2. The values of the variable X and the probabilities of inclusion and their logarithms with base 10 for a 2.5% simple random sample from the artificial generated population with $N = 72\,500$.

The sets of weights $\{w_j\}$ and $\{cw_j\}$ are equivalent for any positive constant c—only the relative sizes of the weights matter. Most estimators that use weights do not depend on c. The dispersion of the weights is therefore more practical to measure on the log scale, as we have the identity $\mathrm{var}\{\log(w)\} = \mathrm{var}\{\log(cw)\}$.

Example 6. To play out the scenario of sampling and estimation and compare a range of alternative estimators based on trimming and shrinkage of weights, we generate an artificial population of size $N = 72\,500$ and values of a variable X in the range $(0, 8.12)$, with high skew. In our realisation, about 43% of the values are equal to zero and a further 18.5% are smaller than 1.0. For a survey with expected sample size $\mathrm{E}(n) = 500$, we devised a sampling design with independent inclusions and probabilities of inclusion, p, correlated with the values of X (correlation 0.35). Figure 3.2 plots the values of X against p and $\log_{10}(p)$ for a simple random sample with probability 0.025. Plotting all the points would totally cover a large part of the plotting area with black ink, and we would not be able to see the relative densities of the values. With the SRS sample and a bit of random noise added to each point to avoid overprinting, the density of the points with $X = 0$ can be clearly discerned.

The probabilities of inclusion range from $2 \cdot 10^{-5}$ to 0.030, and their distribution is highly skewed; their mean is $\mathrm{E}(n)/N = 0.0069$ and median 0.0060. We replicated 1000 times the sampling process with the given probabilities of inclusion and independent inclusions, followed by evaluation of estimators with trimming and shrinkage of the weights. The weights were trimmed at 100, 50, 20, 10, 7.5, and 5 times the median of the weights $1/p$, and the log-probabilities were shrunk toward their mean with coefficients ranging from

Table 3.1. Empirical summaries of the estimators of the population means with trimmed and shrunken sampling weights. The minimum root-MSEs for either method are highlighted.

	Trimming (at multiple of med($w.$))						
	None	100	50	20	10	7.5	5
Bias	−0.0033	−0.0039	−0.0058	−0.0131	−0.0263	−0.0353	−0.0545
Variance	0.0133	0.1245	0.1130	0.0096	0.0083	0.0079	0.0072
Root-MSE	0.1154	0.1116	0.1064	0.0985	*0.0948*	0.0955	0.1007

	Shrinkage (of log-weights)						
	0.05	0.10	0.15	0.20	0.25	0.30	0.35
Bias	−0.0006	0.0037	0.0093	0.0163	0.0244	0.0336	0.0438
Variance	0.1150	0.1023	0.0093	0.0087	0.0083	0.0080	0.0078
Root-MSE	0.1071	0.1011	0.0970	0.0948	*0.0943*	0.0956	0.0988

0.05 to 0.35 in steps of 0.05. The results are summarised in Table 3.1. They show that the smallest MSE is achieved by trimming at the threshold equal to ten times the median weight and by shrinking the log-weights with coefficient 0.25. The sampling weights exceed ten times the median for about 3000 members of the population (4%) and 7.5 times the median for more than 4500 members (6%). (Note that in a sample, the sample median of the weights is used and it is biased for the population median.) The result about shrinkage indicates that a considerable amount of shrinkage should be applied, reducing the population variance of the weights about seven times, from 1.5×10^6 to 0.21×10^6.

In this example, trimming and shrinkage are about equally efficient, *if* we can find the ideal level of trimming or of shrinkage. This would be easy if we had an enumeration of the population, but then the survey would be unnecessary. Nowadays, it is not a computationally excessive task to generate an artificial population of even several million members and conduct a simulation that assesses alternative schemes of weight adjustment. The difficulty is in collecting intelligence about the population to be surveyed that would enable us to make such a simulation realistic. The rewards can be considerable. In our example, we reduced the root-MSE by about 20%, from 0.1154 to 0.0943. Equivalently, we could have reduced the sample size of the planned survey by about 35%. In practice, we are unlikely to hone in on the optimal level of trimming or shrinkage; however, the simulation exercise is well worth it, even if we realise only half the gains. In our example, we can achieve that by setting the trimming threshold in the range of 4 to 40 times the median weight or the shrinkage coefficient in the range 0.10 to 0.40. Investment in computing (analysis) at the planning stage can be more than compensated by savings at the data collection stage.

3.6 Sample Size Calculation

A grossly simplified version of the task of setting the sampling design involves calculating the smallest sample size for a specified class of designs, for which the sampling variance of a key estimator would be smaller than a prescribed value. A typical large-scale survey is used for making inferences about a multitude of population and subpopulation quantities, so its sampling design is a compromise of statistical efficiency, cost-effectiveness, feasibility, the available expertise and capacity, and management's constraints and preferences, which include the existing organisational structures and contractual arrangements. No formal sample calculation can take all these realities fully into account. Nevertheless, even the calculation for a greatly simplified setting can provide a useful guide and can serve as a starting point in planning a survey.

For an entire-domain (population) quantity μ, we may insist on a particular level of sampling variance of its unbiased estimator $\hat{\mu}$ and calculate the sample size that would assure it. The sampling weights (or the inclusion probabilities) are very difficult to take into account in such a calculation because they are not constant and may be correlated with the target variable. In a more practical approach a particular design effect is assumed and the relevant problem is solved for a reference design, such as simple random sampling with replacement.

A commonly considered problem is that of allocating a fixed sample size n to the strata $h = 1, \ldots, H$, as $n = n_1 + \cdots + n_H$, with the aim of estimating the population mean μ with the smallest possible MSE. Suppose the within-stratum designs are set, except for their sample sizes n_h. Each within-stratum population mean μ_h would be estimated without bias by $\hat{\mu}_h(n_h)$, an estimator that depends on the within-stratum sample size. Suppose its sampling variance is $v_h(n_h) = u_h/n_h + t_h$ for some positive constants u_h and t_h. We denote $\mathbf{n} = (n_1, \ldots, n_H)$. The sampling variance of the (national) estimator $\hat{\mu} = (N_1\hat{\mu}_1 + \cdots + N_H\hat{\mu}_H)/N$ is

$$\mathrm{var}(\mu; \mathbf{n}) = \frac{1}{N^2} \sum_{h=1}^{H} N_h^2 \left(\frac{u_h}{n_h} + t_h \right), \tag{3.14}$$

and it can be minimised subject to fixed sample size $n = \mathbf{n}^\top \mathbf{1}$ by the method of Lagrange multipliers or by substituting $n_1 = n - n_2 - \ldots - n_H$. Either way, we obtain the solution

$$n_h^* = n \frac{N_h \sqrt{u_h}}{\sum_{h'=1}^{H} N_{h'} \sqrt{u_{h'}}}.$$

The realistic nature of this calculation can be enhanced by assuming fixed total costs

$$C = B + \sum_{h=1}^{H} n_h C_h$$

(instead of fixed overall sample size n), yielding a similar solution

$$n_h^* = n \frac{N_h \sqrt{u_h/C_h}}{\sum_{h'=1}^{H} N_{h'} \sqrt{u_{h'}/C_{h'}}},$$

which reflects higher costs C_h by reduced within-stratum sample sizes n_h. Note that the quantities n_h^* have to be rounded. The result might rule out sampling within a stratum h in which data collection is very costly, but then $\mathrm{var}(\hat{\mu}) = +\infty$. The design should be adjusted so that this is avoided.

A similar approach can be applied to allocating the sample size to strata when all the within-stratum population means are to be estimated. The design cannot be optimised separately for each stratum because greater subsample size in one stratum comes at the expense of smaller subsample sizes in one or more other strata. This problem is resolved by specifying a *priority* P_h for estimating each target μ_h. The priority of a target is a positive constant that describes the relative importance of its estimation. The linear combination of the sampling variances, with the coefficients equal to the priorities,

$$\sum_{h=1}^{H} P_h \mathrm{var}\,(\hat{\mu}_h) \,, \tag{3.15}$$

is minimised. If an estimator $\hat{\mu}_h$ is biased, its variance in (3.15) is replaced by $\mathrm{MSE}(\hat{\mu}_h ; \mu_h)$. High priority P_h inflates the contribution of the corresponding $\mathrm{var}(\hat{\mu}_h)$ to (3.15), and so the solution prefers to allocate greater subsample size to such a stratum h. This is easy to confirm by finding the minimum of (3.15). This can be done by the same methods as for minimising (3.14). We obtain the condition

$$P_h \frac{u_h}{n_h^2} = \mathrm{const}\,,$$

so that the optimal sample sizes are proportional to $\sqrt{u_h\, P_h}$. Hence

$$n_h^* = n \frac{\sqrt{u_h\, P_h}}{\sum_{h'=1}^{H} \sqrt{u_{h'}\, P_{h'}}}. \tag{3.16}$$

The priorities P_h may be set by negotiation among the parties with a stake in the survey and its analysis. When this is not feasible a class of proposal priorities may be adopted. One such class is given by the powers $P_h = N_h^q$ for nonnegative exponents q. The exponent $q = 0$ corresponds to equal priorities, and high q results in allocating almost all the available sample size to the most populous stratum. By setting $q = 2$, we obtain the allocation that is efficient for estimating the population mean. When it is desirable to improve the estimation for the least populous strata more than for the more populous ones, a setting with $q < 2$ is appropriate.

Whenever $q \neq 2$, optimal estimation of the within-stratum means is accompanied by reduced efficiency of the national estimator $\hat{\mu}$. We may associate $\hat{\mu}$ with a priority P and incorporate the desire for efficient estimation of μ by supplementing the criterion in (3.15) with the term $P\mathrm{var}(\hat{\mu})$ or $P\,\mathrm{MSE}(\hat{\mu}; \mu)$. By differentiating the expression in (3.14) we obtain the condition

$$P_h \frac{u_h}{n_h^2} + \frac{P}{N^2} \frac{N_h^2 u_h}{n_h^2} = \text{const},$$

which yields the solution

$$n_h^* = C\sqrt{u_h}\sqrt{P_h + P\frac{N_h^2}{N^2}},$$

for a constant C that ensures the planned sample size $n_1^* + \cdots + n_H^* = n$. This is the same solution as when we do not care about estimating the population mean ($P = 0$), but the priorities P_h for the subpopulation means are adjusted to $P_h + PN_h^2/N^2$. Only the relative sizes of the priorities have any meaning, because the choices $\{P_h\}$ and $\{cP_h\}$ lead to the same solution for every positive constant c. Greater P brings the allocation closer to optimality of estimating μ, paying less attention to estimating the stratum means μ_h. The 'overall' priority P has a meaningful interpretation only in relation to the total of the stratum-priorities $\sum_h P_h$. With the stratum-level priorities $P_h = N_h^q$ for $q < 2$ fixed, the solution has the expected effect of bringing the allocation of sample sizes to the strata closer to proportionality with the stratum sizes N_h as the domain-priority P increases.

The method described can be extended to more complex formulae for the sampling variances or MSEs, although its application is very difficult when they cannot be expressed analytically. In particular, they are difficult to apply when trimming, shrinkage, or some other adjustment of the weights is planned. However, if the MSEs of the estimators are reduced by approximately the same fraction, the error committed may be inconsequential.

3.7 Using Auxiliary Information

The HT and related estimators are *direct*—they use data only for the domain and the variable concerned. In this section, we explore how the values of other variables and direct estimators from other domains could be exploited in the service of estimating a population quantity more efficiently. Using other variables can be motivated by the following example. Suppose the target is related to variable Y but we have much more abundant information about a closely related variable Z (e.g., its enumeration or, possibly from a different data source, a precise estimator of its population mean). It would be highly desirable to make use of such *auxiliary* information. At an extreme, we might abandon the survey altogether and rely on an estimator based entirely on Z, derived from a different source. Such an estimator may be biased for the target related to Y, but its sampling variance is much smaller and would be evaluated at a fraction of the cost.

Difference and Ratio Estimators

Suppose the target of estimation is the mean μ_Y of a variable Y, and the value of the corresponding target for a related variable X, denoted by μ_X, is known. In the survey, the values of both X and Y are observed on a sample of subjects. The following estimation strategy for μ_Y makes use of μ_X and the values of X recorded in the survey. The survey-based (direct) estimates of μ_X and μ_Y, $\hat{\mu}_X$ and $\hat{\mu}_Y$, respectively, will inform us about how μ_X and μ_Y are related, and we derive an estimator of μ_Y by applying this estimated relationship to μ_X. In effect, the observed estimation error $\hat{\mu}_X - \mu_X$ is used to adjust the direct estimator $\hat{\mu}_Y$. The result is the *difference estimator* $\mu_X + \hat{\mu}_Y - \hat{\mu}_X$. It is very efficient when the variable $Y - X$ has a small population variance, because then $\hat{\mu}_Y - \hat{\mu}_X$ has a small sampling variance. The *ratio estimator* $\mu_X \hat{\mu}_Y / \hat{\mu}_X$ is motivated similarly. It is very useful when the ratio Y/X has small variance, the values of X are nonnegative, and none or only a small fraction of them are close to zero, so that $\mathrm{var}\,(1/\hat{\mu}_X)$ is not excessive.

The difference and ratio estimators are examples of exploiting the similarity of the target and an *auxiliary variable*. This can be done most effectively by relating the target and auxiliary variables by means of a model. The next section develops methods for fitting models to survey data, which is a prerequisite for *model-assisted* estimation.

3.7.1 Fitting Models to Survey Data

Large-scale surveys involve populations of sizes that can be regarded as infinite and models for infinite populations often provide attractive ways of describing the associations among the studied variables. For fitting such models, the reference to a superpopulation is often invoked, and some or all the sampling design features are taken into account in the model. For example, clustering can be represented by random effects, assuming that each cluster has its own regression,

$$Y^{(k)} = \mathbf{X}^{(k)}\boldsymbol{\beta}^{(k)} + \boldsymbol{\varepsilon}^{(k)},$$

and these cluster-specific regressions vary according to a pattern summarised by a cluster-level variance matrix $\boldsymbol{\Sigma}_B = \mathrm{var}\,(\boldsymbol{\beta}^{(\bullet)})$. The pairwise probabilities of inclusion play no role in such models, but they are eliminated also from design-based formulae because sampling designs for such populations have very small sampling fractions n/N and often also very small within-cluster fractions $n^{(k)}/N^{(k)}$. More details of random-effects models are given in Chapter 9.

Here we describe an approach that adheres much more closely to design-based estimation and is less burdened with the caveat of model validity. We consider the problem of estimating the fit of a particular model, such as ordinary regression, to the data for the entire population. We disregard the issue of appropriateness of the underlying model on the grounds that evidence against any model in a very large population is easily found, given a survey with sufficiently large sample size. No large population behaves according to a simple mechanism. The model fit is described by a function $f(\mathbf{X}) = f\{t(\mathbf{X})\}$, where $\mathbf{X}$ is the population matrix of the values of all the relevant variables, and t is a set of sufficient *population-statistics*; that is, they would be statistics (evaluable summaries) if the population were enumerated.

We distinguish between the design-based perspective, in which $\mathbf{X}$ is fixed and $f(\mathbf{X})$ is a constant or a vector of constants, and model-based perspective, in which $\mathbf{X}$ is the realisation of a data-generating process and $f(\mathbf{X})$ is a random variable or vector; the values underlying $f(\mathbf{X})$ could be established only if the superpopulation version of $\mathbf{X}$ were available. We adhere to the design-based perspective to avoid a divide between direct and model-assisted estimation. We have to draw a distinction between the uncertainty due to the population being a 'sample' drawn from the superpopulation and the uncertainty due to sampling from the population. The former source is a population quantity, and therefore can itself be a target of estimation (for instance, to assess to what extent the posited model is suitable), whereas the latter is a characteristic of the sampling process.

Assuming that the sought function $f(\mathbf{X})$ has a short list of sufficient population-statistics $t(\mathbf{X})$, we require (unbiased) estimators of these quantities, $\hat{t}(\mathbf{x})$, and an estimator of their sampling variance matrix. We restrict our development to statistics t that can be described as totals of variables, observed or constructed. For example, the sufficient statistics for ordinary regression parameters are the totals (or means) of squares and crossproducts of the outcome variables and covariates.

We estimate the values of the sufficient population-statistics $t(\mathbf{X})$. Denote by $\hat{t}(\mathbf{x})$ their estimators based on the survey data $\mathbf{x}$. The population-model fit is estimated by $f\{\hat{t}(\mathbf{X})\}$. Adjustment may be applied to reduce or eliminate the bias arising by the nonlinear transformations involved in f. The sampling variance (matrix) of $f\{\hat{t}(\mathbf{X})\}$ is estimated with the aid of the Taylor expansion. An alternative approach to estimating the sampling variance (matrix) is based on simulation from the joint sampling distribution of $\hat{t}(\mathbf{x})$. It can be formulated as a missing data problem (Chapter 5) and is related to the method of multiple imputation (Section 5.5).

Estimation of the sufficient statistics is conducted componentwise. We handle the estimation of the covariances in $\mathrm{var}(\hat{t})$ by extending the results in sampling theory to vectors of variables. All the results for sampling variation carry over directly by replacing the squares x^2 and $(x-\hat{\mu})^2$ with the respective matrices $\mathbf{x}\mathbf{x}^\top$ and $(\mathbf{x} - \boldsymbol{\mu})(\mathbf{x} - \boldsymbol{\mu})^\top$. For example, the multivariate version of the identity (3.6) is

$$\text{var}(\hat{\boldsymbol{\mu}}) = -\frac{1}{2N^2} \sum_{i=1}^{N} \sum_{i'=1}^{N} (p_{ii'} - p_i p_{i'}) \left(\frac{1}{p_i}\mathbf{X}_i - \frac{1}{p_{i'}}\mathbf{X}_{i'}\right) \left(\frac{1}{p_i}\mathbf{X}_i - \frac{1}{p_{i'}}\mathbf{X}_{i'}\right)^\top,$$

where $\mathbf{X}_i$ is the row vector of the values of the variables in $\mathbf{X}$ for member i. (Some clash with the notational conventions is unavoidable.)

Example 7. Fitting Ordinary Regression. The sufficient population-statistics for the ordinary regression of a variable Y on a $p \times 1$ vector of regressors $\mathbf{X}$ are the totals of squares and crossproducts $(\mathbf{X}\ \mathbf{Y})^\top(\mathbf{X}\ \mathbf{Y})$. Let $\mathbf{T}$ be the $\frac{1}{2}(p+1)(p+2) \times 1$ vector of the unique elements in this $(p+1) \times (p+1)$ matrix, and let $\hat{\mathbf{T}}$ be their (design-based) estimator with estimated sampling variance matrix $\mathbf{V} = \widehat{\text{var}}(\hat{\mathbf{T}})$. A smooth function of the population-model fit $g(\mathbf{T})$ is estimated by $g(\hat{\mathbf{T}})$, and its sampling variance is derived from the Taylor expansion:

$$g(\hat{\mathbf{T}}) \doteq g(\mathbf{T}) + \frac{\partial g}{\partial t}^\top \left(\hat{\mathbf{T}} - \mathbf{T}\right),$$

so that

$$\text{var}\left\{g\left(\hat{\mathbf{T}}\right)\right\} \doteq \frac{\partial g}{\partial t}^\top \text{var}\left(\hat{\mathbf{T}}\right) \frac{\partial g}{\partial t}, \tag{3.17}$$

with the partial derivatives evaluated at $t = \mathbf{T}$. The variance matrix is estimated naively, by substituting $\hat{\mathbf{T}}$ for $\mathbf{T}$ in (3.17).

3.7.2 Regression Estimators of the Population Mean

With a given sampling design, the population mean is estimated with greater precision for variables with smaller dispersion. This provides a motivation for exploiting auxiliary information in the form of values of variables that are related to the target variable, are recorded in the survey, and their population totals are known or are estimated with high precision (from a register or another survey).

Let X be the target variable and $\mathbf{Z}$ a vector of auxiliary variables with known population mean (row) vector $\boldsymbol{\mu}_\mathbf{Z}$. Let ε be the variable formed as the residual of the population-regression of X on $\mathbf{Z}$; the vector of its values, $\boldsymbol{\varepsilon}$, would be available if X and $\mathbf{Z}$ were enumerated. With X and $\mathbf{Z}$ observed on a sample (survey data), we fit the ordinary regression of X on $\mathbf{Z}$. The sample-residuals $\hat{\boldsymbol{\varepsilon}} = \mathbf{x} - \mathbf{Z}\hat{\boldsymbol{\beta}}$ are evaluated using the estimated regression coefficients $\hat{\boldsymbol{\beta}}$. (Here $\mathbf{Z}$ is the matrix of the values of $\mathbf{Z}$—we cannot avoid using the same symbol $\mathbf{Z}$ for two distinct objects.) The population mean of X is then estimated by adjusting the HT estimator of μ for the difference between $\boldsymbol{\mu}_\mathbf{Z}$ and its direct estimator based on the survey:

$$\hat{\mu}^\mathrm{R} = \hat{\mu} + (\boldsymbol{\mu}_\mathbf{Z} - \hat{\boldsymbol{\mu}}_\mathbf{Z})\hat{\boldsymbol{\beta}}, \tag{3.18}$$

where the superscript R denotes 'regression estimator'. Thus, the regression estimator anticipates that the error in estimating the means of the covariates, μ_Z, is similar to the error of the direct estimate, $\hat{\mu} - \mu$, of the target variable. If the regression fit were exact this error would be predicted with precision, and the correction would be perfect. The adjustment would certainly be useful if the population-regression parameter vector β were known; the uncertainty in estimating β reduces the usefulness. We can ensure that the balance is on the side of more efficient estimation of μ by using regression models with few covariates (parsimony) that reduce the residual variance substantially. The population means are rarely known for many variables, so parsimony is often forced upon the analyst. However, a good plan anticipates which variables Z might be useful and makes provisions for recording their values.

Two sources of uncertainty contribute to the sampling variation of $\hat{\mu}^R$: sampling variation and uncertainty about the regression parameters β. Combining the two analytically is rather complex. A simpler, even though computationally more demanding alternative is based on the method of multiple imputation introduced in Section 5.5. We regard the regression estimator in (3.18), with β instead of $\hat{\beta}$, as the complete information and β as the missing data. We draw several replicates from the estimated sampling distribution of $\hat{\beta}$. These so-called plausible regression parameters are denoted by $\tilde{\beta}^{(m)}$, $m = 1, \ldots, M$. Then we evaluate $\hat{\mu}^R$ and its complete-data sampling variance (assuming β to be known and equal to $\tilde{\beta}^{(m)}$) with each $\tilde{\beta}^{(m)}$ and average the M plausible estimates and complete-data sampling variances, with an inflation by the between-imputation variance of the latter, according to equations (5.9) and (5.10). The resulting (multiple-imputation) estimator is denoted by $\hat{\mu}^{R,MI}$. If the plausible estimates $\tilde{\beta}^{(m)}$ differ a great deal, that is, there is a large between-imputation variance, then a lot of missing information is due to uncertainty about the regression parameters β. A likely reason for this is that too many covariates are used in the regression. Using a more parsimonious model may resolve this problem and make the estimator $\hat{\mu}^{R,MI}$ more efficient.

The difference estimator is a special case of the regression estimator, with one covariate, no intercept, and unit slope. The ratio estimator can be derived as the regression estimator with the model

$$\frac{y}{\sqrt{x}} = \beta\sqrt{x} + \varepsilon,$$

where ε is a random sample from a centred normal distribution. The model has the alternative description as $y \sim \mathcal{N}(\beta x, \sigma^2 x)$.

Even the unity as a constant can be used as auxiliary information. The corresponding ratio estimator of the population mean is equal to

$$\frac{\sum_{j=1}^n w_j y_j}{\sum_{j=1}^n w_j},$$

which has the form of a weighted average. It does not involve the population size N, and so it can be applied even when N is not known. In fact the denominator, $\sum_j w_j$, is the HT estimator of the population size. When the values of Y are nearly constant the ratio estimator has a small variance even with sampling designs with random sample size. In this respect, it is superior to the HT estimator.

In some settings, it is practical to apply a sampling design in which the probability of inclusion is approximately proportional to the value of the (positive) target variable Y. In this case, the probability p, or the weight W, can be regarded as the auxiliary information, yielding the estimator

$$\bar{w}\,\frac{\sum_{j=1}^{n} w_j y_j}{\sum_{j=1}^{n} w_j^2}\,,$$

where $\bar{w}$ is the sample mean of the weights. The fraction in this estimator has the form of an ordinary least squares estimator of the regression slope of Y on W, with the regression through the origin. This facilitates a natural interpretation of the estimator. Note that the sampling variance of this estimator cannot be derived as in ordinary regression because the weights w are random. Approximations using the Taylor expansion lead to some unwieldy expressions; simulations may be more effective, even if they do not yield an analytical expression.

3.8 Small-Area Estimation

Increasing demand for inferences about the geographical details of the domain (a country) has, over the last few decades, stimulated the development of a wide range of methods for indirect estimation of the population means for subdomains (districts). These methods are collectively referred to as *small-area estimation*. Many of the methods draw on empirical Bayes models as a way of *borrowing strength* across the districts. Random coefficient models (Chapter 9) are models for analysis of covariance in which the groups are associated with random effects. By declaring these 'effects' as random, maximum likelihood estimation yields shrinkage estimators of population and model quantities associated with the districts.

A seemingly model-free rationale for these methods compares two estimators. The *direct estimator* is based on the data solely for the variable and the district involved. Usually it is (approximately) unbiased but its variance may be so large as to render the estimate of limited or no use. As an alternative to the direct estimator, the estimator of the domain (national) mean, $\hat{\mu}$, may be considered. It is biased for the district in question but, being based on the entire sample, its sampling variance is much smaller. If the districts of the country are similar, the national mean estimator may be efficient also for the district. Instead of choosing the direct or national estimator, we combine the two (alternative) estimators,

$$\tilde{\mu}_d = (1 - b_d)\hat{\mu}_d + b_d \,\check{\mu}_d, \tag{3.19}$$

with the positive constant b_d set, in ideal circumstances, so as to minimise the MSE of $\tilde{\mu}_d(b_d)$ in estimating μ_d. We add the argument b_d to $\tilde{\mu}_d$ to emphasise its dependence on b_d. In practice, b_d depends on the target μ_d itself and so can at best only be estimated. The dependence on μ_d, or more precisely on the squared deviation $(\mu_d - \mu)^2$, is removed by using the *between-district variance* σ_B^2, which is the mean of the squared deviations $(\mu_d - \mu)^2$ over the districts. This variance is not known and has to be estimated. However, being based on the data for all the districts, it is estimated with much greater precision than the values $(\mu_d - \mu)^2$ for most districts d.

Estimation of the district-level means can be improved by drawing on auxiliary information. Districts may differ substantially, but these differences may be reduced after an adjustment by regression with one or several covariates. The adjustment has to be flexible, allowing for some systematic differences among the districts. But such auxiliary information can be exploited without using empirical Bayes models. We motivate this by a simple example.

Suppose the population comprises a majority and a minority group. The two groups are distributed unevenly across the districts and are not completely segregated, so that some economic, social, and environmental phenomena affect both groups, even if to somewhat unequal extent. A direct estimator for the minority group is in most districts unsatisfactory because the group is represented in the sample very sparsely. If the district-level differences of the means between the majority and minority groups vary only modestly we could estimate the minority-group means by adjusting the estimates for the majority group in the same district. This can further be improved by estimating the minority-group means by linear combinations of the two direct estimators. The logical progression leads to a multivariate version of the estimator in (3.19), which can be interpreted as exploiting the similarity across the groups as well as across the districts. Further applications of this idea draw on information from registers, past surveys and other variables recorded in the same survey.

Let $\hat{\boldsymbol{\theta}}_d$ be a vector of estimators unbiased for the district-level population vector $\boldsymbol{\theta}_d$, and let $\hat{\boldsymbol{\theta}}$ and $\boldsymbol{\theta}$ be their domain (national) counterparts. For example, the first component of $\boldsymbol{\theta}_d$ may be the target, and the remaining component may be associated with auxiliary information. To estimate the linear combination $\theta_d = \boldsymbol{\theta}_d^\top \mathbf{u}$ for a vector of specified coefficients $\mathbf{u}$, we seek the combination

$$\tilde{\theta}_d(\mathbf{b}) = (\mathbf{u} - \mathbf{b})^\top \hat{\boldsymbol{\theta}}_d + \mathbf{b}^\top \hat{\boldsymbol{\theta}} \tag{3.20}$$

that has the smallest MSE. We have

$$\mathrm{MSE}\left\{\tilde{\theta}_d(\mathbf{b}); \theta_d\right\} = (\mathbf{u} - \mathbf{b})^\top \mathbf{V}_d(\mathbf{u} - \mathbf{b}) + \mathbf{b}^\top \mathbf{V}\mathbf{b} + 2(\mathbf{u} - \mathbf{b})^\top \mathbf{C}_d \mathbf{b}$$
$$+ \mathbf{b}^\top \mathbf{D}_d \mathbf{D}_d^\top \mathbf{b},$$

where $\mathbf{V} = \mathrm{var}(\hat{\boldsymbol{\theta}})$, $\mathbf{V}_d = \mathrm{var}(\hat{\boldsymbol{\theta}}_d)$, $\mathbf{C}_d = \mathrm{cov}(\hat{\boldsymbol{\theta}}_d, \hat{\boldsymbol{\theta}})$, and $\mathbf{D}_d = \boldsymbol{\theta}_d - \boldsymbol{\theta}$. This MSE is a quadratic function of $\mathbf{b}$, and its quadratic (matrix) coefficient

$$\mathbf{Q}_d = \mathbf{V} + \mathbf{V}_d - \mathbf{C}_d - \mathbf{C}_d^\top + \mathbf{D}_d \mathbf{D}_d^\top = \mathrm{E}\left\{ \left(\hat{\boldsymbol{\theta}}_d - \hat{\boldsymbol{\theta}} \right) \left(\hat{\boldsymbol{\theta}}_d - \hat{\boldsymbol{\theta}} \right)^\top \right\}$$

is positive definite. The MSE therefore has a unique minimum. The minimum is found by differentiation or by completing the squares, and it yields the solution

$$\mathbf{b}_d^* = \mathbf{Q}_d^{-1} \mathbf{P}_d \mathbf{u}, \tag{3.21}$$

where $\mathbf{P}_d = \mathbf{V}_d - \mathbf{C}_d$. This vector of 'ideal' coefficients depends on several (unknown) sampling-process quantities and has to be estimated. Estimation of $\mathbf{D}_d$ is particularly problematic because it depends on the target $\boldsymbol{\theta}_d$. We avoid this dependence by substituting for $\mathbf{D}_d \mathbf{D}_d^\top$ its average over the districts, the district-level variance matrix

$$\boldsymbol{\Sigma}_\mathrm{B} = \mathrm{E}_{(d)} \left(\mathbf{D}_d \mathbf{D}_d^\top \right).$$

(The subscript (d) with E indicates that the expectation, or *averaging*, is taken over the districts d.) We estimate $\mathbf{b}_d$ naively, using unbiased estimators of $\mathbf{V}_d$, $\mathbf{V}$ and $\mathbf{C}_d$, and $\boldsymbol{\Sigma}_\mathrm{B}$. We assume that the districts coincide with the strata, so that sampling within districts is independent. If the national estimator $\hat{\boldsymbol{\theta}}$ is a linear combination of the district-level direct estimators $\hat{\boldsymbol{\theta}}_d$, the covariance matrix $\mathbf{C}_d$ can be expressed in terms of $\mathbf{V}_d$:

$$\mathrm{cov}\left(\hat{\boldsymbol{\theta}}_d, \hat{\boldsymbol{\theta}} \right) = \mathrm{cov}\left(\hat{\boldsymbol{\theta}}_d, \frac{1}{M} \sum_{d'=1}^{D} M_{d'} \hat{\boldsymbol{\theta}}_{d'} \right) = \frac{M_d}{M} \mathrm{var}\left(\hat{\boldsymbol{\theta}}_d \right),$$

irrespective of the perspective adopted, design- or model-based. (In most settings, $M = N$ and $M_d = N_d$.) Estimating $\mathbf{V}_d = \mathrm{var}(\hat{\boldsymbol{\theta}}_d)$ is a standard task; its complexity is related to the sampling design within district d. When there are many districts, the variances in $\mathbf{V}$ are much smaller than their counterparts in $\mathbf{V}_d$, and $\mathbf{V}$ can be ignored in $\mathbf{Q}_d$. Then $\mathbf{C}_d$ is also small in relation to $\mathbf{V}_d$ and can also be ignored, reducing (3.21) to

$$\mathbf{b}_d^* \doteq \left(\mathbf{V}_d + \boldsymbol{\Sigma}_\mathrm{B} \right)^{-1} \mathbf{V}_d \mathbf{u},$$

after substituting $\boldsymbol{\Sigma}_\mathrm{B}$ for $\mathbf{D}_d \mathbf{D}_d^\top$. This can be interpreted as weighing (in a multivariate way) the two estimators $\hat{\boldsymbol{\mu}}_d$ and $\hat{\boldsymbol{\mu}}$ by their (matrix) precisions. Thus, it remains only to discuss estimation of $\boldsymbol{\Sigma}_\mathrm{B}$.

We estimate $\boldsymbol{\Sigma}_\mathrm{B}$ by the method of moments. We form a statistic similar to the expression for $\boldsymbol{\Sigma}_\mathrm{B}$,

$$\mathbf{S}_\mathrm{B} = \sum_d G_d (\hat{\boldsymbol{\theta}}_d - \hat{\boldsymbol{\theta}})(\hat{\boldsymbol{\theta}}_d - \hat{\boldsymbol{\theta}})^\top, \tag{3.22}$$

evaluate its expectation, and then solve the equation that matches the (matrix) statistic $\mathbf{S}_B$ with its expectation. The method can be motivated as follows. For a suitable choice of the scalar coefficients G_d, $\mathbf{S}_B$ would recover the target $\mathbf{\Sigma}_B$ if $\hat{\boldsymbol{\theta}}_d$ and $\hat{\boldsymbol{\theta}}$ were precise, if we had $\mathbf{V}_d = \mathbf{V} = \mathbf{0}$. When $\mathbf{V}_d \neq \mathbf{0}$, $\mathbf{S}_B$ is inflated due to the sampling variation of $\hat{\boldsymbol{\theta}}_d$. Therefore we estimate $\mathbf{\Sigma}_B$ by adjusting $\mathbf{S}_B$ for the sampling variation of $\hat{\boldsymbol{\theta}}_d$, $d = 1, \ldots, D$.

Instead of (3.22), we can solve the (univariate) problems separately for each element of $\mathbf{\Sigma}_B$. Then we do not have to assume that the same set of coefficients G_d applies for each element of $\boldsymbol{\theta}_d$. This is useful when the sampling variances of the elements of $\hat{\boldsymbol{\theta}}_d$ have disparate magnitudes. For example, the elements of $\hat{\boldsymbol{\theta}}_d$ may be based on different surveys (data sources), with different distributions of sample sizes to the districts.

For the diagonal element (k, k) in $\mathbf{\Sigma}_B$ (a variance), denoted by $\Sigma_{B,kk}$, we have

$$
\mathrm{E}(S_{B,kk}) = \sum_{d=1}^{D} G_{kk,d} \left\{ V_{kk,d} + V_{kk} - 2C_{kk,d} + (\theta_{k,d} - \theta_k)^2 \right\}
$$

$$
= \sum_{d=1}^{D} \left(1 - \frac{2N_d}{N} \right) G_{kk,d} V_{kk,d} + V_{kk} \sum_{d=1}^{D} G_{kk,d}
$$

$$
+ \sum_{d=1}^{D} G_{kk,d} (\theta_{k,d} - \theta_k)^2 .
$$

By replacing each squared deviation $(\theta_{k,d} - \theta_k)^2$ with its district-level expectation $\Sigma_{B,kk}$, this reduces to

$$
\sum_{d=1}^{D} \left(1 - \frac{2N_d}{N} \right) G_{kk,d} V_{kk,d} + (V_{kk} + \Sigma_{B,kk}) \sum_{d=1}^{D} G_{kk,d} .
$$

Matching this averaged expectation of $\mathrm{E}(S_{B,kk})$ to $S_{B,kk}$ yields the estimator

$$
\hat{\Sigma}_{B,kk} = \frac{S_{B,kk} - \sum_{d=1}^{D} \left(1 - 2\frac{N_d}{N} \right) G_{kk,d} V_{kk,d}}{\sum_{d=1}^{D} G_{kk,d}} - V_{kk} .
$$

A similar estimator is obtained for a covariance in $\mathbf{\Sigma}_B$.

Note that the matrix $\hat{\mathbf{\Sigma}}_B$ is involved in some nonlinear transformations in $\hat{\mathbf{b}}_d^* = \hat{\mathbf{Q}}_d^{-1} \hat{\mathbf{P}}_d \mathbf{u}$, and so the method is effective only when its elements are estimated with high precision. This condition is satisfied in the analysis of a large-scale survey of a country with many districts, many of which are represented in the survey by substantial subsamples. Difficulties arise when attempting to use many auxiliary variables because of the accumulated uncertainty about the elements of Σ_B and the impact of this uncertainty on $\mathbf{Q}_d$ and $\mathbf{b}_d^*$. Absence of a district in the sample is no hindrance to estimation of its population mean. Simply, we set its components of $\hat{\boldsymbol{\theta}}_d$ that are based on the survey sample to arbitrary values, and the corresponding sampling variance submatrix of $\mathbf{V}_d$ to a diagonal matrix with very large variances (representing $+\infty$).

In the vector $\boldsymbol{\theta}_d$, we can include estimators from the same analysed survey, estimators derived from other surveys (even if the elementary data are not available), and even known (population) quantities. In this way, we can combine information from several sources, surveys, administrative registers or observations made on the districts directly, such as their levels of urbanity and population sizes. Thus, a survey of unemployment can be supplemented with information from the register of persons claiming unemployment benefit, and a recent survey can be supplemented with the same survey in the recent past, say, from one, two, and three quarters ago. The surveys use one definition of unemployment, for which inferences are desired. The register uses a different definition, so its summaries are biased, but without any sampling variance, unless we represent administrative errors by (a small) sampling variation. The bias cannot be substantial because the variables recorded in the two sources are bound to be very similar, and so are their district-level summaries. Further, the district-level unemployment rates could not have changed substantially over a year or two, even if changes in unemployment status over such a period of time can be expected for many members of the labour force. A large component of the trend in the rates may be uniform across the districts. All these factors make the registers and the past surveys effective sources of auxiliary information with a great potential to reduce survey costs and increase the precision of estimation.

Suggested Reading

Two classic texts, [95] and [20], are invaluable resources both for the basic theory and as practical guides to all aspects of survey sampling. A carefully compiled comprehensive text on sampling theory with emphasis on exploiting auxiliary information is [168]. A more specialised monograph, [196], focuses on estimation of the sampling variance in surveys. The original paper on the Horvitz–Thompson estimator is [83], although similar estimators have an even longer history. For small-area estimation, [48] is a landmark paper. The multivariate composite estimator given by (3.20) is introduced in [116].

Problems and Exercises

3.1. In the software of your choice, construct a (finite) population of size $N = 10\,000$ as a random sample from a continuous distribution that is distinctly not normal (e.g., log-normal) and apply simple random sampling schemes with replacement with fixed and binomially distributed sample sizes.
Hint: Use a random sample from the uniform distribution as a source of events with specified probabilities.

3.2. Replicate a sampling scheme with sample size $n = 20$ or $E(n) = 20$ from the previous exercise many times, evaluate the HT estimator $\hat{\mu}$ of the population mean, and verify that the estimator is unbiased and that the expression for its sampling variance is correct. Assess whether the estimator is (approximately) normally distributed.

3.3. Apply the systematic sampling scheme with step length 20 in the population generated in Exercise 3.1 and evaluate the (obvious) estimator of the population mean. List all 20 possible values of the estimator and calculate the sampling variance of the estimator. Repeat the exercise on the same population after ordering it according to the values of the outcome variable. What kind of reordering of the members would yield the smallest and largest possible values of the sampling variance?

3.4. Implement on the computer the general systematic sampling design illustrated in Figure 3.1.

3.5. Discuss the problems with and devise some improvements on the following scheme for sampling from a population of size $1\,000\,000$ represented by a perfect sampling frame. The sample size is fixed at 1000. We proceed through the sampling frame, draw for each member a random number from $\mathcal{U}(0, 1)$ and include the member in the sample if the value drawn is smaller than 0.001. We stop if we make the 1000th inclusion before reaching the end of the sampling frame. If by the end we have not selected the full quota of 1000 subjects we return to the top of the sampling frame and continue the selection by the same rule, skipping members that have already been selected.

3.6. Suppose a population comprises $N^{(2)}$ households with sizes given by the following table:

	Household size							
	1	2	3	4	5	6	7	Total
Number of households	20	75	283	412	216	97	9	1112

(The population size is $N = 4392$). In a setting of your choice, discuss the merits of sampling designs for this population, which are

- simple random
- stratified, with the seven strata defined by the household size;
- clustered, with the households as clusters, and with each selected cluster enumerated;
- stratified clustered, with household size defining the strata, households the clusters, and simple random sampling within households.

3.7. Draw a pair of subjects (a sample of size $n = 2$) from the population comprising 12 members with values $\mathbf{X} = (0, 0, 0, 1, 1, 2, 2, 2, 4, 5, 7, 10)$ with probabilities $(3 + X_i)/70$ of drawing the sample comprising members i and $i + 1$; if $i = 12$, the members 12 and 1 are selected. Write down the HT estimator and define some other estimators of the population mean. Replicate the sampling and estimation processes many times and compare the mean squared errors of these estimators. Is this design proper?

3.8. *Quota sampling* is defined by an instruction to interviewers to collect responses to the survey questionnaire from a given number of subjects. The interviewers may be assigned to specific locations, such as the central square of a city, the departure hall of an airport, a commuter train, or the like, on given dates and at particular times of the day. The instructions may be 'stratified', for example, to recruit given numbers of men and women, in specific age groups and from nationalities or ethnic groups. Discuss the merits of such a design for surveys with the following agenda:

- voting intention;
- preference for a particular brand of a consumer product;
- allocation of funds to public services;
- popularity of a personality or a sports team.

3.9. Discuss the problems with implementing a sampling design (devising a sampling mechanism) with given (unequal) probabilities of selection p_i, fixed sample size n, and without replacement.

3.10. On an example of a small population, say 20 members, with a proper sampling design that is easy to implement but has unequal inclusion probabilities, compare equation (3.3) with some alternatives motivated by the equation for the sampling variance of the sample mean of a random sample from an infinite population, such as

$$\mathrm{var}_\dagger(\hat{\mu}) = \frac{1}{w_+ - 1} \sum_{j=1}^{n} w_j \left(x_j - \hat{\mu}\right)^2,$$

where w_+ is the sample total of the sampling weights. Study the proposals made in [148] and apply the proposed adjustments of this formula.

3.11. For a population of your choice (e.g., generated as a random sample from a superpopulation), compare the MSEs of the HT estimator and the estimator

Table 3.2. The subsample sizes and sample totals of sampling weights in the eight categories of a partition of a population.

				Category				
	Total	1	2	3	4	5	6	7	8
N_k	16 020	26 730	86 470	105 880	69 910	34 100	11 540	27 920	378 570
n_k	63	102	417	659	356	207	27	144	1975
$w_+^{(k)}$	13 750	19 820	92 060	111 010	70 050	46 570	5990	32 050	391 300

$$\hat{\mu}' = \frac{1}{w_+} \sum_{j=1}^{n} w_j x_j$$

for the simple random sampling designs without replacement, with fixed and binomially distributed sample sizes. Repeat the comparison for a range of (expected) sample sizes. Discuss the differences between the inferences about the population and about the superpopulation.

3.12. Construct the enumeration of an artificial country that comprises 30 districts with population sizes in the range 1 000 to 12 000, with log-normally distributed values of the target variable within each district. Set the parameters of the within-district distributions so that both the expectations and variances within the districts would be moderately positively correlated with the population size. Summarise the collection of the within-district populations by a suitable graph. Discuss the rationale for using the districts as strata in a national survey in which the constructed variable is of interest and compare it with a clustered sampling design with the districts as clusters. Implement a stratified sampling design with simple random sampling within each district. Set the two stages of a clustered sampling design to simple random sampling designs, and implement this design. Study the variance of the sample size as a function of the sampling designs at the two stages.

3.13. Table 3.2 summarises the sampling weights for a partition of a population into its eight categories (subsample sizes n_k and subtotals of weights $w_+^{(k)}$, $k = 1, \ldots, 8$). The subpopulation sizes for these categories are listed in the table (N_k). Describe how you would adjust the sampling weights by post-stratification, so as to make their totals agree with the subpopulation sizes. What might be the reasons for the difference of the totals $\sum_k N_k$ and $\sum w_+^{(k)}$? Study by replications of some simpler sampling schemes the differences that can be expected between N_k and $w_+^{(k)}$.

3.14. The dataset EX7a.dat on www.sntl.co.uk/BookA/Data contains the records of the sample of subjects in a survey of professional athletes who retired between one and two years ago. The outcome variable is their income from employment in the tax year that has just concluded. Apply the various proposals for trimming and shrinkage of the sampling weights and assess their impact on the HT estimator. Discuss what grounds you might have for selecting a weight adjustment that yields a (nearly) efficient estimator of the mean income. Would your conclusion be different if the target was the proportion of those with income below a certain level?

3.15. Construct a population of size $N = 25\,000$ as a random sample from a superpopulation in which variable X has a continuous uniform distribution on $(1, 6)$ and Y is generated according to the ordinary regression model, $Y = \beta_x X + \varepsilon$, with $\beta_x = 0.85$ and $\text{var}(\varepsilon) = 0.25$. Suppose the values of X are available for every member of the population and Y is the target variable. Discuss the rationale for a stratified sampling design with the strata defined by cut points for the values of X. For example, there could be ten strata defined by the ranges $[1, 1.5)$, $[1.5, 2)$, $\ldots$, $[5.5, 6)$ of values of X. What are the advantages and drawbacks of similar stratifications with much finer or cruder divisions of the support of X, $(1, 6)$?

Implement the following sampling design, called *semi-systematic*. Represent each member by a segment of length equal to its value of X, and join these segments as in Figure 3.1. Draw a random number u_1 from the uniform distribution on $(50, 150)$ and include in the sample the member whose segment covers the location u_1. Then draw independently another random number u_2 from $\mathcal{U}(50, 150)$ and include in the sample the member whose segment covers the location $u_1 + u_2$. Continue in this fashion until the total $\sum_j u_j$ exceeds the population total $X_+ = X_1 + \cdots + X_N$. Relate this sampling design to systematic sampling. Describe the distribution of the sample sizes of this design. Discuss the difficulties in calculating the pairwise inclusion probabilities $p_{ii'}$. Could the estimator of the sampling variance of the HT estimator, given by (3.3), be applied if these probabilities were available?

3.16. For the population in the previous exercise, define $p_i = 0.01/(1 + 2X_i)$. Implement the sampling design with these probabilities of inclusion and independent inclusions. Calculate the variance of the HT estimator. Replicate the sampling process and evaluation of the HT estimator sufficiently many times, so that you could check reliably that the equation for the variance is correct. Experiment with the constants a and b in the formula for the inclusion probabilities, $p_i = a/(1 + bX_i)$, subject to the constraint of a set expected sample size $p_1 + \cdots + p_N = n$, and find a design for which the HT estimator is (nearly) efficient.

3.17. A small country comprises two regions, A and B, with respective subpopulation sizes $N_1 \ll N_2$. A survey is planned for this population, with a stratified sampling design, with the regions as the strata, and simple random sampling designs in both strata. The unit costs of sampling in the two regions are $c_1 \gg c_2$. The targets are the population percentages of a particular indicator that are unlikely to be outside the range 10 to 25% in either region. The parties that have a stake in the results of the survey agree on the inferential priorities $P_1 = 5$, $P_2 = 1$ for the respective regions, and on $P = 5$ for the national estimator of the percentage. Suppose the total funds available for the conduct of the survey are C. Propose suitable sampling fractions for the two regions for the general setting or for some realistic choices of N_1, N_2, c_1, c_2, and C.

3.18. A national survey collected the values of the target variable Y on a sample of about 5000 subjects. Of interest are the population means μ_d of this variable in the $D = 87$ districts of the country. A national organisation maintains a register that contains the values of a variable X closely related to Y. The dataset EX7b.dat on www.sntl.co.uk/BookA/Data contains the HT estimates $\hat{\mu}_d$, $d = 1, \ldots, D$, of the district-level means μ_d, the estimators of the sampling variances of these estimators, and the district-level means of X. Estimate the district-level means μ_d by the estimator related to (3.20), with the register summaries as the auxiliary information. Assume that the direct (within-district HT) estimators are independent and ignore the variance matrix $\mathbf{V}$ of the national estimators as well as the covariance matrix $\mathbf{C}_d$ of the district-level and national means. Regard the register-based quantities as being free of any sampling variation, or associate each of them with a token sampling variance, such as 0.0001. Assess the value of the information from the register by comparing the coefficients of the direct estimator with the coefficients of the register-based means in the composite estimator. Relate them (e.g., the ratios or differences of the coefficients) to the within-district sample sizes or sampling variances of the HT estimators.

3.19. In the setting of the previous exercise, discuss the fallacy of the following proposal. We relate the within-district HT estimates to the corresponding register-based quantities by a linear model. If the model fits well and appears to be valid we estimate the means μ_d by their model-based predictions. (Assume that the model could incorporate the heteroscedasticity due to unequal within-district sample sizes.)

4

The Bayesian Paradigm

In the previous chapters, we regarded the population quantities as unknown fixed constants and the observations or records as outcomes of a random process. In Chapter 3 the sampling process and in Chapters 1 and 2 the data-generating process, as described by a model equation or a class of joint distributions, were the sole sources of randomness. This chapter introduces a radically different approach in which the observed quantities (data) are fixed and all unknown quantities are random and described by their joint *posterior distribution*—the conditional distribution of the target given what is known.

To distinguish between the *Bayesian* approach described in this chapter and the methods that make references to hypothetical replications, we refer to the latter as *frequentist*. We can classify frequentist methods as design-based, which deal with a sampling process applied to a finite population and model-based, which search for one or a few parameters that govern the joint distribution (model) according to which the recorded data are generated.

4.1 The Updating Mechanism

Suppose our target is a parameter θ that governs the process by which the vector of outcomes $\mathbf{y}$ has been generated. If the value of θ were known the data-generating process would be described by the density $f(\mathbf{y}; \theta)$. For maximum likelihood estimation, we exchange the roles of $\mathbf{y}$ as the argument and θ as a fixed (unknown) parameter.

The Bayesian approach adopts the following perspective of the analyst. Everything that the analyst knows and has complete information about it is regarded as fixed. Quantities of interest, focal (important) or peripheral (of secondary importance), the values of which are not known, are regarded as random, and the incompleteness of the information about them is characterised by their joint distribution. Thus, in the setting of an already observed vector of outcomes $\mathbf{y}$ and a single unknown parameter θ, we regard θ as random, so it is more appropriate to write $f(\mathbf{y} \mid \theta = \theta_0)$ instead of $f(\mathbf{y}; \theta)$, and regard f, after $\mathbf{y}$ has been recorded, as a function of the parameter value θ_0 in the condition. We refer to $f(\mathbf{y}\,|\,\theta)$ as the *data-generating distribution*. With greater rigour, we should call it the class of conditional data-generating distributions, because for each value of θ there is a conditional distribution according to which the data would have been generated. The information we have about θ is described by a *prior distribution*; let its density be $p(\theta)$. We assume that the prior is a continuous distribution over a finite or infinite interval of feasible values of θ. Our goal is the posterior distribution of θ, defined as the conditional distribution of θ given the data $\mathbf{y}$.

The posterior distribution is linked to the prior and the data-generating distributions by the *Bayes theorem*, which for continuous (conditional) densities f and continuous prior densities p states that

$$g(\theta\,|\,\mathbf{y}) = \frac{f(\mathbf{y}\,|\,\theta)p(\theta)}{\int f(\mathbf{y}\,|\,\theta')p(\theta')\,\mathrm{d}\theta'}\,. \tag{4.1}$$

For discrete data-generating distributions, this identity remains valid after the densities f are replaced by the conditional probabilities $\mathrm{P}(\mathbf{Y} = \mathbf{y}\,|\,\theta)$. Any inferential statement about θ can be based on the posterior distribution. Any summary or feature of this distribution is called *posterior*. For example, we may quote its expectation or median, which might be regarded as estimates of θ. Its variance is a sample quantity similar in its nature to the sampling variance, but the two variances, posterior and sampling, should not be confused. A sampling variance is usually unknown and is estimated; it is a sampling-process quantity, the value of which could be recovered only after a large number of replications of the study. In contrast, the posterior variance is a known quantity, although its value depends on the data. However, in the Bayesian perspective, all operations and statements are conditional on the data, which are regarded as fixed.

The range of likely values of θ can be described by a so-called *tolerance interval* $(C_{\mathrm{L}}, C_{\mathrm{H}})$ that covers a high percentage (say, 95%) of the posterior distribution:

$$\mathrm{P}\,\{\theta \in (C_{\mathrm{L}}, C_{\mathrm{H}})\} = 1 - \alpha$$

for a small value α, such as $\alpha = 0.05$. Tolerance regions are defined similarly, as subsets of the support of θ that cover the posterior distribution with high probability. Among tolerance intervals for a parameter, we prefer those that have shorter lengths, although one-sided intervals are useful in some contexts. Obvious parallels can be drawn with (frequentist) confidence intervals.

4.1.1 Setting the Prior

The prior distribution plays an important role in the analysis. In an idealised setting, it is the posterior distribution obtained by the previous analysis related to the same target θ. More generally, it is a synthesis of all the information available about θ. Therefore, a Bayesian analysis, which evaluates

(4.1), can be regarded as an updating of the information about the target. In practice, there is no straightforward way of setting the prior distribution, especially when no single study conducted in the recent past can be identified as the sole and definitive source of information about θ prior to recording $\mathbf{y}$ in the current study. The full potential of the analysis can be realised only by a careful synthesis of what is known, conjectured, or believed. This entails eliciting information from experts who are not necessarily well acquainted with Bayesian methods, or statistical methods in general, and the quantification of their statements (expert judgement) can rarely be conducted according to a formal protocol.

Different parties may specify different prior distributions, because beliefs about θ have a rightful place among the inputs used in forming the prior distribution for θ. This *subjective nature* of the analysis is by no means a weakness of the approach. In the frequentist perspective, the prior distribution and the data can be regarded as two data sources; the data are common to all the parties that might conduct an analysis in pursuit of the value of θ. In contrast, the prior is a source specific to the client, and it is their responsibility to contribute to its formulation.

In practice, a default prior distribution is often specified, which bypasses the need for synthesis of the prior information about the target. Such a *noninformative* prior is intended to represent the state of total ignorance about θ or of no prejudice for or against any region of the support of θ prior to data inspection. For example, if the support of θ as a random variable is the interval $(0, 1)$, then the standard uniform distribution is the default prior. With constant $p(\theta)$, the (Bayesian) posterior distribution $f(\theta \,|\, \mathbf{y}) = C(\mathbf{y})f(\mathbf{y} \,|\, \theta)p(\theta)$ is proportional, and therefore for all purposes equal, to the (frequentist) likelihood $L(\theta; \mathbf{y}) = f(\mathbf{y}; \theta)$. Thus, the uniform prior can be interpreted as a Bayesian attempt to reproduce the results of the frequentist likelihood analysis. Of course, the two approaches yield inferential statements in different formats, but the mode of the posterior with the uniform prior coincides with the maximum likelihood estimator.

Using the uniform as the default prior entails an inconsistency. If instead of θ we considered $\eta = \sqrt{\theta}$ as the model parameter, the uniform prior for θ would correspond to the prior $g_\eta(x) = 2x$. This prior would seem to prefer large values of η at the expense of small values—it no longer appears to be noninformative. Noninformativeness is not invariant with respect to nonlinear transformations; it is well defined only in connection with a particular parameterisation. This is in conflict with the reasonable expectation that 'total ignorance' would require no such qualification.

For a parameter with unbounded support, such as $(0, +\infty)$ for the variance σ^2 of a random sample from a normal distribution, a noninformative prior cannot be defined; there is no distribution with constant density on $(0, +\infty)$. We can side-step this problem by defining a noninformative prior for a transformation of σ^2 that is supported on a finite interval. For example, we may specify the prior $\tau \sim \mathcal{U}(0, 1)$ for $\tau = \sigma^2/(1 + \sigma^2)$. It corresponds to the prior density

$$p_{\sigma^2}(x) = \frac{1}{(1+x)^2}$$

for σ^2. The arbitrariness of the transformation τ highlights the lack of a universal default prior for σ^2.

An alternative resolution of this problem is to specify a prior that is uniform on $(0, \sigma_\circ^2)$, where $\sigma_\circ^2$ is the largest plausible value of σ^2. This upper bound cannot be determined unambiguously, but a sensitivity analysis may assess the impact of the details of how $\sigma_\circ^2$ is set. On the one hand, smaller $\sigma_\circ^2$ is advantageous because it represents more (focussed) prior information, expected to yield a posterior distribution with smaller variance; on the other hand, a larger $\sigma_\circ^2$ is more conservative, making it less likely that some plausible values of σ^2 would be ruled out.

Yet another solution is to use in the role of the prior density a function that does not integrate to unity. For example, we may use the constant function $p(\sigma^2) = 1$ for variance $\sigma^2 \in (0, \infty)$. Such a prior is called *improper*. If the updating formula (4.1) yields a function that is a density, we declare it as the posterior for σ^2; otherwise we have to resort to a different prior. This is an unsatisfactory feature of the method, because a prior is meant to represent our knowledge about the data-generation process or the target prior to the conduct of the current study, and its specification should not be affected by any computational contingencies.

The difficulties with specifying a prior should not be regarded as a drawback of a Bayesian analysis. The prior and its incorporation in the analysis offer an opportunity to exploit all the relevant information that the analyst can access. However, in the frequentist analysis, we could represent the prior distribution as a *pseudo-observation*, independent of the (genuine) observations in the study and maximise the corresponding log-likelihood. Bayesian analysis does not have a monopoly over using prior information.

For extensive data, the prior has next to no impact on the posterior; with the same data and model, very different priors yield very similar posteriors. In contrast, the posterior may not differ substantially from the prior for a small dataset. The posterior is a *synthesis* of the two sources of information, the prior and the data, and their relative impacts are a reflection of their informational content.

A posterior is defined for a parameter, and in multiparameter models the posterior is a multivariate distribution. The posterior can be defined for a single parameter, or more generally for a (univariate) function of the parameter vector. The well-established rules for operating with distributions apply. For example, the posterior distribution for the component θ_1 of the parameter vector $\boldsymbol{\theta} = (\theta_1, \theta_2, \ldots, \theta_H)$ is the marginal of the joint posterior,

$$f(\theta_1 \,|\, \mathbf{y}) = \int \ldots \int f(\boldsymbol{\theta} \,|\, \mathbf{y}) \, \mathrm{d}\theta_2 \ldots \mathrm{d}\theta_H.$$

Model specification, setting the class of densities $f(\mathbf{y} \mid \theta)$, has a direct counterpart in the frequentist (model-based) approach. If several (finitely many) models M_k, $k = 1, \ldots, K$, are contemplated as alternatives, a Bayesian version of combining the single-model-based posteriors is by specifying a prior distribution for the models. This is a discrete distribution, with probabilities p_k for the alternative models; the probabilities add up to unity. Let the posteriors for a target θ be f_k, $k = 1, \ldots, K$; we called them *single-model-based* posteriors. The marginal posterior for the collection of the models is

$$f(\theta \mid \mathbf{y}) = \sum_{k=1}^{K} p_k f_k(\theta \mid \mathbf{y}). \tag{4.2}$$

The same vector of prior probabilities $(p_1, \ldots, p_K)$ applies to any target. In the frequentist approach, we combined single-model-based estimators, not densities, similarly, but the coefficients were derived from the estimated biases and the covariance structure of the estimators. This suggests an improvement on (4.2) by informing the choice of the prior probabilities p_k by the joint distribution of the single-model-based posteriors. However, it is difficult to specify a Bayesian analogue of the bias that would result from using an inappropriate model.

A drawback of the marginal posterior in (4.2) is that the weights accorded to the single-model-based posteriors are not informed by the data; the outcomes may provide more support for some models and less for others. Indeed, without any input from the data, the probabilities p_k would in most settings be very difficult to set because they would have to synthesize expertise about the data-generating process with the analyst's understanding of the models. Instead of using model-specific posteriors $f_k(\theta \mid \mathbf{y})$, we may include the model as part of the condition in the density f:

$$f_k(\theta \mid \mathbf{y}) = f(\theta \mid \mathbf{y}; M_k).$$

The posterior probability of model M_k is

$$b_k = P(M_k \mid \mathbf{y}) = \frac{p_k f_k(\theta \mid \mathbf{y})}{f(\theta \mid \mathbf{y})},$$

with the denominator given by (4.2). These probabilities are commonly referred to as *Bayes factors*. They can be used to address model uncertainty in several ways. First, the model with the greatest Bayes factor may be adopted; this would ignore model uncertainty altogether and commit the analyst to the most plausible model. As a solution, we dismissed it in the frequentist context in Chapter 2, and the argument presented there carries over to the Bayesian analysis directly. Next, we may regard the factors as measures of plausibility of each model and quote the single-model-based conclusions together with the associated factors b_k, or with some less formal assessments of plausibility. When there are many alternative models, a cutoff $b^{(0)}$ for the factors b_k may be chosen and only conclusions for models with b_k exceeding $b^{(0)}$ listed and discussed. Finally, the single-model-based posterior densities may be combined, with the Bayes factors as the coefficients, giving greater weight to models judged as more plausible:

$$f(\theta \mid \mathbf{y}) = \sum_{k=1}^{K} b_k f(\theta \mid \mathbf{y}, \mathrm{M}_k).$$

The summation can be curtailed to models with $b_k > b^{(0)}$; then the Bayes factors for the retained models have to be standardised so that they would add up to unity.

Example 8. Suppose we realised a random sample from a normal distribution with unit variance and unknown mean μ that we want to estimate. Let the observed values be $\mathbf{y} = (y_1, \ldots, y_n)^{\top}$.

We set the prior for μ to $\mathcal{N}(10, 10)$; μ is likely to be in the range $(0, 20)$ and values close to 10 are regarded as most probable. The posterior distribution of μ is obtained by standardising the product of the data-generating and prior densities:

$$f(\mu \mid \mathbf{y}) = C \exp\left\{-\frac{1}{2}\sum_{j=1}^{n}(y_j - \mu)^2\right\} \exp\left\{-\frac{1}{20}(\mu - 10)^2\right\},$$

where C is the positive constant for which $\int f(\mu \mid \mathbf{y})\mathrm{d}\mu = 1$. The density is the exponential of a quadratic function of μ, so it can be matched with a normal distribution. We obtain the (normal) posterior distribution directly, without having to evaluate the denominator in the Bayes theorem. The logarithm of the posterior density is

$$\log\{f(\mu \mid \mathbf{y})\} = c(\mathbf{y}) - \frac{1}{2}\left(n + \frac{1}{10}\right)\left\{\mu - \frac{1}{n + \frac{1}{10}}\left(1 + \mathbf{y}^{\top}\mathbf{1}_n\right)\right\}^2,$$

where $c(\mathbf{y})$ does not depend on μ. This density is matched by the normal distribution with mean $10(1 + \mathbf{y}^{\top}\mathbf{1}_n)/(1 + 10n)$ and variance $10/(1 + 10n)$. The impact of the prior on the posterior is the same as of an additional observation equal to 10, with variance 10, independent of the remaining (genuine) observations. Thus, the mean of the posterior is the convex combination of the prior mean and the sample mean $\bar{y} = \mathbf{y}^{\top}\mathbf{1}_n/n$, with the coefficients proportional to the respective precisions (reciprocals of the variances) in estimating μ.

The impact of the prior diminishes with increasing n; the posterior has the same limit as $\mathcal{N}(\bar{y}, 1/n)$. A (normal) prior with a very large variance has only a slight impact on the posterior even when the sample size n is small. A prior with a small variance is accorded substantial weight in the convex combination and the posterior variance is then much smaller than $1/n$. Our confidence about μ is rewarded by smaller posterior variance. This highlights the need for integrity in the specification of the prior. There exists a prior for any (normal) posterior distribution that a dishonest analyst might want to obtain.

4.1.2 Conjugate Priors

Although the prior distribution for a parameter should be selected solely based on the available information, there is often a considerable leeway in the choice to make the evaluation of the posterior in (4.1) tractable. One important class of such priors, for particular data-generating distributions, is such that the posterior distributions belong to the same class. As an example, let y be the number of successes in a sequence of independent binary trials with common probability of success r, so that the data-generating process is

$$f(y \mid r) = \binom{n}{y} r^y (1 - r)^{n-y}.$$

We specify the prior p by the density of the beta distribution with parameters $a > 0$ and $b > 0$;

$$p(r) = \frac{\Gamma(a + b)}{\Gamma(a)\,\Gamma(b)}\, r^{a-1}(1 - r)^{b-1}.$$

Its expectation and variance are $\dfrac{a}{a + b}$ and $\dfrac{ab}{(a + b)^2(a + b + 1)}$, respectively.

The posterior density of r is

$$f(r \mid y) = C r^{y+a-1}(1 - r)^{n-y+b-1},$$

where C is the standardising constant. We do not have to evaluate C by integration because $f(r \mid y)$ is the density of the beta distribution with parameters $y + a$ and $n - y + b$. Its expectation and variance are

$$\bar{r} = \frac{y + a}{n + a + b} \quad \text{and} \quad \frac{\bar{r}(1 - \bar{r})}{n + a + b + 1},$$

respectively. Thus, the prior can be motivated as adding a successes and b failures in $a + b$ independent trials to the n that were realised.

The beta distribution is the conjugate also for the geometric distribution given by the probabilities $r(1 - r)^y$, $y = 0, 1, \ldots$. Another important class of conjugate priors are the gamma distributions for the Poisson and gamma data-generating distributions. The normal prior is conjugate for the normal data-generating distribution, as is the continuous uniform for itself.

4.2 Computational Issues

In the frequentist approach, maximum likelihood involves maximisation of a complex function. The solution is relatively simple when the log-likelihood function is quadratic. For example, fitting ordinary regression by least squares is equivalent to maximum likelihood (except for an adjustment for $\hat{\sigma}^2$). More generally, computations are relatively simple when all the distributions involved are normal because the class of multivariate normal distributions is closed with respect to taking margins, conditioning, and similar operations. The likelihood in many other settings requires iterative maximisation that entails complexities and may require some improvisation. The sampling distribution of the estimators is estimated from the inverse of the information matrix, involving further nontrivial operations of differentiation, expectation and matrix inversion.

In the Bayesian approach, the main difficulty is in evaluating the denominator in (4.1). The integral is the standardising constant for the numerator; its role is to ensure that the result is a density, with the property that $\int f(\theta \mid \mathbf{y}) \, \mathrm{d}\theta = 1$. Thus, the posterior is proportional to the product of the data-generating (model) and prior densities, representing the two (independent) sources of information. The standardising constant can be evaluated analytically or guessed from the form of the numerator only in some simple settings, such as when a conjugate prior is used.

An integral $\int_A^B f(x) \, \mathrm{d}x$ can be approximated by a wide range of numerical methods that partition the support (A, B) into a sequence of intervals. The integrand $f(x)$ is approximated within each interval (a, b) by a function that can be easily integrated analytically. The constant and linear functions are the obvious choices for such an approximation. Suppose the limits A and B are finite. Then

$$\int_A^B f(x) \, \mathrm{d}x = \sum_{h=1}^H \int_{a_h}^{b_h} f(x) \, \mathrm{d}x, \qquad (4.3)$$

where the values $a_1 < b_1 = a_2 < b_2 = \ldots = a_H < b_H$ define the partitioning of (A, B), so that $A = a_1$ and $B = b_H$. Each integrand on the right-hand side of (4.3) is approximated by a constant, a linear or another function $g(x)$ for which the integral over the range (a_h, b_h) is easy to evaluate. This yields the approximation

$$\int_A^B f(x) \, \mathrm{d}x = \sum_{h=1}^H \int_{a_h}^{b_h} g(x) \, \mathrm{d}x.$$

For $g(x)$ constant, a practical choice is based on points $c_h \in [a_h, b_h]$ at which the function $f(x)$ is evaluated, and $g(x)$ is set to $f(c_h)$ throughout (a_h, b_h). Then

$$\int_A^B f(x) \, \mathrm{d}x \doteq \sum_{h=1}^H (b_h - a_h) f(c_h).$$

For approximation by linear functions, the obvious choice in the range (a_h, b_h) is

$$g(x) = f(a_h) + \frac{x - a_h}{b_h - a_h} \left\{ f(b_h) - f(a_h) \right\},$$

which matches f at a_h and b_h. This yields

$$\int_A^B f(x)\,\mathrm{d}x \doteq \frac{1}{2}\sum_{h=1}^{H} (b_h - a_h)\{f(b_h) + f(a_h)\}\,.$$

In general, a finer grid of points $(a_1,\ldots,a_H)$ and linear approximating functions g yield better approximations. More complex approximations may be well suited for particular functions f. For example, quadratic functions g may fit f better, although finding a quadratic approximation requires solving a set of three linear equations for each interval (a_h, b_h).

The cut points $(a_1,\ldots,a_H)$ can be chosen uniformly, to split (A,B) to intervals of equal length. When we know that the function f has substantial curvature in some regions and is well approximated by a linear function elsewhere, the cut points can be set more densely in the former and less densely in the latter regions. As an alternative, the integrand f may be transformed and uniformly distributed cut points can be chosen on the transformed scale.

The integral in (4.3) can be approximated as an expectation, using a distribution from which a large random sample can be drawn easily and with computational economy. We express the integral as

$$\int f(x)\,\mathrm{d}x = \int u(x)g(x)\,\mathrm{d}x = \mathrm{E}_g(U)\,, \tag{4.4}$$

where $g(x)$ is the density of a suitable distribution, $u(x) = f(x)/g(x)$, and $U = u(X)$ is the variable defined by transforming a variable X with density g. We refer to g (and the corresponding distribution) as the *generating* density (distribution). The expression in (4.4) converts the integral to an expectation that can be approximated empirically as

$$\int f(x)\,\mathrm{d}x \doteq \frac{1}{n}\sum_{j=1}^{n} u(x_j)$$

for a random sample from the distribution with density g. This method is called *importance sampling*. The density g has to be selected with care. The ideal choice for g is a density similar to f, so that the ratios $u(x) = f(x)/g(x)$ do not involve very large or very small values, and relatively small samples can estimate the integral with high precision.

The generating density g has to have the same support as f. The choice of g is more difficult when the support of f is the entire real axis. Matching g so that it would have relatively large values in the region where f has large values is usually easy, but finding a density g that has similar behaviour to f in the proximity of $\pm\infty$ is often not trivial.

Example 9. As a simple illustration, we evaluate the gamma integral

$$\int_0^{+\infty} x^2 \mathrm{e}^{-x}\,\mathrm{d}x \tag{4.5}$$

using the exponential distribution with the density e^{-x} as the generating distribution. Thus, we evaluate $E(X^2)$. With a random sample of size $10\,000$, we obtained the estimate 2.040. In this setting, we can derive the result analytically: $E(X^2) = 2$. Moreover, we can derive the sampling variance of the estimator;

$$\text{var}\left(\frac{1}{n}\sum_{i=1}^{n}X^2\right) = \frac{1}{n}\left\{4! - (2!)^2\right\} = \frac{20}{n},$$

so for $n = 10\,000$ the standard error of the estimator of the integral in (4.5) is $1/\sqrt{500} \doteq 0.045$. Although $n = 10\,000$ might seem excessive, the associated computation takes only about two-hundredths of a second, so even much higher precision could easily be afforded, even in conjunction with several other computations of similar complexity.

For an integrand f defined in $(-\infty, +\infty)$, we may find a distribution with suitable tail behaviour in the vicinity of $-\infty$, another in the vicinity of $+\infty$, and a third in another range, such as near the sole maximum of f, where matching the behaviour of f is essential. Let these densities be g_1, g_2, and g_3 and suppose the values of each of them is very small in the two other important ranges: $g_1 \gg g_2$ and $g_1 \gg g_3$ in the vicinity of $-\infty$, $g_2 \gg g_1$ and $g_2 \gg g_3$ in the vicinity of $+\infty$, and $g_3 \gg g_1$ and $g_3 \gg g_2$ in the vicinity of the maximum of f. Then the mixture density $r_1 g_1 + r_2 g_2 + r_3 g_3$ is a suitable generating density for f; all three weights r_m should be distant from zero, but they do not have to be identical.

Rejection sampling is a method for drawing samples from a given density f. To apply it, we have to find another density g and a positive constant c, such that $cg \geq f$. We draw a random sample $(x_1, \ldots, x_n)$ from the distribution with density g and select each value x_k into a subsample with probability $f(x_k)/\{cg(x_k)\}$. This subsample is a random sample from the density f.

The ideal choice for the density g and constant c is such that the ratio $f(x)/g(x)$ is close to unity. When these ratios have values in a wide range and the probability that $f(x)/g(x)$ is small is substantial, a large sample from the density g is required to generate a subsample of a given size; a large fraction of the sample is *rejected*. Finding a density g with a suitable behaviour in the tails is often a problem, just like with importance sampling. The problem can be addressed with mixtures of tractable distributions in a similar manner.

4.2.1 Sampling from Multivariate Distributions

A standard task in Bayesian analysis, associated with summarising the posterior distribution in (4.1), is to draw a random sample from a joint distribution of the parameter vector $\boldsymbol{\theta}$. Often we can draw values straightforwardly only from the univariate conditional distributions $(\theta_h \mid \boldsymbol{\theta}_{-h})$, given all the other components. Until the advent and proliferation of powerful computers and computational software to harness their power, generating draws from multi-variate distributions was an insurmountable task in most settings. Nowadays the problem is resolved by the *Monte Carlo Markov chain* (MCMC) method, which generates a draw from an approximation to the sought joint distribution. The method is computationally intensive, involving many iterations, but its programming is relatively simple.

We describe a special case of MCMC called the *Gibbs sampler*. To generate a sample from the distribution of $\boldsymbol{\theta}$, we start with an arbitrarily set initial value $\boldsymbol{\theta}^{(0)}$ of $\boldsymbol{\theta}$ within its support. Next we draw a single value from the conditional distribution $(\theta_1 \mid \boldsymbol{\theta}_{-1} = \boldsymbol{\theta}_{-1}^{(0)})$; that is, we draw a value of the first component, conditionally on the current values of the other components. Similarly, we draw values of each component $h = 2, 3, \ldots, H$ in turn, conditioning in draw h on the values of the components $1, 2, \ldots, h - 1$ generated earlier, and on the initial values of components $h + 1, \ldots, H$. At the end of this cycle, each component of $\boldsymbol{\theta}$ has been updated once; the result is denoted by $\boldsymbol{\theta}^{(1)}$. This cycle of H univariate draws is repeated many times, generating values $\boldsymbol{\theta}^{(2)}, \boldsymbol{\theta}^{(3)}, \ldots, \boldsymbol{\theta}^{(M)}$. The concluding vector $\boldsymbol{\theta}^{(M)}$ yields a value that can be regarded as a sample from the joint distribution of $\boldsymbol{\theta}$ with the specified univariate conditional distributions.

The theory supporting this procedure claims that the distribution of $\boldsymbol{\theta}^{(m)}$ converges to the joint distribution of $\boldsymbol{\theta}$ as m diverges to infinity. The convergence is often slow and the number of cycles M required for the approximation to be satisfactory is very large, often in tens of thousands. However, the many cycles (iterations) do not take up a lot of computing time, and the programming effort to implement the procedure is quite modest. In practice, we need many draws from the distribution of $\boldsymbol{\theta}$, so the sequence of M cycles has to be repeated. For the second and subsequent draws we may use the previous draw $\boldsymbol{\theta}^{(M)}$ in the role of the initial value $\boldsymbol{\theta}^{(0)}$. Thus, to generate n draws, the cycle is repeated nM times, and the values after cycles $M, 2M, \ldots, nM$ are extracted. Usually the consecutive values $\boldsymbol{\theta}^{(m)}$ and $\boldsymbol{\theta}^{(m+1)}$ are highly correlated. It is therefore essential to maintain a substantial distance (M) between consecutive draws from the approximate distribution of $\boldsymbol{\theta}$; otherwise the draws may be far from being independent. Similarly, to remove any dependence on the initial values $\boldsymbol{\theta}^{(0)}$, the first M_0 cycles are discarded. These cycles are referred to as the *burn-in*. The convention is to set M_0 to a fraction of M, but M_0 is usually still in the thousands.

Example 10. Suppose a random vector $\mathbf{X} = (X_1, X_2, X_3)$ has the normal distribution $\mathcal{N}\left(\boldsymbol{\mu}, \sigma^2 \mathbf{I}_3 + \tau \mathbf{1}_3 \mathbf{1}_3^\top\right)$, with $\boldsymbol{\mu} = (1, 0, 3)^\top$, $\sigma^2 = 1.5$, and $\tau = 0.6$. We generate a random sample from this distribution by MCMC, using the three univariate conditional distributions $(X_k \mid \mathbf{X}_{-k})$.

Denote $\mathbf{V}_m = \sigma^2 \mathbf{I}_m + \tau \mathbf{1}_m \mathbf{1}_m^\top$. The conditional distribution of X_1 given the values $X_2 = x_2$ and $X_3 = x_3$ is also normal,

$$\mathcal{N}\left\{\mu_1 + \tau \mathbf{1}_2^\top \mathbf{V}_2^{-1} \begin{pmatrix} x_2 - \mu_2 \\ x_3 - \mu_3 \end{pmatrix}, \sigma^2 + \tau - \tau^2 \mathbf{1}_2^\top \mathbf{V}_2^{-1} \mathbf{1}_2\right\}.$$

The inverse of $\mathbf{V}_2$ is

$$\mathbf{V}_2^{-1} = \frac{1}{\sigma^2} \left(\mathbf{I}_2 - \frac{\tau}{\sigma^2 + 2\tau} \mathbf{1}_2 \mathbf{1}_2^\top \right)$$

and $\mathbf{V}_2^{-1} \mathbf{1}_2 = (\sigma^2 + 2\tau)^{-1} \mathbf{1}_2$. Hence

$$(X_1 \mid X_2 = x_2, X_3 = x_3)$$

$$\sim \mathcal{N} \left\{ \mu_1 + \frac{\tau}{\sigma^2 + 2\tau} (x_2 + x_3 - \mu_2 - \mu_3), \ \sigma^2 \left(1 + \frac{\tau}{\sigma^2 + 2\tau} \right) \right\}. \quad (4.6)$$

The univariate conditional distributions for the other components are obtained by the appropriate exchange of the components 1, 2, and 3.

Starting with the vector $\mathbf{0}$, we executed $100\,000$ cycles of MCMC and extracted every 100th intermediate vector $\mathbf{X}$ to obtain a sample of size 1000. Its sample mean vector and variance matrix are

$$\begin{pmatrix} 0.93 \\ 0.05 \\ 2.94 \end{pmatrix} \quad \begin{pmatrix} 2.05 \ 0.51 \ 0.63 \\ 0.51 \ 2.01 \ 0.64 \\ 0.63 \ 0.64 \ 2.10 \end{pmatrix}.$$

They are close to their population counterparts but, of course, they are not equal to them. For example, the sampling variance of the sample mean of size 1000 is 0.0021 (standard deviation 0.046). Univariate normality is checked by the normal quantile plots. A concern more relevant than proximity of the sample summaries to the population summaries is whether the consecutive values in the sample are (nearly) independent. This can be checked by plotting the sequences of values of the components, as done in Figure 4.1 for the first 200 values. Constants -1, 9, and 17 have been added to the three sequences to separate them in the diagram. No trend can be observed for either sequence. Independence of the sequence of the generated values can be assessed more formally by checking that the sample variance matrix of the differences $\mathbf{x}_2 - \mathbf{x}_1$, $\mathbf{x}_4 - \mathbf{x}_3, \ldots, \mathbf{x}_M - \mathbf{x}_{M-1}$, for M even, is close to $2(\sigma^2 + \tau)\mathbf{I}_3$.

We emphasise that Examples 9 and 10 have no practical use in Bayesian analysis and are presented solely for illustration. It is easy to check that they yield appropriate results because the problem they solve is tractable without any simulations.

4.3 Coherence

The Bayes theorem (4.1) for updating the prior by the data to form the posterior is the focal equation in Bayesian inference, applicable to every problem. Secondary tasks involve evaluation of the properties of the posterior. The compact description of Bayesian inference by (4.1) is regarded as an advantage; improvisation is involved only in the evaluation (or approximation) to

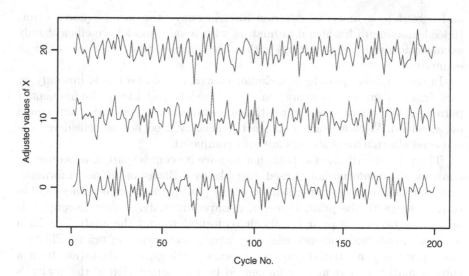

Fig. 4.1. Sequences of the draws from the normal distribution with mean $\mu = (0, 10, 20)^\top$ and variance matrix $1.5\mathbf{I}_3 + 0.61_3 1_3^\top$, using MCMC with burn-in $M_0 = 100$ and sampling frequency $M = 100$.

the posterior. It is therefore very easy to identify the analytical (computational) equipment that a Bayesian analyst requires—evaluation of densities and analytical or numerical integration.

Adherents to the Bayesian paradigm refer to this compact formulation as *coherence* of the Bayesian approach. Those who favour frequentist methods can point out that likelihood maximisation has a similar focal role in how they conduct inference. Admittedly, some other methods, such as ordinary least squares, are often used, but they coincide in their principal features and outcomes with maximum likelihood. A major point of departure is sampling theory (Chapter 3), but it could be regarded as a separate paradigm, competing with the Bayesian and the frequentist. In sampling theory the population is regarded as fixed, whereas in maximum likelihood only its summaries are.

With a noninformative prior, a Bayesian analysis is comparable to the maximum likelihood analysis using the same model for data generation, because the presumed advantage of exploiting prior information in the Bayesian analysis is set aside. In this setting, Bayesian analysis has a unique answer in the form of the posterior. Frequentist analysis has a comparable answer, presented in a different format, in terms of an estimated asymptotic (approximate) sampling distribution. The frequentist paradigm has alternatives to the maximum likelihood with the assumed model, but none of them is universal; they are useful only in some relatively narrow classes of problems. We defined estimator as *any* function of the data; thus, we never contemplated coherence. Instead of a procedural definition of inference we instituted flexibility and agreed to a universal criterion for efficiency—the mean squared error. Indeed, maximum likelihood estimators with a valid model are efficient only asymptotically; in some settings with finite samples, there are more efficient estimators.

In the Bayesian paradigm, a similar contract could be made, but only by sacrificing coherence; there are competing models, just like in the frequentist paradigm, but there is no competition for estimation once a prior and model are specified. Without such a contract, efficiency need not be considered because no alternative posteriors are ever compared.

The prior distribution appears not to have its counterpart in a frequentist analysis. Prior information is used, just like by a Bayesian, in model formulation, but the frequentist specification of the parameter space is rather rigid in comparison with the prior. However, a Bayesian analysis often foregoes this advantage because a prior is difficult to formulate and the analysis is for a wide or unspecified audience who may have a wide range of priors. Eliciting one's prior is a nontrivial process. In some settings, the elicitation from a subject-matter expert may be influenced by the formulation of the analyst's questions, and a misunderstanding may result in an inappropriate prior. Often the prior is subject to substantial uncertainty—even the expert may be uncertain, especially about some less familiar population summaries, such as regression parameters in a multiple regression, and the conclusion about the prior may to a large extent be arbitrary.

The frequentists have an obvious recourse to specifying a prior within their likelihood. Simply, some pseudo-observations are added to the data. The pseudo-observations and the genuine observations are independent, so their (joint) likelihood is equal to the product of their densities, as in the numerator of (4.1). Pseudo-observations can be motivated by the Bayes prior and their joint density set to the prior. Then the frequentist's task coincides with finding the mode of the posterior, without having to evaluate the denominator in (4.1).

As an alternative, the current data may be analysed jointly with past data in a single estimation process. The two datasets are independent, so their joint likelihood is easy to construct, if the constituent (dataset-specific) likelihoods are available. A set of minimal sufficient statistics for such a likelihood can be compiled by concatenating sets of minimal sufficient statistics for each of the constituent likelihoods. This reveals a problem with the general formulation of a Bayes prior. Suppose there is no single sufficient statistic for a parameter in the past study that is involved also in the current study. The frequentist view suggests that when no single summary of the prior information (the past study) is sufficient, neither is a one-parameter prior distribution. In brief, there may be prior information that cannot be presented in terms of a single prior distribution.

The frequentist alternative to the Bayes posterior is the sampling distribution of the estimator. The posterior is a single distribution. In contrast, the sampling distribution often depends on some (unknown) model parameters, so the assessment of its quality is not straightforward. An estimator may have some (frequentist) strengths and weaknesses. Although these are often difficult to explore, they open up possibilities to tailor the choice of an estimator to the specific needs of the analysis, responding to the assumed consequences of estimation errors. The Bayes prior can be interpreted as averaging (smoothing) over the strengths and weaknesses of the (maximum likelihood) estimator. The client is rewarded by an answer that is simpler (a single distribution), but a more complex answer, in terms of a distribution for each plausible value of the parameter, might inform more completely about the quality of the estimator.

A prior distribution may be degenerate, informing the analysis that the values of some of the parameters or of their combinations are known. A univariate prior is called highly concentrated if its variance is very small. A multiviarate prior is called *highly concentrated* if some of its marginals are highly concentrated. If the target is known then the data are redundant. If only the values of some other (nuisance) parameters are known, or pretended to be known, the posterior distribution is a proper distribution. Exploration of the posteriors for a range of such degenerate or highly concentrated priors is closely related to studying the sampling distribution of an estimator. However, a posterior for a parameter with a degenerate prior is also degenerate, so the Bayesian cannot explore how well a parameter would be estimated given that it has a particular value.

The frequentist's replication principle provides a universal way of learning about properties of estimators in a wide range of congenial and adverse conditions. Although much of statistical theory is about properties of estimators in congenial conditions, with a valid model, the integrity of any analysis is enhanced by sensitivity analysis—exploring the properties of the engaged estimator in plausible adverse conditions. There are obvious Bayesian counterparts of the sensitivity analysis, but they are outside the confines of coherence. The only way to bypass insurmountable analytical problems of evaluating a posterior with an inappropriately specified density $f(\mathbf{x}; \boldsymbol{\theta})$ is by borrowing the frequentist principle—replication.

Frequentist thinking is full of 'what might have happened' because of the ubiquitous reference to replications. For any given dataset, the frequentist may have different optimal estimators depending on the (sampling) design. For example, if simple random sampling design is applied, the sample mean has no credible alternative as an estimator of the population mean. However, if the sampling design is known to prefer units with larger values of the target variable, a different estimator is optimal. Thus, we cannot condition on data and on the distribution of the variable in the population, because other details of the data collection process, the sampling design in particular, are essential.

Suppose a random sample from an unknown distribution is recorded in a study. The sample size n is variable. The target is the data-generating distribution. For simplicity, suppose it is described by a single parameter θ. The frequentist would contemplate replications of the study, and these may yield samples of different sizes. But common sense suggests that the realised value of the sample size n should not be ignored. Any analysis that is conditional on this sample size, that is, that considers only replications with the same sample size, borrows a bit of the Bayesian paradigm, which conditions on *everything* that has been recorded. The orthodox frequentist approach, which does not condition on the sample size, would have an insurmountable problem if zero sample size had a positive probability. As the value of the estimator is not defined when $n = 0$, neither is any property of the estimator without ruling out such an outcome. In practice, some other resolution of this problem would be improvised; for example, resources might still be available if no data were collected, and the study would be replicated. Of course, the study plan may anticipate this problem and rule it out by design.

4.4 Bayesian Study Design

In Bayesian analysis, the posterior is a function of the data; a different dataset would yield a different posterior. The inference, encapsulated by the posterior, is subjective (prior-specific) and private to the analyst—a replication of the study will yield a different posterior, but the variation of such replicate posteriors is not a concern in the analysis of the single realised dataset.

In this perspective, planning a study does not fit comfortably into the Bayesian framework: the Bayes theorem is a clear prescription for dealing with a realised dataset, but it offers no immediate clues as to how to conduct a study so that the posterior would be sufficiently concentrated. Yet the design is indispensable, both for arranging that the analysis is (likely to be) satisfactory and for the conduct of the analysis itself. The design is reflected in the model for data generation. For example, independence and identical distributions of a sequence of observations are ensured by the design. If we regard these features as observations, then the design is treated on par with the data. In the frequentist analysis, there is a clear distinction: the design is always fixed, common to all replications, but the data (outcomes) are random.

The statistical design of any study is based on the anticipated conclusions. Thus, we consider the posteriors $f(\theta \mid \mathbf{y})$. For a particular data-generating process, we may consider the average posterior,

$$\int \cdots \int f(\theta \mid \mathbf{y}) g(\mathbf{y}) \, \mathrm{d}y_1 \ldots \mathrm{d}y_n \,,$$

where g is the joint density of $\mathbf{y}$. Of course, g depends on the unknown θ and sometimes also on some other parameters. This we could address by another round of averaging,

$$g(\mathbf{y}) = \int g(\mathbf{y} \mid \theta) p(\theta) \, \mathrm{d}\theta \,,$$

but that would merely yield our starting point, the prior.

We can explore the posteriors more directly. Let $V(\mathbf{y})$ be the posterior variance, expressed as a function of $\mathbf{y}$. For instance, in Example 8,

$$V(\mathbf{y}) = \frac{\tau}{1 + n\tau},$$

where τ is the variance of the prior; $\tau = 10$ in the example. We can ensure that the posterior variance does not exceed a given value v_0 by solving the inequality $V(\mathbf{y}) < v_0$; the solution is

$$n > \frac{\tau - v_0}{v_0 \tau}.$$

The lower bound is negative when $\tau < v_0$; we do not need any observations if the prior variance is already smaller than v_0.

The design in this setting is easy because the posterior variance does not depend on the data $\mathbf{y}$ and depends on only one design feature, the sample size n. For the general setting, we use the notation $V(\mathbf{y}, \boldsymbol{\xi})$ for the posterior variance; $\boldsymbol{\xi}$ are the features of the design that we can control. At the design stage, we have to address the uncertainty about $\mathbf{y}$. This we can do only by considering a 'prior' for $\mathbf{y}$, the distribution of the outcomes without conditioning on the model parameters. This is the denominator in (4.1),

$$\int f(\mathbf{y} \mid \theta) p(\theta) \, d\theta.$$

We do not have to evaluate this integral when $\mathbf{V}$ depends on $\mathbf{y}$ only through one or a few functions of $\mathbf{y}$, when

$$V(\mathbf{y}; \boldsymbol{\xi}) = V^* \{t(\mathbf{y}); \boldsymbol{\xi}\}.$$

Then we require a prior only for the summary $t(\mathbf{y})$. Setting the design now entails solving the inequality

$$\int V^* (t; \boldsymbol{\xi}) \, \psi(t) \, dt < v_0,$$

where ψ is the prior density of the statistic $t(\mathbf{y})$. In most settings, $\boldsymbol{\xi}$ is univariate, equal to the sample size n, so we seek the smallest sample size for which the average posterior variance would be smaller than a set standard. A small number of alternative designs can be compared straightforwardly.

Example 11. Suppose a single observation is generated according to the binomial distribution with n trials and probability of success equal to r. We set the prior distribution to beta with parameters $a > 0$ and $b > 0$. Earlier we established that the posterior distribution for p is also beta, with parameters $a + y$ and $n - y + b$. Its variance is

$$V(\mathbf{y}; n) = \frac{(a + y)(n - y + b)}{(n + a + b)^2 (n + a + b + 1)}.$$

We could avoid any complex computations by finding an upper bound for V that does not depend on y:

$$V(\mathbf{y}; n) \leq \frac{1}{4(n + a + b + 1)},$$

exploiting the inequality $r(1 - r) \leq \frac{1}{4}$ for any probability r. Hence, setting $n > 1/(4v_0) - a - b - 1$ would ensure that the posterior variance does not exceed the threshold variance v_0. This is a stronger result than we set out to obtain: the posterior variance will be smaller than v_0 not only in expectation, but for any possible outcome y. The frequentist version of this result is that we need sample size $n > 1/(4v_0)$ to ensure that the sampling variance of the proportion of successes falls below v_0, irrespective of the underlying probability r. Of course, these calculations are quite crude when, in the frequentist perspective, r is distant from $\frac{1}{2}$ and, in the Bayesian perspective, the prior places a lot of weight on r being either distant from $\frac{1}{2}$ or in the vicinity of $\frac{1}{2}$, in brief, when $a + b$ is large.

For a more refined calculation, we derive first the prior distribution for y. This is

$$f(y) = \int \binom{n}{y} p^y (1-p)^{n-y} \frac{\Gamma(a+b)}{\Gamma(a)\,\Gamma(b)} p^{a-1} (1-p)^{b-1} \, dp$$

$$= \binom{n}{y} \frac{\Gamma(y+a)\,\Gamma(n-y+b)}{\Gamma(a+b+n)} \frac{\Gamma(a+b)}{\Gamma(a)\,\Gamma(b)}.$$

The expected posterior variance is

$$\sum_{y=0}^{n} V(y; n)\, f(y). \tag{4.7}$$

Suppose $v_0 = 0.001$. Then the sample size of $1/(4v_0) = 250$ would certainly be sufficient, but we may be able to do with a much smaller study, depending on the parameters a and b or the prior. Before exploring a few settings, we discuss evaluation of (4.7). For large n, the summation in (4.7) involves many terms of small magnitude. Each term involves values of gamma functions, and some of them are so large that a computer would fail to conclude the calculation because of an overflow. Working with the logarithm of the gamma function is more practical, but a more direct approach involves logarithms of beta functions. The beta function is defined as $B(a, b) = \Gamma(a)\,\Gamma(b)/\Gamma(a+b)$, so that

$$f(y) = \frac{B(y+a, n-y+b)}{B(a,b)\,B(y, n-y)}.$$

Many of these expressions are very small numbers, so a direct computation is likely to fail. The problem can be avoided by evaluating $\log\{f(y)\}$, involving logarithms of beta functions. Most software packages evaluate $\log\{B(a,b)\}$ directly, without the intermediation of $B(a, b)$.

For $a = 6$ and $= 10$, which represents a fairly focussed prior (expectation 0.375 and standard deviation 0.12), we require the sample size of at least 205.

This figure can be found by the Newton method, although trial and error is only slightly less effective. For the noninformative prior, $a = b = 1$, the minimum sample size is only 165. The explanation for this seeming paradox is that probabilities r close to zero and unity are plausible, so the posterior variance could be quite small. This exposes a weakness of our sample size calculation: the value of the expected posterior variance as a criterion for study design diminishes with increasing dispersion of the posterior variance. We can resolve this problem by adopting a more conservative criterion, that a specified high quantile, such as 0.95, of the prior distribution of the posterior variances should not exceed v_0. The posterior variance is highest for $y = \frac{1}{2}(n+a+b) - a$ when $n + a + b$ is even, and for $y = \frac{1}{2}(n + a + b \pm 1) - a$ otherwise, and is symmetric around the maximum (or the mean of the two maxima). Therefore, the quantile is found by adding up the probabilities for the outcomes near the maximum until we reach the complement of the quantile (say, 0.05). The posterior variance at this value of the outcome is the sought quantity.

The function $r(1-r)$ is quite flat in a wide range around $r = 0.5$, so we are likely to reach the complement of the quantile for r such that $r(1-r) \doteq 0.25$. Therefore, we can calculate the required sample size simply by assuming that $r(1 - r) = 0.25$. For more focussed priors, which effectively rule out values of r in the neighbourhood of 0.5, the required sample size can be based on the plausible value of r that is closest to 0.5. For example, we may use the 0.95-quantile of the prior distribution that has its focus within $(0, 0.5)$ and the 0.05-quantile of the prior that has its focus within $(0.5, 1)$.

Costs can be incorporated in the analysis as a function P of the design features $\boldsymbol{\xi}$. We define gain G as a decreasing function of the posterior variance V, and seek to maximise the expected profit

$$\int G\left[V^* \{t(\mathbf{y}); \boldsymbol{\xi}\}\right] \psi(t) \, dt - P(\boldsymbol{\xi})$$

(ψ is the prior density of t). The maximum is unique when the costs increase with sample size or, generally, with the extent of the study. Setting the functions G and P is rarely straightforward, and it may be more constructive to explore a few realistic proposals and choose a compromise among the corresponding maxima.

4.5 Model Diagnostics and Prediction

It is a good practice to look back after evaluating the posterior and assess whether the specified model is appropriate. The rationale for this is essentially the same as in the frequentist perspective. The model assumptions cannot be confirmed, but their contradiction with the observed data might raise a doubt about them and justify their revision. In a Bayesian analysis, we make two assumptions: the prior and the data-generating distributions.

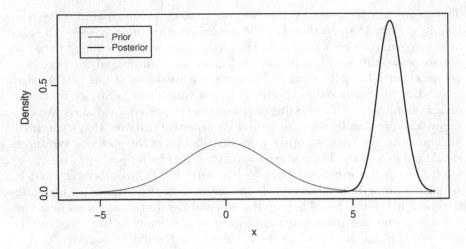

Fig. 4.2. Example of a conflict between the prior and posterior distributions, $\mathcal{N}(0,3)$ and $\mathcal{N}(6.5, 0.25)$, respectively.

We may have a good reason for revising the prior or for revisiting the process that led to its declaration, when most of the probability of the posterior distribution is in a region where the prior has a small probability. For example, suppose the prior is $\mathcal{N}(0,3)$ and the posterior is $\mathcal{N}(10, 0.25)$; see Figure 4.2. With a large dataset we need not be concerned about this conflict because the prior has been effectively ignored. With a smaller dataset we should be concerned that a prior that better reflects the information available at the time would yield a posterior substantially different from the one obtained originally.

Another source of potential conflict is between the observed data $\mathbf{y}$ and the posterior distribution. For example, the empirical distribution of $\mathbf{y}$ may be highly skewed, even though the posterior distribution is normal. In this case, we may revise the specification of the data-generating model, for instance, questioning the assumption of normality. For a given posterior, we can predict (anticipate) what another observation, or a dataset, generated by the same process would be. The *posterior predictive* distribution is defined by the density

$$f^*(\mathbf{u}) = \int f(\mathbf{u}\,|\,\theta)\,f(\theta\,|\,\mathbf{y})\,\mathrm{d}\theta\,;$$

it is the marginal data-generating distribution after averaging over the posterior distribution. We use the argument $\mathbf{u}$ to distinguish it from the observed vector $\mathbf{y}$. We have to use both qualifiers, posterior and predictive, because we can define the *prior predictive density* as

$$f(\mathbf{u}) = \int f(\mathbf{u}\,|\,\theta)\,p(\theta)\,\mathrm{d}\theta\,; \tag{4.8}$$

it describes the data we would expect before the actual data has been collected. The posterior predictive distribution is informed by the data, whereas the prior is not.

We can search for a conflict between the data and the posterior predictive distribution by comparing their summaries, such as the histogram of the data and the density of the posterior predictive distribution. A much more effective approach is based on simulations from the posterior predictive distribution. We define a feature, such as a graph, a table, a function of the data, or their combination, and evaluate it on both the observed data and a large number (19, 49, or 99) of simulated datasets from the posterior predictive distribution. If among these (20, 50, or 100) features, one realised and the remainder simulated, the realised feature stands out, we have evidence of a conflict. This approach, introduced in Chapter 1, has a frequentist (replication) flavour, but is equally well suited in the Bayesian context. We may forego the integration in (4.8) and generate a replicate vector $\mathbf{u}$ in stages as follows. First we draw a value of the parameter θ from the posterior distribution, and then we draw a realisation from the data-generating process with this parameter θ. This approach is closely related to numerical integration.

An important component of the method is the choice of the feature that is to be explored. It has to be informed by our a priori concerns about particular aspects of model validity. For example, with the normal posterior distribution we may be concerned about symmetry. Then we can proceed as in Section 1.3.1 by constructing a statistic that serves as a measure of asymmetry. We compare the values of this statistic on the realised and simulated datasets and conclude with evidence against the data-generating model if the realised value stands out among the simulated values.

If we approach the analysis without confidence, prepared to apply an extensive battery of diagnostic checks and act upon their results by reviewing the prior or the data-generating distributions, we should be less confident in the posterior-based inference than if we approached the analysis with justified confidence that all the specifications are appropriate. The lack of confidence should be reflected in our inference even if all diagnostic checks turn out to be negative and the original posterior is accepted. At present, this problem does not have a satisfactory solution and the advice on the extent of diagnostic checks to be applied is ambiguous at best. Pretending confidence when it is not justified is not a good solution.

Suggested Reading

The Bayes theorem is named after the Reverend Thomas Bayes, the author of [5]. Prior to the introduction of personal computers, Bayesian analysis was principally a theoretical and partly philosophical discipline, but the ideas espoused in the 1960s and earlier by [88], [63], [102], [32], and [10] have built a solid foundation for the modern Bayesian statistics. A more modern theoretical introduction is given by [66], and [150] is more practically oriented and up-to-date with regard to computational technology. Bayesian inference became a practical proposition after the advent of modern computing and the simulation-based methods for generating samples from multivariate distributions ([55], [183], and [57]). A very readable introduction to MCMC is given by [16]. All the essential elements of Bayesian computing, including efficient simulation-based sampling from multivariate distributions, are implemented in the software winbugs; see www.mrc-bsu.cam.ac.uk/bugs. Other influential texts on Bayes analysis are [7], [189], [8], and [56]. Important references on Bayes factors include [92], [139], and practically oriented [79]. The theoretical support for the simulation-based diagnostics using features is given in [160].

Problems and Exercises

4.1. Prove the Bayes theorem.
Hint: Recall that a conditional density $f(\mathbf{y} \mid \theta)$ is related to the joint density $f(\mathbf{y}, \theta)$ by the identity

$$f(\theta \mid \mathbf{y}) = \frac{f(\mathbf{y}, \theta)}{f(\mathbf{y})},$$

where f is the density of the distribution implied by its argument. Further, a marginal distribution is derived from the joint distribution by integration:

$$f(\mathbf{y}) = \int f(\mathbf{y}; \theta) \, d\theta.$$

Carefully state the conditions necessary in the proof. Derive a version of the Bayes theorem for discrete distribution of θ. What changes are required when $\mathbf{y}$ is discrete?

4.2. Suppose the posterior distribution for a parameter θ is exponential, with the density $u^{-1}e^{-u\theta}$ for a given value of the parameter $u > 0$. Find the 95% tolerance interval of the shortest length. Compare it with the tolerance interval that has limits equal to the 2.5 and 97.5 percentiles of the distribution.

4.3. Prepare for the analysis of a survey of employment in your region by formulating the prior for the rate of unemployment. This rate is defined as the percentage of the labour force who are not in employment at present but are actively seeking employment and would be prepared to take up an offer and start working in a matter of days or as the offer stipulates. What information would you draw on and how would you search for it? Suppose each student in a class has this assignment and the students share all the information they collect. Why could the students' priors differ? If the priors do differ, how would you try to reconcile them and formulate a prior that represents the entire class?

4.4. In a study, a random sample from a power distribution on $(0, 1)$, given by the density $a^{-1}x^{a-1}$ for a parameter $a > 0$, is observed. Suppose the exponential distribution with density $3e^{-a/3}$ is declared as the prior for a. Derive the posterior distribution of a. Compare it with the sampling distribution of the maximum likelihood estimator of a (which ignores the prior information). Explore ways of incorporating the prior information in the maximum likelihood analysis.

4.5. Suppose the data in a study are generated as a random sample of size n from the continuous uniform distribution on $(0, \theta)$ and a noninformative prior is to be declared for θ. Explore how this prior can be declared, and compare the posteriors for some of your proposals. Discuss whether the inefficiency (if any) of the maximum likelihood estimator of θ is reflected in the Bayesian analysis.

4.6. Describe the problem of estimating the mean of a group in the standard setting of ANOVA. Specify a common prior for the mean of each group and the noninformative prior for the two contending models:

A. the groups have identical means;
B. the groups do not have identical means.

Consider several distributions for the priors and discuss how convenient they are for the computations. Compare the solutions with the synthetic estimators derived in Chapter 1.

4.7. The class of *negative binomial* distributions is defined by the probabilities

$$P(X = k) = \binom{m + k - 1}{m - 1}(1 - r)^m r^k,$$

where m is an integer, r a probability (parameter), and $k = 0, 1, \dots$. The geometric distributions are a special case, with $m = 1$. A negative binomial distribution arises as the number of trials with a positive outcome until the mth trial with a negative outcome in a sequence of independent binary trials with a constant probability r. Solve the problem of estimating r with a random sample from this distribution with known m. Choose a conjugate prior for r. Suppose it is not known whether $m = 2$ or $m = 4$. Compare the posterior distributions for these two settings, and combine the posteriors using Bayes factors. Use the noninformative prior for m. As an alternative to Bayes factors, consider the problem of simultaneous estimation of m and p. Should the priors for p and m be correlated?

4.8. Apply importance sampling to evaluate the integral

$$\int_0^{+\infty} \sqrt{x^2 + \frac{1}{2}} \, \exp\left(-x^4 - 2x^2\right) dx.$$

Hint: Complete the squares under the square root and the exponential and relate an upper bound for the integrand to the density of the normal or gamma distribution (after a change of variable in the integral).

4.9. Evaluate the integral

$$\int_0^1 \frac{1 + 3x + e^{-x}}{2 + x + e^x}\, dx$$

by importance sampling.

4.10. Apply rejection sampling to generate a random sample from the distribution with the polynomial density $f(x) = c(1 + 3x - 2x^2 + 4x^3)$ on $(0, 1)$ for the appropriate constant c. Use random draws from the uniform distribution. As an alternative, generate a random sample by a direct method. For example, you could derive the distribution function $F(u) = \int_0^u f(x)\, dx$ and numerically approximate its inverse, the quantile function F^{-1}. Then, for a uniformly distributed variable X, $F^{-1}(X)$ has the sought distribution. Compare the two procedures for the amount of computing and programming (and mental) effort they require, and check on large samples $(n \geq 1000)$ generated by the two methods that the underlying distributions are similar (identical).

4.11. Suppose a bivariate distribution is given by its conditional distributions $(X_1 \mid X_2)$ and $(X_2 \mid X_1)$ with exponential densities with respective parameters (reciprocals of the means) $3 + x_2/10$ and $4 + x_1/10$. Apply MCMC to generate a random sample of size 250 from this bivariate distribution. Choose a sampling frequency to avoid any perceptible dependence of consecutive draws. Discuss what (you think) might happen if a distribution with the specified conditional distributions did not exist.

4.12. Explain why the Bayesian sample size calculation in Example 11 with a binomial outcome yields a lower minimum sample size, $1/(4v_0) - a - b - 1$, than its frequentist counterpart, $1/(4v_0)$, even for the uniform prior $(a = b = 1)$. Is the Bayesian approach inherently superior?

4.13. Apply the sample size calculations to a study with a negative binomial outcome with a given number m of failures (see Exercise 4.7). Use a conjugate prior for the probability r.

4.14. Generate two independent random samples, with sample sizes in hundreds, from distinct normal distributions, such as $\mathcal{N}(\mu_1, 3)$ and $\mathcal{N}(\mu_2, 2)$, $\mu_1 \neq \mu_2$, and regard their union as a single dataset. (If μ_1 differs a lot from μ_2, then the underlying distribution may even be bimodal.) Suppose the data-generating and the prior distributions are (inappropriately) declared as a random sample from $\mathcal{N}(\mu, 3)$ and $\mathcal{N}(0, 5)$. Apply suitable diagnostic procedures that would identify a conflict between the data and the assumptions, those of normality of the data-generating distribution in particular.

4.15. Collect all your arguments that support the statement:

The posterior variance is never greater than the variance of the prior.

Relate your arguments to the frequentist version of this statement:

Two independent estimators of the same target θ can always be combined so that the result would have a smaller mean squared error than either constituent estimator.

4.16. Suppose a study in which a random sample from a normal distribution is observed has the outcomes

$$0.972, \ 0.998, \ 1.015, \ 0.983, \ 1.047, \ 1.020, \ 0.961, \ 0.998, \ 1.009, \ 1.107.$$

Discuss how the (Bayesian and frequentist) inferences about the mean of this sample would differ if we knew that

1. the sample size is fixed;
2. the sample size is in the range 8 to 12 and is set by a known mechanism (e.g., with probabilities equal to 0.2 for each size) before the first observation is made;
3. the study is concluded when the first observation that exceeds 1.10 is recorded;
4. the study is concluded as soon as the first observation outside the range $(0.9, 1.1)$ is recorded or 20 observations are made.

4.17. Recall an example of ordinary regression that you fitted in the past and discuss how you would set the prior distribution for its residual variance σ^2, with the limited resources at your disposal (a day or two, which does not permit you to communicate with anybody familiar with the substantive background and details of the study). In particular, why would it make sense to define a prior with a bounded support that rules out very large values of σ^2? Can a similar argument be presented about a regression slope?

5

Incomplete Data

In the previous chapters we assumed that the observational units are selected by a sampling design, usually simple random, and that the values of the relevant variables are recorded with precision for each selected unit. A sound principle in conducting studies is to ensure good representation of the relevant population by a planned (deliberate) design, a controlled sampling mechanism, and to collect all the data as planned. This chapter describes methods applicable when the data collection exercise is imperfect—when, contrary to the plan, some data are not collected or the sampling and data recording processes depart from the protocol in some other way. At the outset, we consider a sampling design with good representation and collection of the values of a set of variables from each selected unit. Later we expand the scope of the methods by defining ideal sampling and measurement processes that were not intended to be implemented, but for which the analysis would have been simple and manageable. We adapt the analysis to this less congenial setting. Further exploitation of this idea, entailing ingenuity in what is declared as 'missing' from the ideal dataset, substantially widens the horizon of problems that can be analysed efficiently and with integrity. Chapters 6 and 7 present two such applications of methods for incomplete data.

5.1 Terminology and Notation

Suppose a study design intends to represent a population $\mathcal{P}$ by a sample s drawn by a given sampling design, and the values of each of a set of variables are recorded for every subject. A population quantity θ that is a function of the values of these variables is to be estimated. Denote by $\mathbf{X}^{**}$ the $N \times p$ matrix of the values of the variables in the population and by $\mathbf{X}^*$ the corresponding $(n \times p)$ matrix for the planned sample. If $\mathbf{X}^{**}$ were available, θ could be established with precision. We obtain $\mathbf{X}^*$ only when the study is executed perfectly, with no deviation from the plan to apply the sampling design (or the data-generating process). We consider settings in which another process or

Table 5.1. Illustration of complete, incomplete (recorded), and missing datasets, $\mathbf{X}^*$, $\mathbf{X}$, and $\mathbf{X}_{\mathrm{mis}}$, respectively.

	$\mathbf{X}^*$			$\mathbf{X}$			$\mathbf{X}_{\mathrm{mis}}$		
Id.	X_1	X_2	X_3	X_1	X_2	X_3	X_1	X_2	X_3
1	2.6	4	0.25	2.6	4	0.25			
2	3.1	4	0.31	?	4	0.31	3.1		
3	2.7	2	0.40	2.7	2	?			0.40
4	1.9	1	0.11	1.9	1	0.11			
5	2.4	2	0.52	?	?	0.52	2.4	2	
6	3.7	3	0.56	?	?	?	3.7	3	0.56
7	3.0	5	0.42	3.0	5	0.42			
8	2.6	3	0.32	2.6	3	0.32			
9	2.5	4	0.44	2.5	?	0.44		4	

mechanism intervenes between sampling and estimation and further reduces the data and, with it, the information collected. We call this the *nonresponse mechanism* but, apart from noncooperation of a subject (nonresponse in a narrow sense of its meaning), it includes many other reasons for failing to collect every planned item of data. For example, the subject may have provided a response, but it was misinterpreted or mishandled and ended up not being recorded. The dataset obtained after the losses due to nonresponse is denoted by $\mathbf{X}$. We denote by $\mathbf{X}_{\mathrm{mis}}$ the missing data; this is a matrix of the same dimensions as $\mathbf{X}^*$, with entries defined (but unknown) only when the corresponding value of X_{jk} was not recorded, contrary to the plan. We loosely write $\mathbf{X}^* = (\mathbf{X}, \mathbf{X}_{\mathrm{mis}})$, although this identity should not be interpreted as two matrices attached to one another, but rather as two matrices overlaid in such a way that the defined value always appears on top. A small example is given in Table 5.1.

We refer to the planned dataset $\mathbf{X}^*$ as the *complete data* and to $\mathbf{X}$ as the *incomplete data*. Apart from a reference to the plan, these terms are meant to indicate that the analysis of $\mathbf{X}^*$ would be a relatively simple task, using methods we can implement, such as those in Chapters 2 and 3, whereas the analysis of $\mathbf{X}$ is much more complex. We could even regard the matrix $\mathbf{X}^{**}$ as the complete data and $\mathbf{X}^*$ as the incomplete data. Calculation of a population quantity from $\mathbf{X}^{**}$ would then be the standard task and its estimation based on $\mathbf{X}^*$ a task we do not want to address directly. In this chapter, we assume that estimation based on $\mathbf{X}^*$ would be a standard task if $\mathbf{X}^*$ were available, but estimation based on $\mathbf{X}$ is not. In brief, the terms 'complete' and 'incomplete' are relative, related to our analytical ability and equipment.

Both $\mathbf{X}^*$ and $\mathbf{X}$ have two forms, as random objects, prior to execution of the study and as structured sets of fixed values after the data are collected. Whereas $\mathbf{X}^*$ is (usually) a matrix of values, $\mathbf{X}$ is an irregular object. It is convenient to regard it also as a matrix, using a special code for the missing values, such as the question mark in Table 5.1. Several such codes may be used to record distinct circumstances related to the nonresponse, such as 'subject not available', refusal, illegible handwriting, uncodable or ambiguous response, and the like. Together with a code for 'response', these codes define a separate categorical variable.

In a typical setting, a particular sampling design is planned in conjunction with a specific analysis or a set of analyses that evaluate one or several estimators and other statistics (sample quantities). These statistics, as random variables, are called *complete-data statistics* (estimators and the like). For example, if a survey has the plan to collect the values of a variable on 1000 subjects, the sample mean of such a (randomly selected) set of subjects is a complete-data statistic. The same statistic applied to the incomplete dataset is called an incomplete-data statistic. We use the notation in which the dataset is indicated as an argument. Thus, for an estimator $\hat{\theta}$ we distinguish between its complete-data version $\hat{\theta}(\mathbf{X}^*)$ and its incomplete-data version $\hat{\theta}(\mathbf{X})$. This distinction is essential because the distributions of $\hat{\theta}(\mathbf{X}^*)$ and $\hat{\theta}(\mathbf{X})$ differ, and they both differ from the conditional distribution of $\hat{\theta}(\mathbf{X}^*)$ given $\mathbf{X}$. This conditional distribution is relevant after data collection, when $\mathbf{X}$ becomes available, but the plan to evaluate $\hat{\theta}(\mathbf{X}^*)$ has been undermined by nonresponse. Another conditional distribution to consider is $\{\hat{\theta}(\mathbf{X}) \mid \mathbf{X}^*\}$, which describes the variety of incomplete-data estimates for a given complete dataset, that is, the impact of the nonresponse mechanism.

Note that $\hat{\theta}$, originally defined and planned to be applied on $\mathbf{X}^*$, may require some adaptation so that $\hat{\theta}(\mathbf{X})$ could be evaluated at all, because mathematical operations that involve a missing value either are not defined or their result is defined as 'missing'. In most cases, $\hat{\theta}(\mathbf{X})$ is defined by applying $\hat{\theta}$ on an object obtained from $\mathbf{X}$ by some form of data reduction, commonly by discarding all rows of $\mathbf{X}$ that have a value missing. As an alternative, elementary operations with missing values, such as summation and multiplication, may be defined that do not result in missing values. They include defining a 'default' value for each missing item. The default may depend on the variable and subject involved. This is an example of *imputation* or *data completion*.

The Extent and Pattern of Nonresponse

We define an object with the same dimensions as $\mathbf{X}^*$, which indicates whether a particular element of the dataset has been recorded. This object is called the *response indicator* and is denoted by $\mathbf{R}$. When it is a matrix, its element, called the *response status* (of subject j and variable k), is denoted by R_{jk}, row, called the *response pattern*, by $\mathbf{r}_j$ and column by $\mathbf{R}_k$; $R_{jk} = 1$ when X_{jk} is available and $R_{jk} = 0$ otherwise.

The *response rate* for a variable X is defined as the proportion of the subjects for whom the value of X is recorded; $\eta_k = \mathbf{R}_k^\top \mathbf{1}/n$ for variable X_k. The extent of nonresponse for variable X_k is defined as $1 - \eta_k$. A variable is said to be observed completely if its value is recorded for every subject. The proportions $\eta_1, \eta_2, \ldots, \eta_p$ do not provide all the information about the missing values, because nonresponse may be concentrated in a small group of subjects, or dispersed across many of them, with many subjects having only a few missing values each.

The extent of nonresponse is a sample quantity, but we could also define its population version. For this definition to be meaningful, we require the assumption of *response stability*, that each pair of member i and variable k would result in the same response status R_{jk} if member i became the subject j in a sample. A weaker assumption is that each member is associated with a distribution of the response patterns $\mathbf{r}$, and, when the member is included in the sample, a random draw from this *response distribution* determines how the complete record is reduced to an incomplete one (or is left complete). In most settings, it can reasonably be assumed that these draws are independent across subjects. Note that subjects do exercise influence over one another, for instance, when they are from the same household or neighbourhood, but the result of that is that the distributions of their vectors $\mathbf{r}$ are similar. Lack of independence of the draws means that one subject's *realised value* of $\mathbf{r}$ has an impact on the realised value of another.

It is very difficult to learn about the individual subjects' distributions $\mathbf{r}$, because each subject provides only one realisation, a vector $\mathbf{r}_j$. Thus, a subject's distribution could be degenerate (the subject would have the same response pattern in every replication), some of its marginals could be degenerate, or none of them. Further, the response status for one question may be correlated with the response status for other questions, the next and previous question in particular.

We can classify subjects according to their response patterns $\mathbf{r}_j$ as having complete records (no missing items, $\mathbf{r} = \mathbf{1}^\top$), empty records (none of the data items available, $\mathbf{r} = \mathbf{0}$), and partial records (some items missing and some available). The p indicators in the response pattern $\mathbf{r}_j$, each equal to zero or unity, can be 'glued' together and tabulated. For example, when $p = 5$, the code for an empty record is 00000 and for a complete record it is 11111; the code 01110 is for a partial record in which the values of the the first and fifth variables are not recorded. Figure 5.1 summarises graphically the response patterns for an imaginary sample of 749 subjects and $p = 5$ response items. The response rates η_k are given at the top and the numbers of subjects with each response pattern at the right-hand margin. The subjects are reordered so that those with the same pattern are in contiguous records, and the patterns are ordered according to the number of subjects that have them. The patterns could be displayed in any other meaningful order, such as in the alphanumeric order, 00011, 01110, 10111, 11100, 11110, 11111 in the case of the example. For data with many variables and many patterns, patterns with very few subjects

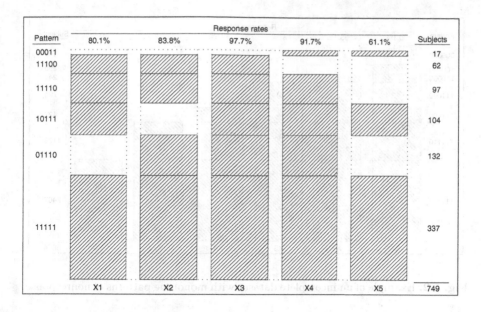

Fig. 5.1. A graphical summary of the response patterns in a survey. An artificial example.

could be dropped or displayed in a separate diagram drawn on a different scale. Also, the diagram may be easier to comprehend when similar patterns are clumped together.

We can distinguish between *unit nonresponse*, when a subject is not contacted or refuses to cooperate at the outset or there is another single reason for no response to any of the items (response pattern 00...0), and *item nonresponse*, which gives rise to partial records. In survey databases in which the variables are organized in sections, such as the responses to blocks of questions, we can define response patterns for sections and section-level nonresponse. Similarly, in surveys with clustered sampling design, it is meaningful to consider cluster-level nonresponse. For example, in surveys in which households or schools are the clusters, the entire household or the entire school may refuse to cooperate.

In longitudinal and panel surveys, in which subjects are contacted on several occasions, it is practical to define response patterns associated with each occasion. When there are only two patterns for the occasions, complete response (pattern 11...1) and total nonresponse (pattern 00...0), we can define the occasion-level response pattern in which each occasion is represented for a subject by a unity for complete response and zero for total nonresponse. Among these response patterns, the *drop-out* and *drop-in* are often the most frequent incomplete patterns. In a drop-out pattern, such as 11100, a sequence of responses is followed by a sequence of nonresponses; the subject cooperates

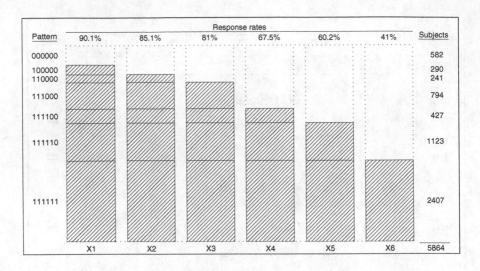

Fig. 5.2. Example of an incomplete dataset with monotone patterns of nonresponse.

up to a point and provides no responses thereafter. In a drop-in pattern, such as 00011, the first response is obtained from a subject on a later occasion, but the subject cooperates from then on until the last occasion. It is expedient to regard the complete and empty response patterns as drop-out (and also as drop-in). Completion of a long questionnaire can be treated like a longitudinal survey in which each question (a block of questions or a page of the questionnaire) corresponds to an occasion. In such surveys, the drop-out pattern may occur when a subject who proceeds through the questionnaire sequentially stops completing it at some point.

The response patterns are said to be *monotone* if the variables can be ordered in such a way that the corresponding response patterns are all drop-out. When there are K variables, there are 2^K possible response patterns in general, but among monotone patterns there are at most $K+1$ patterns. With the appropriate ordering of the variables and response patterns, the graphical summary of the patterns looks like a staircase; Figure 5.2 gives an example.

For each record, we consider its (possibly empty) *available* and *missing parts* as the subvectors of the record for the variables that were recorded and those that were not. These two parts may be considered as both fixed (after data collection) and random (prior to data collection). In the latter case, they have variable lengths.

5.2 Dealing with Incomplete Data

It is much easier to deal with complete datasets because they have a regular shape and all the usual (matrix) arithmetic operations are well defined for them. For incomplete data, we have to make special arrangements: define operations that involve a missing value or avoid missing values altogether. Any analysis conducted with incomplete data has to incorporate the fact that for a missing value we do not know its counterpart in the complete dataset—the value that would have been recorded had the survey been executed perfectly. However, it may be too pessimistic to act as if no information were available about the value at all. The available part of the record may provide some clues about the missing value. For example, in a longitudinal survey of employment status, in which some members of the labour force are contacted every quarter, the status on any particular occasion is very likely to be unchanged from the previous occasion, especially for those middle-class middle-aged subjects who are known to have recently held permanent jobs since several years ago. Thus, if they are not contacted on an occasion, copying the status from the previous occasion is an attractive proposition. It is not correct to do so, but the rate of error with this procedure is likely to be low. In contrast, a similar arrangement for young men and women is not advisable because a much greater percentage of them change their status within a quarter, as they complete education, decide to return to education or training, leave the labour force for other reasons, including end of tenure of a temporary or seasonal employment and child-bearing or looking after the family.

The difficulty of evaluating $\hat{\theta}(\mathbf{X})$ can be overcome in two distinct ways. The first discards all the incomplete records, so that $\hat{\theta}$ is in fact evaluated on the set of subjects with complete records, denoted by $\mathbf{X}_-$. This method is called *data reduction*, and $\mathbf{X}_-$ is said to have been obtained by *listwise deletion*. The term *complete-case analysis* is also used for evaluating $\hat{\theta}(\mathbf{X}_-)$. The method is highly problematic when there are many partial records, because a lot of valuable information they contain is discarded. Variants of this method discard only records that have incomplete subrecords for the variables used in evaluating $\hat{\theta}$, or that are incomplete for particular calculations involved in evaluating $\hat{\theta}$. When $\hat{\theta}$ depends on $\mathbf{X}^*$ only through a few summaries, data reduction may be applied separately for each summary. Such approaches remain deficient because they ignore any information about the missing values that is contained in the available data. Apart from this drawback, the (incomplete) sample associated with a reduced dataset may not be a good representation of the population, even if the complete sample would have been.

An *imputation* method completes the dataset by substituting a value for each missing item. Such a substitute can be regarded as an estimate of the value. Imputation methods are defined by the details of such estimation. The estimators can be chosen so as to take advantage of the intelligence available about the population and the data-collection process. Simple methods for imputation include copying the value, possibly after a transformation, of another variable and imputing the sample mean (median or mode) or the summary of the variable for a suitable subsample. A dataset completed by imputation is denoted by $\mathbf{X}_+$. The apparent advantage of an imputation is that the estimator $\hat{\theta}$ can be applied straightforwardly to $\mathbf{X}_+$. However, the sampling distributions of $\hat{\theta}(\mathbf{X}^*)$ and $\hat{\theta}(\mathbf{X}_+)$ are bound to differ because $\mathbf{X}_+$ contains less information than $\mathbf{X}^*$; except for some trivial settings, it is impossible to recover what has been lost by imperfect execution of the data-collection process.

By analysing $\mathbf{X}_+$ with the response status ($R = 1$ or $R = 0$) discarded, we pretend that we have in fact observed $\mathbf{X}_+$. Had we observed $\mathbf{X}_+$ as a complete dataset, with no values missing, we would have been more confident about the inferences made. However, the two analyses, of the same dataset $\mathbf{X}_+$, regarded as a completion in one case and as the complete dataset in the other, yield identical results. This suggests that we should not estimate the mean squared error MSE$\{\hat{\theta}(\mathbf{X}_+); \theta\}$ by applying the estimator $s^2(\mathbf{X}^*)$ of MSE$\{\hat{\theta}(\mathbf{X}^*); \theta\}$ with $\mathbf{X}_+$ substituted for $\mathbf{X}^*$, that is, by $s^2(\mathbf{X}_+)$. This is not appropriate because the uncertainty of the imputation process (of the attempted recovery of $\mathbf{X}^*$) is ignored. Apart from underestimating MSE$\{\hat{\theta}(\mathbf{X}_+); \theta\}$, $\hat{\theta}(\mathbf{X}_+)$ may be inefficient and biased, even when $\hat{\theta}(\mathbf{X}^*)$ is (or would have been) efficient and unbiased.

By way of an example, suppose we wish to estimate the population variance of a variable X. If we impute the sample mean for each missing value of X, the sample variance of the completed set of values of X will underestimate the population variance because the completed sample contains more observations that do not deviate from the sample mean than the complete data would have. As another example, suppose a missing value x is estimated by zero, with sampling variance known to be equal to unity. If this value contributes to a particular summary by its square, $0^2 = 0$ would be substituted. However, in view of the sampling variance of the estimator involved, substituting 1.0, the value of the unbiased estimator $(\hat{x})^2 + \widehat{\mathrm{var}}(\hat{x})$ of x^2, would seem to be better suited. This example confirms that efficiency is not maintained by nonlinear transformations.

A more general criticism of this approach, based on efficient estimation of each individual missing value, is provided in Section 5.4. It will suggest that the imputed values should represent missing values not only on average but also by their distribution and by their dispersion at least.

Imputation methods may involve some randomness; such methods are called *stochastic*. A replication of a stochastic method on the same incomplete dataset would yield different imputed values; the imputed values would have *between-imputation variance*. Imputation methods that involve no between-imputation variance are called *deterministic*.

The following scheme is an example of a stochastic imputation. We generate substitute values of a variable X according to the model

$$\hat{x} = \bar{x} + \varepsilon, \qquad (5.1)$$

where $\bar{x}$ is the (sample) mean of X for the subjects with the value of X recorded, the values of ε are drawn independently from $\mathcal{N}(0, \hat{\sigma}^2)$ and $\hat{\sigma}^2$ is an estimate of the population variance σ^2 of the values of X. Note that this model differs from

$$\hat{x} = \mu + \varepsilon,$$

where μ is the population mean of X and $\varepsilon \sim \mathcal{N}(0, \sigma^2)$. The former model uses estimates ($\bar{x}$ and $\hat{\sigma}^2$) and the latter uses the corresponding targets (μ and σ^2). The imputations based on these two models have different sampling properties, because the mean used in the first, $\bar{x}$, as well as the variance $\hat{\sigma}^2$, would vary across replications, whereas their counterparts in the second, μ and σ^2, would not.

Yet another modelling possibility is

$$\hat{x} = \tilde{\mu} + \varepsilon, \tag{5.2}$$

where $\varepsilon \sim \mathcal{N}(0, \tilde{\sigma}^2)$ and $(\tilde{\mu}, \tilde{\sigma}^2)$ are a random draw from the estimated joint distribution of the estimator $\{\hat{\mu}(\mathbf{X}), \hat{\sigma}^2(\mathbf{X})\}$. The methods based on (5.1) and (5.2) do not aim to reproduce the values lost by nonresponse. In the method based on (5.2), we inject random (between-imputation) variation in the imputed values—the sets of imputed values are generated in such a way that there are some systematic differences among them. The substitute values generated by a stochastic imputation are called *plausible values*. The randomly drawn values of the model parameters in (5.2) and in similar (more complex) models are called *plausible parameter values*. Ideally, the empirical distribution of the plausible parameter values in replications based on the same incomplete dataset would match the sampling distribution of the parameter estimator (vector). Of course, this is difficult to arrange because the sampling distribution itself can only be estimated. But relying on one value of the parameter vector, such as its estimate, amounts to pretending that the value is known. It is far better to use an estimated (approximate) sampling distribution, admittedly, pretending that it is known.

Imputation methods can be identified with models such as (5.2). They relate the missing values ($\hat{x}$) to the recorded values and their summaries, with a random deviation (ε). Inasmuch as we seek more realistic models, including a random deviation in them is essential. Deterministic imputation methods can be described by models that relate missing values to observed values with no random deviation. For example, in a longitudinal dataset, the imputation based on the rule 'bring last value forward' (BLVF), according to which the recorded outcome x_k on occasion k is imputed for the missing outcome x_{k+1} on occasion $k + 1$, corresponds to the model

$$\hat{x}_{k+1} = x_k.$$

For continuous outcomes, $\hat{x}_{k+1} = x_k + \varepsilon$ and $\hat{x}_{k+1} = \beta_0 + \beta_1 x_k + \varepsilon$, with appropriate distributions for ε, are the obvious adaptations that make the model more realistic. More complex regression models, including those introduced in later chapters, can be used for the imputation model.

For categorical longitudinal outcomes, a natural deterministic model is $\hat{x}_{k+1} = x_k$, and its obvious adaptation defines the conditional (*transition*) probabilities $P(\hat{x}_{k+1} = h_1 \,|\, x_k = h_0)$. The conditional probabilities of no change, $P(\hat{x}_{k+1} = h \,|\, x_k = h)$, may be quite large, but they do not reach unity. When an ordering of the categories, from 0 or 1 to H, is meaningful, the transitions to the neighbouring states, from h to $h+1$ and $h-1$ may have higher probabilities than the transitions to states further apart.

5.3 Nonresponse Mechanisms

The sampling mechanism can be perceived as reducing the population to a sample. The *nonresponse mechanism* can be regarded similarly, as reducing the complete dataset to an incomplete dataset by deleting some of the items that were planned to be recorded. We might consider a separate mechanism for each variable, but these processes are usually correlated, so it is more appropriate to think of them as a single multivariate process. We could then borrow the terminology of sampling processes for nonresponse processes. One crucial difference between them is that a typical sampling process is under the study designer's control, whereas the details of a typical nonresponse process are not known and can, at best, be only conjectured.

The simplest nontrivial nonresponse process is related to the simple random sampling design. Values of a variable are missing for a set of subjects selected at random from the sample. Data are said to be *missing completely at random* (MCAR) when the (multivariate) distribution of the response pattern $\mathbf{r}$ does not depend on the complete data:

$$(\mathbf{r} \,|\, \mathbf{X}^* = \mathbf{x}) \sim (\mathbf{r}).$$

It implies that nonresponse for each variable is like a simple random sampling process. We use the acronym MCAR also for the nonresponse process in which data are MCAR. As simple random sampling is a very special process, one can hardly expect that the circumstances beyond our control would arrange the event of nonresponse to be independent of any of the variables.

A much more general class of nonresponse processes is derived from stratified sampling designs. The population is split into strata, and a different MCAR process acts in each stratum. For example, young subjects may be more reluctant to respond to a survey than the middle-aged or elderly, but the nonresponse processes are MCAR within each age group. If the age category is known for every subject, such data are said to be *missing at random* (MAR). MAR is qualified by the stratification or *conditioning variables*, such as age group in the previous example, although more than one variable can be involved in general. Stratification can be extended to continuous variables, by a limiting argument referring to strata defined by narrow intervals of values, or by defining conditional processes given the values of the conditioning variables $\mathbf{Z}$. That is, conditionally on $\mathbf{Z} = \mathbf{z}$, with $\mathbf{z}$ observed, the process of nonresponse is MCAR:

$$(\mathbf{r} \mid \mathbf{X}^* = \mathbf{x}, \mathbf{Z} = \mathbf{z}) \sim (\mathbf{r} \mid \mathbf{Z} = \mathbf{z}).$$

In principle, $\mathbf{r}$ for a subject may be related to the values of the variables on other subjects, and so the definition of MAR includes all processes in which the missing data are conditionally independent of the response indicator, given the recorded data:

$$(\mathbf{R} \mid \mathbf{X}^*) \sim (\mathbf{R} \mid \mathbf{X}); \tag{5.3}$$

the values that were not recorded contain no information about the nonresponse process. MCAR is a special case of MAR, in which the conditioning is redundant even on $\mathbf{X}$:

$$(\mathbf{R} \mid \mathbf{X}^*) \sim (\mathbf{R}).$$

Any nonresponse process that is not MAR is called NMAR—data are not missing at random. (Logically it is more exact to refer to them as missing *not at random*.) It includes a vast variety of idiosyncratic processes in which the probability of nonresponse depends on the values that are missing. Such nonresponse mechanisms are called *nonignorable* or *informative*. The informative nature of a nonresponse process can rarely be gleaned from the incomplete (collected) data without making some unverifiable assumptions.

For example, in a survey of drug use, occasional (recreational) drug users may be more reluctant to respond. Suppose subjects respond to all questionnaire items, but most of the occasional users who took some drugs the previous week would not respond to the item about drug use during that week. If such use cannot be inferred or predicted from the other responses, then the recorded data would generate an impression that occasional drug users tend to take drugs less frequently than they do in reality. Inferences based on estimators efficient for the complete-data design and that ignore the impact of the nonresponse mechanism are then distorted.

The characterisation of MAR in (5.3) plays a key role in the analysis of incomplete data. An analysis is much easier when the nonresponse mechanism is MAR, and the chances of attaining MAR in a particular setting are improved (or, more precisely, not worsened) by extending the list of conditioning variables. When nonresponse is anticipated in a survey the values of some variables may be collected specifically for the purpose of promoting MAR in the key analyses. Thus, identifying and recording suitable variables for this purpose is an important element of survey design. However, dealing with incomplete data should be regarded as a damage control measure, inferior to collecting complete data. Therefore, expertise in imputation methods is no substitute or excuse for reduced attention to eliciting responses, the more complete the better, from survey subjects.

5.3.1 Models for Incomplete Data

As the data-generating (sampling) and nonresponse processes may be correlated, they should be modelled jointly. The joint distribution of the complete
data and the response indicator can be partitioned in two ways, as

$$f(\mathbf{X}^*, \mathbf{R}) = f(\mathbf{X}^* \mid \mathbf{R}) f(\mathbf{R}) \tag{5.4}$$

and

$$f(\mathbf{X}^*, \mathbf{R}) = f(\mathbf{R} \mid \mathbf{X}^*) f(\mathbf{X}^*), \tag{5.5}$$

where f is the density or probability of the (conditional) distribution indicated by its argument. In (5.4), each pattern $\mathbf{r}$ is associated with a conditional
distribution $(\mathbf{X}^* \mid \mathbf{R} = \mathbf{r})$, so the joint distribution is a mixture of the pattern-
specific distributions $(\mathbf{X}^* \mid \mathbf{r})$. Such models are called *pattern-mixture models*.
Without some constraints, a pattern-mixture model is not identified, because
for some incomplete patterns $\mathbf{r}$ certain components are never observed. Constraints have to be imposed, for instance, so that the conditional distributions
$(\mathbf{X}^* \mid \mathbf{r})$ have some parameters in common.

In (5.5), the conditional distribution $(\mathbf{R} \mid \mathbf{X}^*)$ is specified for the response
pattern given complete data, together with the marginal distribution of the
complete data. The conditional distribution can be interpreted as a selection
mechanism that reduces the complete dataset. Such models are called *selection models*. In general, there is no straightforward correspondence between
pattern-mixture and selection models. Under an NMAR mechanism, the models given by (5.4) and (5.5) may differ essentially; a model for one partitioning
may not have an obvious counterpart in the other. Under MCAR, the conditioning in (5.4) and (5.5) is redundant, and their equivalence is obvious.

The set of variables in $\mathbf{X}^*$ can be split into those that are always observed
completely, $\mathbf{Z}$, and those subject to nonresponse, $\mathbf{Y}$. The former include variables associated with the sampling design and attributes of the units to which
subjects belong, such as the neighbourhood or area (e.g., urban/rural). In
models (5.4) and (5.5), $\mathbf{X}^*$ can be replaced by $\mathbf{Y}^*$, the complete-data counterpart of $\mathbf{Y}$, and $\mathbf{Z}$ relegated to conditioning, or dropped altogether.

The joint distribution of the incomplete data $\mathbf{X}$ and the response indicator
$\mathbf{R}$ is obtained from the joint distribution of $\mathbf{X}^*$ and $\mathbf{R}$ by integration over the
distribution of the missing values:

$$f(\mathbf{X}, \mathbf{R}) = \int f(\mathbf{X}^*, \mathbf{R}) \, dF(\mathbf{X}_{\text{mis}}),$$

and similarly for the distribution of $\mathbf{X}$,

$$f(\mathbf{X}) = \int f(\mathbf{X}^*) \, dF(\mathbf{X}_{\text{mis}}),$$

which, in principle, can be obtained by summing over all the possible values of
$\mathbf{R}$. Under MAR, we can replace in the selection model (5.5) the conditioning
on $\mathbf{X}^*$ with the conditioning on $\mathbf{X}$; then

$$f(\mathbf{X}^*, \mathbf{R}) = f(\mathbf{R} \mid \mathbf{X}) f(\mathbf{X}^*).$$

Hence

$$f(\mathbf{X}, \mathbf{R}) = \int f(\mathbf{R} \mid \mathbf{X}) f(\mathbf{X}^*) \, dF(\mathbf{X}_{\mathrm{mis}}).$$

When $f(\mathbf{R} \mid \mathbf{X})$ and $f(\mathbf{X}^*)$ have unrelated parameters, not connected by any constraints, then $f(\mathbf{R} \mid \mathbf{X})$ can be extracted from the integral and the joint density $f(\mathbf{X}, \mathbf{R})$ can be expressed as the product

$$f(\mathbf{X}, \mathbf{R}; \psi, \theta) = f(\mathbf{R} \mid \mathbf{X}; \psi) \, f(\mathbf{X}; \theta), \qquad (5.6)$$

where ψ and θ are the respective parameter vectors for the selection, $(\mathbf{R} \mid \mathbf{X})$, and the outcomes $\mathbf{X}$. A pair of parameter vectors ψ and θ is said to be *separated* in a model if their joint parameter space is the product $\mathbf{\Psi} \times \mathbf{\Theta}$ of their respective parameter spaces ($\psi \in \mathbf{\Psi}$ and $\theta \in \mathbf{\Theta}$); that is, none of the constraints on the parameters, if there are any, involves an element of both ψ and θ. When the parameter vectors are separated in this way and the nonresponse process is MAR, the nonresponse is said to be *ignorable*. Ignorability confers an important advantage on the analysis of $\mathbf{X}$. Owing to the factorisation in (5.6), the complete-data model parameters can be estimated by maximising the likelihood for $\mathbf{X}$, ignoring the nonresponse mechanism.

5.4 EM Algorithm

We assume now that MAR applies. The likelihood for $\mathbf{X}$ can be partitioned according to the response patterns as

$$L(\theta; \mathbf{X}) = \prod_{\mathbf{r}} L_{\mathbf{r}}(\theta; \mathbf{X}_{\mathbf{r}}),$$

where $\mathbf{X}_{\mathbf{r}}$ denotes the incomplete data for subjects with pattern $\mathbf{r}$. The likelihoods $L_{\mathbf{r}}$ cannot be maximised separately because they share some or all of the components of θ as their arguments. When incomplete data involves several response patterns, direct maximisation of this likelihood is much more complex than the corresponding problem for the complete dataset. The *EM algorithm* is a method for likelihood maximisation that takes advantage of the availability (and relative simplicity) of a procedure for maximising the complete-data likelihood $L^*(\theta; \mathbf{X}^*)$.

The incomplete-data likelihood is related to its complete-data counterpart L^* by the identity

$$L(\theta; \mathbf{X}) = \int L^*(\theta; \mathbf{X}^*) \, dF(\mathbf{X}_{\mathrm{mis}}).$$

Suppose $\mathbf{s} = \mathbf{s}(\mathbf{X}^*)$ is a vector of linear sufficient statistics for θ in the complete-data model. That is, the complete-data log-likelihood depends on

$\mathbf{X}^*$ only through $\mathbf{s}$ and is a linear function of $\mathbf{s}$. When missing data are involved in $\mathbf{s}(\mathbf{X}^*)$, these statistics cannot be evaluated.

The EM algorithm is an iterative procedure for fitting the incomplete-data model. Each iteration comprises two steps. In the first step, the *estimation* or E-step, the conditional expectation of $\mathbf{s}(\mathbf{X}^*)$ is evaluated, given the incomplete data and model parameters, with the model parameters on which it depends replaced by their current (provisional) estimates. This step is usually much simpler when MAR is assumed.

In the second step, the *maximisation* or M-step, the complete-data likelihood is maximised, with the linear sufficient statistics $\mathbf{s}(\mathbf{X}^*)$ replaced by their estimates $\mathrm{E}\{\mathbf{s}(\mathbf{X}^*) \mid \mathbf{X}, \boldsymbol{\theta} = \hat{\boldsymbol{\theta}}\}$ obtained in the preceding E-step. The pairs of E- and M-steps are iterated (applied repeatedly) until the parameter estimates are changed by updating in the M-step by less than a set threshold. A practical implementation of this is based on the Euclidean distance,

$$\left\| \hat{\boldsymbol{\theta}}_{h+1} - \hat{\boldsymbol{\theta}}_h \right\| = \sqrt{\left(\hat{\boldsymbol{\theta}}_{h+1} - \hat{\boldsymbol{\theta}}_h \right)^\top \left(\hat{\boldsymbol{\theta}}_{h+1} - \hat{\boldsymbol{\theta}}_h \right)},$$

between the estimates obtained in successive iterations h and $h+1$. When it is smaller than the threshold, such as 10^{-5}, the iterations are terminated.

Although the M-step uses the algorithm for complete-data analysis, the algorithm has to be adapted, by replacing the linear sufficient statistics with their estimates calculated in the preceding E-step. This suggests that a (complete-data) algorithm that might in the future be applied as the M-step of an EM algorithm should be constructed in the form of two modules, one to calculate the linear sufficient statistics and the other to evaluate the estimators as their functions. In an EM algorithm, the first module is replaced by the E-step and the second can be used intact, with its arguments provided by the result of the preceding E-step.

In some applications, the EM algorithm converges very slowly. The rate of convergence is related to *the fraction of the missing information*, defined for a univariate target as the complement of the ratio of the sampling variances of its estimator in the complete- and incomplete-data analyses:

$$1 - \frac{\mathrm{var}\left\{ \hat{\theta}^*(\mathbf{X}^*) \right\}}{\mathrm{var}\left\{ \hat{\theta}(\mathbf{X}) \right\}}.$$

An asterisk is added to $\hat{\theta}$ to emphasise that the complete- and incomplete-data estimators differ; they are different functions of their respective arguments $\mathbf{X}^*$ and $\mathbf{X}$. When a lot of information is missing the EM algorithm converges very slowly.

As EM is an iterative algorithm, it requires an initial set of estimates for the first application of the E-step. Any reasonable provisional vector of estimates is usually suitable, such as the complete-data estimates based on the reduced dataset $\mathbf{X}_-$, $\hat{\boldsymbol{\theta}}^*(\mathbf{X}_-)$. Except for some very complex problems, the EM algorithm requires at most a handful of iterations to get on the right track from a poor initial solution. Each iteration of the EM algorithm increases the value of the log-likelihood, although, like all other maximisation algorithms, it may converge to a local extreme that is not a global maximum.

An approximation to the maximum likelihood estimator is obtained by the concluding M-step. (The level of precision is controlled by the set threshold.) If the complete-data estimator implemented in the M-step is accompanied by an estimator of the sampling variance $s^2(\hat{\theta})$, it could be evaluated at convergence. The result, $\hat{s}^2(\hat{\theta})$, estimates the complete-data sampling variance, $\mathrm{var}(\hat{\theta}^* \mid \mathbf{X}^*)$, that is, the variance that would be attained if the complete dataset were available. The MSE of the (EM) maximum likelihood estimator, $\mathrm{MSE}(\hat{\theta} \mid \mathbf{X})$, is greater because it is based on less data.

The EM algorithm requires that the parameter space be convex, the complete-data likelihood be smooth, and its expected information matrix be positive definite. In general, convergence is attained at a local maximum, so we have to verify that this maximum is also global.

Example 12. Suppose we wish to fit the ordinary regression of Y on X for (X, Y) with a bivariate normal distribution, but some of the values of $\mathbf{x}^* = (x_1, x_2, \ldots, x_n)^\top$ and $\mathbf{y}^* = (y_1, y_2, \ldots, y_n)^\top$ in the complete bivariate sample $(x_1, , y_1)$, $\ldots$, (x_n, y_n) have not been recorded. Suppose these values are missing at random (MAR). The linear sufficient statistics for the regression slope β_1 are the totals of crossproducts $\mathbf{x}^{*\top}\mathbf{y}^*$ and squares $\mathbf{x}^{*\top}\mathbf{x}^*$ and the totals $\mathbf{x}^{*\top}\mathbf{1}$ and $\mathbf{y}^{*\top}\mathbf{1}$. The latter two totals are linear functions of $\mathbf{x}^*$ and $\mathbf{y}^*$, so they are 'estimated' in the E-step by substituting for each missing item its conditional expectation, given the available data and current values of the model parameter estimates:

$$\mathrm{E}\left(\mathbf{x}^{*\top}\mathbf{1} \mid \mathbf{x}, \mathbf{y}; \boldsymbol{\theta} = \hat{\boldsymbol{\theta}}\right) = \mathbf{x}^\top\mathbf{1} + \mathrm{E}\left(\mathbf{x}^*_{\mathrm{mis}} \mid \mathbf{x}, \mathbf{y}; \boldsymbol{\theta} = \hat{\boldsymbol{\theta}}\right)^\top\mathbf{1} \qquad (5.7)$$

where $\boldsymbol{\theta}$ collects all the parameters involved in the joint distribution of X and Y.

For a subject's contribution to $\mathbf{x}^{*\top}\mathbf{y}^*$, we distinguish three cases. First, if both X and Y are recorded, the contribution is established with precision. Next, if one of the values is recorded and the other is missing, the contribution $x_j y_j$ is a linear function of the missing value, so its estimated conditional expectation can be substituted:

$$\hat{x}_j = \mathrm{E}\left(x_j^* \mid \mathbf{x}, \mathbf{y}; \boldsymbol{\theta} = \hat{\boldsymbol{\theta}}\right),$$

or $\hat{y}_j$ derived by analogy. Finally, when both x_j and y_j are missing, the conditional expectation of the contribution is estimated by

$$\mathrm{E}\left(x_j y_j \mid \mathbf{x}, \mathbf{y}; \boldsymbol{\theta} = \hat{\boldsymbol{\theta}}\right) = \hat{x}_j \hat{y}_j + \mathrm{cov}\left(x_j, y_j \mid \mathbf{x}, \mathbf{y}; \boldsymbol{\theta} = \hat{\boldsymbol{\theta}}\right). \qquad (5.8)$$

So the product of the conditional expectations has to be 'adjusted' by the conditional covariance. As the pairs (x_j, y_j), $j = 1, \ldots, n$, are mutually independent, the conditioning in the covariance in (5.8) is redundant and the unconditional covariance σ_{xy} can be used instead. A similar adjustment is necessary for the contribution to $\mathbf{x}^{*\top}\mathbf{x}^*$ when x_i is not recorded:

$$\mathrm{E}\left(x_j^{*2} \,|\, \mathbf{x}, \mathbf{y}; \boldsymbol{\theta} = \hat{\boldsymbol{\theta}}\right) = (\hat{x}_j)^2 + \mathrm{var}(x_j \,|\, \mathbf{x}, \mathbf{y}; \boldsymbol{\theta} = \hat{\boldsymbol{\theta}}).$$

The conditional expectations and variance required are

$$\mathrm{E}\left(x_j^* \,|\, \mathbf{x}, \mathbf{y}; \boldsymbol{\theta}\right) = \mu_x + \frac{\sigma_{xy}}{\sigma_y^2}\left(y_j - \mu_y\right),$$

$$\mathrm{E}\left(y_j^* \,|\, \mathbf{x}, \mathbf{y}; \boldsymbol{\theta}\right) = \mu_y + \frac{\sigma_{xy}}{\sigma_x^2}\left(x_j - \mu_x\right),$$

$$\mathrm{var}\left(x_j^* \,|\, \mathbf{x}, \mathbf{y}; \boldsymbol{\theta}\right) = \sigma_x^2 - \frac{\sigma_{xy}^2}{\sigma_y^2}.$$

Estimation of the residual variance σ^2 requires also the sum of squares $\mathbf{y}^{*\top}\mathbf{y}^*$; it is estimated in analogy with $\mathbf{x}^{*\top}\mathbf{x}^*$.

In each E-step, these quantities are evaluated with the current estimates in place of the population means μ_x and μ_y and (co-)variances σ_x^2, σ_y^2, and σ_{xy}. In each M-step, these moments are estimated using the current estimates of the linear sufficient statistics. In the concluding M-step, the complete-data sampling variance matrix of the model parameters could be estimated by substituting parameter estimates for their targets in the complete-data formula. This matrix estimates the sampling variance of the model estimators in the hypothetical setting of the complete data. It estimates the incomplete-data sampling variance with bias, because it ignores the uncertainty associated with the estimation of the sufficient statistics in the E-step.

For nonresponse mechanisms that are NMAR, the E-step can be adjusted, although the nature of the departure from MAR has to be known. Even though the EM algorithm is a very general prescription for dealing with missing values, it cannot be applied universally, because it relies on the availability of a shortlist of sufficient statistics and on our ability to evaluate, analytically or numerically, their conditional expectations.

5.5 Multiple Imputation

Many large-scale (national) surveys are conducted to make inferences about numerous population quantities, often by several parties (secondary analysts) who have limited expertise in handling missing values and rely on standard software and complete-data methods. As they wish to apply the programmes (estimators) that implement these methods without any alterations, treating them as a 'black-box', the EM algorithm is not suitable. The data constructors may do their best to impute the value of an efficient estimator of each missing value, but such efficiency will not be translated to efficient estimation of population quantities and unbiased estimation of the associated MSEs by the secondary analysts.

The method of multiple imputation (MI) was designed for such a setting. A small number M of *plausible complete datasets*, also called *completed datasets*, are generated by completing the recorded dataset. They are denoted by $\mathbf{X}_{[1]}$, $\mathbf{X}_{[2]}$, ..., $\mathbf{X}_{[M]}$. These completions are replicates of a process in which the uncertainty about the missing values (conditionally, given the recorded values) is reflected. The complete-data analysis is applied, without any alterations, on the completed datasets $\mathbf{X}_{[m]}$, yielding *plausible estimates* $\hat{\theta}_{[m]} = \hat{\theta}\left(\mathbf{X}_{[m]}\right)$. The complete-data estimator of the sampling variance $\mathrm{var}\{\hat{\theta}(\mathbf{X}^*)\}$, denoted by $\hat{s}^2$, applied to the completed dataset $\mathbf{X}_{[m]}$, is denoted by $\hat{s}^2_{[m]}$; that is, $\hat{s}^2_{[m]} = \hat{s}^2\left(\mathbf{X}_{[m]}\right)$.

We assume that the method of analysis, represented by the pair of estimators $\{\hat{\theta}, \hat{s}^2(\hat{\theta})\}$, is efficient and honest in the following sense: $\hat{\theta}(\mathbf{X}^*)$ is a (nearly) unbiased and efficient estimator of the target θ and $\hat{s}^2(\mathbf{X}^*)$ is an unbiased estimator of its sampling variance $\mathrm{var}\{\hat{\theta}(\mathbf{X}^*)\}$. Then, under conditions described later, each plausible estimator $\hat{\theta}_{[m]}$ is nearly unbiased for θ, and so is their average

$$\tilde{\theta} = \frac{1}{M} \sum_{m=1}^{M} \hat{\theta}_{[m]}, \tag{5.9}$$

called the *MI estimator*. The sampling variance of $\tilde{\theta}$ is estimated with small or no bias by

$$\tilde{s}^2 = \frac{1}{M} \sum_{m=1}^{M} \hat{s}^2_{[m]} + \frac{M+1}{M(M-1)} \sum_{m=1}^{M} \left(\hat{\theta}_{[m]} - \tilde{\theta}\right)^2. \tag{5.10}$$

The latter equation can be described and motivated as

$$\tilde{s}^2 = \hat{W} + \left(1 + \frac{1}{M}\right)\hat{B}, \tag{5.11}$$

where $\hat{W}$ estimates the complete-data sampling variance $\mathrm{var}\{\hat{\theta}(\mathbf{X}^*)\}$ and $\hat{B}$ estimates the variance inflation attributable to the missing values; it is equal to the between-imputation variance. There is an additional variance inflation, by B/M, which could be made arbitrarily small by using sufficiently many replicate completions or letting $M \to +\infty$. That is, B/M represents the lack of efficiency of the MI estimator, and $B/(W + B)$ is the fraction of the information contained in the missing data.

5.5.1 Modelling Nonresponse

The method of MI is devised in such a way that secondary analysts do not have to face any nonstandard tasks and need not be informed about the details of the process used to generate the completed datasets or about the (assumed or real) response mechanism. The dataset completions are generated by the data constructor prior to releasing the data and are based on a model for nonresponse which relates the missing values to the recorded values by means of a class of conditional distributions $(\mathbf{X}_{\text{mis}} \mid \mathbf{X}, \mathbf{Z})$. In most practical settings, this model is for MAR, which can be promoted by sufficiently rich conditioning, that is, by including several suitably selected variables in $\mathbf{Z}$ as well as $\mathbf{X}$. That calls for a careful selection of variables to be recorded in the survey; the selection should be informed by the planned analyses and the likely response patterns.

One completion is generated by simulating from a *plausible distribution* of the missing values. Such a distribution is drawn using the estimated sampling distribution of the model parameters. Thus, suppose the vector of parameters θ in the model for nonresponse is estimated by $\hat{\theta} \sim \mathcal{N}(\theta, \Sigma_\theta)$. Then a plausible distribution is given by $\tilde{\theta}$ drawn at random from $\mathcal{N}(\hat{\theta}, \Sigma_\theta)$ when Σ_θ is known. When Σ_θ is estimated a random draw $\tilde{\Sigma}_\theta$ from the estimated (joint) distribution of $\hat{\Sigma}_\theta$ is used instead of Σ_θ, and $\tilde{\theta}$ is then drawn from $\mathcal{N}(\hat{\theta}, \tilde{\Sigma}_\theta)$.

By using the fitted distribution $\mathcal{N}(\hat{\theta}, \hat{\Sigma}_\theta)$, we would pretend that the model parameters are known and would underrepresent the uncertainty about θ. The substitutes for the missing values, called the *plausible values*, are simulated from the plausible conditional distribution of the missing values.

Another set of plausible values is generated by replicating this process. Thus, another plausible distribution is drawn, via a vector of plausible parameter values $\tilde{\theta}$, independently of the previous draw(s), and a set of plausible values is drawn from this plausible distribution, independently of the previous set(s) of plausible values. The key feature of this process is the faithful reflection in the plausible values of the uncertainty about the missing values for which they are substituted (*imputed*). A process of generating sets of plausible values is said to be *proper* if it satisfies this condition. Properness of the plausible values is an essential assumption of the method of MI. In practice, it is difficult to establish that it is satisfied, and so it may seem that MI is not practical. However, most single imputation methods can be described as trivial versions of MI, denying one or both sources of uncertainty (about the parameters in the model for nonresponse and about the missing value given the model parameters). A more constructive way of considering MI is as an improvement over a single imputation (SI) method.

5.5.2 Working with Plausible Values

The completions can be organised as separate datasets with the same layout. The recorded values in such a database are duplicated, so a lot of storage space is required. However, storage is quite cheap nowadays and there are all manner of devices for external storage, so that this can no longer be regarded as a constraint. The secondary analyst then has to apply the planned complete-data analysis once on each completion and average the estimates and estimated complete-data sampling variances with an inflation of the latter according to equation (5.10).

Alternatives that are more storage-efficient include the incomplete dataset with a code for missing values and a separate dataset with $M+2$ columns, the first two identifying the missing item (record/subject and variable), and the remaining M columns containing the plausible values for the missing item. The second column can be dropped if the plausible values within a record are placed in the same order as in the incomplete dataset, and the first column can also be dropped if the order of the subjects is the same in the two datasets. Instead of the sets of plausible values the data constructor may provide only a programme that generates them, and it could be integrated in the planned complete-data analysis. When values are missing for only a few variables the sets of plausible values can be included in a single dataset, together with the completely recorded variables, as M separate variables.

We emphasise that it is not appropriate to analyse the dataset generated by averaging the completions—that would destroy the between-imputation variation which is essential for (approximately) unbiased estimation of the incomplete-data sampling variance. Moreover, the efficiency of the complete-data analysis would not carry over to the incomplete-data analysis. As a simple example to reinforce this point, suppose the plausible values for a missing item are drawn independently from the normal distribution with $\mathcal{N}(0,1)$. Averaging $M = 5$ plausible values is equivalent to drawing from $\mathcal{N}(0,0.2)$. Suppose the contribution to a sufficient statistic made by a subject is the square of the missing item. If we ignore the uncertainty altogether, we would impute zero, the square of the expectation. If we average the five plausible values, we would impute 0.2 on average. Only with the plausible values that are not averaged would we impute the correct contribution on average, equal to 1.0, the expectation of the square.

How Many Sets of Plausible Values?

The fraction of the missing information $B/(W+B)$, as well as the inefficiency of MI, represented in (5.11) by B/M, depend on the target of estimation. For convenience, we prefer to have fewer sets of plausible values M, but the more of them we have the smaller the variance inflation B/M. The concern about M is about the size of the database and the amount of computing involved. The former concern can be dismissed, as storage capacity is cheap and easy to expand nowadays. The amount of programming required to implement MI for a particular setting does not depend on M because the complete-data method is simply placed in a loop over the completions. The computing time is also hardly a hindrance, as other activities can be attended to while the programme runs. Thus, there is little incentive to be sparing about M, except for the analysis of extremely large datasets.

The established practice has been to use $M = 5$ sets of plausible values. Even when $B = W$, so that half the complete-data information is contained in the missing values, five sets of plausible values result in an inflation by $B/5$ over $B+W = 2B$, that is, by 10%. This percentage is halved with $M = 10$ sets of plausible values. The fraction of missing information is usually much smaller than 50%. It is usually smaller than the percentage of missing values (e.g., averaged over the variables involved), because some information is always available about the missing values.

The between-imputation variance estimator $\hat{B}$ has a distribution related to χ^2_{M-1}, approximately, and can be interpreted as being based on $M-1$ degrees of freedom. Estimation of B, the MI sampling variance $W + B(1 + 1/M)$, or the ratio $B/(B + W)$, is more precise for smaller B. A given number of completions may be sufficient for near efficient estimation of θ, but sufficiently precise estimation of $\mathrm{var}(\hat{\theta})$ may require more completions.

5.5.3 Monotone Response Patterns and Chained Equations

The advantage with the monotone response patterns is not only that the number of patterns is small, $K + 1$ at most, but mainly that sets of plausible values can be generated using models for univariate outcomes. With monotone patterns, MI can be organised into K separate univariate imputations, corresponding to the factorisation of the density

$$f(\mathbf{X}) = f(X_1) f(X_2 \mid X_1) f(X_3 \mid X_1, X_2) \ldots f(X_K \mid X_1, X_2, \ldots, X_{K-1}).$$
$$(5.12)$$

First we generate the plausible values for X_1, the variable observed most frequently, conditioning on the completely recorded variables (if any). Conditioning on variables $X_2, \ldots, X_K$ is redundant, because all their values are missing whenever X_1 is not recorded. Plausible values are then generated for the second variable, using a model that conditions on the (recorded or imputed) values of the first variable and the completely recorded variables, and so on, concluding with generating plausible values for X_K, conditioning on the (recorded or imputed) values of all the other variables. The factorisation in (5.12) applies generally, but the sequence of univariate imputations it implies can be used only with monotone response patterns. When imputing for missing values of a variable X_k, we use all the information, because when X_k is not recorded neither are the 'later' variables $X_{k+1}, \ldots, X_K$.

Whereas the multivariate normal distribution has all possible covariance structures, similarly rich multivariate distributions with other univariate marginals are hard to come by and are less well explored, and algorithms for fitting them are much more complex. Therein lies the advantage of generating plausible values using univariate models—we have at our disposal a much wider array of tractable models.

When the monotone patterns of nonresponse are spoilt by only a few records, items in these records may be deleted temporarily, so that univariate methods for MI could be implemented. After generating the requisite sets of plausible values, the values of the deleted items may be restored. A problem that may arise by such restoration is that some pairs or bigger groups of variables have implausible or outright impossible combinations of values. For example, when the body mass of some (human) subjects is missing much more frequently than their height, we may delete the body mass for the few subjects for whom height is not available. For a subject, a plausible height of 200 cm may be generated, but it is not plausible if the subject's (missing) body mass is only 50 kg; the values of both variables are plausible, but not their combination.

Chained equations is a method for generating plausible values for incomplete data with arbitrary response patterns. It is iterative, with each iteration comprising a univariate imputation for each incompletely recorded variable. First, a default value is provisionally imputed for each missing item. The value may be specific to each variable and, in principle, even for each subject. Next, plausible values are generated for the missing values for X_1, to replace the values provisionally imputed for X_1. The imputation model for X_1 conditions on all the remaining variables $\mathbf{X}_{-1} = (X_2, X_3, \ldots, X_K)$, using their recorded or imputed values. Plausible values are then generated, in sequence for $X_2, \ldots, X_K$ similarly. For X_k, the provisionally imputed values of X_k are discarded and ignored, and the conditioning in the imputation model is on the values of all the recorded or imputed values of all the other variables, $\mathbf{X}_{-k}$. These K univariate imputations constitute one iteration. The sequence of provisional imputations for the K variables, for one of them at a time, is repeated, with the imputations from the previous iteration used as provisional values.

A small number of iterations, up to ten, usually suffices. Convergence is not straightforward to ascertain because each univariate imputation is stochastic, and of interest is convergence in distribution. The sample distributions of the imputed values (or just their means and variances) for each variable should be monitored, and the iterations can be terminated when these are altered only as much as one would expect owing to the stochastic nature of the imputation. Since this is not straightforward to judge, it is prudent to apply a few iterations after the one at which we are satisfied that convergence has been achieved. At convergence, we have obtained one completion. The iterative process is then replicated to obtain further completions.

5.5.4 Sensitivity Analysis with Respect to NMAR

Sensitivity analysis is a general term for assessing the performance of an estimator, or any other outcome of an analysis, when some of its assumptions may not be satisfied. Sensitivity analysis is often formulated as an exploration of how distant the reality could be from the assumption before the estimate, or another concluding statement of an analysis, is altered appreciably.

A typical analysis of incomplete data relies on the usually unverifiable assumption of MAR. This assumption should be subjected to scrutiny. Instead of completions based on the assumption of MAR, we generate plausible values according to an NMAR mechanism. A practical way of implementing a wide range of NMAR mechanisms is by altering the MAR-based plausible values in a systematic way.

Sensitivity analysis is most effective when employed to challenge a particular conclusion. For example, when the difference between two groups, A and B, without any adjustments, is estimated, the obvious way to challenge the conclusion is by altering the plausible values for subjects in A in one direction and the plausible values for subjects in B in the other, aiming to reduce the estimated difference between the sample means of A and B.

5.6 MI for Categorical and Longitudinal Data

To complete a record that has some of its items missing, it is natural to look for similar records that are complete and 'borrow' their values for the missing subvector. A wide range of such procedures can be devised, based on different definitions of similarity. With categorical data, we may define similarity as agreement of the values of all the categorical variables that are recorded for both subjects. Such a definition may be too stringent when data comprises many variables. It can be relaxed by reducing the list of variables used for matching, aggregating some of the categories, and allowing one or a few discrepancies, either on a subset or for any of the variables. More generally, we may define a distance between any two records and define similarity as distance shorter than a set threshold.

The class of *nearest-neighbour* imputation methods is based on such definitions of similarity. For the missing part of a subject's incomplete record, we impute the corresponding subrecord of its nearest neighbour; in case of a tie we select a neighbour at random from the pool of candidates. Such methods aim to estimate the missing subrecords efficiently, and as we discussed in Section 5.2, this goal is not in accord with making efficient incomplete-data inferences when the complete-data estimators (linear sufficient statistics) involve some nonlinear functions of the missing data.

The hot-deck method is an improvement on these methods, inasmuch as it seeks to represent the variety of plausible subrecords for substitution. In hot deck, each incomplete record $\mathbf{x} = (\mathbf{x}_{rec}, \mathbf{x}_{mis})$ is associated with a *pool of donors*. The subject with the incomplete record is called a *recipient*, indicating that his or her completion will be based on a subrecord obtained from a donor. The pool of donors comprises subjects with complete records whose subrecords corresponding to $\mathbf{x}_{rec}$ are similar to the recipient's subrecord. A donor is then drawn at random and the recipient's record is completed by this donor's subrecord that corresponds to $\mathbf{x}_{mis}$. In a practical implementation, the recipients are also grouped, according to their response patterns and the values of $\mathbf{x}_{\mathrm{rec}}$ within the response patterns, so that the groups of recipients share pools of donors.

The pools have to be large enough to ensure that their subrecords, which are on offer for donation, represent the entire variety of plausible subvectors. Hot deck is a stochastic imputation method; its replication yields a different completion, unless there is no variety within the pools of donors. Even when MAR applies, hot deck is not a proper imputation method. To see this, suppose a particular pool of donors comprises $h_1, \ldots, h_P$ records with respective vectors of values $\mathbf{v}_1, \ldots, \mathbf{v}_P$. Let $h_+ = h_1 + \cdots + h_P$. Then the donated subrecord can be described as a random draw from the multinomial distribution with probabilities $p_1 = h_1/h_+, \ldots, p_P = h_P/h_+$. Each completion would be based on the same set of probabilities. In this application of the hot deck, we have ignored the uncertainty about the probabilities; the quantities $p_1, \ldots, p_P$ are merely estimates of the probabilities we should use. Given that these probabilities are unknown, we should represent our uncertainty about them by drawing plausible sets of probabilities $\tilde{p}_1, \ldots, \tilde{p}_P$ from their estimated (joint) sampling distribution and use a different (replicate) set of plausible probabilities for each completion of the dataset. This improvement of the hot deck is called the *approximate Bayes bootstrap* (ABB).

To implement ABB, we estimate the distribution of the estimators $\hat{\mathbf{p}} = (\hat{p}_1, \ldots, \hat{p}_P)^\top$, where $\hat{p}_k = h_k/h_+$. (This has to be done separately for each pool of donors.) Assuming an infinite underlying population and simple random sampling, this estimator is unbiased for the underlying vector of probabilities $\mathbf{p}$, and its sampling variance matrix is given by

$$\mathrm{var}\,(\hat{\mathbf{p}}) = \frac{1}{h_+} \left\{ \mathrm{diag}(\mathbf{p}) - \mathbf{p}\mathbf{p}^\top \right\}.$$

This is a singular matrix: $\hat{\mathbf{p}}^\top \mathbf{1} = 1$, and so $\mathbf{1}^\top \mathrm{var}(\hat{\mathbf{p}})\mathbf{1} = 0$. In practice, we have to rely on asymptotic normality of $\hat{\mathbf{p}}$; this is problematic when some of the counts h_k are small. The problem is not serious when there are only a few such counts among many, but when the counts of such categories add up to a nontrivial fraction of the donor pool, the variety of the candidate donations in the pool will not be well represented. Such pools of donors are ineffective for another reason. If there are many sparse categories in a pool, we cannot have confidence that there are categories absent from the pool that would be present in a replication of the study or, indeed, in the complete dataset. Then the variety of the pool is underrepresented by the realised pool.

With incomplete longitudinal data, hot deck and ABB can be developed from the deterministic imputation by BLVF. For categorical outcomes, copying the previous value corresponds to the model $P(X_t = k \mid X_{t-1} = k) = 1$ for the outcomes on occasions $t - 1$ and t. A more realistic model estimates this and other conditional (transition) probabilities $P(X_t = k \mid X_{t-1} = h)$ and reflects the uncertainty about them. If the uncertainty is ignored, imputation based on this model is equivalent to hot deck with matching on the outcome on the previous occasion.

Conditioning can be extended to the occasion preceding the last one, $t-2$, for imputations for occasions $t = 3, \ldots, T$. Then the donor pool comprises subjects who match the recipient on X_{t-2} and X_{t-1} and have their values of X_t recorded. The potential donors need not have complete records; outcomes at the earlier occasions need not be available. In fact, nonresponse at an occasion may be part of the matching criterion. For example, for a recipient with X_1 missing, $X_2 = 1$, $X_3 = 3$, and X_4 missing, we may include in the pool of donors all subjects with X_1 missing, $X_2 = 1$, $X_3 = 3$, and X_4 recorded. Of course, it is better to impute for X_1 and X_4 simultaneously, but if X_1 is not involved in any planned analysis, then imputing for it is unnecessary.

The BLVF method for continuous outcomes can be treated similarly. Instead of the implied unrealistic model $X_t = X_{t-1}$, we admit that some change takes place, $X_t = X_{t-1} + \varepsilon$, with a suitable centred distribution for ε. This can be extended to simple regression, $X_t = \beta_{0t} + \beta_{1t} X_{t-1} + \varepsilon$, with the usual assumptions of normality and homoscedasticity, or to the regression on two or more previous outcomes. Transforming X may be necessary for the ordinary regression to be appropriate. The log-transformation should always be considered for outcomes that describe growth or reduction, because it may be on a multiplicative scale.

In some settings with continuous outcomes, no change, $X_t = X_{t-1}$, has a positive probability. This can be accommodated by mixture models that assume that the sample is partitioned into several subsamples, and the corresponding population to the corresponding subpopulations, and each subpopulation is governed by a different model. For a subject, his or her subpopulation need not be known.

For one subpopulation we specify the model $X_t = X_{t-1}$ and for the other a linear regression. After fitting such a mixture model, we draw first from the plausible binary distribution (indicating whether any change took place at all), and if the outcome is positive, another draw is made from the plausible conditional distribution given that change did take place. Combining the two sources of incompleteness, whether change took place and nonresponse, generates no problems additional to dealing with each source on its own. Section 5.7.1 deals with mixture models in greater detail.

5.7 Other Applications of the Missing-Data Idea

In the applications of the EM algorithm and MI, missing data is the difference between the complete data, the data we intended to collect, and the incomplete data, what we managed to collect. More generally, we can declare any hypothetical dataset as the complete data, irrespective of the study plan, and the realised dataset as the incomplete data. The complete dataset should be relatively easy to analyse and should not involve an excessive amount of missing information. If the EM algorithm is applied, the sufficient statistics for the E-step should be easy to calculate; in MI, the model for 'nonresponse', used for generating sets of plausible values, should be easy to work with.

We sketch here two generic applications of missing-data methods, which are discussed in greater detail in Chapters 6 and 7. Suppose we want to estimate a population summary that involves a variable X^*, but it is a *latent variable*—its values cannot be recorded with precision. Instead, the values of its manifest version X are recorded. We declare an analysis in which we would like to use the values of X^* as the complete-data analysis, and the values $\mathbf{x}^*$ of X^* as the missing data. A set of plausible values $\tilde{\mathbf{x}}^*$ is generated, for the entire vector $\mathbf{x}^*$, from a plausible conditional distribution of $\mathbf{x}^*$ given $\mathbf{x}$. If we can observe the process of distortion, which alters a value of X^* to X, then we can estimate the conditional distribution $(\mathbf{X} \mid \mathbf{X}^* = \mathbf{x}^*)$. From it, we can infer about the conditional distribution $(\mathbf{X}^* \mid \mathbf{X} = \mathbf{x})$, from which plausible values of $\mathbf{X}^*$ can be generated, and the method of MI applied straightforwardly.

Randomisation is an important principle in study design, which enables an unbiased comparison of educational, medical, or other treatments. But what should we do when randomisation is not feasible or, simply, was not applied? As an example, suppose we want to compare the quality of two schools, A and B. For each student, we consider the pair of outcomes Y_A and Y_B that would result after attending the alternative schools A and B. If both outcomes were available the analysis would be straightforward, for instance, by comparing the means of Y_A and Y_B. Let W be the school attended, so that Y_W is the recorded outcome variable—it is a 'mix' of Y_A and Y_B. We declare Y_W as the incomplete and (Y_A, Y_B) as the complete data. Imputation then involves generating plausible outcomes Y_A for students who attended school B and Y_B for those who attended A.

The remainder of this section outlines other applications of the EM algorithm and MI. They show how a limited range of models that we can fit can be extended and how we can attend to various data imperfections other than nonresponse.

5.7.1 Finite Mixtures

Suppose a population $\mathcal{P}$ comprises a small number K of subpopulations with distinct distributions of a target variable X. Although inferences are desired about these K distributions, the subpopulation is not identified for any of the n subjects in the sample. In other words, we observe a *mixture* of a finite number K of distributions, and we wish to make inferences about each component distribution. For simplicity, we assume that the number of components K is known. In practice it is not, but the problem is solved for several values of K and one or several plausible solutions are presented, together with an assessment of how plausible they are.

In the terminology of the EM algorithm, we regard the indicator of each subject's subpopulation (group or component) as the missing information and estimate it in the E-step. The outcome of the E-step is the subjects' conditional probabilities of belonging to each component; for the sample, this is an $n \times K$ matrix with its rows adding up to unity. In the M-step, we estimate the parameters of each distribution. In estimating the parameters for component k, the indicator of belonging to component k is replaced by its conditional expectation, equal to the subject's conditional probability of belonging to component k. The E- and M-steps are then iterated until convergence is achieved.

Let $f_k(x)$ be the density of component k and p_k the probability of the component. Then the (mixture) density is

$$f(x) = p_1 f_1(x) + p_2 f_2(x) + \cdots + p_K f_K(x). \tag{5.13}$$

Suppose the current estimates of the component distributions at iteration h are $\hat{f}_k^{(h)}(x)$ and the estimated marginal probabilities of the components are $\hat{p}_k^{(h)}$, $k = 1, \ldots, K$. The next E-step evaluates the estimated probabilities

$$\hat{r}_{jk}^{(h+1)} = \frac{\hat{p}_k^{(h)} \hat{f}_k^{(h)}(x_j)}{\hat{p}_1^{(h)} \hat{f}_1^{(h)}(x_j) + \cdots + \hat{p}_K^{(h)} \hat{f}_K^{(h)}(x_j)}$$

for subject j and component k. In the subsequent M-step, the estimates of the marginal probabilities $\hat{p}_k$ are updated as the within-component averages of $\hat{r}_{jk}^{(h+1)}$,

$$\hat{p}_k^{(h+1)} = \frac{1}{n} \left(\hat{r}_{1k}^{(h+1)} + \cdots + \hat{r}_{nk}^{(h+1)} \right),$$

and the parameters for component k are estimated by the complete-data method. For example, the expectation of the kth distribution is estimated as the weighted mean

$$\hat{\mu}_k^{(h)} = \frac{\sum_{j=1}^{n} \hat{r}_{jk}^{(h)} x_j}{\sum_{j=1}^{n} \hat{r}_{jk}^{(h)}}.$$

The components may involve models of differing complexity. For example, some components may comprise unconditional distributions and others may involve regression.

Mixtures of distributions can be useful even when the population does not comprise any interpretable subpopulations with distinct distributions. Suppose the population distribution is difficult to estimate directly. We can approximate it by a mixture of distributions from a specified class with which estimation is much simpler. This class can be regarded as a basis, providing the building blocks. For example, any continuous distribution can be approximated with arbitrary precision by a mixture of normal distributions, but also by a mixture of uniform distributions, and even by a mixture of degenerate distributions. We prefer approximations by mixtures of a few rather than many components. Therefore, if we know or assume that the target distribution is continuous and does not have more than, say, two modes, approximation by

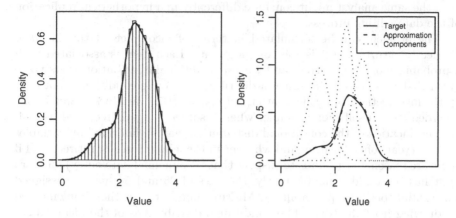

Fig. 5.3. Approximation of a distribution by a mixture of normal distributions.

a mixture of a few normals may be suitable. Figure 5.3 gives an illustration. Its left-hand panel contains the density with a histogram superimposed. In the right-hand panel, the component densities, $\mathcal{N}(2.0, 0.17)$, $\mathcal{N}(2.4, 0.08)$, and $\mathcal{N}(3.0, 0.14)$, are drawn by dots, their mixture, with respective probabilities 0.50, 0.35, and 0.15, by dashes, and the target by the solid line.

Mixtures can be applied also to multivariate distributions. There is a paucity of classes of distributions that could serve as the basis, and we have to rely on the multivariate normal distributions. Nevertheless, this basis, together with transformations of the outcomes, provides a powerful tool for approximating distributions and for widening the horizon of models that we can work with.

5.7.2 Outliers and Contaminants: Data Editing

Outliers are observations that spoil the good fit of a model. They are candidates for exclusion from the sample on account of possibly not being members of the relevant population (being included in the sample erroneously) or of having incorrectly recorded values. When there is an obvious resolution, such as contacting the subject again to check the recorded values or the nature of the error is obvious (using different units, resulting in the values being, say, 1000 times greater than they should be), the appropriate correction (*data editing*) can be made and the item regarded as if it were recorded according to the original protocol.

In many settings, the outlier status or the incorrectness of a value cannot be established with certainty. Sometimes, the status of an item is assessed subjectively, and the verdict of outlier/no outlier or plausible/implausible is far too coarse, as another analyst might come to a different conclusion, and even the same analyst might conclude differently in a hypothetical replication of the data-editing process.

The problem can be formulated in terms of incomplete data; the ideal (perfectly clean) dataset is the complete data. Each item is associated with a probability of being correct and with a conditional distribution of its value given that it is not correct. Such a distribution may be conditioned not only on the incorrectness or outlier status, but also on other variables as well as the recorded value itself. For example, when a subject's age is recorded as 254, the specification of the conditional distribution may be informed by variables such as (years of) education and whether in the labour force or retired, and if there are reasonable grounds to suspect that (in a manual data entry) an extra digit has been added inadvertently, the ages of 25 and 54 may be assigned substantial (positive) probabilities. Multiple imputation is then implemented by drawing from the (plausible) conditional distributions of the ideal values. The key advantage of MI is that the uncertainty about the outlier status or correctness is reflected by the between-imputation variation. With a single editing, no idiosyncrasies among the amended records are introduced, even if some idiosyncrasies do occur among the records that were left intact—the edited records look 'too good'. As a consequence, the inferences based on the edited (completed) dataset project more confidence than is justified.

5.7.3 Balanced Complete Data

Some analyses are much easier to conduct when the data have a balanced structure, such as equal number of subjects in each cluster. When the realised (incomplete) data do not have such a structure, but would have it if appropriately supplemented, e.g., by additional observations, we can declare such a supplemented dataset as the complete dataset. When it can be reasonably assumed that the distribution of the studied attribute does not depend on the cluster size, the data can be regarded as missing completely at random. Otherwise care has to be exercised in specifying a model that relates the values we regard as missing to the recorded values for the subjects in the same cluster. This approach is useful only when a completion can be achieved by adding a small number of records to the data; otherwise the fraction of the missing information is very large.

Suggested Reading

A much more detailed and comprehensive text on missing data is the monograph [110]. The terminology and other background were originally set out in [158]. The original reference for the EM algorithm is [33], although there are several earlier applications of its principle, such as [71] and [141]. Further developments and extensions of EM, with an emphasis on speeding up its convergence, can be traced in [162] and [136]. A suitable textbook on the

EM algorithm is [134]. Estimation of the incomplete-data standard errors is addressed by [131] and [197]; [135] and [87] explore ways of accelerating the convergence of the EM algorithm. The theory of MI is developed in [165]; [164] reiterates the arguments for MI for large-scale incomplete data. Models for missing data are developed and motivated in [107]–[109]. The monograph [169] is an excellent text on the applications of MI, with a detailed treatment of computational issues. Further instructional material is presented in [170]. Part I of [122] gives a condensed account of the theory, discusses several case studies, and outlines some less standard applications of MI. Readable journal articles on applications of missing data include [75], [173], [74] [167], and [125]. Data augmentation, a Bayesian adaptation of the EM algorithm, is described in [190]. The original reference for the method of chained equations is [14]. A sensitivity analysis accompanying an application of MI is presented in [129]. An important reference on poststratification is [80].

SOLAS is a software package for MI, suitable for instruction and less demanding analysis (www.statsol.ie). A comprehensive suite of functions in R/Splus accompanies the monograph [169]; see

www.stat.psu.edu/~jls/misoftwa.html.

Software for the method of chained equations can be downloaded from

web.inter.nl.net/users/S.van.Buuren/mi/docs.

Most established statistical packages have modules for some of the elements of MI. See [82] for a review of these and some other packages.

Problems and Exercises

5.1. Discuss the difference between the following two studies. The datasets, A and B, obtained by the studies have the same variables. Dataset A has sample size 900 obtained by simple random sampling from a population $\mathcal{P}$. Every record in the dataset is complete; every subject responded to all the questionnaire items. Dataset B also contains 900 complete records; they are from the respondents in a survey with a simple random sampling design in $\mathcal{P}$ and planned sample size of 1200. No information is available from the 300 nonrespondents. Would you apply the same analysis to both datasets? If not, which dataset is easier to analyse and why? For which dataset would you have more confidence in the results?

5.2. Write a programme (e.g., a function in Splus or R) to summarise the extent of missing data in an incomplete dataset. It should calculate the numbers and percentages of missing values for each variable, tabulate the subjects' response patterns, and present them according to the number of missing values in a record. The programme should have an option to draw a diagram similar to Figure 5.1. It could be developed further to incorporate some of the suggestions made in Section 5.1. Use a dataset of your choice for debugging and refining the programme.

5.3. For the dataset used in Exercise 5.2, find a permutation of the variables that brings about the patterns of nonresponse as close as possible to being monotone. In the solution, consider deleting individual values, discarding subjects, discarding variables, and splitting the variables into subsets so that the patterns are (almost) monotone in each subset. Further, these steps can be combined. Automate these steps by a suitable programme or function.

5.4. Summarise the problems related to sampling and nonresponse in the following setting. A survey of environmental awareness plans to take advantage of the time that departing passengers have in departure halls of major U.S. airports. On days of the week and times of the day selected to ensure good representation and to be balanced across the locations, every twentieth person passing the security check will be asked to complete a short questionnaire in a language of his or her choice. The passenger can either respond straightaway or send the responses by mail on a card in a self-addressed envelope provided.

5.5. In a longitudinal study of diet, adult subjects are contacted once a year and requested to complete the same questionnaire that comprises so-called frequency items. The items have the common preamble:

In the last twelve months, how frequently did you eat the following foods:

For each food item, such as bread, biscuits, or eggs, there are ten response options, ranging from 'Never' to 'Every day'. The items are presented in blocks that relate to food types, such as 'Fruit and vegetables', 'Meat, fish, and poultry', and 'Baked products'. Describe the various kinds of nonresponse related to the structure of the collected information (years, blocks, and items) and the response patterns that are likely to occur. Consider that subjects may also skip and leave out the response to an odd item because of distraction.

5.6. Discuss some intuitively motivated imputation schemes for a dataset anticipated in the study of diet in the previous exercise. Why would any data reduction be particularly disadvantageous? How would you justify imputation by 'bringing the last value forward' (BLVF) from the previous year? (This exercise is suitable when you start studying the chapter, but it could be revisited at the end of the study.)

5.7. Suppose a single normally distributed variable X was planned to be recorded on a simple random sample of n subjects (sample size fixed by design), but the values were recorded only for a subsample of size n_0. Assume that the nonresponse is MCAR. Apply the sample mean $\bar{x}$ as an estimator of the population mean and the obvious estimator $\hat{s}^2$ of its sampling variance. Apply these estimators to the complete dataset, the incomplete dataset, and datasets completed by (deterministic and stochastic) single-imputation methods of your choice. To the extent that it is possible, compare the results analytically and draw conclusions about the completed-data analyses.

5.8. Construct a population of large size (several thousands) and generate the values of a variable according to a normal distribution. Replicate the processes of sampling, nonresponse, and estimation that were considered in the previous exercise and confirm your results empirically (by replications).

5.9. In a longitudinal study of lifestyle and health, the body mass of each subject is measured once a year. Subjects may refuse the measurement or may be unavailable for a visit by the nurse who would like to come and conduct the interview with a questionnaire about illnesses, changes in occupation, activities pursued in free time, and mode of transportation used most often in the last year. Compile a list of plausible reasons for nonresponse and discuss what information they contain, if any, possibly in conjunction with some of the recorded information (age, state of health, occupation, and the like) about the change in body mass since last year. Based on this discussion, propose models for imputation for body mass. Adapt to multiple imputation any of those that involve single imputation.

5.10. For the setting of Example 12, specify an NMAR mechanism that is easy to simulate (implement) and revise all the details, including equations (5.7) and (5.8), for this mechanism.
Hint: In one such mechanism, the conditional expectation of the missing value x_j^* is greater by a fixed (known) constant than what the conditional expectation would be if MAR applied. (The conditional variance is the same.)

5.11. Describe and implement the multiple imputation version of the EM algorithm in Example 12. That is, replace the calculations of the conditional expectations and variances by generating plausible values of the missing items. Compare the complexity of the procedures (EM and MI) and how easy they are to implement. What is the point of applying the EM algorithm but following it up by generating plausible completed datasets?

5.12. Compile a table that would relate the proportion of missing information to the number of completions required to reduce the inefficiency of MI to $f = 5\%$. Write a programme to generate such a table for an arbitrary percentage f.
Hint: The inefficiency is defined as the percentage that B/M forms in $W + (1 + 1/M)B$.
Assess the resources required and the effort and inconvenience to yourself as the analyst involved in doubling the number of data completions in the context of Example 12 or a similar problem. Consider this issue for the various ways in which the plausible values or the completions might be stored and delivered to the secondary analyst(s).

5.13. The Labour Force Survey in the United Kingdom (LFS) is conducted every quarter and a subject is retained in the sample for five consecutive quarters. For example, a subject who was included for the first time in the first quarter (Q1) of 2006 is retained for Q2–Q4 of 2006 and is 'retired' from the sample after Q1 of 2007. In any one quarter, approximately one-fifth of the sample is interviewed for the first time, one-fifth a second time, and so on, and about one-fifth for the last time. A principal outcome variable is the employment status, coded as E — employed, U — unemployed, and N — economically inactive (not in the labour force). Discuss the rationale for using BLVF to impute for missing outcome in an interview when there is an earlier interview in which the outcome is recorded. How can such an imputation be improved? Discuss how hot deck could be applied effectively. Look up details of imputation procedures for the LFS on www.statistics.gov.uk/labour_market/lfs or on the web site for a similar survey in your country.

5.14. In a study of alcohol dependence, subjects were interviewed on one of the first days of every month in 2004. They were asked to recall what kind and quantity of alcoholic beverages they consumed in the previous month, in what settings (home, friends' home, public house, restaurant, and the like) and how much their life was disrupted during the month (absence from work, running out of money for everyday necessities, inability to attend to everyday tasks, such as care for children, and having to sleep or rest several hours during the day). Discuss why the interview-level nonresponse is likely to be nonignorable. How suitable would be imputation by BLVF or by its improvements? How would you alter your answers if the subjects were aware that they would receive rewards if the assessment based on their responses indicated reduced dependence? Would you draw any distinction between interview- and item-level nonresponse? The former is due to not turning up for an interview, while the latter is due to an error in the interview procedure (an item inadvertently skipped or subject's refusal to respond). Would you draw any distinction between nonresponse to an isolated item and dropping out from the interview (no response to the remainder of the questionnaire)?

5.15. Many large-scale surveys use sampling weights set by design, which are then adjusted for imperfections of the sampling frame, nonresponse, and other problems with the data collection by relating some sample summaries to their known population versions; see Section 3.5.1 (poststratification). Obtain the data from a national survey (e.g., from a social science data archive or a national statistical office) and the accompanying documentation. Find out how the sampling weights are adjusted, and summarise the adjustments with suitable diagrams. Discuss the problems associated with poststratification and propose some alternatives. Compare the estimates of some key quantities using estimators based on the original and adjusted sampling weights.

5.16. For the analysis of a planned study, compile a protocol for dealing with outliers (how they would be identified, what action would be taken about them, and so on). Borrow the setting from a dataset or analysis that you are familiar with. Adapt the protocol to allow for the possibility that the analyst might be uncertain as to whether an observation is an outlier or not.

Revisit the definition of the term 'outlier', and discuss it in greater detail. For example, is being an outlier a population or a sample property? (Is the labelling of a subject as an outlier associated with any uncertainty?) Could a subject be an outlier in one sample but not in another? Consider defining an index for every subject on the scale from 0 (definitely not an outlier) to 1 (certainly an outlier), which could be interpreted as the probability of being an outlier. Draw up a proposal for how to analyse a dataset supplemented with the values of such an index.

5.17. As a matter of convenience, experiments on a particular piece of equipment in a manufacturing process are usually conducted in sets of eight, although in some cases the sets are smaller. Dataset `EX6a.dat` on

    `www.sntl.co.uk/BookA/Data`

contains the results of ten sets of experiments. To estimate the mean for a set of experiments and for the collection of sets, apply a missing-data method that uses as the complete dataset the 10×8 records that would be realised if each set comprised all eight experiments. Compare the advantages and drawbacks of the EM algorithm and multiple imputation for this problem. Compare the solutions based on the balanced complete-data analysis and on the direct analysis of the recorded data.

5.18. Construct a population that comprises two disjoint subpopulations of sizes $N_1 \neq N_2$ in thousands. A variable X has different normal distributions in the two subpopulations, say, $\mathcal{N}(10, 1)$ and $\mathcal{N}(14, 2)$. Draw a simple random sample of substantial size (several hundreds) from the population and, using the EM algorithm, fit the model that assumes that the distribution of X is a mixture of two normals. Study the subjects' estimated probabilities of belonging to a subpopulation and compare them with the reality, which was assumed not to be known in the estimation process. Carefully consider how you associate an estimated distribution with one of the population distributions.

5.19. The dataset listed in file `EX6b.dat` on `www.sntl.co.uk/BookA/Data` is an enumeration of the pool of applicants for a high-profile appointment. The important variables recorded are age (A), number of years in education (E), number of years of relevant working experience (W), and current annual salary (S). The question about W was misunderstood by some applicants and they entered either zero or the same response as to item E. Confidentiality and time constraints make it impossible to get in touch with these applicants to check whether their records are correct. How would you rescue the situation? Carefully state the assumptions you make.

Hints: Impute multiply for W where its value is in doubt. Start with some simple schemes, and add useful features (complications) to them, so long as you can cope with the computations. You can bypass some problems if you work with a categorical version of the salary by defining suitable cut points for the categories.

Imperfect Measurement

The developments in the earlier chapters assumed that the values of the variables involved in an analysis are obtained with precision. More often than not, this is an unrealistic or even patently flawed assumption, but one without which our ability to make inferences would be severely curtailed. This chapter deals with the general problem of imperfect measurement, which includes measurement with error and using a variable that is a substitute for the one we would ideally like to have recorded.

An instinctive way of addressing this problem is by estimating each value of the ideal variable separately and then conducting the desired analysis as if the estimated values were the ideal ones. We dismiss this approach as deficient. We consider first the problem of measurement with normally distributed variables and then its counterpart for categorical variables, which we refer to as *misclassification*.

We refer to the ideal variable, with which the planned analysis would be simpler, as the *latent* variable, and its substitute, which is recorded or constructed, as the *manifest* variable. A study may involve several latent variables, but we will assume that each of them is associated with one manifest variable. By a *naive analysis* or the naive version of an analysis, we mean the analysis as planned for the latent variables or one that would be well suited for them, but in which each variable is replaced by its manifest version.

6.1 The Measurement Process

The values of a latent variable may be obtained, sometimes only in principle, but there are numerous examples in which the latent variable is merely a concept defined in abstraction. For instance, our state of health, or even the function of a vital organ, such as the heart, can at best be assessed, by an expert using specialised equipment, subject to an 'error' that may be perfectly acceptable given the purpose of the assessment and the state of the art in making the relevant medical diagnosis.

A student's ability is assessed by an exam. But the outcome of such an exam is much more accurately described as performance on the day, affected by a myriad of minor distractions, elements of preparation, and coping with the artificial setting of the examination (dealing with the time constraint, attitude to taking risks when not certain about which of the offered response options is correct, and the like). The representation of the domain (curriculum) by the questions and the way the responses are marked (both the general instructions and the idiosyncrasies of the rater who marks the exam papers), are further nuisance features that contribute to the deviation of the recorded result from what it is meant to stand for.

Among the manifest variables for a latent variable, we can distinguish variables that are defined with precision and those that entail some uncertainty due to measurement or, more precisely, due to determination of the value. For example, age of an individual is recorded with precision, but it is an imperfect substitute (manifest variable) for maturity or experience, in whichever reasonable way these traits may be defined. In contrast, the systolic blood pressure of a patient at a time point has a clinical definition, but its measurement entails some uncertainty; had it been measured for the same patient at the same time point in a hypothetical replication, by different equipment, a different nurse, or even the same nurse, the outcome might have been slightly different. In this case, we can talk about the *measurement process*, which describes how the value of the latent variable becomes distorted (tainted), so that the recorded differs from the ideal.

We can consider convolutions of these two kinds of imperfection, such as imperfect measurement of an alternative variable. One such example is recording the age group, as guessed by the interviewer, instead of age. The imperfection need not have a stochastic nature. For instance, rounding can be regarded as an imperfection. For a given ideal value, each (hypothetical) replication would in this case yield the same value.

To draw parallels with the notation in Chapter 5, we denote the latent variable by X^* and its manifest variable by X. In Section 6.5, we develop an approach in which the values of the latent variable are regarded as the missing data. Inferences that involve latent variables can then be formulated as dealing with incomplete information and the problem can be delegated to the methods developed in Chapter 5.

Since measurement is concerned with reproducing a particular value of X^*, we define the process of measurement by the conditional distributions of X given the values of X^*. Parsimony of this description is achieved by stating what the conditional distributions $(X \mid X^* = x)$ for the values x in the support of X^* have in common. A simple example is

$$(X \mid X^* = x) \sim \mathcal{N}\left(x, \sigma_\delta^2\right) ;$$

it states that the manifest value differs from the latent value by a random draw from a particular centred normal distribution. An alternative description of X is that

$$X = X^* + \delta, \tag{6.1}$$

with the deviation $\delta \sim \mathcal{N}(0, \sigma_\delta^2)$ independent of X^*. This suggests a particular mechanism of how X^* is distorted and 'converted' to X, by adding a random 'error' (*white noise*) to the value of the latent variable. This model may be appropriate even when no such mechanism can be identified. Its obvious generalisations allow the variance σ_δ^2 to depend on the value of X^* and the mean of the deviation δ to differ from zero and to depend on X^*. Further, δ need not be normally distributed. The model in (6.1) is often regarded as a definition of measurement error in a narrow sense.

We say that a measurement process is *unbiased* if $E(X - X^*) = 0$; otherwise it is called *biased*. An unbiased measurement process may become biased when the measurement refers to a different scale. As an example, suppose g is a nonlinear monotone function. Then $g(X)$ can be regarded as a manifest version of $g(X^*)$. The measurement process may be biased with regard to $g(X^*)$ when it is unbiased with regard to X^* because, in general, $E\{g(X) - g(X^*)\} \neq g\{E(X - X^*)\}$.

The property of unbiasedness is related also to the population. The restriction of an unbiased measurement variable to a subpopulation may be biased; simply, the subpopulation-specific biases may average out. The manifest variable X in (6.1) is unbiased for each subpopulation (stratum) defined by a value of X^* or an interval of values; that is, $E(X \mid X^* = x) = x$ for each x. We say that such a manifest variable is *pointwise unbiased*. Being pointwise unbiased for every x in the support of X^* is a much more stringent condition than being unbiased without any qualification.

Historically, the difference between the manifest and latent versions of a variable has been referred to as *measurement error*. This term is motivated by applications involving physical measurement, regarding the value of the latent variable as being within our grasp. We do not use this term and refer to 'deviation' (from the latent value), distortion, or imperfect measurement instead, to avoid the connotation that an avoidable mistake was committed in the conduct of the study. A deviation is often anticipated and cannot be avoided. In some settings, the value of the latent variable could be established, but doing so is very expensive and would reduce the resources that might be allocated more productively to other activities in the study. For example, with the precise measurement, the study could afford a sample of only a much smaller size. More generally, the trade-off between precise measurement (quality) and number of subjects (quantity) is an important consideration in studies in which there are several options for measurement.

The cost of measurement, expressible not necessarily solely in financial terms, is an important consideration. For example, a detailed discussion of the subject's income in a lifestyle survey may erode the motivation, patience, and goodwill of many subjects, and some of them may terminate the interview prematurely or would not agree to a follow-up interview in the future. This example reaffirms that we should also drop the term 'measurement', because we intend to deal with all forms of eliciting and recording information.

A case in point is estimation of the unemployment rate. The extensive option is to contact each subject of a random sample of the members of the labour force and, after a suitable introduction, ask them the relevant question directly. As an alternative that involves no direct contact with the subjects, the register of those claiming unemployment benefit may be consulted and the rate of unemployed based on the number of registrations and the size of the labour force. By direct contact and interview, we establish the value of the latent variable with precision (assuming that all subjects give valid responses), but do so only for a sample from the population. By inspecting the register, we establish the value of a related (manifest) variable but obtain it for every member of the population. (Not being registered is interpreted as being employed or not being in the labour force.) The two variables, the employment status as established by the interview and by the unemployment register, differ; some unemployed have income, are not qualified for benefit, or do not wish to claim it for some other reason, and there may be some fraudulent claims and administrative errors in the register, e.g., due to delays in reporting and recording changes in the employment status, as well as deaths and migration. Assuming that each subject would give the same response in a hypothetical replication of the interview, the deviation of the manifest from the latent variable in this example is not stochastic. An analytical challenge is to combine the information in the survey and register, to make inferences that are superior to those based solely on either source of information.

Another instructive example is the assessment of the success of a medical procedure, such as a surgery. If we waited for a few years we could establish whether it was successful or not, except for a few patients who have in the meantime died of causes unrelated to the surgery. However, an assessment is required in a more timely fashion, for instance, in a clinical trial or to prescribe a suitable follow-up treatment, including discharge. Making an (independent) assessment by a medical consultant a few days after the surgery is a practical proposition even though it may entail some sacrifice of precision.

An advantage of the mechanistic description by a model, such as (6.1) or its various extensions, is that it can be explored by simulations. However, some properties and associations of X and X^* can be derived analytically. First, $E(X) = E(X^*) + E(\delta)$ in (6.1), highlighting how useful it is that $E(\delta)$ vanishes—X and X^* have identical expectations. However, $\mathrm{var}(X) = \mathrm{var}(X^*) + \sigma_\delta^2$, so X is dispersed more than X^*. Further, $\mathrm{cov}(X, X^*) = \mathrm{var}(X^*)$, which we denote by σ_*^2, so that

$$\mathrm{cor}(X, X^*) = \sqrt{\frac{\sigma_*^2}{\sigma_*^2 + \sigma^2}} \, .$$

An alternative description of the measurement process is by the joint distribution of X^* and X. For example, the model in (6.1) corresponds to

$$(X^*, X) \sim \mathcal{N}_2 \left\{ \mu_* 1_2, \begin{pmatrix} \sigma_*^2 & \sigma_*^2 \\ \sigma_*^2 & \sigma_*^2 + \sigma_\delta^2 \end{pmatrix} \right\}, \tag{6.2}$$

where $\mu_* = \mathrm{E}(X^*)$. The conditional distribution of X, given that $X^* = x$, is derived straightforwardly, and it confirms equivalence with (6.1).

6.1.1 Information About the Measurement Process

Information about the measurement process can be gathered by observing X^* precisely when this is possible and affordable, together with X, as pairs of observations of (X^*, X). This does not have to be done on every subject in the study; it suffices to observe (X^*, X) on a random subsample of the subjects in the study, or even of the subjects in a different study, so long as the two studies use representative samples from the same population. As soon as the populations differ or the subsampling of one of the samples is not representative, caution is in order, because the properties of a measurement process may be closely connected with the population involved.

An indirect but often much more affordable alternative is to observe the subjects or their subsample twice, that is, observe variables $X^{(1)}$ and $X^{(2)}$ that are related to X^* by the same model and are conditionally independent, given the value of X^*. The model for these three variables is

$$X^{(k)} = X^* + \delta^{(k)},$$

$k = 1, 2$, where $\delta^{(1)}$ and $\delta^{(2)}$ are independent variables with the same distribution $\mathcal{N}(0, \sigma^2)$. This is equivalent to

$$\left(X^*, X^{(1)}, X^{(2)} \right) \sim \mathcal{N}_3 \left\{ \mu_* 1_3, \begin{pmatrix} \sigma_*^2 & \sigma_*^2 & \sigma_*^2 \\ \sigma_*^2 & \sigma_*^2 + \sigma_\delta^2 & \sigma_*^2 \\ \sigma_*^2 & \sigma_*^2 & \sigma_*^2 + \sigma_\delta^2 \end{pmatrix} \right\}.$$

The variables $X^{(1)}$ and $X^{(2)}$ can be regarded as replicates of the measurement process or as replicate manifest variables. In fact, a population of measurements can be considered, of which $X^{(1)}$ and $X^{(2)}$ are two members (realisations). In this perspective, σ_δ^2 is the replication variance.

The assumptions about the measurement process imply that the difference $X^{(1)} - X^{(2)}$ has zero expectation and variance $2\sigma_\delta^2$. Good measurement can therefore be identified with small variance σ_δ^2. However, two measurement processes can be meaningfully compared by their variances σ_δ^2 only when both processes are unbiased. Extensions to more than two and to unequal numbers of replications are straightforward. They include the setting in which only a random subsample of subjects is involved in any replications, and, in general, when the number of replications K is variable. In the latter case, some complexities are avoided by arranging that the number of replications is independent from X^*.

We can define the average of the replicate manifest variables, $X^{[K]} = \left(X^{(1)} + \cdots + X^{(K)}\right)/K$ for K replications as another manifest variable. Since $\text{var}\left(X^{[K]}; X^* = x\right) = \sigma_\delta^2/K$, $X^{[K]}$ is preferred as a manifest variable for X^* to either of the replicates $X^{(k)}$; however, when $X^{(k)}$ is (pointwise) biased, $X^{[K]}$ 'inherits' the (pointwise) bias of $X^{(k)}$:

$$\text{B}\left(X^{[K]}; X^* \mid X^* = x\right) = \text{E}\left(X^{(k)} \mid X^* = x\right) - x. \tag{6.3}$$

Unlike the replication variance, the bias cannot be reduced by replications. Neither can it be inferred from $X^{(1)}, X^{(2)}, \ldots, X^{(k)}$, because each $X^{(k)}$ is unbiased for another latent variable, $X^\dagger = X^* + B$, where B is the bias in (6.3).

6.2 Attributes of a Good Manifest Variable

Unbiasedness and small variance σ_δ^2 of the deviations are clearly desirable properties of a measurement process. However, the ultimate measure of the quality of a manifest variable is how good are the inferences conducted with it as a substitute for the latent variable, and so the assessment of the quality may depend on the intended analysis. Ideally, we would like to recover the inference that would have been obtained had the values of the latent variable X^* been recorded perfectly and, as second best, we would like to estimate the population quantities of interest with as small inflation of MSE as possible.

For example, unbiased measurement is advantageous for estimating the population mean of X^*, because the mean of the values of X for a random sample is unbiased: $\text{E}(\bar{X}) = \text{E}(\bar{X}^*) = \mu_*$. If X^* were observed on a random sample of n subjects the sampling variance would be $\text{var}(\bar{X}^*) = \sigma_*^2/n$. When only the manifest variable is observed, the sampling variance is greater: $\text{var}(\bar{X}) = (\sigma_*^2 + \sigma_\delta^2)/n$. For a manifest variable with bias B, we have

$$\text{MSE}(\bar{X}; \mu_*) = \frac{1}{n}\left(\sigma_*^2 + \sigma_\delta^2\right) + B,$$

so we should not dismiss biased measurements, especially when estimation (of the population mean μ_*) is based on a small sample and the bias is small. The appropriate criterion for a good measurement in this context is small value of $\sigma_\delta^2/n + B$, and it depends on the sample size n.

6.2.1 Impartiality

A highly desirable property of a measurement process is that all variables other than X^* are associated with X only through X^*. A measurement process with this property is called *impartial*. The condition can be expressed in terms of conditional distributions as

$$(X \mid X^*, \mathbf{Z}) = (X \mid X^*) \tag{6.4}$$

where $\mathbf{Z}$ is a vector of specified attributes; they are irrelevant to how X^* is distorted into X.

For example, in a judicial system, in which fairness of the assessment is paramount, the penalty X meted out to an accused should depend only on the crime committed (U) and, conditionally on this, should be unrelated to sex, race, age, or political allegiance $(\mathbf{Z})$ of the accused. In this setting, $X^* = g(U)$ is the penalty that should be given (including full exoneration, $X^* = 0$). The system may operate imperfectly, that is, with positive $E\{(X - X^*)^2\}$. Note that impartiality is qualified by the variables in $\mathbf{Z}$. By adding variables to $\mathbf{Z}$ it becomes a more stringent criterion.

Similarly, conditionally on the latent ability, a student's grade in an exam should not be related to the student's ability in other subjects, or to any elements of his or her background, socioeconomic background in particular, that are meant to be irrelevant to the educational process. Such a criterion for a fair exam or assessment may be a tall order and is not trivial to check, because the student's ability in the academic subject concerned can be assessed only by an exam like the one that we are subjecting to scrutiny. In an examination that comprises several elements (items, or questions), it is reasonable to insist that the score given for the response to each element should be impartial. Then, presuming that most of the items are impartial, summaries for a partial item would stand out. For instance, one group of examinees would perform on this item more poorly than another, even after matching on the scores attained on the remaining items.

Impartial manifest variables are in general pointwise biased. Often the bias cannot be defined unambiguously because the underlying variable is defined only subject to a class of monotone transformations. For example, the ability to drive a motor vehicle does not have an unambiguous definition, even though the driving test may be graded according to a well-defined scale. But a desirable property of the test score is that better drivers tend to attain higher scores. This property is in general referred to as *validity*. Impartiality is a necessary condition for validity, but it is not sufficient. One particular interpretation of the term validity is that any decision based on the value of the manifest variable (test score) is the same as would be made if the latent score were available. In most settings, this is an unrealistic assumption, even when the decision depends only on a coarsened version of the latent variable, for instance, when it is required to classify each examinee as 'good enough' or not.

Impartiality, absence of bias, and validity are *absolute* criteria. In most settings, they are unlikely to be satisfied, but it would suffice if departures from them were only slight, not undermining the purpose for which the manifest variable is intended. Such variables may provide a more economic and practical solution than variables recorded by the more precise (and more resource-intensive) measurement of the same latent variable.

Suppose variable X is manifest for X^* and Z is another variable, and they are jointly normally distributed. The manifest variable is then related to the other two as

$$X = a + bX^* + cZ + \delta, \qquad (6.5)$$

where δ is a centred normally distributed variable, independent of both X^* and Z. We prove this assertion by construction. No generality is lost by assuming that the means of all three variables vanish; otherwise we use their centred versions $X - \mathrm{E}(X)$, $X^* - \mathrm{E}(X^*)$, and $Z - \mathrm{E}(Z)$ and absorb the differences that arise in the constant a. Let $\mathbf{U} = (X^*, Z)^\top$ and assume that var$(\mathbf{U})$ is positive definite. We set $a = 0$ and

$$(b, c) = \mathrm{cov}(X, \mathbf{U}) \{\mathrm{var}(\mathbf{U})\}^{-1}.$$

Then

$$\mathrm{cov}\{X - (b, c)\mathbf{U}, \mathbf{U}\} = \mathbf{0},$$

so for this choice of a, b, and c, $\delta = X - (b, c)\mathbf{U}$ is correlated with neither X^* nor Z. For normally distributed variables, independence and no correlation are equivalent conditions, hence the assertion in (6.5). When var$(\mathbf{U})$ is singular, X^* and Z are linearly related, so $X^* = dZ$ for some constant d, since $\mathrm{E}(X^*) = \mathrm{E}(Z) = 0$. The assertion is then obtained by setting $c = 0$ and applying the preceding proof to univariate $U = X^*$. The assertion has an obvious generalisation for a vector $\mathbf{Z}$ with a multivariate normal distribution.

Impartiality in (6.5) corresponds to $c = 0$ and absence of bias to

$$(1 - b)\mathrm{E}(X) = a + c\mathrm{E}(Z).$$

The model in (6.1) is a special case of impartiality, which arises when $a = 0$ and $b = 1$.

6.3 Linear Regression with Manifest Variables

In this section, we consider the problem of estimating the regression of a latent variable Y^* on a perfectly measured variable X and the regression of a perfectly measured variable Y on a latent variable X^*, when the latent variables are represented by their manifest versions, by Y in the former and X in the latter case. In both cases, we assume that all three variables involved are normally distributed. We show that different properties of the manifest variable are desirable in these two problems.

6.3.1 Latent Outcome Variable

Suppose the target is the slope β_1 of the regression $\mathrm{E}(Y^* \mid X = x)$, but instead of Y^* we observe only the values $\mathbf{y}$ of a manifest variable Y. By substituting Y for Y^*, we obtain the estimator of the vector of regression parameters β

$$\hat{\boldsymbol{\beta}}^{\dagger} = \left(\mathbf{X}^{\top}\mathbf{X}\right)^{-1}\mathbf{X}^{\top}\mathbf{y};$$

$\mathbf{X}$ is composed of the intercept column $\mathbf{1}$ and the values of X, denoted by $\mathbf{x}$, and they are assumed to be fixed in replications.

Assuming the representation $Y = a + bY^{*} + cX + \delta$, as in (6.5), the bias of $\hat{\boldsymbol{\beta}}^{\dagger} = \left(\hat{\beta}_0^{\dagger}, \hat{\beta}_1^{\dagger}\right)^{\top}$ is

$$\mathrm{E}\left(\hat{\boldsymbol{\beta}}^{\dagger} \mid \mathbf{x}\right) - \boldsymbol{\beta} = \left(\mathbf{X}^{\top}\mathbf{X}\right)^{-1}\mathbf{X}^{\top}\mathrm{E}\left(a + by^{*} + cx \mid \mathbf{x}\right) - \boldsymbol{\beta}$$

$$= \left(\mathbf{X}^{\top}\mathbf{X}\right)^{-1}\mathbf{X}^{\top}\left\{a + (b-1)\beta_0\,\mathbf{1}, (b-1)\beta_1\mathbf{x} + c\mathbf{x}\right\}$$

$$= \left\{a + (b-1)\beta_0\,,\, c + (b-1)\beta_1\right\}\,.$$

Therefore, apart from the special case when $c + (b-1)\beta_1 = 0$, $\hat{\beta}_1^{\dagger}$ is unbiased for β_1 only when $b = 1$ and $c = 0$, that is, when Y is pointwise unbiased for Y^{*}. We are less concerned about the bias in estimating β_0 because that corresponds to adding the same (unknown) constant to each predicted value of Y^{*} and it does not affect any comparisons or differences of the predictions $\hat{Y}^{*}$ for different values of X. In any case, the additional condition for $\hat{\beta}_0^{\dagger}$ to be unbiased is that $a = 0$.

Denote by σ_{ε}^2 the residual variance in the regression of Y^{*} on X. The sampling variance matrix of $\hat{\boldsymbol{\beta}}^{\dagger}$ is

$$\mathrm{var}\left(\hat{\boldsymbol{\beta}}^{\dagger} \mid \mathbf{x}\right) = \left(\mathbf{X}^{\top}\mathbf{X}\right)^{-1}\mathbf{X}^{\top}\left(\sigma_{\delta}^2 + b^2\sigma_{\varepsilon}^2\right)\mathbf{I}\,\mathbf{X}\left(\mathbf{X}^{\top}\mathbf{X}\right)^{-1}$$

$$= \left(\sigma_{\delta}^2 + b^2\sigma_{\varepsilon}^2\right)\left(\mathbf{X}^{\top}\mathbf{X}\right)^{-1},$$

to be compared with $\sigma_{\varepsilon}^2\left(\mathbf{X}^{\top}\mathbf{X}\right)^{-1}$, its counterpart if the values of Y^{*} were recorded. It may seem paradoxical that the regression parameters could be estimated with smaller variance using the manifest than the latent outcome variable. This happens when $|b|$ is so small that $\sigma_{\delta}^2 + b^2\sigma_{\varepsilon}^2$ is smaller than σ_{ε}^2. On reflection, this is not a surprising result; when Y is dispersed much less than Y^{*}, its regression on X is estimated with smaller sampling variance than if it were widely dispersed. In any case, we should be concerned with MSEs of estimators, not with their variances. In this regard, $\hat{\beta}_1^{\dagger}$ fares much worse when β_1 is substantial because of the large bias $c + (b-1)\beta_1$.

In summary, when the variables X, Y^{*}, and Y are jointly normally distributed, naive estimation of the regression parameters in $\mathrm{E}(Y^{*} \mid X)$, based on a manifest variable Y, is unbiased when Y is pointwise unbiased for Y^{*}. Given choice, and other factors held fixed, manifest variables with smaller coefficients b are preferred, although with large samples the squared bias becomes the dominant contributor to MSE, and the proximity to pointwise unbiasedness, $b = 1$ and $c = 0$, becomes more important.

6.3.2 Latent Regression Variable

We consider next the problem of estimating the regression parameters in the linear model

$$\mathbf{y} = \mathbf{X}^*\boldsymbol{\beta} + \boldsymbol{\varepsilon}, \qquad\qquad (6.6)$$

with $\mathbf{X}^*$ comprising the intercept $\mathbf{1}$ and the values of the normally distributed latent variable X^* observed through its manifest version

$$X = a + bX^* + cY + \delta.$$

We assume that $\delta \sim \mathcal{N}(0, \sigma_\delta^2)$, independently of X^*, Y, and ε. We reuse the notation from the previous section, but the values of the associated quantities in the previous and this section are unrelated.

The model in (6.6) is not in accord with the assumption that the values of the latent variable X^* are fixed or set by design. (Setting the values of a latent variable is a logical contradiction.) Nonetheless, it is meaningful to consider the model as a description of how Y and X^* are related. The estimator of $\boldsymbol{\beta}$ in (6.6) with the substitute manifest variable is

$$\hat{\boldsymbol{\beta}}^\dagger = \left(\mathbf{X}^\top\mathbf{X}\right)^{-1}\mathbf{X}^\top\mathbf{y}.$$

Instead of considering the bias and MSE of this estimator, which cannot be expressed analytically, we study the crossproducts $\mathbf{X}^\top\mathbf{X}$ and $\mathbf{X}^\top\mathbf{y}$ separately. For the elements of $\mathrm{E}\left(\mathbf{X}^\top\mathbf{X}\,|\,\mathbf{x}^*\right) = \begin{pmatrix} A_1 & A_{12} \\ A_{12} & A_2 \end{pmatrix}$, we have

$$A_1 = n,$$

$$A_{12} = \mathrm{E}\left[\left\{\mathbf{X}^*\begin{pmatrix} a \\ b \end{pmatrix} + c\mathbf{X}^*\boldsymbol{\beta} + c\boldsymbol{\varepsilon} + \boldsymbol{\delta}\right\}^\top \mathbf{1}\,\Big|\,\mathbf{x}^*\right]$$

$$= \boldsymbol{\gamma}^\top\mathbf{X}^{*\top}\mathbf{1},$$

$$A_2 = \mathrm{E}\left[\left\{\mathbf{X}^*\boldsymbol{\gamma} + c\boldsymbol{\varepsilon} + \boldsymbol{\delta}\right\}^\top\left\{\mathbf{X}^*\boldsymbol{\gamma} + c\boldsymbol{\varepsilon} + \boldsymbol{\delta}\right\}\right]$$

$$= \boldsymbol{\gamma}^\top\mathbf{X}^{*\top}\mathbf{X}^*\boldsymbol{\gamma} + n\left(c^2\sigma_\varepsilon^2 + \sigma_\delta^2\right),$$

where $\boldsymbol{\gamma} = \{(a, b)^\top + c\boldsymbol{\beta}\}$ and $n = \mathbf{1}^\top\mathbf{1}$ is the sample size. Further,

$$\mathrm{E}\left(\mathbf{X}^\top\mathbf{y}\,|\,\mathbf{x}^*\right) = \left(\mathbf{1}\ \ \mathbf{X}^*\boldsymbol{\gamma}\right)^\top\mathbf{X}^*\boldsymbol{\beta}.$$

If $\mathbf{x}^*$ were available, the 'latent' counterparts of these objects would be $\mathbf{X}^{*\top}\mathbf{X}^*$ and

$$\mathbf{X}^*\,\mathrm{E}(\mathbf{y}\,|\,\mathbf{x}^*) = \mathbf{X}^{*\top}\mathbf{X}^*\boldsymbol{\beta}.$$

Apart from some esoteric settings, $\mathrm{E}\left(\mathbf{X}^\top\mathbf{y}\,|\,\mathbf{x}^*\right)$ and $\mathbf{X}^{*\top}\mathbf{y}$ coincide only when $a = 0$, $b = 1$, and $c = 0$, that is, when X is pointwise unbiased. The matrices

$\mathbf{X}^{*\top}\mathbf{X}^*$ and $\mathrm{E}\left(\mathbf{X}^\top\mathbf{X}\,|\,\mathbf{x}^*\right)$ differ even when X is pointwise unbiased for X^*; in that case,

$$\mathrm{E}\left(\mathbf{X}^\top\mathbf{X}\,|\,\mathbf{x}^*\right) = \mathbf{X}^{*\top}\mathbf{X}^* + \begin{pmatrix} 0 & 0 \\ 0 & n\sigma_\delta^2 \end{pmatrix}.$$

So, in expectation, the total of crossproducts $\mathbf{x}^\top\mathbf{x}$ is an inflated version of $\mathbf{x}^{*\top}\mathbf{x}^*$—the expected difference, $n\sigma_\delta^2$, is positive, unless the manifest and latent variables coincide.

In conclusion, except for some esoteric cases that are of no practical importance, the slope of the regression $\mathrm{E}(Y\,|\,X^*)$ is estimated with bias when X^* is replaced by a manifest variable X in the ordinary least squares estimator. In contrast, the slope of the regression $\mathrm{E}(Y^*\,|\,X)$ is estimated without bias, but with an inflated sampling variance, when Y is pointwise unbiased for Y^*. We note in passing that, even when we estimate the two factors, $\mathbf{X}^{*\top}\mathbf{X}^*$ and $\mathbf{X}^{*\top}\mathbf{y}$, without conditional bias (given $\mathbf{x}^*$), some bias arises due to the nonlinear operations applied in forming $\left(\mathbf{X}^\top\mathbf{X}\right)^{-1}\mathbf{X}^\top\mathbf{y}$.

Suppose manifest X is generated from latent X^* according to the pointwise unbiased model in (6.1). By centring X^*, we could arrange that $\mathbf{X}^{*\top}\mathbf{X}^*$ is diagonal. Then the substitution estimator of the slope, $\hat{\beta}_1^\dagger = \mathbf{x}^\top\mathbf{y}/\mathbf{x}^\top\mathbf{x}$, is likely to underestimate its target β_1, because the numerator estimates its latent counterpart $\mathbf{x}^{*\top}\mathbf{y}$ (conditionally on $\mathbf{y}$) without bias, whereas the denominator overestimates its positive target $\mathbf{x}^{*\top}\mathbf{x}^*$. This phenomenon, called *attenuation*, is addressed by subtracting the estimated bias from the denominator, that is, using $\mathbf{x}^\top\mathbf{x} - n\hat{\sigma}_\delta^2$. The resulting estimator $\mathbf{x}^\top\mathbf{y}/\left(\mathbf{x}^\top\mathbf{x} - n\hat{\sigma}_\delta^2\right)$ is unbiased only approximately, but the bias, arising from the nonlinear transformations, is negligible when the sample size is moderate or large.

Figure 6.1 gives an illustration with an artificially generated dataset. The outcomes are related to the latent covariate X^* by the simple regression $Y = \beta_0 + \beta_1 X^* + \varepsilon$, with $\beta_0 = 0.0$, $\beta_1 = 0.35$, and $\sigma^2 = 0.08$. The manifest variable X is generated according to the model $X = X^* + \delta$ with the deviations δ drawn at random from $\mathcal{N}(0, 0.30)$, independently of X^* and Y. In the left-hand panel, the 'latent' pairs (X^*, Y) are highlighted, with their fitted regression drawn by dashes, whereas in the right-hand panel the 'manifest' pairs (X, Y) are highlighted, with their regression marked by dots.

If we regard each value of X as an estimate of the underlying value X^*, then the results of this section can be interpreted as follows. When we would like to evaluate a function $g(\mathbf{x}^*; \mathbf{y})$, its manifest counterpart $g(\mathbf{x}; \mathbf{y})$ is suitable only when g is a linear function of $\mathbf{x}^*$. Substituting estimates for each value in $\mathbf{x}^*$ is not efficient, even if $g(\mathbf{x}^*)$ would have been efficient for the intended target. In the next section, we derive an estimator of $\mathbf{x}^*$ that differs from $\mathbf{x}$ but it is also poorly suited for naive estimation, as a substitute for $\mathbf{x}^*$.

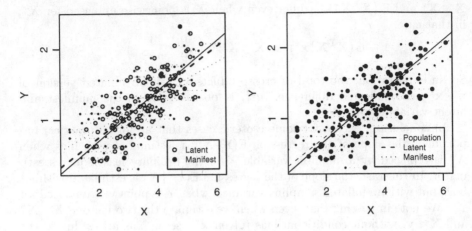

Fig. 6.1. Attenuation in simple regression. Latent values and the regression on them are highlighted in the left-hand panel and manifest values and their regression in the right-hand panel.

6.3.3 Estimating the Latent Values

Suppose the latent and its manifest variable have an arbitrary joint bivariate normal distribution

$$\begin{pmatrix} X^* \\ X \end{pmatrix} \sim \mathcal{N} \left\{ \begin{pmatrix} \mu^* \\ \mu \end{pmatrix}, \begin{pmatrix} \sigma_{x^*}^2 & \sigma_{x^*x} \\ \sigma_{x^*x} & \sigma_x^2 \end{pmatrix} \right\}.$$

The values of X^* can be estimated from their manifest counterparts as the conditional expectations $\hat{x}^* = \mathrm{E}(X^* \mid X = x)$. We have

$$\mathrm{E}(X^* \mid X = x) = \mu^* + \frac{\sigma_{x^*x}}{\sigma_x^2}(x - \mu),$$

with the (constant) conditional variance $\mathrm{var}(X^* \mid X = x) = \sigma_{x^*}^2 - \sigma_{x^*x}^2/\sigma_x^2$. For the model in (6.1), this is

$$\hat{x}^* = \mathrm{E}(X^* \mid X = x) = \mu + \frac{\sigma_{x^*}^2}{\sigma_{x^*}^2 + \sigma_\delta^2}(x - \mu). \tag{6.7}$$

In a practical setting, the parameters μ^*, $\sigma_{x^*}^2$, and $\sigma_\delta^2 = \mathrm{var}(\delta)$ are not known and have to be replaced by their estimates.

Suppose all our information about μ^*, σ^2, and σ_δ^2 is contained in the manifest values $\mathbf{x}$ for a random sample of n subjects. Then $\mathbf{x}$ are dispersed more widely than $\mathbf{x}^*$; $\mathrm{var}(X) = \mathrm{var}(X^*) + \sigma_\delta^2$. In contrast, the estimated values $\hat{x}^*$ are dispersed less;

$$\mathrm{var}(\hat{x}^* \mid x^*) = \frac{\sigma_{x^*}^4}{\sigma_{x^*}^2 + \sigma_\delta^2},$$

ignoring the fact that μ and the variances have to be estimated. The estimators in (6.7) can be interpreted as *shrinking* each manifest value $\mathbf{x}$ toward the population mean μ, or as combining two estimators of x^*, x and μ. The population mean μ is a trivial estimator, with bias $\mathrm{B}(\mu; x^*) = x^* - \mu$, so its mean MSE, after taking expectation of the squared bias, is $\sigma_{x^*}^2$. The manifest value has MSE σ_δ^2. The shrinkage estimator $\hat{x}^*$ combines these two estimators according to their precisions (reciprocals of MSEs).

We can estimate x^* so that the estimates would have the variance $\sigma_{x^*}^2$;

$$\tilde{x}^* = \mu + (x - \mu)\sqrt{\frac{\sigma_{x^*}^2}{\sigma_{x^*}^2 + \sigma_\delta^2}}$$

has this property but is less optimal for other purposes, including estimation of the individual values x^*. No single estimator is efficient for all targets related to x^*.

6.4 Categorical Manifest Variables

Suppose a categorical latent variable X^*, with support on the integers $1, 2, \ldots, H$, is observed through a manifest variable X with the same support. We say that X arises by misclassification of X^*. The misclassification process is described by the $(H \times H)$ *transition matrix* $\mathbf{T}$ comprising the elements $T_{h,h^*} = \mathrm{P}(X = h \mid X^* = h^*)$ for all pairs of integers h (row) and h^* (column) in $1, \ldots, H$. The rows of $\mathbf{T}$ add up to unity, $\mathbf{T1} = \mathbf{1}$, so $\mathbf{1}$ is a right-hand eigenvector of $\mathbf{T}$ and the corresponding eigenvalue is 1.0. As the eigenvectors that correspond to other right-hand eigenvalues are orthogonal to $\mathbf{1}$, all such eigenvectors $\mathbf{v}$ of $\mathbf{T}$ have zero totals; $\mathbf{v}^\top \mathbf{1} = 0$. Further let $\mathbf{p}^*$ be the distribution of X^*; its elements are the probabilities $p_h^* = \mathrm{P}(X^* = h^*)$. The manifest probabilities $\mathbf{p}$, with elements $p_h = \mathrm{P}(X = h)$, are related to the latent probabilities $\mathbf{p}_h^*$ by the identity

$$\mathbf{p} = \mathbf{Tp}^*.$$

The deviations $X - X^*$ and their variance are meaningful quantities only when the categories $1, \ldots, H$ are ordered, so that a deviation by one point is appropriately regarded as smaller than a deviation by two or more points. In misclassification processes of particular interest in such a setting, X and X^* do not differ by more than one point; the transition matrix has positive entries only on the diagonal and immediately below and above it.

To explore when $\mathbf{p} = \mathbf{p}^*$, we look for circumstances in which $\mathbf{p}^* = \mathbf{Tp}^*$, that is, when $\mathbf{p}^*$ is a right-hand eigenvector of $\mathbf{T}$ with unit eigenvalue. We consider a single category, 1, and collapse all the other categories into another single one, denoted by 2. Let the corresponding transition matrix be $\mathbf{T}'$, with elements T'_{hh^*}, $h, h^* = 1, 2$. A solution of the equation $\mathbf{p}^{*\prime} = \mathbf{T}'\mathbf{p}^{*\prime}$ has to be a scalar multiple of an eigenvector of $\mathbf{T}'$, that is, either $c\left(\frac{1}{2}, \frac{1}{2}\right)$ or $c\left(\frac{1}{2}, -\frac{1}{2}\right)$, where c is a nonzero constant. Only the former solution is admissible, because it has to comprise probabilities. Hence $p_h = p_h^*$ only when $p_h^* = \frac{1}{2}$. Furthermore, $T_{12}' = T_{21}'$. Therefore, the settings in which the manifest and latent variables have identical distributions are: $H = 2$, $\mathbf{p}^* = \frac{1}{2}\mathbf{1}$, and $\mathbf{T}$ symmetric; $T_{12} = T_{21}$.

Next we consider the discrete analogues of the regression. Suppose Z is a dichotomous variable with support on $(1, 2)$ and X^* is impartial for X with respect to Z, that is,

$$P(X = k \mid X^* = h, Z = z) = P(X = k \mid X^* = h) = T_{hk} \qquad (6.8)$$

for all possible combinations of categories h, k, and z. We explore when

$$P(X = 1 \mid Z = 1) = P(X^* = 1 \mid Z = 1).$$

By conditioning on the value of X^* and using the identity in (6.8), we obtain

$$P(X = 1 \mid Z = 1) = T_{11}P(X^* = 1 \mid Z = 1) + T_{12}P(X^* = 2 \mid Z = 1)$$
$$= T_{12} + P(X^* = 1 \mid Z = 1)(T_{11} - T_{12}).$$

Combined with the analogous equation for $P(X = 1 \mid Z = 2)$, this yields

$$P(X = 1 \mid Z = 1) - P(X = 1 \mid Z = 2)$$
$$= (T_{11} - T_{12})\{P(X^* = 1 \mid Z = 1) - P(X^* = 1 \mid Z = 2)\}$$
$$\leq T_{11} - T_{12},$$

with equality only when either $P(X = X^*) = 1$ or X^* and Z are independent. The latter case also requires that $T_{11} = T_{12}$, that is, $P(X = 1 \mid X^* = 1) = P(X = 1 \mid X^* = 2)$, or that X and X^* are independent. Thus, the contrast $P(X^* = 1 \mid Z = 1) - P(X^* = 1 \mid Z = 2)$ would be estimated by using X instead of X^* with bias, akin to attenuation, with any imperfect impartial manifest variable X, unless X^*, X, and Z are independent.

The substitution of X for X^* in the condition of the 'reverse' probability $P(Z = 1 \mid X^* = 1)$ can be explored similarly. Let

$$\Delta_* = P(Z = 1 \mid X^* = 1) - P(Z = 1 \mid X^* = 2)$$

and $\Delta_x = P(Z = 1 \mid X = 1) - P(Z = 1 \mid X = 2)$ its manifest version. The Bayes theorem implies that

$$P(Z = 1 \mid X = k) = P(X = k \mid Z = 1)\frac{P(Z = 1)}{P(X = k)},$$

$k = 1, 2$. We expand the conditional probability on the right-hand side and make use of impartiality to derive

$$P(Z = 1 \mid X = k) = P(Z = 1) \sum_{h=1}^{2} \frac{P(X = k \mid X^* = h)}{P(X = k)} P(X^* = h \mid Z = 1)$$

$$= P(Z = 1) \sum_{h=1}^{2} P(X^* = h \mid X = k) \frac{P(X^* = h \mid Z = 1)}{P(X^* = h)}$$

$$= \sum_{h=1}^{2} P(X^* = h \mid X = k) P(Z = 1 \mid X^* = h).$$

Hence the difference $\Delta_x - \Delta_*$ is equal to

$$P(Z = 1 \mid X^* = 1) \{ P(X^* = 1 \mid X = 1) - P(X^* = 1 \mid X = 2) - 1 \}$$
$$+ P(Z = 1 \mid X^* = 2) \{ P(X^* = 2 \mid X = 1) - P(X^* = 2 \mid X = 2) + 1 \}$$
$$= - \Delta_* \{ P(X^* = 2 \mid X = 1) + P(X^* = 1 \mid X = 2) \} .$$

Therefore, replacing X^* with X results in no change only when either X^* and Z are independent ($\Delta_* = 0$) or the classification is perfect:

$$P(X^* = 2 \mid X = 1) = P(X^* = 1 \mid X = 2) = 0,$$

that is, $\mathbf{T} = \mathbf{I}$; these are both trivial cases. In brief, there is no good substitute for a latent categorical variable.

6.5 Measurement Error as Incompleteness

Correction for attenuation in ordinary regression can be motivated as an application of the EM algorithm. In the E-step, we estimate the totals of the crossproducts that involve the latent variable, and in the subsequent M-step we apply the complete-data analysis, with these totals of crossproducts replaced by their estimates. The reference to the EM algorithm is not necessary in this application, but in others, in which the latent variable is involved in the analysis in more convoluted ways, or the measurement process is more complex than (6.1), the specification of the problem in terms of incomplete data can be very constructive.

We regard the values $(\mathbf{x}^*, \mathbf{x}, \mathbf{z})$ of (X^*, X, Z) on a sample of subjects as the complete data and the values of (X, Z) as the incomplete data. It is of no consequence that $\mathbf{x}$ is not involved in the complete-data analysis. If the complete-data analysis is by maximum likelihood and it involves the missing data $\mathbf{x}^*$ only through a short list of linear sufficient statistics, then the EM algorithm can be applied. Otherwise, sets of plausible values of $\mathbf{x}^*$ can be generated by multiple imputation (MI). The application is in general easier than for missing values because the process of 'nonresponse' (distortion) can be observed by replications of the measurement or, when circumstances permit, by recording the values of both X^* and X for some subjects.

For simplicity, we assume that X^* and X are independent across subjects, so that the MI method can be described in terms of univariate distributions. We observe, or posit, a model for the measurement process, given by conditional probabilities $P(X = x \mid X^* = x^*; \boldsymbol{\theta})$ or densities $f(x \mid X^* = x^*; \boldsymbol{\theta})$, usually involving one or several parameters $\boldsymbol{\theta}$. First a plausible vector $\tilde{\boldsymbol{\theta}}$ is drawn from the estimated sampling distribution of $\hat{\boldsymbol{\theta}}$. Then a set of plausible values, denoted by $\tilde{\mathbf{x}}^*$ to indicate that they differ from the values $\mathbf{x}^*$, is generated from the plausible conditional distribution $(X^* \mid X = x; \tilde{\boldsymbol{\theta}})$, derived by the Bayes theorem:

$$f\left(x^* \mid X = x; \tilde{\boldsymbol{\theta}}\right) = \frac{1}{f\left(x; \tilde{\boldsymbol{\theta}}\right)} \int f\left(x \mid \mathbf{X}^* = x^*; \tilde{\boldsymbol{\theta}}\right) f\left(x^*; \tilde{\boldsymbol{\theta}}\right) \, \mathrm{d}x^*$$

for continuous variables, and similarly, with the integral replaced by summation, for categorical variables. A set of plausible values $\tilde{\mathbf{x}}^*$ is based on one draw of $\tilde{\boldsymbol{\theta}}$, and other sets on replicates of such a draw. The number of these sets (completions) is denoted by M. The complete-data analysis is carried out for each completion $(\tilde{\mathbf{x}}^*, \mathbf{y}, \mathbf{z})$, yielding M (replicate) completed-data results, which are then averaged as in (5.5), with the appropriate inflation of the estimated sampling variance, which involves the between-imputation variance.

Example 13. As an illustration, we implement the method of MI for ordinary regression, with a single covariate X^* observed with the distortion given by (6.1). Further, we generate $r = 50$ pairs of replicate values of $X = X^* + \delta$, which we will regard as the sole information about $\sigma_\delta^2 = \mathrm{var}(\delta)$. Suppose these pairs are observed on units different from those involved in the regression. The solution derived in Section 6.3.2, by correcting for attenuation, is much more practical for this setting, but it gives us an opportunity to make a direct comparison with MI, which is applicable much more widely.

We generate a set of $n = 120$ values of the single regressor X^* and corresponding values of the outcome $Y = \beta_0 + \beta_1 X^* + \varepsilon$, with $\beta_0 = 0$, $\beta_1 = 0.35$, and $\sigma_\varepsilon^2 = 0.08$, as in Figure 6.1. We also set $\sigma_\delta^2 = 0.30$, to agree with the example in the diagram, but in all estimation we pretend that β_0, β_1, σ_ε^2, and σ_δ^2 are not known. We evaluate the estimator based on the latent values (this would in practice not be possible), based on the manifest values, with the measurement error ignored, with the correction for attenuation, using the estimated measurement-error variance $\hat{\sigma}_\delta^2$, and several MI estimators that we describe next.

Correction for attenuation implies generating plausible values of X^* from a plausible conditional distribution $(X^* \mid X)$. Thus, we generate plausible values of the variances σ_δ^2 and σ_x^2, followed by a plausible value of the mean μ_x of X^*. The distributional identity

$$r \frac{\hat{\sigma}_\delta^2}{\sigma_\delta^2} \sim \chi_r^2,$$

implies that for a random draw χ^2 from χ^2_r,

$$\tilde{\sigma}^2_\delta = r\frac{\hat{\sigma}^2_\delta}{\chi^2}$$

generates a plausible value of σ^2_δ. As $\mathrm{var}(X) = \sigma^2_* + \sigma^2_\delta$, a plausible value of σ^2_* can be obtained by adjusting the sample variance of X,

$$\widehat{\mathrm{var}}(X) = \frac{1}{n-1}\left(\mathbf{x}^\top\mathbf{x} - n\bar{x}^2\right).$$

For χ^2 drawn at random from χ^2_{n-1},

$$\tilde{\sigma}^2_* = (n-1)\frac{\widehat{\mathrm{var}}(X)}{\chi^2} - \tilde{\sigma}^2_\delta.$$

A plausible value of μ_x is generated by a random draw from $\mathcal{N}(\hat{\mu}_x, \tilde{\sigma}^2_* + \tilde{\sigma}^2_\delta)$. Having generated a plausible value of each parameter, a plausible value of x^*_j is generated as a random draw from its plausible distribution:

$$\tilde{x}^*_j \sim \mathcal{N}\left\{\tilde{\mu}_x + \frac{\tilde{\sigma}^2_*}{\tilde{\sigma}^2_* + \tilde{\sigma}^2_\delta}(x_j - \tilde{\mu}_x),\; \frac{\tilde{\sigma}^2_*\tilde{\sigma}^2_\delta}{\tilde{\sigma}^2_* + \tilde{\sigma}^2_\delta}\right\}.$$

The complete-data method is then applied to the completion $(\tilde{\mathbf{x}}^*, \mathbf{y})$, and the process of generating $\tilde{\sigma}^2_\delta$, $\tilde{\sigma}^2_*$, $\tilde{\mu}_x$, and $\tilde{\mathbf{x}}^*$, followed by the complete-data analysis of the completion, replicated $M - 1 = 9$ times. Finally, the ten sets of results are averaged, with the inflation of the sampling variance according to (5.10).

It may come as a surprise that this method yields rather disappointing results. Although the plausible values of $\mathbf{x}^*$ have the appropriate sampling variance, their covariance with Y is smaller (closer to zero) than it should be. The reason for this is that the outcomes Y contain information about X^*, and this is not reflected in how we generate plausible values of $\mathbf{x}^*$. Although the mechanisms for generating X and Y involve independent random terms, δ and ε, respectively, X and Y are correlated through their connection with X^*.

The problem can be resolved by generating plausible values of X^* from the conditional distribution $(X^* \mid X, Y)$. This is more complex because we have to work with a trivariate normal distribution, and it turns out that the conditional distribution of X^* involves the targets β_0, β_1, and σ^2.

The joint distribution of (X^*, X, Y) is

$$\begin{pmatrix} X^* \\ X \\ Y \end{pmatrix} \sim \mathcal{N}\left\{\begin{pmatrix} \mu_x \\ \mu_x \\ \beta_0 + \beta_1\mu_x \end{pmatrix},\; \begin{pmatrix} \sigma^2_* & \sigma^2_* & \beta_1\sigma^2_* \\ \sigma^2_* & \sigma^2_* + \sigma^2_\delta & \beta_1\sigma^2_* \\ \beta_1\sigma^2_* & \beta_1\sigma^2_* & \beta^2_1\sigma^2_* + \sigma^2_\varepsilon \end{pmatrix}\right\}.$$

$$(6.9)$$

Hence the conditional distribution of X^* given X and Y has expectation

$$\mathrm{E}(X^* \mid X, Y) = \mu_{\mathrm{x}} + \begin{pmatrix} \sigma_*^2 \\ \beta_1 \sigma_*^2 \end{pmatrix}^{\mathsf{T}} \boldsymbol{\Sigma}_{-1,-1}^{-1} \begin{pmatrix} X - \mu_{\mathrm{x}} \\ Y - \beta_0 - \beta_1 \mu_{\mathrm{x}} \end{pmatrix},$$

where $\boldsymbol{\Sigma}_{-1,-1}$ is the variance matrix in (6.9), with its first row and column removed. The corresponding conditional variance is

$$\mathrm{var}(X^* \mid X, Y) = \sigma_*^2 - \sigma_*^4 \begin{pmatrix} 1 \\ \beta_1 \end{pmatrix}^{\mathsf{T}} \boldsymbol{\Sigma}_{-1,-1}^{-1} \begin{pmatrix} 1 \\ \beta_1 \end{pmatrix}.$$

Elementary operations lead to the identities

$$\begin{pmatrix} 1 \\ \beta_1 \end{pmatrix}^{\mathsf{T}} \boldsymbol{\Sigma}_{-1,-1}^{-1} = \frac{1}{\sigma_*^2 \sigma_\varepsilon^2 + \beta_1^2 \sigma_\delta^2 \sigma_*^2 + \sigma_\delta^2 \sigma_\varepsilon^2} \begin{pmatrix} \sigma_\varepsilon^2 \\ \beta_1 \sigma_\delta^2 \end{pmatrix}$$

and

$$\begin{pmatrix} 1 \\ \beta_1 \end{pmatrix}^{\mathsf{T}} \boldsymbol{\Sigma}_{-1,-1}^{-1} \begin{pmatrix} 1 \\ \beta_1 \end{pmatrix} = \frac{\sigma_\varepsilon^2 + \beta_1^2 \sigma_\delta^2}{\sigma_*^2 \sigma_\varepsilon^2 + \beta_1^2 \sigma_\delta^2 \sigma_*^2 + \sigma_\delta^2 \sigma_\varepsilon^2}.$$

With these expressions, the sought conditional mean and variance are

$$\mathrm{E}\left(X^* \mid X, Y\right) = \mu_{\mathrm{x}} + \frac{1}{v} \left\{ X - \mu_{\mathrm{x}} + \beta_1 \frac{\sigma_\delta^2}{\sigma_\varepsilon^2} (Y - \beta_0 - \beta_1 \mu_{\mathrm{x}}) \right\},$$

$$\mathrm{var}\left(X^* \mid X, Y\right) = \frac{\sigma_\delta^2}{v},$$

where

$$v = 1 + \beta_1^2 \frac{\sigma_\delta^2}{\sigma_\varepsilon^2} + \frac{\sigma_\delta^2}{\sigma_*^2}.$$

As indicated earlier, these expressions involve β_0, β_1, and σ_ε^2, for which we only have biased estimators, derived by assuming that X and X^* coincide, that is, $\sigma_\delta^2 = 0$. (At this stage, we do not want to use the estimators derived by correcting for attenuation.)

We implement the following procedure in which MI is applied several times. First, we generate plausible values of β_0, β_1, and σ_ε^2 using the false assumption of no measurement error. With these (multiple sets of) values $\tilde{\beta}_0$, $\tilde{\beta}_1$, and $\tilde{\sigma}_\varepsilon^2$ and plausible values of the variances σ_*^2 and σ_δ^2, we generate (multiple sets of) plausible values of $\mathbf{x}^*$ and carry out the completed-data analyses, yielding, by averaging, provisional MI estimates and the associated estimates of the sampling variances.

From the results of this improperly applied MI, we generate plausible values of β_0, β_1, and σ_ε^2 and reuse the plausible values of σ_*^2 and σ_δ^2 to generate new sets of plausible values of X^*, carry out the completed-data analyses and average them, and obtain updated MI estimates and the associated estimates of the sampling variances. We could keep iterating this procedure until we reach stability, when the estimates are changed only slightly. However, it turns out that iterations of this procedure beyond the second or third yield only negligible improvements.

It remains to assess the efficiency of the various estimators. For this, we apply the estimators in a simulation study comprising $H = 1000$ replications. The H sets of replicate values of the estimates of β_0, $\beta_{1,}$, and σ_ε^2 are summarised by their empirical biases, sampling variances, and MSEs. We prefer to use the square roots of the latter two, to have them on the same scales (units of measurement) as the target and bias. Taking the square root of the sampling variance and MSE moderates their sizes, avoiding the printing of many decimal or trailing zeros.

The results are summarised in Table 6.1. The seven methods (sets of estimators) described in the caption of the table are compared. Each method estimates the intercept β_0, slope β_1, and the residual variance σ_ε^2. For each estimator $\hat{\theta}$, we calculate from its replicate values the empirical bias, $\hat{B}(\hat{\theta}; \theta)$, the square root of its sampling variance, $\sqrt{\widehat{\text{var}}(\hat{\theta})}$, and the root-MSE (rMSE). Further, for the intercept and slope, their sampling variances are estimated directly by the method applied, based on a single replication. The means of these quantities assess whether the method estimates the MSE without a negative bias. These figures, with the square root applied after averaging, are given in the table in row 'Internal rMSE'. The root-MSE is not listed for the residual variance for which it is of limited importance.

For example, the empirical bias of the complete-data estimator of the intercept is 0.001. We know that the estimator is unbiased, so the discrepancy of 0.001 can be attributed to chance, having executed 'only' 1000 replications. The discrepancy between the empirical and internal root-MSE, also by 0.001 (0.095 vs. 0.096), is negligible. The regression based on the manifest X (MAN), with the measurement error ignored, is grossly dishonest (0.027 vs. 0.089), a consequence of overrating the quality of the data. By correcting for attenuation (COR), we reduce the absolute bias substantially, but the standard errors are still grossly underestimated (0.027 vs. 0.046); they estimate without bias the standard errors of the complete-data estimators (LAT). The MI method MIx, which ignores the information about $\mathbf{x}^*$ contained in $\mathbf{y}$, performs very poorly. The iterative MI methods, $MI1$, $MI2$, and $MI3$, improve with iterations. Their biases and rMSEs are reduced substantially by the second iteration, and further iterations are not helpful; although the bias is reduced, the sampling variance is inflated slightly. $MI2$ and $MI3$ are honest—their internal and replication-based estimates of MSE agree. Based on this, we would recommend $MI2$ for settings similar to this example.

In all MI procedures, we used $M = 10$ completions. From Table 6.1, we can assess whether this would be sufficient. The sampling variance of the complete-data estimator of the slope is 0.027^2, whereas its counterpart in $MI2$,

Table 6.1. Summary of the simulations of several estimators for the simple regression model with measurement error. The methods are: *LAT*—using complete data (latent values); *MAN*—using manifest values, ignoring measurement error; *COR*—correction for attenuation; *MIx*—MI based on the conditional distribution $(X^* \mid X)$; *MIk*—MI based on the conditional distribution $(X^* \mid X, Y)$; k iterations, $k = 1, 2, 3$. Ten sets of plausible values are used in each MI procedure and 1000 replicates of each procedure.

	Method						
	LAT	*MAN*	*COR*	*MIx*	*MI*1	*MI*2	*MI*3
Intercept (β_0)							
$B(\hat{\beta}_0 ; \beta_0)$	0.001	0.294	−0.012	0.290	0.116	0.057	0.025
$\sqrt{\widehat{\mathrm{var}}(\hat{\beta}_0)}$	0.096	0.094	0.161	0.098	0.116	0.129	0.138
$\sqrt{\widehat{\mathrm{MSE}}(\hat{\beta}_0 ; \beta_0)}$	0.096	0.309	0.162	0.306	0.164	0.141	0.140
Internal rMSE	0.095	0.097	0.094	0.150	0.138	0.143	0.145
Slope (β_1)							
$B(\hat{\beta}_1 ; \beta_1)$	0.000	−0.085	0.004	−0.084	−0.033	−0.015	−0.007
$\sqrt{\widehat{\mathrm{var}}(\hat{\beta}_1)}$	0.027	0.026	0.046	0.027	0.033	0.037	0.039
$\sqrt{\widehat{\mathrm{MSE}}(\hat{\beta}_1 ; \beta_1)}$	0.027	0.089	0.046	0.088	0.047	0.040	0.040
Internal rMSE	0.027	0.027	0.027	0.042	0.039	0.040	0.041
Residual variance (σ_ε^2)							
$B(\hat{\sigma}_\varepsilon^2 ; \sigma_\varepsilon^2)$	−0.001	0.025	−0.003	0.047	0.015	0.008	0.004
$\sqrt{\widehat{\mathrm{var}}(\hat{\sigma}_\varepsilon^2)}$	0.010	0.014	0.017	0.016	0.014	0.014	0.014
$\sqrt{\widehat{\mathrm{MSE}}(\hat{\sigma}_\varepsilon^2 ; \sigma_\varepsilon^2)}$	0.010	0.029	0.017	0.050	0.021	0.016	0.015

0.040^2 is about $1.5^2 = 2.25$ times greater. Therefore, the between-imputation variance B is about $2.25/(1 + 1/10) \doteq 1.15$ times greater than the complete-data variance W, and the inflation of the variance due to using only $M = 10$ completions is about $0.11W$, that is, about 5% of the overall sampling variance $W + B(1 + 1/M)$. Another ten completions would cut this inflation to half, gaining very little, but the amount of programming and computing to achieve it is minute nevertheless.

This extended example may at first be discouraging, as it involves much computing. The appropriate gauge for such an assessment is always the value (gain, profit, or the like) of more efficient estimation and the better decision made as a result of the analysis. Note that most of the complexity is due to the generation of the plausible values $\tilde{\mathbf{x}}^*$; the complete-data analysis is elementary in comparison. However, for a more complex complete-data analysis, the same process of generating plausible values is required. In fact, the same set of completions could be used for several analyses. In our implementation, the completions are not stored, so it might be more practical to generate them separately for each analysis. The extra computational load is only slight; after all, we replicated the imputation and estimation processes 1000 times in the simulation.

Most of this computing should be done at the design stage to select a method of analysis and set its details. By doing so without having an opportunity to inspect the values of the outcome variable we forego any suspicions that the method of analysis has been selected to promote a particular result, confusing an estimator with a mixture of estimators. Also, if we prepare the computer programmes in advance of data collection the analysis can be completed soon after the data become available. In the process, the methods can be put to various tests regarding the assumptions made, in the spirit of sensitivity analysis (Section 5.5.4). The assumption of multivariate normality is particularly problematic, but experience shows that imputation methods perform reasonably well even with substantial departures from normality. For instance, in Example 13 we generated the values of X^* not from a normal distribution but as $2 + 3U^{1.1} + 0.4S$, where U has standard uniform and S standard normal distribution. The negative aspect of this approach is that the *real* data may inform us about a more efficient estimator than the one selected without the benefit of data inspection. However, such input into the analysis is tainted with the possibility of distortions in the inferences.

6.6 Simulation–Extrapolation

The method described in the previous section can be applied whenever we can estimate the relevant sampling distributions and draw samples from the conditional distributions involved. This is relatively easy when working with the multivariate normal distributions but much more complex otherwise, encouraging us to look for shortcuts which, although introducing some loss of efficiency, would make the programming and computational load manageable.

This section describes an alternative method that is also computationally intensive, but its programming is relatively easy, based on multiple applications of the complete-data method. It is not as universal as MI and involves very different complexities. To make the comparison easier, we discuss it using the setting of Example 13.

Suppose we know the value of the measurement-error variance σ_δ^2. We can fit the manifest regression $(Y \mid X)$, as done by method MAN in Table 6.1. We can increase the measurement-error variance by adding further distortion to X. The distorted variable $X' = X + \eta$, with $\eta \sim \mathcal{N}(0, \sigma_+^2)$ independently of X and Y, has measurement-error variance

$$\text{var}(X' \mid X^*) = \sigma_\delta^2 + \sigma_+^2.$$

We can fit manifest regression for a range of nonnegative values of σ_+^2 and observe, subject to the variation associated with generating the values of X', how the regression $\mathrm{E}(Y \mid X')$ depends on σ_+^2 or on the total measurement-error variance $\sigma_\delta^2 + \sigma_+^2$. The inferential question posed, translated to this perspective, is: what would the regression be if the measurement-error variance were equal to zero? Setting aside the uncertainty associated with the generation of the distorted sets of values $\mathbf{x}'$ for each selected value of σ_+^2, this amounts to extrapolation, because with the original observations $\mathbf{x}$ we can realise no measurement error with variance smaller than σ_δ^2.

For the selected positive values of σ_+^2, we generate several sets of values $\mathbf{x}'$, to reduce the impact of the vagaries of the additional distortion (from $\mathbf{x}$ to $\mathbf{x}'$). The method is known by the acronym $SimEx$, motivated by its two parts— simulation of estimates using manifest variables with extra measurement error and extrapolation to the setting of no measurement error.

An example implementing this method is drawn in Figure 6.2, using the setting of Example 13, with a computer-generated dataset, for which the latent values $\mathbf{x}^*$ are available. The variances σ_+^2 were set to 0.1, 0.2, 0.3, 0.4, and 0.5, and the process of generating $\mathbf{x}'$ and estimation with it was replicated 100 times for each value of σ_+^2. In panel A, each estimate of the slope β_1 is represented by a dot and the mean within each value of the overall measurement-error variance $\sigma_\delta^2 + \sigma_+^2$ by a dash. The target β_1, which corresponds to σ_δ^2, is marked by a thin horizontal line. The estimate $\hat{\beta}_1$ based on the latent values is marked by the black box. The panel suggests that the task of extrapolation is difficult because of the curvature involved.

Panel B presents the same information, except that the vertical axis is on the reciprocal scale, plotting $1/\hat{\beta}_1$. Extrapolation is now straightforward, because the dependence of $1/\mathrm{E}(\hat{\beta}_1)$ on σ_+^2 is linear. Usefulness of the transformation becomes obvious when we examine how the correction for attenuation works. The regression slope is estimated as

$$\hat{\beta}_1^{(c)} = \frac{(\mathbf{x} - \bar{x}\mathbf{1})^\top (\mathbf{y} - \bar{y}\mathbf{1})}{(\mathbf{y} - \bar{y}\mathbf{1})^\top (\mathbf{y} - \bar{y}\mathbf{1}) - n\sigma_\delta^2} .$$

Hence

$$\frac{1}{\hat{\beta}_1^{(c)}} = \frac{(\mathbf{y} - \bar{y}\mathbf{1})^\top (\mathbf{y} - \bar{y}\mathbf{1})}{(\mathbf{x} - \bar{x}\mathbf{1})^\top (\mathbf{y} - \bar{y}\mathbf{1})} - \frac{n\sigma_\delta^2}{(\mathbf{x} - \bar{x}\mathbf{1})^\top (\mathbf{y} - \bar{y}\mathbf{1})} ,$$

so long as the denominator (covariance) differs from zero. Therefore, for fixed $\mathbf{x}$ and $\mathbf{y}$, $1/\hat{\beta}_1^{(c)}$ is a linear function of the measurement-error variance σ_δ^2.

Panel C displays the results for estimating the residual variance σ_ε^2. The extrapolation on the original scale is just as difficult as for the slope β_1, but now there is no obvious transformation of the estimates $\hat{\sigma}_\varepsilon^2$ that would simplify the task. Panel D shows that taking the reciprocal is not helpful. A suitable transformation can be found by inverting the formula for the estimator of the residual variance.

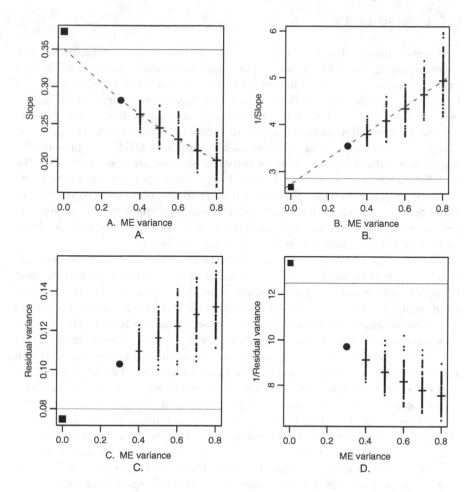

Fig. 6.2. Illustration of the SimEx method on the setting of Example 13 (simple regression with $\beta = (0, 0.35)^{\top}$, $\sigma_{\varepsilon}^2 = 0.08$, and $\sigma_{\delta}^2 = 0.30$). Estimating the slope β_1 (the top panels) and the residual variance σ_{ε}^2 (bottom panels).

The SimEx method is restricted on several counts. First, the simulation part can be implemented only with measurement processes with which **x** can be made more distorted. Next, the extrapolation task is in general difficult, and a suitable transformation to make it easier is not always easy to identify. Finally, the selection of the parameter values at which simulation is conducted is not obvious either, although much can be accomplished by trial and error. Extrapolation in problems with two or more dimensions is particularly challenging.

6.7 Coarse Data

The questionnaire design of many surveys has to strike a delicate balance between asking for a lot of detail and minimising the response burden. For example, a survey of annual household income may ask the subjects (heads of households) for the relevant details from their tax returns, for rounded figures (say, in thousands of UK£) for income from various sources (employment, self-employment, pensions, rents, savings, sales of property, and the like), for a single figure (total, also rounded to thousands of UK£), or present the respondent with a small number of response options, such as below £10 000, £10 000–19 999, ..., and above £100 000. The last response format represents the least response burden. Subjects are more likely to respond to it and less likely to be discouraged from responding to further questions. However, the response is poorer for information content than the response to one of the more detailed questions would be *if* all subjects responded.

We can regard the process that distorts the exact (ideal) household income, as would be declared for the given year on the tax return(s) in good faith, into an income category as *coarsening*. It is a process akin to measurement error, except that, conditionally on the ideal value X^*, it entails no randomness. Since it has a deterministic description, we refer to this process as a mechanism. The original variable has been *coarsened*, and the resulting variable is said to be *coarse*. In general, a coarsening mechanism applied to a variable X^* is defined as any known function on the support of X^*. One-to-one and constant functions are trivial cases of coarsening. One-to-one functions correspond to no coarsening; the original values of X^* can be recovered by the inverse transformation. Constant functions annihilate all the information about the original variable; they represent the other extreme. Nontrivial coarsening mechanisms for categorical variables correspond to aggregation of some categories. For example, the number of political parties represented on the city councils of a country may be recoded to three categories: one party, two parties, and more than two parties.

For continuous variables, a wide variety of coarsening mechanisms can be conceived, but those of any practical importance can be described as follows. A (finite or infinite) ordered set of *cut points* $c_1 \leq c_2 \leq \ldots \leq c_H$ is defined, complemented with $c_0 = -\infty$ and $c_{H+1} = +\infty$ or the respective minimum and maximum of the support. The values c_h, $h = 1, \ldots, H$, are such that no three of them are identical; that is, no pair of successive inequalities are both 'equal to'. Each interval $[c_h; c_{h+1})$ for which $c_h < c_{h+1}$ is associated with a *typical value* v_h such that $c_h \leq v_h < c_{h+1}$; when $c_h = c_{h+1}$ we set $v_h = c_h$. The intervals $[c_h; c_{h+1})$ are sometimes referred to as *bins* and the corresponding coarsening process as *binning*.

A coarsening mechanism f_1 is said to be *cruder* than another coarsening mechanism f_2 if the result of applying f_1 is equivalent to the application of f_2 followed by another coarsening mechanism, say, f_3; that is, $f_1 = f_3(f_2)$. For continuous variables, the cut points of a cruder mechanism are a subset of the cut points of the finer (less crude) mechanism. Crudest mechanisms, for which there are no nontrivial cruder mechanisms, result in a binary variable, defined by a single cut point.

Histograms are perhaps the most common examples of coarsening. The impact of coarsening of a variable is easy to explore. Too little coarsening leaves details in the histogram that obscure the main features of the distribution, whereas too much coarsening obliterates some of the important features.

The cut points and typical values of a coarsening mechanism are usually set by design and are always known. The population (and therefore the sample) may be partitioned into strata and a different coarsening mechanism applied in each stratum. We regard such a composition of coarsening mechanisms also as a single coarsening mechanism, so long as the stratum is known for each subject. One of the constituent mechanisms in such a composition may involve no coarsening. For example, some subjects in a survey of diet may provide exact details of all the food and drink they consume in a designated week, whereas others indicate the quantities by the coarse response options provided in the questionnaire.

A coarse variable X is often regarded in an analysis as if it were the original variable X^*—the distortion by coarsening is ignored. It is easy to show that this is inappropriate, for any choice of the typical values v_h. A choice that is suitable for one analysis, such as estimating the population mean of X^*, is poorly suited for another, such as estimating its variance. The typical values can be regarded as estimates of the original values, and the (average) efficiency of such estimation is not closely related to the efficiency of the completed-data analyses conducted with them.

The original variable may be observable in principle, such as the income reported on the tax return, or it may not be. An example of the latter case is the level of satisfaction with a particular service. It can be thought of as being on a continuum, but its recording is practical only with a discrete ordinal scale, such as the *Likert scale*, in which the extreme categories 1 and 5 represent total dissatisfaction and full satisfaction, respectively, category 3 is neutral (neither satisfied nor dissatisfied), and categories 2 and 4 represent intermediate levels of (dis-)satisfaction. The Likert scale can be used for questions about preference, level of agreement, willingness to take part in an activity, and the like. Of course, in most such cases the cut points defining the coarsening are not known, because the original variable is not defined. It may be defined by reference to the cut points, but its values are usually impossible to establish.

6.7.1 Inference with Coarse Variables

We assume that the complete-data analysis involves the original variable and adopt the strategy of Section 6.5. We generate several sets of plausible values of the original variable and apply the complete-data analysis to each of them.

We consider the simplest nontrivial setting in which only one (coarsened) variable is recorded.

Let the density of the original (continuous) variable X^* be f and the corresponding distribution function F; they may involve some unknown parameters $\boldsymbol{\theta}$. The definition of coarsening implies that

$$P(X = v_h; \boldsymbol{\theta}) = F(c_{h+1}; \boldsymbol{\theta}) - F(c_h; \boldsymbol{\theta}).$$

Therefore, estimation of $\boldsymbol{\theta}$ entails matching the sample distribution of X with the probabilities $F(c_{h+1}; \boldsymbol{\theta}) - F(c_h; \boldsymbol{\theta})$.

The conditional density of X^* given the value v_h of its coarse version X is

$$f(x^* \mid X = v_h) = \frac{f(x^*)}{P(X = v_h; \boldsymbol{\theta})}, \tag{6.10}$$

for $x^* \in (c_h, c_{h+1})$. Thus, we require methods for drawing random samples from such distributions. This may involve some approximations.

When the interval (c_h, c_{h+1}) is narrow enough that the density in it is well approximated by a constant, the conditional distribution in (6.10) is uniform and drawing samples from it is simple. The corresponding unconditional distribution has a piecewise constant density. Such a distribution of X^* may be unrealistic, but any smooth continuous distribution (density) can be approximated arbitrarily closely by such distributions (densities).

Suppose both c_0 and c_{H+1} are finite. The distribution of X^* can then be approximated by the distribution of the mixture

$$U = \sum_{h=0}^{H} I_h U_h,$$

where each variable U_h has a uniform distribution in the interval $[c_h; c_{h+1})$ and I_h is the multinomial indicator of the category: $I_h = 1$ if $X^* \in [c_h; c_{h+1})$ and $I_h = 0$ otherwise. Let $p_h = P(I_h = 1)$. Then for distinct cut points $h_1 \neq h_2$, $\text{cov}(I_{h_1}, I_{h_2}) = -p_{h_1} p_{h_2}$, because the categories (bins) are disjoint. The expectation and variance of U are

$$E(U) = \sum_{h=0}^{H} p_h \, E(U_h),$$

$$\text{var}(U) = \sum_{h=0}^{H} p_h \, \text{var}(U_h) + \sum_{h=0}^{H} p_h \left\{ E(U_h) - E(U) \right\}^2. \tag{6.11}$$

Before proving these identities, we discuss what they imply. The result for the expectation is natural and suggests that we should choose the midpoints as the typical values, that is, set v_h to the conditional expectation within bin h, and in the absence of any substantial asymmetry, set $v_h = \frac{1}{2}(c_{h+1} + c_h)$. If we do so, then the result for the variance indicates that the variance of the coarse variable, the second summation on the right-hand side, is smaller than the variance of the original variable by the weighted total of the within-interval variances. Thus, in addition to smoothness, the dispersion of the distribution of X^* is also distorted by coarsening.

The expectation in (6.11) follows from the linearity of the expectation and independence of I_h and U_h. We decompose the variance first as

$$\mathrm{var}(U) = \sum_{h=0}^{H} \mathrm{var}(I_h\,U_h) + 2 \sum_{h_1=0}^{H} \sum_{h_2=0}^{h_1-1} \mathrm{cov}\,(I_{h_1}\,U_{h_1}\,,I_{h_2}\,U_{h_2})\,. \qquad (6.12)$$

For each variance on the right-hand side, we use the identity

$$\mathrm{var}(I_h\,U_h) = \mathrm{E_I}\,\{\mathrm{var}(I_h\,U_h\,|\,I_h)\} + \mathrm{var_I}\,\{\mathrm{E}(I_h\,U_h\,|\,I_h)\}$$
$$= p_h\,\mathrm{var}(U_h) + p_h\,(1-p_h)\{\mathrm{E}(U_h)\}^2\,,$$

where the subscript I denotes expectation or variance over the distribution of I_h. Each covariance in (6.12) is equal to the negative product of the expectations

$$\mathrm{cov}\,(I_{h_1}\,U_{h_1}\,,I_{h_2}\,U_{h_2}) = -p_{h_1}\,\mathrm{E}(U_{h_1})\,p_{h_2}\,\mathrm{E}(U_{h_2})\,,$$

because $\mathrm{E}(I_{h_1}\,I_{h_2}) = \mathrm{P}(I_{h_1}\,I_{h_2} = 1) = 0$. With these identities for the variances and covariances, we have

$$\mathrm{var}(U) = \sum_{h=0}^{H} p_h\,\mathrm{var}(U_h) + \sum_{h=0}^{H} p_h(1-p_h)\,\{\mathrm{E}(U_h)\}^2$$
$$- 2 \sum_{h_1=0}^{H} \sum_{h_2=0}^{h_1-1} p_{h_1}\,\mathrm{E}(U_{h_1})\,p_{h_2}\,\mathrm{E}(U_{h_2})$$
$$= \sum_{h=0}^{H} p_h\,\mathrm{var}(U_h) + \sum_{h=0}^{H} p_h\{\mathrm{E}(U_h)\}^2 - \left\{\sum_{h=0}^{H} p_h\,\mathrm{E}(U_h)\right\}^2\,,$$

from which the second identity in (6.11) follows immediately.

Working with the uniform conditional distributions is very easy because plausible values of X^* are generated directly, without having to generate any plausible parameters, as implied by (6.10). The conditional distributions can be approximated alternatively by distributions with linear densities,

$$f(x) = a_h + b_h\,\frac{x - c_h}{c_{h+1} - c_h}\,,$$

$$f(x) = a_h + b_h\,\frac{c_{h+1} - x}{c_{h+1} - c_h}\,,$$

for constants a_h and b_h, for which $f(x)$ is a density. However, estimating such densities or choosing among them is in general not straightforward.

When a class of distributions is specified for X^* and we do not want to apply any approximations, the distribution (or the parameters it involves) can be estimated by the *method of moments*. The method looks for a match of the expectation of X^* and possibly other summaries of the distribution, such as the variance, with its estimate based on (6.11) and similar identities. For example, the expectation of X^* is estimated as

$$\hat{\mu}^* = \sum_{h=0}^{H} \hat{p}_h v_h, \qquad (6.13)$$

where $\hat{p}_h$ is the fraction of the sample with observations in the interval $[c_h, c_{h+1})$. In this formula, the typical values v_h can be replaced by the estimated or approximated conditional expectations. The method can be used iteratively as follows. Starting with (6.13), we estimate $E(U_h)$ from $\hat{\mu}^*$ using (6.10); this may involve numerical integration or sampling from the relevant conditional distribution. Then we re-estimate μ^* using (6.13), with v_h replaced by the estimates of $E(U_h)$. The iterations are terminated when convergence is achieved. This should not take more than a few iterations.

When the variance of the (normal) distribution of X^* is not known either, it can be estimated similarly, using the second equation in (6.11). This is somewhat more complex because of the intervening term $\sum_h p_h \text{var}(U_h)$. We may start by evaluating $\text{var}(U_h)$ for the uniform distribution. This implies a moment matching estimate of $\text{var}(U)$, which can then be used to update $\text{var}(U_h)$, as well as the expectations $E(U_h)$ and $E(U)$. In fact, estimation of the expectation and variance of U should be meshed in one; that is, one iteration of moment matching should update estimates of both $E(U_h)$ and $\text{var}(U_h)$ for all h.

Note that a sample distribution of X, given by the proportions $\hat{p}_h$, can strongly contradict a particular distributional assumption about X^*. For example, a distinctly bimodal categorical variable X cannot be a rounded version of a normally distributed variable X^*.

6.7.2 Bootstrap

Finally, we discuss estimation of the sampling variance of the parameters associated with X^*. We apply a general method called *bootstrap*, which is based on repeated applications of the estimator to samples drawn from the original sample. Suppose the observations x_j, $j = 1, \ldots, n$, are independent and n is sufficiently large. Bootstrap proceeds by the following steps. First draw a simple random sample of size n, with replacement, from the n observed units and apply the estimator(s) on this sample, resulting in estimate $\hat{\theta}^{(1)}$. Replicate this process (sampling and estimation) to obtain a large number (M) of so-called *bootstrap* replicate estimates $\hat{\theta}^{(m)}$, $m = 1, \ldots, M$. The bias and sampling variance of the estimator $\hat{\theta}$ are estimated by their sample versions evaluated on the bootstrap replicates:

Table 6.2. Summary of the annual income in a survey. Monetary values are in thousands of Euros. Sample size $n = 12\,000$.

	Income category (thousand Euros)							
From	0	10	20	30	40	50	75	100
To	10	20	30	40	50	75	100	$+\infty$
Typical value	5	15	25	35	45	62.5	87.5	200
Subjects	43	1347	3068	2890	1943	2081	470	158

$$\hat{B}\left(\hat{\theta};\theta\right) = \hat{\theta} - \bar{\hat{\theta}}\,,$$

$$\widehat{\mathrm{var}}\left(\hat{\theta}\right) = \frac{1}{M-1}\sum_{m=1}^{M}\left(\hat{\theta}^{(m)} - \bar{\hat{\theta}}\right)^2,$$

where $\bar{\hat{\theta}} = \left(\hat{\theta}^{(1)} + \cdots + \hat{\theta}^{(M)}\right)/M$. Bootstrap is an example of applying the computer's power and speed to make up for our analytical inadequacies.

Example 14. A survey of the annual income of the labour force of a European country in year 2003 concluded with the summary given in Table 6.2. We describe how a set of plausible values of the income is generated based on this table. The coarse variable, with eight categories and typical values given in the third row of the table, has sample mean 40 708 Euro and sample standard deviation 25 591 Euro.

We assume that the values of income have a log-normal distribution. This assumption is often well supported for variables in monetary units, such as house prices, income, the values of assets and liabilities of companies, and the like. Thus, the logarithm of the income is assumed to be normally distributed. We estimate the mean and standard deviation of this distribution by maximising the log-likelihood

$$\log(n!) - \sum_{h=0}^{H}\log(n_h!) + \sum_{h=0}^{H} n_h \log\left\{\Phi\left(\frac{c_{h+1} - \mu}{\sigma}\right) - \Phi\left(\frac{c_h - \mu}{\sigma}\right)\right\}, \quad (6.14)$$

where n_h are the counts in Table 6.2, Φ is the distribution function of the standard normal distribution, and $\mathcal{N}(\mu,\sigma^2)$ is our target, the original normal distribution. We can ignore $\log(n!)$ and the first summation in (6.14), which do not involve the parameters μ and σ. The remainder is relatively easy to evaluate, yet its derivative is not. We therefore search for the maximum by evaluating the log-likelihood over a grid of values of μ and σ, locate the provisional maximum, and then refine the grid, find the maximum on it, and continue until the grid is so fine that the maximum is located with sufficient precision. We start with the values $\mu = 10.4, 10.41, \ldots, 10.5$ and

Table 6.3. Estimates of the conditional means and standard deviations within the eight income categories indicated in Table 6.2. Based on the uniform and the fitted normal distribution on the log-scale.

	Income category (thousand Euros)							
From	0	10	20	30	40	50	75	100
To	10	20	30	40	50	75	100	$+\infty$
Means $\hat{E}(U_h)$								
Uniform	—	9.616	10.127	10.463	10.714	11.043	11.379	—
ML fit	9.065	9.695	10.128	10.453	10.704	10.989	11.342	11.676
Standard deviations $\sqrt{\widehat{\text{var}}(U_h)}$								
Uniform	—	0.200	0.117	0.083	0.064	0.117	0.083	—
ML fit	0.135	0.164	0.114	0.083	0.064	0.113	0.080	0.149

$\sigma = 0.40, 0.41, \ldots, 0.50$ and find that the maximum value of the log-likelihood is attained for $\mu = 10.46$ and $\sigma = 0.47$. In the second round, we evaluate the log-likelihood in the range 10.45–10.47 for μ and 0.46–0.48 for σ, finding the provisional maximum at $\mathcal{N}(10.464, 0.470^2)$. By the next round, we conclude the search at $\mathcal{N}(10.4643, 0.4696^2)$; the attained maximum, equal to $-20\,877.91$ (with the functions of the factorials in (6.14) omitted), is of no importance on its own but is useful for comparisons with the log-likelihood at other points (μ, σ).

The fitted log-normal distribution has expectation 39 126 and standard deviation 19 437; see Section A.10.1 for the relevant formulae. Given the sample size, this is a substantial change from the sample mean and standard deviation of the coarse variable X, which are unduly affected by the typical values set for the extreme bins.

Table 6.3 gives the within-category (conditional) means and standard deviations based on the uniform distribution and the maximum likelihood fit. It shows that the uniform distribution fits well in the mid-range of the values but is problematic near the tails. In fact, uniform distributions cannot be fitted to the extreme categories because they both correspond to infinite intervals on the log scale.

For generating a set of plausible values of income, we require an estimate of the sampling distribution of the estimator of $\left[E\{\log(X^*)\}, \sqrt{\text{var}\{\log(X^*)\}} \right]$. This we obtain by bootstrap. We replicate 1000 times the processes of resampling from the sample given in Table 6.2 and estimation by iterated moment matching. The mean of the bootstrap estimates is (10.4643, 0.4696) for the mean and standard deviation, respectively. It agrees with the maximum likelihood estimate to four decimal places, indicating that the bias of the moment-matching estimator is small or none. The bootstrap estimates of the standard errors are 0.00451 and 0.00338. The former figure can readily be translated to the original scale. As $\exp(1 + \alpha) = \alpha$ when $|\alpha|$ is small, it indicates that the standard error corresponds to approximately 0.45% of the mean. The pairs of bootstrap replicate estimates are correlated very weakly, so plausible values of the mean and standard deviation can be generated independently. The bootstrap replicates can be plotted to check that their distribution is very close to (bivariate) normality; we omit the details to conserve space. To conclude, plausible parameters of the log-normal distribution are drawn from the bivariate normal distribution with mean $(10.4643, 0.4696)^\top$ and variance matrix $10^{-6} \begin{pmatrix} 4.51^2 & 0 \\ 0 & 3.38^2 \end{pmatrix}$.

Having fitted a complete-data distribution using, in essence, an unverified assumption of log-normality, we can now look back and assess whether the fitted, or indeed, plausible, distributions are realistic for the observed distribution of the coarse variable given in Table 6.2. A method based on hypothesis testing compares the observed proportions $\hat{p}_h$ with the fitted probabilities $\hat{r}_h = F(c_{h+1}; \hat{\boldsymbol{\theta}}) - F(c_h; \hat{\boldsymbol{\theta}})$, where F is the distribution function of the fitted log-normal distribution, the exponential transform of $\mathcal{N}(10.4643, 0.4696)$. The test statistic is

$$\sum_{h=0}^{H} n_h \frac{(\hat{p}_h - \hat{r}_h)^2}{\hat{r}_h}, \tag{6.15}$$

and under the hypothesis that the distribution given by F does generate the proportions $\hat{r}_h$ it has, asymptotically, the χ^2 distribution with H degrees of freedom. The approximation due to asymptotics is not a problem in this instance ($n = 12\,000$), but, asymptotically, most hypotheses of special cases are rejected because the test has a very high power and detects even a minute deviation from the hypothesis. In our case, the value of the test statistic is 1.15, and it would be compared with the 0.95-quantile of χ^2_7, equal to 14.1. The fit is extremely good. The largest contribution to (6.15) is 0.49 for category 30 000–40 000 Euro, for which the recorded count is 1943 and the fit is 1974.

A more suitable method is based on generating datasets from the fitted distribution; see Section 1.3.1. We replicate this process 19 times, creating, together with the recorded table of counts, a 20×8 matrix of counts. A set of such counts is displayed in Figure 6.3, with the realised counts drawn by thick dashes. The counts are on the log scale to reduce their disparities. The realised counts do not stand out, so we have found no contradiction with the assumption of log-normality.

It may at first appear that a rather extravagant amount of computing is involved in this example. The amount and intricacy of programming might be a better gauge of the analytic effort. In any case, modern computers and software are very efficient. All the computing for this example took about 20 seconds on a laptop computer. Of course, the programming took much longer, but the expenditure of time (a few hours) is minor in comparison with the

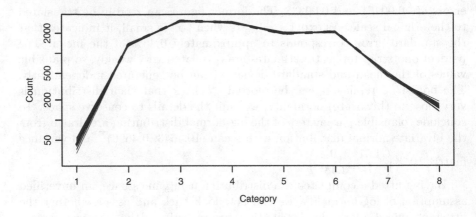

Fig. 6.3. The realised and simulated counts in Example 14. The realised counts are drawn by thick dashes (largely obscured).

effort of collecting the data and the importance of the inferences made based on numerous analyses planned to be conducted with the survey data.

Suggested Reading

The subject of imperfect measurement, with normally distributed distortions in particular, is treated comprehensively by [54]. Impartiality is defined and motivated and its importance in clinical trials discussed in [149]. The SimEx method was introduced by [23]. A practically oriented textbook on measurement errors for more complex models is [15]; it deals with SimEx extensively. Classic texts on the methods for latent and manifest variables in psychometrics (assessment of mental skills) are [130] and [29]. A collection of applications in educational testing, some of them dealing with distortion due to the subjective nature of the assessment, is presented in [115]. Methods for coarse data are reviewed by [73], and [75] presents an original example that studies the uncertainty brought about by coarsening. Studying the impact of rounding in an analysis has a very long history; the so-called Sheppard's correction is attributed to [182]. Another reference of historical importance is [47]. In the literature, coarse data are often referred to as *grouped* data.

Censored data arise when the time of an event is not recorded with precision but is known to have exceeded a recorded limit (e.g., the time when the study was concluded). Such data can be regarded as coarsened so that the latent value is recorded whenever censoring is not applied and is in a special 'bin' otherwise. There is an extensive literature on censored data, especially in connection with survival analysis. A seminal paper on survival analysis is

[26]; [91] and [28] are standard texts on the subject that have withstood the passage of time. A comprehensive reference to bootstrap is [46].

Problems and Exercises

6.1. A study is planned in which the outcome variable will be recorded on a simple random sample from a large population with a known positive measurement-error variance σ_e^2. The measurement process is pointwise unbiased. Suppose each measurement involves a unit cost. Show that the population mean of the variable is estimated with greater precision if a single measurement is applied on a sample of Kn subjects than K replicate measurements on each of a sample of n subjects. Revise this conclusion if the second and consecutive replicates involve a lower unit cost, say, by $Q\%$, and the same overall funds are available in each scenario.

6.2. A study intends to collect information about a (latent) variable X^*. Options for the measurement of X^* include a so-called gold standard, which establishes the value of X^* with precision, but the largest sample size that such a study could afford is n_0. With a different instrument, the sample size $n_1 > n_0$ could be afforded, but the measurement process, although pointwise unbiased, would have the variance σ_1^2. With a third instrument, $n_2 > n_1$ observations could be afforded, but the measurement process has variance σ_2^2 and its bias is known to be in the range $(-B, B)$. The positive constants B, σ_1^2, and σ_2^2 are known, as is the population variance $\sigma_*^2 = \text{var}(X^*)$. Which instrument would you select (and in what circumstances) for estimating the population mean of X^*?

6.3. Implement the general solution of the problem in Exercise 6.1 in a computer programme and expand it in the following direction. The measurement variances are not known and would be estimated by replications of the measurement process on a random sample of subjects. This would be done in advance, and its results would inform the design of the study. You may have some idea of the size of the variances (say, in the form of a plausible range for each of them). Experiment with allocation of resources to the replicate measurements and the study proper; the measurements made in the replications may entail the same costs as the measurements with the same instrument in the study proper, or they can be somewhat cheaper (e.g., by 20%).

6.4. A professional organisation has a test that is administered to the applicants for a particular licence. Suppose the test scores are pointwise unbiased and impartial for the ability or skill that is meant to be assessed. Suppose the organisation decides to permit appeals. An applicant can re-sit for the test once if he or she presents a credible explanation for the poor performance. There are several options for how to score the responses from the second test (the re-sit):

1. the first score is ignored;
2. the better of the two scores is adopted;
3. an a priori set 'penalty' is subtracted from the score of the re-sit.

Discuss what happens to the properties of pointwise unbiasedness and impartiality when one of these scoring schemes is adopted. In this setting, relate the idea of 'fairness' to impartiality. Do they represent the same property?

6.5. Consider the following variation of Example 12 in Chapter 5. Whenever a value of X is missing an alternative (second-rate) measurement of X, denoted by X', is made. The variables X' and X are related by the model

$$X' = X + \delta$$

with δ distributed according to $\mathcal{N}(0, \sigma_x^2)$; see (6.1). Similarly, a substitute measurement Y' is made whenever Y is not observed and Y' is related to Y by an analogous model, with a different measurement-error variance σ_y^2. Discuss how the substitute measurements could be used for estimating the regression $E(Y \mid X)$ and implement the procedure for a simulated or real dataset. (You may use a real dataset, but delete some observations in it and replace them by simulated values of X' and Y'.)

6.6. *Transformed measurement-error processes.* Suppose a manifest variable X is related to its latent version X^* by the pointwise unbiased model (6.1), with the usual assumptions of normality and independence. Suppose the target variable is a monotone transformation of X^*, $g(X^*)$. For a variety of functions g (logarithm, power, a distribution function, and the like), explore the properties of $g(X)$ as a manifest for $g(X^*)$. Do this analytically whenever possible and empirically otherwise.

6.7. This exercise is suitable for group discussion. Review the syllabus of a subject you studied in the last term and the questions on its final exam. Define carefully the curriculum (domain) of the subject and assess each exam question whether and to what extent it might be partial. Compile a list of issues on which you have failed to agree and summarise your recommendations for preparing exam papers in the future. How is impartiality of the grade for the exam related to the impartiality of the scores for the individual questions? Are there subjects for which impartial exams are more difficult to prepare than for others?

6.8. Revisit the proof of the identity in (6.5) and generalise it to a vector $\mathbf{Z}$ with an arbitrary trivariate normal distribution. Can the identity be generalised to a vector (with a multivariate normal or another joint distribution) of arbitrary length?

6.9. For the assessment of a recovering patient by a consultant, consider the various types of replications: the same patient at the same time, assessed by the same or a different consultant; the same patient at a different time (say, a few hours earlier or later) assessed by the same or a different consultant. The latent variable is dichotomous: appropriateness to discharge in two days' time or not. Discuss how in some types of replication the assessment may be biased and in others not. Rephrase the problem for the setting with the outcome that indicates successfully solving or failing to solve a problem (of a particular kind) in an exam.

6.10. Illustrate the phenomenon of attenuation in simple regression on a real or simulated dataset; see Figure 6.1. Generate a diagram with several panels with gradually increasing measurement-error variances applied to the same 'latent' dataset. As a more ambitious alternative, produce an animated graph by redrawing the 'manifest' points and the fitted line in the same graph with a time delay that would generate the desired effect.

6.11. Derive the necessary and sufficient conditions for a misclassification process among the ordered categories 1, 2, 3, and 4 to be unbiased.
Hint: Express the condition in terms of the transition matrix $\mathbf{T}$.
What condition(s) have to be added for pointwise unbiasedness?

6.12. Explain how the conclusion that $\mathbf{p} = \mathbf{p}^*$ only when $\mathbf{p}^* = (\frac{1}{2}, \frac{1}{2})$ in Section 6.4 is extended to variables with more than two categories.

6.13. In the setting of a simple regression on a latent variable X^* represented by a manifest variable X related to X^* by the model in (6.1), explore the consequences of correcting for attenuation using an incorrect or estimated value of the measurement-error variance σ_δ^2.
Hint: Follow the outline of a similar exploration in Section 1.1.1.

6.14. Express the estimator of the residual variance $\hat{\sigma}^2$ of an outcome variable Y on a manifest covariate X in the simple regression in terms of the values of the latent covariate X^*. Find a transformation of $\hat{\sigma}^2$ that is linear in the total of squares $\mathbf{x}^\top \mathbf{x}$ of the values of the manifest variable. Estimate σ^2 by SimEx using a linear extrapolation based on this transformation. Show that the naive estimator of the residual variance (which ignores the measurement error) is, in expectation and with some approximation, an increasing function of the measurement-error variance σ_δ^2.

6.15. Explain the origin of the rule that states that the variance of the rounded version of a variable is smaller by $\Delta^2/12$ than the variance of the original variable X^*; Δ is the width of the interval (bin) that is rounded to the same value. For example, $\Delta = 0.1$ when rounding to one decimal place is applied. Discuss when the rule is suitable and when it is not.
Hint: Assume that the conditional distribution of X^* within each bin is uniform.

6.16. Explain how a random sample from the conditional density in (6.10) could be drawn by rejection sampling. Implement the method for several common distributions (normal, exponential, power, and the like) of the latent variable.

6.17. In the assessment of a feature of a residential property (a house or a flat), such as the foundations, roof, windows, and the like, surveyors use the ordinal scale of integers from 0 to 10. The interpretation of score k is that $10k\%$ of the replacement cost of the feature would be required for the repairs or improvements to bring the feature up to the prevailing standard. In a survey of single-household residential properties of a country, a random subsample of the properties is assessed twice. The two surveyors who assess a property do not know about one another's involvement or the score assigned. Describe a realistic model for misclassification that takes account of two kinds of discrepancies. One is such that the surveyor assigns a score that neighbours on the ideal score; with the other, a randomly selected score is given as a result of a gross error. Describe how the scores from the twice-surveyed properties could be used for estimating the parameters of this misclassification process. Derive the relevant moment-matching equations.

6.18. Suppose two normally distributed latent variables X^* and Y^* are observed through their coarse versions X and Y. Explore by simulations the differences between the regressions $E(Y^* \mid X^*)$ and $E(Y \mid X)$ for a range of settings of the cut points (their numbers and locations and typical values), and draw up a set of guidelines for coarsening for which the difference would be sufficiently small.

6.19. In a study concerned with recovery from a disease, the concentration of a compound in the bloodstream of each patient is measured twice at the beginning of a period of intensive treatment and once at the conclusion two weeks later. The sets of three measurements are listed in dataset EX4a.dat on www.sntl.co.uk/BookA/Data; they are in log-units per ml. Fit the ordinary regression of the concentration at the conclusion on the concentration at the beginning of the study. Take account of the uncertainty about the measurement-error variance at the beginning by multiple imputation of plausible values of the variance. Assuming that the measurement-error variance at the conclusion is similar to the variance at the beginning, discuss how useful it would be to have a replicate measurement also at the conclusion.

6.20. Find information about the use of plausible values for the students' proficiencies in the National Assessment of Educational Progress (web site www.nces.ed.gov/pubsearch). They represent the unknown 'true' scores (abilities) of the survey subjects (students) and are derived from the fit of a complex item-response model. Relate these plausible values to the measurement-error framework presented in this chapter.

6.21. Explore some analytical alternatives to maximising the likelihood in (6.14), the Newton method in particular.

6.22. Re-analyse the study in Example 14, with the uniform conditional distribution assumed within each bin on the original scale. Compare the plausibility of this assumption with its counterpart in the analysis. To avoid problems with the infinite length of the bin for the highest incomes, impose the upper limit of one million Euro. Devise an improvement on the diagram in Figure 6.3 so that the realised and simulated counts would be much easier to discern.

Experiments and Observational Studies

Experiments and observational studies are two kinds of statistical investigations. Experiments are characterised by tight control over the processes involved. They tend to incur high expenditure per subject (unit), but have greater potential to collect more information in relatively small samples. In contrast, observational studies involve much less control, their expense per unit tends to be lower, but inferences are more difficult to make, and some of the difficulties could not be resolved by increasing the sample size. In many settings, experiments are not feasible, and inferences have to be based on observational studies. Their analysis is more challenging than that of experiments and often has to rely on some unverifiable assumptions.

This chapter presents a framework in which experiments and observational studies are simply 'studies' distinguished by the presence or absence, or in general the level, of the designer's control over the assignment of treatments to units. In several aspects, this approach parallels the sampling theory introduced in Chapter 3. In particular, it makes use of a missing-data formulation of the inferential task.

Experiments and observational studies relate to a population for which inferences are intended. For instructional reasons, we assume at the beginning of this chapter that the studies involve the entire population, so as to set aside any issues related to good representation. These we address later in Section 7.2.2.

7.1 Comparing Treatments

We motivate the development of this chapter by a contrived example. Kevin J., a recent graduate of college A makes a complaint stating that had he attended college B (of the same type as A and involving the same costs), he would have earned better grades, been better prepared for life, had better prospects in further education, and acquired a greater potential to have high income in the future. In ideal circumstances, these claims could be arbitrated by winding the clock back, wiping out all of Kevin's experiences from school, home, and the rest of his life over the four years he spent attending college A, enrolling him in the alternative college B, and then comparing the grades attained and other outcomes in the alternative versions of the reality. An equally unrealisable proposal is to compare two identical copies (clones) of Kevin J., one enrolled in college A and the other in college B.

The two proposals have one important feature in common—they attempt to compare *like with like*. As they are not realistic, we have to consider some compromise on this absolute standard. Kevin J., or his advocates, may point to higher grades attained by graduates of college B than by graduates of college A, but this may be a consequence of the ability of college B to attract students with better background. So we should compare Kevin's grades with the grades of students in college B who were like Kevin when he enrolled in college A.

We relate several key definitions to this story. Attending college A and college B are two *treatments* we wish to compare. In general, there may be more than two treatments (alternatives). The result of a treatment, recorded as a single value, is called the *outcome*. For Kevin J., or *unit i*, we consider the values of two outcomes, $Y_i^{(A)}$ following treatment A and $Y_i^{(B)}$ following treatment B. Their difference, $Y_i^{(B)} - Y_i^{(A)}$, or the variable $Y^{(B)} - Y^{(A)}$, is the unit-level (Kevin J.'s) *effect* of treatment B over treatment A. The fundamental difficulty in establishing this effect, or even estimating it, is that no more than one of the outcomes $Y_i^{(B)}$ and $Y_i^{(A)}$ can be realised and recorded for any unit i. We therefore call them *potential outcomes*.

By W we denote the *assignment* variable; $W_i = $ T if member i is assigned treatment T; in our case, T = A or B. We can recode W to a 0/1 variable, with the understanding that 0 stands for A and 1 for B. Further, by Z we denote the variable that captures the background; usually it is multivariate, but that generates no complexities additional to the univariate case. For simplicity, we assume first that Z is a single categorical variable with a small number of categories.

In one interpretation, Kevin J. is the sole unit because we focus on him as the only student. It is more appropriate to consider a population of units (students) from the catchment area (constituency) of the two colleges, who could conceivably have attended either college. This we can reduce to the subpopulation of those who have the same background as Kevin J. The variables that describe or define the background and what we would regard as 'the same' (background) would have to be defined carefully.

We call the variable $Y^{(B)} - Y^{(A)}$ an effect to emphasise that we want to attribute its deviation from zero to no other *cause* than using, applying, or administering treatment B instead of A. Such an attribution is appropriate only when the (hypothetical) applications of the treatments A and B on a unit differ in no aspect other than the identity of the treatment. Further, the label of the treatment has to be genuine—each application of treatment A (or

B) has to follow the same protocol (procedure), with all its details, without any deviations.

We use the term *effect* exclusively in association with a cause (use of one treatment instead of another with no other circumstance altered). Thus, it implies that although one treatment was applied, the other could equally well have been applied instead. For example, it makes sense to talk about school effect (for one student or a population of students) if, even though they attended one school they could have attended another as an equal alternative. In principle, a study could be designed in which the school to be attended would be assigned by design. The effect of a country on a subject's freedom, happiness, or well-being is more problematic because a person could not be moved from one country to another without altering his or her other circumstances (values of variables), such as proximity of and close communication with family, relatives, and friends, as well as other elements of the social, economic, and physical environment. The effects of gender and age are meaningless terms because the values of these variables cannot be assigned. Conceivably, a person's sex could be changed by surgery, but it would be impossible to discount the experiences and influences exerted on the subject during the life prior to the change. In brief, effect is a meaningful term only when the treatment could conceivably be manipulated in isolation, without influencing any other variables that are well defined at the time of such manipulation, or earlier.

Variables defined after administering the treatment are called *intermediate*. Their values depend on the treatment applied. We can avoid some confusion by defining *potential versions* of such variables by reference to the treatment applied. For example, a summary U of the friendships with classmates is defined assuming that the member attended school A (variable $U^{(A)}$) and school B (variable $U^{(B)}$).

7.1.1 Experimental Design

The population-level effect of treatment B over treatment A is defined as the difference of the expected outcomes, or the expectation of the unit-level effects,

$$\Delta_{AB} = E\left(Y^{(B)}\right) - E\left(Y^{(A)}\right) = E\left(Y^{(B)} - Y^{(A)}\right), \qquad (7.1)$$

where the expectations are taken over the population. It is also called the *average effect*. We assume that each expectation in (7.1) is well defined. (This is an issue only in infinite populations and with outcomes that are not bounded.) For a population of size N, only N of the $2N$ values $Y_i^{(A)}$ and $Y_i^{(B)}$, $i = 1, \ldots, N$, are available, one per member. We can address this problem by imputation—defining substitute values for each missing item in the $N \times 2$ matrix $\left(\mathbf{Y}^{(A)}, \mathbf{Y}^{(B)}\right)$. A well-motivated proposal is to borrow a recorded value of $Y^{(A)}$ for each missing value of $Y^{(A)}$, and similarly for $Y^{(B)}$. How to select such a value is discussed in Section 7.3.1. A seemingly easier method estimates Δ_{AB} by the difference of the observed means,

$$\widehat{\Delta}^{\dagger}_{AB} = \frac{\sum\limits_{i=1}^{N} Y_i^{(B)} I(W_i = B)}{\sum\limits_{i=1}^{N} I(W_i = B)} - \frac{\sum\limits_{i=1}^{N} Y_i^{(A)} I(W_i = A)}{\sum\limits_{i=1}^{N} I(W_i = A)}, \tag{7.2}$$

where I is the indicator function; $I(C) = 1$ if statement C is true and $I(C) = 0$ otherwise. The expectation of this estimator is the difference of the conditional expectations

$$E\left(\widehat{\Delta}^{\dagger}_{AB}\right) = E\left(Y^{(B)} \mid W = B\right) - E\left(Y^{(A)} \mid W = A\right),$$

denoted by $\Delta^{\dagger}_{AB}$. We can ensure that $\widehat{\Delta}^{\dagger}_{AB}$ is unbiased for Δ_{AB}, that is, $\Delta^{\dagger}_{AB} = \Delta_{AB}$, only by arranging that W is independent of $Y^{(A)}$ and $Y^{(B)}$. This is the purpose of *experimental design*. In studies for comparing two treatments A and B, experimental design is a (probabilistic) prescription for controlling the assignment variable W in such a way that W is independent of $Y^{(A)}$ and $Y^{(B)}$. *Randomisation* is the process of assignment in which each member (experimental unit) has the same pair of probabilities (p_A, p_B), with $p_A + p_B = 1$, of being assigned to the respective treatments A and B. We say that such an assignment is *completely at random* (CAR), or *unconfounded*. Under randomisation, $\Delta^{\dagger}_{AB} = \Delta_{AB}$. The variance $\text{var}(\widehat{\Delta}^{\dagger}_{AB})$ is difficult to evaluate in general and requires further discussion of the assumptions made. The CAR assignment mechanism can be related to the MCAR nonresponse mechanism introduced in Section 5.3. In both settings, assignment and nonresponse, we miss some data that would make the analysis much simpler.

In some randomised designs, the assignments are mutually independent. Such an assignment (mechanism) is easy to implement, similarly to selecting a random sample of subjects (who are to be administered treatment A) by simple random sampling without replacement. The within-treatment sample sizes, n_T, T = A or B, are random; $\text{var}(n_T) = N p_T (1 - p_T)$. This may be inconvenient for the management of the study. In small studies, too few units may be assigned a treatment, less than the expected count $N p_T$. We can protect the study against such occurrence by selecting the units for a treatment by simple random sampling with a fixed sample size.

In the perspective we have adopted, the values of $Y^{(A)}$ and $Y^{(B)}$ are fixed for each member of the population, and the assignment W is variable—it is left to chance, under designer's control or otherwise, whether any particular unit is assigned treatment A or B. This is very close to the design-based perspective of Chapter 3, where we regarded the population values of a variable as fixed and the sampling mechanism as the sole source of variation. Assignment can be regarded as sampling from the $2N$ values of the two potential outcome variables.

We use the notation $I_i = I(W_i = A)$ and let

$$p_i = \mathrm{E}(I_i) = \mathrm{P}(W_i = A),$$

$$p_{i,i'} = \mathrm{E}(I_i I_{i'}) = \mathrm{P}(W_i = A \text{ and } W_{i'} = A),$$

for $1 \leq i, i' \leq N$. We assume that the within-treatment subsample sizes $n_A = I_1 + \cdots + I_N$ and $n_B = n - n_A$ are fixed. As I_i are (dependent) binary variables,

$$\mathrm{var}\left(\widehat{\Delta}^{\dagger}_{AB}\right) = \mathrm{var}\left\{\frac{1}{n_A}\sum_{i=1}^{N} I_i Y_i^{(A)} - \frac{1}{n_B}\sum_{i=1}^{N}(1 - I_i) Y_i^{(B)}\right\}$$

$$= \mathrm{var}\left(\sum_{i=1}^{N} I_i Y_i^{(+)}\right)$$

$$= \sum_{i=1}^{N} Y_i^{(+)2} p_i(1 - p_i) + \sum_{i=1}^{N}\sum_{i' \neq i} Y_i^{(+)} Y_{i'}^{(+)} (p_{i,i'} - p_i p_{i'}), \quad (7.3)$$

where $Y_i^{(+)} = Y_i^{(A)}/n_A + Y_i^{(B)}/n_B$. The second line is obtained by exploiting the fact that the total $Y_1^{(B)} + \cdots + Y_N^{(B)}$ is constant. We derived an analogous formula in Section 3.2 for the sampling variance of the estimator of the population total in a survey with the sampling design given by the joint distribution of $(I_1, \ldots, I_N)$. This establishes a direct connection of our problem with sampling methods, and through them with missing data problems. It is now easy to anticipate the difficulties we encounter when the joint distribution of the assignment indicators I_i is not known or is complex and related to the values of some other variables, to values that were not recorded in particular. Before discussing this, we derive some simple cases that are of practical importance.

A constant number of units n_A means that $\mathrm{var}(I_1 + \cdots + I_N) = 0$, or

$$\sum_{i=1}^{N} p_i(1 - p_i) + 2\sum_{i=1}^{N}\sum_{i'=i+1}^{N} (p_{i,i'} - p_i p_{i'}) = 0,$$

and since $I_1 + \cdots + I_N = p_1 + \cdots + p_N = n_A$,

$$2\sum_{i=1}^{N}\sum_{i'=i+1}^{N} p_{i,i'} = -\sum_{i=1}^{N} p_i + \sum_{i=1}^{N}\sum_{i'=1}^{N} p_i p_{i'}$$

$$= n_A(n_A - 1).$$

When each unit has the same probability $p = p_1 = \ldots = p_N$, then $p = n_A/N$. When all the pairwise probabilities are also identical, $p_{i,i'} = p_{(2)}$ for all pairs $i \neq i'$, then

$$p_{(2)} = \frac{n_A(n_A - 1)}{N(N - 1)}.$$

With p and $p_{(2)}$, equation (7.3) reduces to

$$\text{var}\left(\widehat{\Delta}_{AB}^{\dagger}\right) = \frac{n_A(N-n_A)}{N(N-1)}\left\{\sum_{i=1}^{N}Y_i^{(+)2} - \frac{1}{N}\left(\sum_{i=1}^{N}Y_i^{(+)}\right)^2\right\}$$

$$= \frac{n_A(N-n_A)}{N(N-1)}\sum_{i=1}^{N}\left(Y_i^{(+)} - \bar{Y}^{(+)}\right)^2, \tag{7.4}$$

where $\bar{Y}^{(+)} = (Y_1^{(+)} + \cdots + Y_N^{(+)})/N$. This is the sampling variance of the sample total of $Y^{(+)}$ in a survey with simple random sampling design without replacement and fixed sample size n_A; $(N-n_A)/N = 1-f$ is the complement of the finite-population correction.

The variance in (7.4) vanishes when the variable $Y^{(+)}$ is constant. Given that the definition of $Y^{(+)}$ involves the numbers of units, n_A and n_B, this is a rather esoteric condition, implying that $\text{cor}\left(Y^{(A)}, Y^{(B)}\right) = -1$. Much more commonly, the two potential outcomes are positively correlated. In fact, the assumption that the effect $Y^{(B)} - Y^{(A)}$ is close to a constant is often reasonable; then the correlation is close to $+1$.

In the balanced randomised allocation design, N is even, $p = \frac{1}{2}$ and $p_{(2)} = \frac{1}{4}(N-2)/(N-1)$, and $Y^{(+)} = 2(Y^{(A)} + Y^{(B)})/N$. Therefore,

$$\text{var}\left(\widehat{\Delta}_{AB}^{\dagger}\right) = \frac{1}{N(N-1)}\sum_{i=1}^{N}\left(Y_i^{(A)} + Y_i^{(B)} - \bar{Y}^{(A)} - \bar{Y}^{(B)}\right)^2$$

$$= \frac{1}{N-1}\text{var}_{\mathcal{P}}\left(Y^{(A)} + Y^{(B)}\right), \tag{7.5}$$

where subscript $\mathcal{P}$ indicates that the variance is over the members of the population. To find the optimal allocation among the randomised designs, we search for the minimum of the expression in (7.4). Denote $V_T = \text{var}_{\mathcal{P}}\left(Y^{(T)}\right)$ for T = A or B and $C_{AB} = \text{cov}_{\mathcal{P}}\left(Y^{(A)}, Y^{(B)}\right)$, so that, for example,

$$V_A = \frac{1}{N}\sum_{i=1}^{N}\left(Y_i^{(A)} - \bar{Y}^{(A)}\right)^2.$$

Now

$$\text{var}\left(\widehat{\Delta}_{AB}^{\dagger}\right) = \frac{1}{N-1}\left(\frac{N-n_A}{n_A}V_A + \frac{n_A}{N-n_A}V_B + 2C_{AB}\right), \tag{7.6}$$

and this function of n_A attains its minimum when $V_A/n_A^2 = V_B/n_B^2$, that is, when

$$\frac{n_A}{n_B} = \sqrt{\frac{V_A}{V_B}}.$$

Therefore, the optimal allocation is proportional to the population standard deviations of the potential outcomes. The minimum variance attained is

$$\min_{n_A} \text{var} \left(\widehat{\Delta}^\dagger_{AB} \right) = \frac{2}{N-1} \sqrt{V_A \, V_B} \, (1 + \rho_{AB}),$$

where ρ_{AB} is the correlation of the potential outcomes $Y^{(A)}$ and $Y^{(B)}$. Calculation of this quantity for a range of plausible values of ρ_{AB}, V_A, and V_B enables us to anticipate what the sampling variation of $\widehat{\Delta}^\dagger_{AB}$ might be. It is not relevant to discuss what would happen if ρ_{AB} or a variance V_T were reduced because they are population quantities, fixed and outside the control of the study designer.

7.1.2 Assignment and Sampling Designs

The connection between assignment and sampling designs can be made explicit by translating an assignment design directly to a sampling design. The sampling setting is as follows. We have a population of $2N$ members, two for each unit. We denote them by two subscripts, indicating the unit and the treatment, as (i, T), $i = 1, \ldots, n$ and $T = A$ or B. The pairs of members (i, A) and (i, B) form strata. The outcome variable is defined as $X_{i,A} = -2Y_i^{(A)}$ and $X_{i,B} = 2Y_i^{(B)}$, so that the population mean of X is equal to the target $\bar{Y}^{(B)} - \bar{Y}^{(A)}$. Assignment design is equivalent to the stratified sampling design with probabilities $p_{i,A} = 1 - p_{i,B}$ with the pairs as strata, and fixed within-stratum sample sizes equal to unity; $p_{i,A;i,B} = 0$. Fixed within-treatment sample sizes impose a between-stratum dependence.

Thus, an assignment design is an improper sampling design, as some pairwise inclusion probabilities vanish. Further, the within-stratum (within-subject) variances cannot be estimated; that would require at least two observations within some strata. This limits the direct application of the results in Chapter 3 to the context of experiments. However, the designs of experiments, often in small populations, are usually much simpler in relation to sampling designs in large structured populations.

7.1.3 SUTVA Assumptions and Cluster-Randomisation

Not even by applying a treatment (A or B) on the entire population can we compare the treatments with certainty, unless $\rho_{AB} = -1$. That is a consequence of the randomness of the assignment W and the limitation of a single treatment for each unit; the (potential) outcomes $Y^{(T)}$ entail no variation. More explicitly, in our definition of $Y^{(T)}$ we assumed that their values are *stable* and units do not interfere with one another's outcomes. These assumptions, stable unit-treatment and variable assignment, are commonly referred to by the acronym SUTVA.

Examples of violation of SUTVA are studies of intervention, such as smoking cessation or sexual abstinence, in which the units, say, students from the same classroom or school, communicate, discuss the treatment applied to each of them, and are bound to influence one another's behaviour and therefore their outcomes. The solution to this problem is to define units (clusters) that do not communicate, such as schools, and apply the same treatment to each member of a cluster. Such designs are called *cluster-randomised*. For instance, the clusters may be households, schools, general (medical) practices, businesses, or even towns and postcode sectors.

Without such an arrangement, we have to consider more than two potential outcomes, because apart from the treatment the outcome depends also on the assignment of treatments to the other units of the cluster. In practice, this becomes unmanageable for all but very small populations and when interference could occur only among a small subset of the $\frac{1}{2}N(N-1)$ pairs of units.

In some exceptional settings, pairs of (nearly) identical units are available. For example, some studies recruit twins and assign each pair of twins (U_1, U_2), independently, either to the treatment pair (A, B) or to (B, A), with probabilities $p_{AB} = p_{BA} = \frac{1}{2}$. Such an assignment is CAR. Although rarely an issue, we should bear in mind that the conclusions of a twins study are usually aimed at a human population (with particular attributes) and not the population of twins. The difficulties with locating and recruiting twins are a strong disincentive to conducting such studies.

7.1.4 The Scale for Comparison

Potential outcomes $Y^{(A)}$ and $Y^{(B)}$ can be compared by means other than their difference $Y^{(B)} - Y^{(A)}$. In some contexts, the ratio $Y^{(B)}/Y^{(A)}$, or its logarithm, are more appropriate. We say that the outcomes are compared on the *linear scale* by differences and on the *multiplicative scale* by ratios. Ratios are appropriate only for outcomes with positive values that are all distant from zero. The multiplicative scale becomes linear when the outcomes are subjected to the log-transformation. In principle, any other (continuous) monotone transformation can be applied to the outcomes, and the linear scale used after this transformation.

From the purely analytical standpoint, the difference is preferred. However, when we regard the difference as a summary of the pairs of potential outcomes within units, we would like it not to be associated with the actual values of $Y^{(A)}$ and $Y^{(B)}$. That is, a given unit-level effect $\Delta_{AB,i}$ could be interpreted without any reference to $Y_i^{(A)}$ and $Y_i^{(B)}$. For example, when $Y^{(T)}$ is annual income, comparison by means of ratio (percentage) is more appropriate in many contexts. We would like to regard the increase from £10 000 to £10 500 and from £50 000 to £52 500 as the same, equal to 5%. On the linear scale, the values of the increases £500 and £2500 differ a lot. A reference to the values of $Y^{(A)}$ would help to explain the disparity. After taking logarithms, the two contrasts are both equal to $\log(1.05) = 0.049$.

When the outcomes $Y^{(T)}$ are proportions (or percentages), which have to be in the range 0–1 (or 0–100), both the linear and multiplicative scale may be inappropriate. For small percentages, a fixed reduction (subtraction) may lead to a negative percentage, an inadmissible value. Similarly, for percentages close to 100%, a fixed increase may result in exceeding 100%. The odds, defined as $o^{(T)} = Y^{(T)} / \left(100 - Y^{(T)}\right)$, offer a practical solution. The appropriate scale for the odds is multiplicative, using odds-ratios, so that $o^{(T)}$ would be comparable when the roles of 'success' and 'failure' are interchanged and $100 - Y^{(T)}$ is used instead of $Y^{(T)}$. Thus, we should use the log-odds scale,

$$\log\left(\frac{Y^{(T)}}{100 - Y^{(T)}}\right).$$

If we insist on using the linear scale we should apply a continuous monotone transformation g such that the difference $g\left(Y^{(B)}\right) - g\left(Y^{(A)}\right)$ would amount to the same effect, as interpreted substantively, irrespective of the value of $Y^{(A)}$.

An average (additive) effect of treatment B over treatment A is sometimes interpreted as a net addition to the (potential) outcome of treatment A, implying the model

$$Y^{(B)} = Y^{(A)} + \Delta_{AB} + \varepsilon, \tag{7.7}$$

where ε is a random variable with zero mean and is independent of $Y^{(A)}$. The term ε is sometimes referred to as error. In most instances, this is inappropriate because no mistake has been committed; the model simply does not provide a perfect description of how the outcomes are related. Thus, ε is more appropriately regarded as a *deviation* from the very simple and in most cases invalid model of identical unit-level effects.

When the unit-level effects $\Delta_{AB,i}$ are widely dispersed, the average effect Δ_{AB} does not summarise them effectively because many values of $Y^{(B)} - Y^{(A)}$ differ from Δ_{AB} substantially. That reinforces the rationale for a transformation after which the model in (7.7) would be palatable.

7.2 Block-Randomisation

In block-randomisation, separate randomisation schemes are applied in each subpopulation (stratum) into which the population $\mathcal{P}$ is partitioned. These subpopulations do not overlap and cover $\mathcal{P}$. For example, medical treatments A and B may be assigned to patients suffering from a specified condition at random within age groups, denoted by G1, G2, G3, and G4, but the proportions of patients assigned the novel (test) treatment B is highest for the youngest patients (G1) and lowest for the elderly (G4). Such a design may

respond to clinical research priorities or ethical considerations or may be in-
strumental in easier recruitment of patients. The conduct of a study may be
devolved to several *centres*, each of them, in effect, conducting their own sub-
study, although the results are to be analysed only for the units from all the
centres. In this setting, block-randomisation may be used for administrative
convenience. Although in the practical versions of these examples the study
usually involves only a sample from the target population, we assume here
that the entire population takes part in the study, and each of its members is
assigned a treatment.

For motivation, consider the number of months after surgery until requiring another treatment for a particular chronic condition. If younger patients
tend to be healthier and more resilient, their outcomes would be higher on average for both treatments A and B. Thus, any comparison of the realised outcomes would be tainted by the uneven assignment of patients to treatments.
The obvious solution is to compare the treatments within groups, yielding a
comparison for each age group, and then combine the comparisons, to reflect
the composition of the population. In this context, the groups are referred
to as *blocks* and the term *blocking* is used for the separate randomisations
(and analyses) within the blocks. Note the close parallels with stratification
in sampling theory.

Let $n_T^{(k)}$ be the number of units in block (group or centre) $k = 1, \ldots, K$
assigned treatment T = A or B, and set $N^{(k)} = n_A^{(k)} + n_B^{(k)}$. Further, denote
by $V_T^{(k)}$ the subpopulation variance of the potential outcomes $Y^{(T)}$ in block
T, and by $C_{AB}^{(k)}$ their covariance.

The within-block estimators of the treatment effect are

$$\widehat{\Delta}_{AB}^{\dagger,h} = \mathrm{E}\left(Y^{(B)} \mid W = \mathrm{B}, G = k\right) - \mathrm{E}\left(Y^{(A)} \mid W = \mathrm{A}, G = k\right)$$

$$= \frac{1}{n_B^{(k)}} \sum_{i=1}^{N} I(W_i = \mathrm{B})\, I(G_i = k)\, Y_i^{(B)}$$

$$- \frac{1}{n_A^{(k)}} \sum_{i=1}^{N} I(W_i = \mathrm{A})\, I(G_i = k)\, Y_i^{(A)},$$

where G is the variable that identifies the unit's block. These estimators are
unbiased for their respective targets $\Delta_{AB}^{(k)}$ and have variances

$$\mathrm{var}\left(\widehat{\Delta}_{AB}^{\dagger,k}\right) = \frac{1}{N^{(k)} - 1} \left(\frac{n_B^{(k)}}{n_A^{(k)}} V_A^{(k)} + \frac{n_A^{(k)}}{n_B^{(k)}} V_B^{(k)} + 2C_{AB}^{(k)}\right);$$

see (7.6). Hence, the *pooled* estimator

$$\widehat{\Delta}_{AB}^{\dagger,G} = \frac{1}{N} \sum_{k=1}^{K} N^{(k)} \widehat{\Delta}_{AB}^{\dagger,k}$$

is also unbiased and has the variance

$$\text{var}\left(\widehat{\Delta}_{AB}^{\dagger,G}\right) = \frac{1}{N^2} \sum_{k=1}^{K} \frac{N^{(k)^2}}{N^{(k)} - 1} \left(\frac{n_B^{(k)}}{n_A^{(k)}} V_A^{(k)} + \frac{n_A^{(k)}}{n_B^{(k)}} V_B^{(k)} + 2C_{AB}^{(k)} \right). \quad (7.8)$$

7.2.1 When and How to Block

In this section, we explore when blocking is rewarded by greater precision in estimating the effect Δ_{AB}. This amounts to comparing the sampling variances in (7.6) and (7.8). An analytical comparison for a general setting is not feasible, so we restrict our attention to some simple cases. It suffices to consider the case of two blocks ($K = 2$); our conclusions can then be generalised by mathematical induction.

When the blocks are relatively homogeneous and the within-block variances $V_T^{(k)}$ are much smaller than the pooled variances V_T, blocking may be useful even if the assignment proportions $n_A^{(k)}/N^{(k)}$ are similar (or identical). The covariances $C_{AB}^{(k)}$ exert a limited impact on these comparisons because their sizes are constrained by the variances $V_A^{(k)}$ and $V_B^{(k)}$. The within-block variances are much smaller than the pooled variances when the within-block means of the potential outcomes differ across the blocks a great deal.

Next, suppose the within-block variances and covariance depend only on the treatment. Then $V_A^{(k)} = V_A$ for each k, and similarly for V_B and C_{AB}. If the assignment fractions $n_A/N^{(k)}$ are also identical, then

$$\frac{\text{var}\left(\widehat{\Delta}_{AB}^{\dagger,G}\right)}{\text{var}\left(\widehat{\Delta}_{AB}^{\dagger}\right)} = \left(\frac{N_1^2}{N_1 - 1} + \frac{N_2^2}{N_2 - 1} \right) \frac{N - 1}{N^2}.$$

This ratio exceeds unity, since

$$\frac{N_1^2}{N_1 - 1} + \frac{N_2^2}{N_2 - 1} - \frac{N^2}{N - 1} = \frac{N_1}{N_1 - 1} + \frac{N_2}{N_2 - 1} - \frac{N}{N - 1}$$

$$= 1 + \frac{1}{N_1 - 1} + \frac{1}{N_2 - 1} - \frac{1}{N - 1},$$

and this exceeds unity by at least $1/\{\min(N_1, N_2) - 1\}$. Thus, blocking is ineffective and may even be counterproductive (inflating the sampling variance), when the blocks do not differ in their mean outcomes and the within-block assignment fractions are similar. Note that a (completely) randomised assignment design $\mathcal{D}$ differs from the block-randomised assignment design with assignment fractions identical to those in $\mathcal{D}$. Blocking ensures that the assignment fractions are adhered to within blocks, not only overall. By blocking, the variety of assignments W that have positive probability is reduced.

7.2.2 From Sample to Population

Thus far, we assumed that every member of the population (unit) is involved in the study and is subjected to one of the treatments. When only a sample of units is involved, the estimators $\widehat{\Delta}_{AB}^{\dagger}$ and $\widehat{\Delta}_{AB}^{\dagger,G}$ involve two sources of variation: assignment and sampling (engagement in the study). We assume that these two processes do not interfere; the sampling design does not involve the values of the potential outcomes and the assignment does not depend on any aspect of the sampling design other than the sample size and the values of the covariates.

Methods for analysing sample surveys were dealt with in Chapter 3. Here we discuss two key identities related to the problem of extending inferences from a sample s to the target population $\mathcal{P}$. For the population-expectation of an estimator $\widehat{\Delta}$ we have

$$\mathrm{E}\left(\widehat{\Delta}\right) = \mathrm{E}_{\mathcal{P}}\left\{\mathrm{E}_{\mathcal{W}}\left(\widehat{\Delta}\,|\,\mathbf{s}\right)\right\},$$

where the subscript $\mathcal{P}$ indicates expectation (averaging) over the sampling process (samples s), and $\mathcal{W}$ over the assignment process. In particular, if $\widehat{\Delta}$ is conditionally unbiased for every sample s with respect to the assignment design, then it is unbiased also without conditioning and with respect to both the assignment and sampling designs.

For the unconditional sampling variance, we have the identity

$$\mathrm{var}\left(\widehat{\Delta}\right) = \mathrm{E}_{\mathcal{P}}\left\{\mathrm{var}_{\mathcal{W}}\left(\widehat{\Delta}\,|\,\mathbf{s}\right)\right\} + \mathrm{var}_{\mathcal{P}}\left\{\mathrm{E}_{\mathcal{W}}\left(\widehat{\Delta}\,|\,\mathbf{s}\right)\right\};$$ (7.9)

there are two contributions to the unconditional variance of $\widehat{\Delta}$: the average assignment-related variance for a fixed sample and the sampling variance of the average sample-level effects. Even when the bias of $\widehat{\Delta}$ vanishes for every sample the second term in (7.9) may not vanish because the average effects are not constant across samples s.

In a study with cluster-randomisation, the treatment may be applied not to all the units, but only to a sample in each cluster. Then estimators of the within-block average effects involve two sources of uncertainty, the assignment and sampling, just like in a study with no blocking. For each cluster, we may consider a superpopulation of elements; this introduces sampling as an additional source of uncertainty. In principle, a superpopulation may be considered also for the clusters, so that the clusters involved in the study are a sample. We may also consider hypothetical replications in which the clusters are formed by different sets of individuals (schools with different students, neighbourhoods with different households, and the like), but with similar background profiles. The issues of good representation are relevant throughout. A suitable definition of the superpopulation may always resolve it, but only superficially, because the target of inference should be defined at the planning stage. If this was not done then, it should be done later, but without any regard for the sample that was observed.

An extreme form of blocking arises when the units are first paired, and the units (i_1, i_2) in each pair are assigned treatments (A, B) (i_1 to A and i_2 to B) or to (B, A). Such blocking is referred to as *matching*. Twin studies are an example of matching. The discussion earlier in this section suggests that matching is useful when the units within pairs have very similar potential outcomes ($Y_{i1}^{(T)} \approx Y_{i2}^{(T)}$ for T = A and B) and the pairs differ a lot from one another. Note that any matching can be based only on the values of the background variables, prior to the study, and so we often have to face the uncertainty about the usefulness of matching, whether and to what extent similar background implies similar outcomes. This highlights the need for collecting intelligence about background variables at the planning stage and using for matching those that are (believed to be) highly correlated with the outcomes.

The rationale for matching can be formulated in terms of missing data. Suppose unit i_1 is assigned treatment A, $W_{i_1} = A$, and its pair i_2 treatment B. It would be hard to find a substitute better than $Y_{i_2}^{(B)}$ for the missing outcome $Y_{i_1}^{(B)}$. Nonetheless such a substitute is not perfect, because it is likely that $Y_{i_2}^{(B)} \neq Y_{i_1}^{(B)}$.

Intermediate variables should never be used for matching. First, it would amount to matching post hoc, as their values can be established only after administering the treatments. Further, unit i with $U_i^{(A)} = u$, established after having received treatment A, cannot be regarded as a match for unit i' with $U_{i'}^{(B)} = u$, after having received treatment B, because this is a match on neither $U^{(A)}$ nor $U^{(B)}$; the potential intermediates $U^{(A)}$ and $U^{(B)}$ are distinct variables. Matching on either $U^{(A)}$ or $U^{(B)}$ would be appropriate if both values were available for all subjects. This suggests an avenue for using an intermediate variable for matching, by declaring the unobserved values of $U^{(T)}$, T = A, B, as missing and applying a suitable (multiple) imputation method for them.

7.3 Observational Studies

In real life, the assignment variable W is often of keen interest; we select among alternative treatments (schools, jobs, providers of services, shops, employees, and the like), trying to maximise the benefit to us (our future outcome). We base such decisions on the knowledge of our own background (or the background of the unit about to be treated), as well as guesses, not always very good ones, about the values of the potential outcomes. In *observational studies*, the assignment is not controlled and is left to be set by the circumstances, usually by the choices made by the subjects or their representatives. The (joint) distribution of the assignment W is then not known, and neither are any of its summaries, such as the number of units receiving treatment A.

In Section 7.1, we defined the term CAR for assignment designs that are completely randomised. In all but some esoteric settings, it is highly unlikely that the assignment would be CAR, especially when the units (human subjects) are strongly motivated to avoid it. By the time they are making their choices, they cannot influence the values of the background variables Z but may make good (intelligent) guesses about the values of their (future) potential outcomes $Y^{(\mathrm{T})}$. We say that such choices are *informed*.

An assignment that is not CAR may be CAR for each of the subpopulations defined by one or several background variables Z. For example, it may be CAR for all four categories defined by sex (M or F) and immigration status (born in the UK, coded as H, or abroad, as O) in a particular study, but with different pairs of probabilities $(p_{A,G}, p_{B,G})$, where G stands for the combinations MH, FH, MO, and FO. Such an assignment design is said to be *at random* (AR). It is qualified by the background variables (sex and immigration status in this example). The background variables have to be defined prior to assignment and their values have to be known for each unit.

An AR assignment (mechanism) is much more general than CAR, but assuming it is not always appropriate. Rarely is it possible to establish whether a particular assignment mechanism is AR with respect to a given set of variables Z. However, by adding variables to Z we do no harm to our chances of attaining AR. This suggests that we should be liberal in recording background variables in an observational study. The flip side of this suggestion is that recording more variables (increasing the response burden by requesting more detailed information) may discourage full cooperation and bring about other difficulties, such as nonresponse. Anticipating that we would analyse an observational study with assignment design that is AR as a block-randomised experiment suggests some other deficiencies, as discussed in Section 7.2.1. Note the parallels of how we discuss assignment here and nonresponse in Chapter 5.

There are assignment mechanisms that are neither AR nor CAR; we call them 'not at random' (NAR) or *nonignorable*. The latter term can be motivated by the inequality $\mathrm{E}(\hat{\Delta}^{\dagger}_{\mathrm{AB}}) \neq \Delta_{\mathrm{AB}}$. The conditioning on W cannot be ignored, not even when the expectations are restricted to subpopulations defined by the background variables Z. Assignment mechanisms AR and NAR are called *confounded*; AR mechanisms are confounded with Z (and not with Y), whereas NAR mechanisms are confounded with Y, even after conditioning on Z. With CAR, we can make straightforward comparisons without paying any attention to the covariates Z; with AR, the covariates are relevant.

A simple example of NAR assignment is given in Table 7.1. The assignment W is NAR because it depends on the differences $Y^{(\mathrm{A})} - Y^{(\mathrm{B})}$ even within the groups defined by sex and immigration status; treatment A is assigned (selected) with higher probability, 0.8, when the outcome with A is greater than 12 (except for two units) and with lower probability, 0.2, when the outcome of treatment B tends to be smaller than its average. The unit-level effects are graphically represented in Figure 7.1 for the four background categories. For

Table 7.1. Example of a nonignorable assignment.

P(W = A)	Sex	Status	$Y^{(A)}$	$Y^{(B)}$	P(W = A)	Sex	Status	$Y^{(A)}$	$Y^{(B)}$
0.8	M	H	17	14	0.8	F	H	14	12
0.8	M	H	15	12	0.8	F	H	15	10
0.2	M	H	12	10	0.2	F	H	12	12
0.2	M	H	11	12	0.2	F	H	14	11
0.8	M	O	14	13	0.8	F	O	13	10
0.8	M	O	15	13	0.2	F	O	12	10
0.2	M	O	10	11	0.2	F	O	16	12

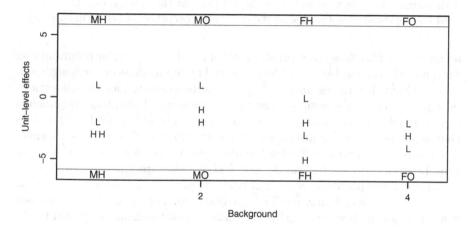

Fig. 7.1. Unit-level effects for the data given in Table 7.1. The effects are marked by symbols 'H' when P(W = A) = 0.8 and 'L' when P(W = B) = 0.8.

MH, MO, and FO, units that are selected to A with high probability (symbol 'H') have smaller average effects than units selected to A with low probability (symbol 'L').

In any one study, we observe only half the 14 × 2 values of the potential outcomes Y, so we could not infer the insidious nature of the assignment process. For example, if we happen to assign treatment A to the seven units that have high probabilities of being assigned A and treatment B to the other seven units, the naive estimator of the average effect, (7.2), is $\widehat{\Delta}^{\dagger}_{AB} = -3.6$, whereas the average effect is $\Delta_{AB} = -2.0$.

With the complete data on the potential outcomes, the bias of $\widehat{\Delta}^{\dagger}_{AB}$ can be established by evaluating the estimator for all the $2^{14} = 16\,384$ possible

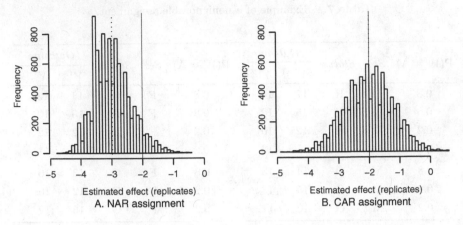

Fig. 7.2. Empirical distributions of the estimator $\widehat{\Delta}^{\dagger}_{AB}$ for the setting of Table 7.1 with assignment design indicated in the subtitles of the histograms. The vertical solid line represents the target and the dots the expectation of the estimator.

assignments. This does not represent a substantial computing or programming task, but if it did, the bias could be estimated by replications of the assignment process. Note that the estimator $\widehat{\Delta}^{\dagger}_{AB}$ cannot be evaluated for the allocations in which every unit is assigned the same treatment. These two assignments can be ruled out, together with some other severely unbalanced assignments that assign one of the treatments to h and the other to $N - h$ units for small h, such as $h = 1$ and $h = 2$. But the assignment can be constrained to have exactly seven units (or 6–8 units) assigned to either treatment.

In general, replications are much easier to program than the enumeration of all the possible assignments. The left-hand panel of Figure 7.2 summarises a set of 10 000 replications of the NAR assignment mechanism applied to the 14 subjects with complete data given in Table 7.1. The target of estimation, $\Delta_{AB} = -2.0$, is marked by the solid vertical line, and the empirical mean of the estimates, $\mathrm{E}(\widehat{\Delta}^{\dagger}_{AB}) \doteq -2.98$, by the dotted vertical line. The bias of nearly -1.0 is a result of the nonignorable assignment process. Only 650 (6.5%) of the replicates yield estimates greater than the target -2.0. The empirical sampling variance of this estimator is 0.373. In the replications we discarded every realised assignment that would have two or fewer units in a treatment group; only 22 such assignments (0.2%) were discarded.

The right-hand panel gives the same summary for a set of 10 000 replications of the CAR assignment mechanism, with $p_A = p_B = \frac{1}{2}$, applied to the same dataset. The estimator $\widehat{\Delta}^{\dagger}_{AB}$ is unbiased; its empirical bias is smaller than 0.001. The empirical sampling variance of this estimator is 0.629. (140 assignments, 1.4%, were discarded because they would result in two or fewer units in a treatment group.)

It should come as no surprise that the NAR design results in smaller sampling variance. As we make the probabilities of assignment more extreme (closer to zero or unity), we reduce the variation among the samples—some samples become more frequent and others rarer. Taking this to its limit, if each assignment probability is either zero or unity, only one sample is realised, and then the sampling variance of the estimator vanishes. We should be concerned with MSE and not the sampling variance or bias on its own. The NAR assignment in Figure 7.2 has MSE equal to $0.373 + 0.980^2 = 1.369$ and the MSE of the CAR assignment is 0.629. If the sample size were greater (or the population were subsumed in a greater population), the overwhelming contribution of the bias might remain, while the sampling variances would be reduced; the advantage of CAR would be more pronounced. The example in Table 7.1 and Figure 7.2 shows that the bias can make a substantial contribution to the MSE even in a small study. With greater sample size, the sampling variance is reduced, but the bias remains intact. This justifies our focus on combating bias by applying CAR and AR assignment whenever possible. When an assignment design with CAR is out of the question, suitable background variables should be recorded, with which the assumption of AR is palatable.

The Sampling Variance of $\widehat{\Delta}_{AB}^{\dagger}$

If the N outcomes and the associated treatments are all the information available for the analysis, the sampling variance of $\widehat{\Delta}_{AB}^{\dagger}$ cannot be estimated without bias. To see this, consider a small experiment with treatments A and B, in which the treatment groups have fixed sizes, $n_A = n_B = 3$. Suppose the recorded outcomes are 3, 5, and 7 following treatment A for one subset of the population and 1, 3, and 2 following treatment B for its complement, so that the value of $\widehat{\Delta}_{AB}^{\dagger}$ is -3.0. In (7.6), we related $\mathrm{var}(\widehat{\Delta}_{AB}^{\dagger})$ to the population variance of the totals $Y^{(A)} + Y^{(B)}$. From the recorded outcomes, we have no way of knowing whether the potential outcomes add up to a constant, $\mathrm{var}(Y^{(A)} + Y^{(B)}) = 0$, in which case $\mathrm{var}(\widehat{\Delta}_{AB}^{\dagger}) = 0$, or $Y^{(A)}$ and $Y^{(B)}$ are perfectly positively correlated, in which case

$$\mathrm{var}\left(\widehat{\Delta}_{AB}^{\dagger}\right) = \frac{1}{N-1}\left(\sqrt{V_A} + \sqrt{V_B}\right)^2.$$

For given within-treatment population variances V_A and V_B, this is the greatest possible value of $\mathrm{var}(\widehat{\Delta}_{AB}^{\dagger})$, so by estimating it without bias, we overestimate $\mathrm{var}(\widehat{\Delta}_{AB}^{\dagger})$ but satisfy the criterion of honesty in the assessment of the precision of $\widehat{\Delta}_{AB}^{\dagger}$. In the complete dataset given in Table 7.1, $V_A = 3.96$, $V_B = 1.65$, and $C_{AB} = \mathrm{cov}_{\mathcal{P}}(Y^{(A)}, Y^{(B)}) = 1.26$, so that the correlation is $\rho_{AB} = 0.49$. Hence, with the within-treatment group sizes fixed at $n_A = n_B = 7$, $\mathrm{var}(\widehat{\Delta}_{AB}^{\dagger}) = 0.626$. If we substitute $\rho_{AB} = 1$ and keep the two variances unchanged, we obtain the upper bound on $\mathrm{var}(\widehat{\Delta}_{AB}^{\dagger})$ equal to 0.825.

We can confirm these derivations on the dataset given in Table 7.1. The empirical variance of $\widehat{\Delta}^{\dagger}_{AB}$ is 0.629; if we restrict the allocation to balance, $n_A = n_B$, the empirical variance is 0.564. The sampling variance of $\widehat{\Delta}^{\dagger}_{AB}$ is estimated from the within-treatment sample variances of the outcomes, assuming $\rho_{AB} = 1$. For the balanced design, the empirical mean of the estimator is 0.815; 79% of the replicate estimates exceed the target of 0.626.

7.3.1 Matching

If the assignment process is AR, it is meaningful, and natural, to make comparisons within strata (subpopulations) defined by the combinations of the values of the background variables. This motivates the general method of matching. For each unit i that was assigned treatment A, we find a unit that has a background as similar as possible to i and was assigned treatment B and 'borrow' his or her value of $Y^{(B)}$. The records of the units that were assigned treatment B can be completed similarly. After such a completion, the two treatments can be compared straightforwardly.

To illustrate the method, suppose the study ended up with the assignment given in Table 7.2. The recorded data are printed with the standard type, and the values printed in smaller type are discussed later. The naive estimate of the average effect is $\widehat{\Delta}^{\dagger}_{AB} = 98/8 - 70/6 = -2.33$. The first two units, both with background MH and treatment A (outcomes 17 and 15), have two matches with treatment B, the next two units (outcomes 10 and 12). For each of the first two units we select a match at random from the other two units. The outcomes of the matches are the imputed (plausible) values of $Y^{(B)}$. To impute values of $Y^{(A)}$ for the third and fourth units, we exchange the roles of the first two and the next two units. To impute values of $Y^{(A)}$ for the sixth and seventh units, we have no other choice than 14, donated from the fifth record, the only match. The donors are selected independently from the relevant pool. There are no rules regarding reciprocity. For example, unit 1 received its plausible value of $Y^{(B)}$ from unit 3; unit 3 happens to have received its plausible value $Y^{(A)}$ from unit 1, reciprocally, but the same value was donated also to unit 4. The values printed in small type are the imputed values for the potential outcomes that were not observed. We emphasise that the purpose of imputation is to facilitate estimation of the average effect, not itemwise estimation of the unobserved potential outcomes.

The variance of the estimator of the effect Δ_{AB} would be underestimated if we regarded the completed dataset as having been observed (recorded). In fact, the complete dataset is without any variation, so a completion, if confused with the complete dataset of the $2N$ values, would be without any variation. Each imputation is associated with uncertainty, and this uncertainty should coincide with the sampling variation. Methods for its assessment were discussed in Chapter 5, where we emphasised the importance of multiple imputation (MI)—replicating the process of completion a few times and estimating the variance inflation from the between-imputation variance.

Table 7.2. The results of a study of the population and outcomes listed in Table 7.1. Imputed values are printed in small font.

W	Sex	Status	Outcome $Y^{(A)}$	$Y^{(B)}$	W	Sex	Status	Outcome $Y^{(A)}$	$Y^{(B)}$
A	M	H	17	10	B	F	H	14	12
A	M	H	15	12	A	F	H	15	12
B	M	H	17	10	A	F	H	12	12
B	M	H	17	12	A	F	H	14	12
A	M	O	14	13	A	F	O	13	12
B	M	O	14	13	A	F	O	12	12
B	M	O	14	11	B	F	O	13	12

MI does not work well in the example given in Table 7.2 because the pools of donors are too small and fail to represent the uncertainty about the missing values by the candidates for plausible values, the donor pools. At the extreme, as when imputing for $Y^{(B)}$ for the background combination FH, the donor pool comprises a single unit, and so the value of 12 is imputed for all three missing items in every completion.

In larger-scale studies, this problem does not arise, although when many background variables are recorded, a fine balance has to be struck between defining relatively small pools by conditioning on many variables and large pools of donors by conditioning on a selection of the variables. The pools of donors can be made larger by coarsening some of the background variables. It is particularly useful to eliminate rare categories by aggregating them with their neighbours.

Intermediate variables should never be involved in conditioning, because their values are affected (tainted) by the treatment applied. Some studies record the values of several intermediate variables, such as the outcome variable recorded at regular intervals during the administration of the treatment. For each intermediate variable, we can define its treatment-specific potential versions. One-half of their values are not recorded, so plausible values have to be generated for them. This is done multiply to reflect our uncertainty about them. The 'true' value of any one of these potential intermediate variables is defined prior to administering the treatment; they are independent of the assignment. They can therefore be treated in conditioning as if they were background variables, except that they are represented by sets of plausible values. Thus, each completed-data analysis is based on a different (replicate) set of such values.

7.4 Imperfect Experiments

The assignment imposed by an experimental design may be violated by mistake or by the human subjects exercising their prerogative to discontinue treatment (abandon participation in the experiment) or switch to the alternative treatment. This section deals with the analysis of such experiments using the following approach. We consider the dataset planned to have been collected as the complete and the recorded data as the incomplete (observed) dataset, and address the problem by a method for missing data, such as MI. The analysis of the complete data may itself require an application of MI, but combining the two MI procedures generates no difficulties. First we outline some alternatives related to data reduction and single imputation and point out their deficiencies.

Treated as per Protocol

We may reduce the analysis to the units that were subjected to the treatments as set out by the protocol and randomisation and ignore the units for which the assigned treatment was applied only partially or not at all. The problem with this approach is that the experiment is no longer regarded as having been conducted on the entire population or a sample drawn according to a specified design, and the units that departed from the assigned treatment may have done so after an informed guess of their potential outcomes. For instance, a patient in a clinical trial may opt out from (further) treatment believing that it is not useful and that another treatment would be more effective. Another patient may drop out from a study because of improvement that in his or her view makes further treatment unnecessary and does not justify the inconvenience involved.

Information about the reasons for dropping out may be useful for an application of MI to (multiply) complete the data. It would narrow the range or distribution of plausible values on which to base the data completion. In some settings the dissenting subjects may provide such information, possibly supplemented by expert opinion.

The Treatment Applied (as Treated)

If a unit switched (or has been switched) from the assigned to another treatment we may estimate the treatment effect by regarding the treatments that were applied as if they were assigned a priori. The deficiency of this approach is that such an *altered* assignment is no longer an assignment by randomisation. A concern is that any switch may have been informed, made in an attempt to obtain a better outcome. Would the same outcome be observed if the subject were assigned the latter treatment originally? If a switch of treatments can occur we have to consider four possibilities: T assigned and T′ administered, where T and T′ are either A or B. The combinations (T

$= A, T' = A$) and ($T = B, T' = A$) need not result in the same values of the outcomes, even though the same treatment is applied. And, of course, the switch is not assigned by randomisation.

Intent to Treat

Finally, we may ignore any violations of the protocol and simply analyse the data as if the protocol had been adhered to in every detail. The obvious deficiency of this approach is the denial—pretending that the study was conducted as intended, when in fact it was not. The missing-data perspective entails a speculation as to what the outcome would have been had the protocol been adhered to.

Randomised assignment is a key design feature in experiments that enables us to make efficient inferences about the treatment effects. Any deviation from randomisation should be reflected by reduced confidence, to maintain the integrity of the analysis. Multiple imputation has a potential to achieve this, and it does so when the uncertainty about the missing values is appropriately reflected in the differences among the sets of completions.

For settings in which the (human) units are aware of the treatment received and its status (e.g., as a novel experimental or as an established treatment), we consider two complementary subpopulations: compliers (C) and noncompliers (N). Let their proportions in the population be p_C and p_N. Compliers would not object to the novel treatment B and would receive it as per protocol. Noncompliers would object and would switch to A if assigned treatment B. Thus, we can identify noncompliers only among the units that were assigned treatment B. We cannot distinguish between compliers and noncompliers among the units assigned treatment A. Therefore, 'as treated' analysis does not compare the treatments on the same (sub)populations.

We could estimate the treatment effect by imputing values for all the missing items—for the noncompliers who were assigned treatment B but refused to take it. For the noncompliers the assignment is irrelevant—they would insist on their preferred treatment. This assumption of irrelevance is referred to as the *exclusion restriction*. It should not be taken for granted in any setting, although it is often quite realistic. In some settings, the roles of the treatments are reversed. When treatment B is more attractive, departures from the protocol occur among units assigned to A who wish to receive the more promising treatment B. In principle, there may be defections in both directions.

Without the exclusion restriction, we have to consider the four potential outcomes, for the combinations (T, T') of treatment assigned and treatment received. One of these, such as A assigned and B received (or vice versa), may not occur. We can avoid having to impute values for each missing item by considering the effect of assigning treatment B over A, denoted by Γ_{AB}. This is different from the effect of (applying) treatment B over A, Δ_{AB}. We have

$$\Gamma_{AB} = p_N \, \Gamma_{AB}^{(N)} + p_C \, \Gamma_{AB}^{(C)}.$$

The left-hand side is estimated directly by the 'Intent to treat' analysis, assuming that no error occurred in implementing the assignment (offering the treatment selected by randomisation). For compliers, assignment is equivalent to treatment, and so $\Gamma_{AB}^{(C)} = \Delta_{AB}^{(C)}$. For noncompliers, $\Gamma_{AB}^{(N)} = 0$, according to the exclusion restriction. Hence

$$\Delta_{AB} = \frac{\Gamma_{AB}}{p_C}.$$

When estimating Δ_{AB} naively we have to be concerned about dividing by an (unbiased) estimator $\hat{p}_C$; p_C can be estimated straightforwardly from the units assigned treatment B, for which noncompliance is identified without uncertainty. This is problematic particularly when $1/p_C$ is estimated with little precision; when $\hat{p}_C$ is small and when the experiment (n) is small. In general, the smaller the fraction p_C the more we have to rely on the exclusion restriction.

7.5 Comparing Institutions

Modern management of services, such as education, health care, and public transport, is invariably connected with targets and competition among the institutions providing the service. Examples of such a trend are the prominently publicised league tables that list the institutions (schools, universities, hospitals, local administrative authorities, and the like) in the order of the summaries of their performances, such as examination results for schools and survival rates and waiting times for surgery for hospitals. In most of these examples, manifest variables are used in place of latent variables, which are difficult to 'measure', or their precise measurement would entail unacceptable disruption of the institutions' core activities. To avoid handling a convoluted problem, we set aside the issue of substitution of a latent variable by a manifest one, dealt with in Chapter 6, even though it is highly relevant in this context.

Schools have students, hospitals have patients and, in general, institutions have clientele or *intake*. A fundamental difficulty in comparing institutions is that their intakes differ. Institutions may deliberately aim to serve or as a result of development end up serving a clientele with a particular distribution of profiles (backgrounds). Inasmuch as these distributions differ, comparison of institution-level summaries is not of like with like. Desired are comparisons for the hypothetical setting in which each institution has the same intake. Therefore, we should first specify this intake, or the distribution of the profiles of the clientele. We could borrow it from an institution or define it as the overall (national) profile. However, neither choice, nor any other, is appropriate because the performance of each institution should be assessed for *its* clientele, not for a clientele they would never contemplate serving.

We regard the act of client i receiving the service of institution A as a treatment and consider the outcome $Y_i^{(A)}$ together with the potential outcomes of the client in response to treatment by other institutions in which the client could conceivably have been treated. These are usually not all the institutions in their population, because the client may not qualify for or may not be interested in being treated by some of them. We define the *constituency* C_T of institution T as the subpopulation of clients who could conceivably be treated by institution T. A client and an institution are said to be *compatible* if the client belongs to the constituency of the institution. A compatible pairing of client and institution is *realised* if the client is or was treated by the institution and is unrealised otherwise.

We say that two institutions are *comparable* if their constituencies have a substantial overlap. The term substantial overlap itself has to be defined. For example, two universities have a substantial overlap if at least a certain percentage (say 80%) of students who attend one university would consider attending the other as an equal alternative, defined as offering similar courses, having similar entry requirements, comparable reputations, and similar fees and other expenses. The constituencies need not be constrained by the catchment areas of the institutions. For example, a patient would not contemplate treatment for a minor ailment in a distant hospital. However, if the catchment areas of the two hospitals are similar in terms of the profiles of their patients—their socioeconomic, environmental, and related conditions—then it is meaningful to define potential outcomes of patients in one area for the distant hospital.

We define the *effect* of institution B over institution A for client i as the difference of the potential outcomes $Y_i^{(B)} - Y_i^{(A)}$. Such an effect is defined only for clients compatible with both institutions. The average (constituency-level) effect of institution B over a comparable institution A is defined as the mean of the client-level effects, averaged over the overlap of the institution's constituencies. We adopt the SUTVA assumptions, so that the effect does not depend on the actual assignment.

In the complete-data setting, with all the defined potential outcomes available, the problem of comparing any two institutions is elementary, involving a comparison of the means of the potential outcomes for the two institutions. This complete-data analysis entails no uncertainty. The incompleteness, having observed only one (or no) potential outcome for each client, is the sole source of uncertainty, placing all the inferential burden on the process of generating (multiple) plausible outcomes for each unrealised compatible client-institution pairing (i, T).

The hot deck and approximate Bayesian bootstrap (Section 5.6) are well motivated methods for generating plausible outcomes. We define a match of the backgrounds of clients as the agreement on their values of selected background variables; these variables may be original or coarsened. For an unrealised compatible client-institution pairing (i, T), we form a pool of realised pairs (i', T) who are a match for client i, draw a client from this pool at random, and use his or her value as the plausible value of $Y_i^{(\text{T})}$. This process of completion, for every unrealised compatible pairing (i, T), is replicated M times, resulting in M comparisons which are then summarised by the rules for the results of completed-data analyses [see Section 5.5 and equation (5.10)] with the within-imputation variance W set to zero.

As an alternative to matching on several background variables, a single variable (an 'index') may be defined, when appropriate, and the match based on its coarsened version. In some settings, institutions have many realised clients and their backgrounds are not available or not accessible, or the analysis of their backgrounds is not feasible for some other reason, such as confidentiality. A random sample of clients may then be used for estimating whether a pair of institutions is comparable, but the resulting uncertainty has to be incorporated in the analysis.

When the background can be represented by a single ordinal variable, such as a university entrance examination score, then the institutions can be ordered by suitable summaries of the backgrounds of their clients. If only within-institution summaries of this background variable are available or the client-level matching exercise is regarded as too complex, *caliper matching* provides a solution. For a set integer K, the $2K$ closest rivals of a given institution T are defined as the K institutions immediately preceding and following institution T in the order of their background summaries. The outcome of the comparison is the rank of the summaries of the outcomes of institution T among its $2K$ closest rivals. Establishing this may itself be an incomplete-data problem, if the background summaries or the outcome summaries are established subject to uncertainty. Some provisions have to be made for the top and bottom K institutions which have too few rivals preceding or following them in the ranking according to the background and are not at the median of the list of their closest rivals. Apart from conceptual simplicity, caliper matching has the advantage of an easy-to-interpret outcome: the score (rank) of 1 is ideal and $2K + 1$ is the worst possible. Although each institution has a score on the same scale, these scores can be compared only for pairs of institutions whose sets of closest rivals have a substantial overlap. For such a pair of institutions, scores can be defined also on the overlap of their closest rivals.

The managements of institutions regard the assessment of their performances as vital for recruitment of staff and clientele, and good assessment may be accompanied by direct (financial) rewards. If they are acquainted with the analysis planned for the summaries of the outcomes, they may manipulate the intake procedures so as to alter the distribution of their clients' backgrounds or set aside some of the clinical priorities in favour of improving the values of the outcome summaries. For example, a university may recruit more intensively among students with backgrounds associated with successful graduation, or a hospital may discourage references from general practices for surgery cases that are likely to entail risks or complications not taken into account by the performance assessment system.

The results of caliper matching cannot be influenced by such manipulation of the intake in any straightforward way because, by changing the distribution of the profile of the intake, the institution changes the composition of the group of its close rivals, and its score is then based on a different set of rival institutions. Ordering the institutions' scores is meaningless because they are scores from different 'contests'. The scores of two institutions can be compared only when they share most of their closest rivals—when they are comparable according to a well-founded definition.

7.5.1 Comparing Performances over Time

A single institution may assess the improvement of the quality of its services by comparing within-period summaries of the outcomes, such as annual success rates of the operations of a particular kind and percentages of students retained (who do not drop out from courses). Comparisons of such summaries are meaningful only when the period-specific constituencies of the institution have a substantial overlap. Although the distribution of the clientele's background changes very little from one period (year) to the next, these distributions may *drift*, move slowly but consistently, so that the profiles of the constituencies several periods apart are substantially different. Therefore, comparability is maintained only for a limited number of periods.

This setting is closely related to comparisons of institutions. Simply, we regard the pairs of the institution in question and period $t = 1, \ldots, T$ formally as separate institutions, with t defining their ordering; time is regarded as capturing all the background of the clientele within the time period. In this setting, comparing only within a 'window of time' corresponds to caliper matching.

When background information about the clientele is available, the period can be compared using multiple sets of plausible outcomes for the overlap of the constituencies of the pairs of periods. If for periods far apart few clients are compatible with the two periods, the comparison is not meaningful—the periods are not comparable.

By way of an example, consider the rates of ruptured abdominal aortic aneurysm (RAAA). It is an accident-like condition requiring immediate (emergency) intensive treatment, and the success rate of treating it is not very high. Many patients die before or during the emergency treatment or within days, and few of those who survive can recover their earlier life style. A (national) health care system may be concerned that the survival rates of RAAA have not been rising over the years, despite improved training, new equipment, accumulated expertise, and greater resources devoted to the treatment.

RAAA can be attributed to the long-term wear and tear of the human organism, exacerbated by various diseases such as heart disease, cancer, and infections. Although these diseases are cured or alleviated by invasive medical procedures, at least temporarily, they impose shocks on the organism that tend to accumulate until the body gives up at its weakest point. This suggests that the relevant background of RAAA patients (more precisely, cases, since a person may in principle suffer RAAA repeatedly) are their medical histories, and invasive surgeries in particular. A typical RAAA patient in the 1970s had a very different medical history than a more recent patient because numerous types of surgeries that are commonly conducted today (or in the recent past) were not available in the 1970s or were in early stages of their development and were conducted with equipment inferior to today's. This makes any comparison of the survival rates over the span of thirty or so years, but probably even over a much shorter time span, misleading, because it is not a comparison of like with like. There may be a few patients in the 1970s or today who are compatible with the other (unrealised) period, but basing a comparison on them may also be misleading because they are exceptional patients in one or both periods.

7.6 Regression Methods

The relevant background variables can be related to the outcomes by a regression model. If the values of the background variables were under the control of the study designer, each regression parameter associated with a continuous variable would have a straightforward interpretation as the expected change in the outcome in response to the change of the value of the background variable by one unit of measurement. In brief, the regression slope of a covariate is equal to the effect of changing its value by a unit of measurement. The values of the background variables usually cannot be prescribed (manipulated), and so such an interpretation is inappropriate. The slope is more appropriately described as the difference between two strata, after an adjustment for the other background variables in the model.

Applying regression models to assess performance of institutions may seem attractive because the outcomes have to be adjusted for background. A lack of such an adjustment was a profound objection to early methods of assessment that compared the mean outcomes, paying no regard to the differences in the within-institution distributions of the background variables. Fitting regression represents an improvement over comparing sample means. Some extensions of regression to structured samples, with units within institutions, are discussed in Chapter 9. When the variables used in the analysis are defined for institutions, not for units, the residuals are interpreted as indicators of performance—high residual as very good performance, low as poor performance.

Such analysis is open to the vagaries of specification of the model. Linearity is assumed, yet it may be problematic, especially when some covariates have a wide support. Obvious nonlinearity is easy to detect with large-scale data (many institutions), but small deviations may not be, yet their impact on the residuals may be decisive. A related argument against applying regression is that the performance of an institution is, in effect, decided by some institutions that are not comparable with it. Institutions with extreme values, or distributions of values, of the background variables exert a stronger influence over the assessment of an institution closer to the middle of the range of the backgrounds than the substance of the problem might suggest. Comparisons based on plausible outcomes respond to this problem much more satisfactorily, although they place the onus on the process of generating plausible values.

Suggested Reading

The theory presented in this chapter was developed by Donald Rubin in several articles; see [157], [161], [163], and [166] and the references in the latter two. An instructive exposition of the so-called Rubin's causal model is given by [81]. For a review of the earlier work on causal inferences from observational studies, see [22] and [19]. The subject is treated in an up-to-date form by the monograph [156]. An alternative and in some aspects complementary approach that addresses causal inference from observational studies is developed by [65]. The monograph [144] is a scientifically rigorous treatise on causality.

A landmark case study in comparing the performance of surgical teams is reported in [185]. Methods for assessing surgical performance are reviewed from a historical perspective by [184]. A study of outcomes of the UK higher educational institutions is reported in [39]. A comprehensive list of guidelines for the construction, use, and interpretation of performance indicators for institutions is compiled and discussed by [9]. The idea of using caliper matching for comparing the performance of institutions is outlined in [128]. A framework for incorporating information from intermediate variables is developed by [52]. The example about ruptured abdominal aortic aneurysm in Section 7.5 is drawn from [86]; see [123] for its critique.

The monograph [96] is an inexhaustible source of profound and commonsense advice on conducting experiments and observational studies. The foundations of experimental design have been laid by [50], [21], and [25].

Problems and Exercises

7.1. Discuss the role that intermediate variables may usefully play in an analysis of the outcomes of a study in which drop-out is anticipated. If you find it helpful, discuss this issue separately for experiments and observational studies.

7.2. The file EX25a.dat on www.sntl.co.uk/BookA/Data contains a complete dataset, with one background variable X and the two potential outcomes,

$Y^{(A)}$ and $Y^{(B)}$, for respective treatments A and B. Implement on the computer the design with randomised allocation of subjects to treatments and two designs with blocked randomisation. In the first, blocking is applied haphazardly, placing the first $\frac{1}{2}n$ subjects into one block and the remainder into the other, and in the second, blocking is based on X: the $\frac{1}{2}n$ subjects with the smallest values of X are placed in one block and the remainder in the other. Replicate the assignment and estimation processes for each design 1000 times and assess their efficiencies.

7.3. In a marketing study, recruited households can choose one of three known brands of washing powder, A, B, and C. At the end of the trial period, they are asked to rate how satisfied they have been with the brand they used. Discuss how the study could have been improved by applying the principles of experimental design. List difficulties this would have entailed. Why might the study designers argue that the choice of brand is governed by CAR? Or by AR, with a short list of background variables?

7.4. In *encouragement studies*, recruited units (individuals or groups) are randomly assigned to two groups. One group receives no treatment, and the other group is encouraged to pursue a particular activity, such as exercise, to consume or stop consuming a particular product, to change diet or some other element of the lifestyle, and the like. All subjects complete a questionnaire at the end of the study period, and a suitable outcome variable is constructed from the responses. Is such a study an experiment or an observational study? Hint: Carefully define what constitutes a treatment.

7.5. Suppose the value of the individual-level outcome in a cluster-randomised study of two treatments is recorded for a simple random sample of $p = 2\%$ of the population of the cluster. Derive the sampling variance of the estimator of the average cluster-level effect. Suppose the costs of administering the treatments and measuring the outcome for a unit are given and the funds available for the study are fixed. How should the percentage p be traded for the cluster-level sample size n to estimate the treatment effect with as high precision as possible?

7.6. Suppose potential outcomes $Y^{(A)}$ and $Y^{(B)}$ differ by a constant c, $Y^{(B)} = Y^{(A)} + c$; the unit-level effect is constant, equal to c. Suppose $Y^{(A)}$ and $Y^{(B)}$ are both positive. Can you anticipate how the variance of the unit-level effects behaves as a function of the power transformation $g\left(Y^{(T)}\right)$ for T = A and B? Use a standardised power transformation $g(u) = u^q/D(q)$, so that a large variance of $U^{(A)} - U^{(B)}$ could not be explained by the large variances of $U^{(T)} = g\left(Y^{(T)}\right)$, T = A or B. Check your intuition analytically or by simulation. Discuss the impact of the distributions of $Y^{(A)}$ and $Y^{(B)}$ on this variance function. With another dataset, how would you search for the power transformation that brings the transformed outcomes closest of all to being a constant apart? Define the target of this search very carefully.

7.7. The principal statement on a death certificate states the 'cause of death'. Find in the appropriate literature its definition and decide whether and in what context this 'cause' is related to any intermediate variables.

Hint: Could poor diet or lack of exercise be declared causes of death?

7.8. Search in the statistical literature for references to studies of the association of smoking and lung cancer and find out how they concluded that smoking causes lung cancer. Describe the design of a hypothetical experiment from which the effect of smoking could be estimated without bias, and list the reasons why it cannot be conducted.

7.9. *Discrimination* of a group (subpopulation) A by or in favour of group B with respect to outcome Y is defined as the effect of group membership in the following sense. There is an authority (or a mechanism) that sets the value of Y for each member of the population $A \cup B$ and a vector of covariates Z that should, apart from some inexplicable (unexplainable) deviations, determine the value of Y. Adjust this definition as you see fit to suit your perception of discrimination in public services, in contracting employment, wages paid, and the like. Relate this definition to impartiality (recall the definition from Chapter 6). Can the group membership be regarded as a cause, even though it cannot be assigned to an individual? Discuss how you would design a study for assessing the presence (and extent) of discrimination in a setting of your choice. How is discrimination related to AR and CAR for a binary outcome variable Y?

7.10. Relate the rules for comparing sports teams in a competition, such as a league, in which each pair of teams play one or two matches, a cup that comprises rounds of matches from which winners proceed to the subsequent rounds, to criteria used for comparing institutions, such as hospitals, universities, or national governments. Assess these rules or criteria by relevance (face validity), fairness, and impartiality. Discuss the consequences of the comparisons (position in the league table) and whether the management of the institutions would conduct their business differently if the consequences were changed.

7.11. Discuss the difficulties of conducting a large-scale experiment to study the effectiveness of vaccination against a disease. Which of these difficulties are resolved by cluster-randomisation?

Hint: Consider the setting with and without a current vaccine and the public perception of the vaccine as a potential solution.

This exercise can be revisited after Chapter 8.

7.12. A world-class sprinter (athlete) requires about 30 metres to reach a speed close to his or her maximum. In outdoor competitions, there are two events for sprinters, 100 metres and 200 metres. There has been a long-standing argument among the connoisseurs of sprinting about who runs at a greater average speed: the 100-metre or the 200-metre runner. That is, whether 200 metres can be run faster than double the time for 100 metres. Check in the appropriate sources the world records for men and women, as well as the national records and recent years' best performances in your country. Discuss the appropriateness of the following comparisons to resolve this issue:

1. Compare the mean of the ten best performances in the world for the two events.
2. Select the ten fastest athletes ever who had no preference between 100 and 200 metres and compare the means of their best performances.
3. Reduce the comparison to athletes who took part in both 100-metre and 200-metre races at the same world championships (or Olympic Games) and compare the means of their best performances in the championships.
4. Set a reasonable 'qualifying limit', such as 10.5 sec for 100 metres and 20.5 sec for 200 metres for men and compare the means of the best performances of the athletes who have surpassed both these limits.

Discuss the hypothetical experiment that would resolve this issue, and what kind of compromise has to be made in each feasible setting. What assumption(s) have to be made in the analysis?

7.13. Discuss whether it is feasible and, if so, how caliper matching might be applied to assess the individual employees of a midsize corporation.

7.14. Compile a list of plausible explanations for the substantially higher number of successful results in the examinations at a particular level in the educational system, such as the SAT scores in the United States or the number of A-level passes in the UK. Classify the explanations into groups according to whether they are associated with improved instruction, instruction better targeted for the examinations, the examination papers becoming easier over time (carefully define what this means), and the like.

7.15. The dataset in file EX25b.dat on www.sntl.co.uk/BookA/Data contains the results of an experiment with a binary outcome, in which some subjects switched their treatment, in most cases from the novel treatment B to the established treatment A. Analyse the data by the three naive methods described in Section 7.4 and by a missing-data approach assuming the exclusion criterion, assuming that treatment A is more attractive than treatment B. Ignore the few switches from A assigned to B taken if it makes the problem simpler.

7.16. Discuss the advantages and drawbacks of the regression analysis using the model

$$Y_W = \beta_0 + X\beta_1 + I(W = B)\,\Delta_{AB} + \varepsilon$$

(W is the allocated treatment and I the indicator function) for the example in Exercise 7.2 with the three allocation designs. Check in the analysis those of your arguments that can be checked, either by the realised (incomplete) data or by the complete dataset. Discuss the circumstances in which the interaction of the covariate X and the treatment would be necessary or useful to add to the model. Apply the estimator of Δ_{AB} in replications for each allocation design and compare its efficiency with its counterpart in Exercise 7.2.

7.17. Organise a discussion of the issues related to gun control in the United States. Formulate the arguments in its favour and against it in terms of effects (such as violent crime and accidents with firearms versus personal security and inalienable rights) and the difficulty of collecting statistical evidence that would provide an effective support for a legislative proposal to ban private ownership of firearms.

8

Clinical Trials

Clinical trials are experiments conducted on human subjects or animals in the process of developing new medical treatments, devices, and procedures. The results of a clinical trial are usually part of a package that supports the developer's a priori stated claim that the proposed treatment has a beneficial effect of a specified kind and for a specified condition. Clinical trials are characterised by the intent to adhere to the principles of experimental design and to ensure that the exposure of vulnerable subjects (humans or animals) to experimentation is as small as possible, and yet sufficient for collecting evidence related to the claim. After setting out the context in which clinical trials are conducted, this chapter discusses the established methods for their design and analysis and then presents some alternatives.

8.1 The Context

Development of a new medical treatment, such as a drug or a procedure for treating a disease, is very a expensive and in its later stages a highly regulated enterprise. Developing a drug can cost several tens of millions of Euro and the process usually takes several years. It comprises several stages, starting with identifying the compound or group of compounds as candidates for the role of the active ingredient of a new drug. Experiments then may be conducted on animals to establish that the compound has the desired effect and to decide what quantity of the active ingredient (dose) would have the desired effect in human subjects, without any undesirable side effects. This entails some extrapolation which may not be perfectly reliable. In the next stage, the set dose, or a range of doses, are tried out on healthy human subjects (volunteers). Finally, the drug is tried out on a group of subjects who have the condition for which the drug is intended.

In this chapter, we are concerned mainly with clinical trials at this final stage, when the details of the drug—its dose, form of delivery (orally, as an injection, or the like), frequency (such as once a day), period of administration (such as two weeks), the condition and its exclusion criteria, that is, the intended population of patients, and other details—are specified. The inferential issue is now reduced to providing evidence that the proposed treatment B has a positive effect over the established treatment A. When there is no established treatment, placebo is used for treatment A. Treatment B is referred to as the novel (studied or tested) treatment and A as the *comparator*.

Subjects for a clinical trial are recruited, usually by agents in the health care system who come into contact with patients who have the condition. Although inferences are sought about a particular population, a design for sampling from it is not feasible, because the population is not accessible and a sampling frame is impossible to construct. Of course, the treatment is intended for administration to patients in the future, and so the target population is not even identified—some are yet to contract the condition. However, the population of current sufferers is likely to represent quite well the population in a few years' time, even if the overlap of the two populations is small. Although we refer to a population of patients, it is more appropriate to consider a population of *cases*, since some diseases are temporary and may be contracted more than once in a lifetime.

Each recruited subject (a parent or carer for a minor) is sought for an *informed consent*, by which the subject agrees to take part in the trial and understands that a treatment will be assigned to him or her at random, without any regard for which treatment might be (judged to be) more suitable. The subjects are made aware that they can withdraw from the trial at any time, without their statutory rights being affected in any way. Patients are regarded as *vulnerable subjects* and the participation of every one of them in a trial is associated with high ethical costs. The design of each trial is subject to an approval process by the agency that regulates the process of testing and distribution of drugs; the best known of these is the Food and Drug Administration in the United States.

Randomisation and blinding are key principles for clinical trials. The sample size (number of patients engaged in the trial) and the extent of exposure to the tested drug (or its alternative) are other important considerations. On the one hand, these should be as small as possible; on the other hand, the chances of arriving at the appropriate conclusions should be high, so that the conduct of the clinical trial would be justified.

8.2 Models and Inference

Suppose the established and novel treatments, A and B, respectively, are to be compared in a clinical trial. Each subject will be administered one of the treatments, assigned at random. Let $n_A = n_B = \frac{1}{2}n$ be the planned within-treatment subsample sizes. Suppose higher values of the outcome variable Y signify better outcomes. Each member of the target population is associated with two *potential outcomes*, denoted by $Y^{(A)}$ and $Y^{(B)}$, the outcomes that will or would be recorded if the respective treatment A and B is applied. Exactly one treatment is applied to each subject, so only half the values of $Y^{(A)}$ and $Y^{(B)}$ on the subjects are recorded. All $2n$ values are well defined because, for any one subject, the randomisation could have yielded the other assignment. Let τ_A^2 and τ_B^2 be the respective population variances of $Y^{(A)}$ and $Y^{(B)}$. We assume that $\tau_A^2 = \tau_B^2 = \tau^2$, unless stated otherwise.

A statistic that might be used for inferences about the population mean treatment effect of B over A is the sample difference of the within-treatment means

$$\hat{\Delta}_{AB}^{\dagger} = \bar{y}_B - \bar{y}_A \,.$$

As evidence is sought that treatment B is superior to treatment A, the hypothesis that the expectations $\mu_A = \mathrm{E}\left(Y^{(A)}\right)$ and $\mu_B = \mathrm{E}\left(Y^{(B)}\right)$ satisfy the inequality $\mu_A \geq \mu_B$ is adopted, so that its rejection would constitute evidence of the claimed properties of the novel treatment B, $\mu_B > \mu_A$. Therefore, the hypothesis is rejected for large values of $\hat{\Delta}_{AB}^{\dagger}$; the critical region $\{\hat{\Delta}_{AB}^{\dagger} > c\}$ is set so that if $\mu_A = \mu_B$, then the probability of the incorrect decision would not exceed a prescribed level α:

$$\mathrm{P}\left(\hat{\Delta}_{AB}^{\dagger} > c \,|\, \mu_A = \mu_B\right) \leq \alpha. \tag{8.1}$$

When $\mu_A > \mu_B$, $\mathrm{P}(\hat{\Delta}_{AB}^{\dagger} > c)$ is smaller than when $\mu_A = \mu_B$, so the size α of the test is maintained. As a matter of convention, without any scientific basis, α is set to 0.05. The assumption of normality of $\hat{\Delta}_{AB}^{\dagger}$ is usually well supported even for moderately large subsample sizes n_A and n_B. Further, we assume that the sample of patients is a simple random sample from the target population. This assumption is contentious and easy to challenge; its discussion is postponed to Section 8.4. With the assumption,

$$\hat{\Delta}_{AB}^{\dagger} \sim \mathcal{N}\left\{0, \left(\frac{1}{n_A} + \frac{1}{n_B}\right)\tau^2\right\},$$

implying the critical region given by

$$c = \tau\sqrt{\frac{1}{n_A} + \frac{1}{n_B}}\,\Phi^{-1}(1 - \alpha) \tag{8.2}$$

(Φ is the distribution function of the standard normal distribution and Φ^{-1} is its inverse, the normal quantile). If the two sample means are normally distributed (and τ is known), this choice of c results in equality in (8.1).

We set a *minimum important difference* $\Delta\mu$ which we regard as the smallest difference of $\mu_B - \mu_A$ that is of any clinical importance. Setting $\Delta\mu$ is a task for a clinical expert who can relate the differences on the scale of the outcomes to the clinical changes in the treated condition. For this value of $\Delta\mu$, we seek subsample sizes n_A and n_B, for which the planned test has a prescribed power, such as $\beta = 90\%$:

$$P\left(\hat{\Delta}^{\dagger}_{AB} > c \,|\, \mu_B = \mu_A + \Delta\mu\right) \geq \beta. \tag{8.3}$$

Just like the value of α, this percentage does not have a firm scientific basis either, but it is a well-established convention. The power cannot exceed $1 - \alpha$; otherwise equality in (8.1) could not be attained.

Equation (8.3) is solved by reference to the standard normal distribution. By applying Φ^{-1} to both sides and substituting for the critical value c from (8.2), we obtain the equivalent equation

$$\Phi^{-1}(1 - \alpha) - \frac{\Delta\mu}{\tau}\left(\frac{1}{n_A} + \frac{1}{n_B}\right)^{-\frac{1}{2}} \leq \Phi^{-1}(1 - \beta).$$

Therefore the subsample sizes have to satisfy the inequality

$$\frac{1}{n_A} + \frac{1}{n_B} \leq \frac{1}{\{\Phi^{-1}(1 - \alpha) + \Phi^{-1}(\beta)\}^2}\frac{\Delta\mu^2}{\tau^2}.$$

When $n_A = n_B$, this implies that

$$n \geq \frac{4\tau^2}{\Delta\mu^2}\left\{\Phi^{-1}(1 - \alpha) + \Phi^{-1}(\beta)\right\}^2. \tag{8.4}$$

When $\tau_A^2 \neq \tau_B^2$, the solution is obtained similarly, although the rationale for equal treatment-group sizes, $n_A = n_B$, is no longer sustained. We may want to minimise the total sample size $n_A + n_B$, in which case the subsample sizes should be proportional to the reciprocals of the standard deviations, $n_A/n_B = \tau_B/\tau_A$. There may be other reasons for assigning a greater proportion of subjects to one of the treatments, for example, to make the participation more attractive. (The informed consent form has to contain information about the randomisation and related details.)

Ethical standards dictate that the sample size n should be as small as possible. Therefore, the sample size should not be set much higher than the right-hand side of (8.4), although some allowance is usually made for withdrawals during the course of the trial. The value of $\Delta\mu$ is rarely without any contention or ambiguity, and the value of τ^2 is usually guessed or estimated from past trials in which the same outcome variable was used and subjects were recruited from the same or a related target population using a similar recruitment process.

Clinical trials described so far are associated with the model

$$Y_{jT} = \mu_T + \varepsilon_{jT}, \tag{8.5}$$

where T is the treatment applied (A or B) and ε_{jT} are a random sample from a centred distribution specific to each treatment T. For each subject j, Y_{jT} is realised only for one treatment. The deviation ε_{jT} should not be confused with measurement error or deviation due to temporal variation or due to the details of how the treatment was administered. Usually the dominant contributor to the within-treatment variance $\text{var}(Y \mid T) = \text{var}(Y^{(T)})$ is the heterogeneity of the patients—they may be at various stages of the treated condition, and the extent and severity as well as the ability to combat the condition differ from patient to patient. The association of the outcomes with some of these factors might be anticipated, but a trial can rarely afford a careful screening among suitable patients, so as to reduce the heterogeneity of those in the sample. In any case, good representation of the population should be a priority, because approval is sought not for the participants in the trial, nor for a particular narrow subpopulation, but for the entire population of sufferers from the specified condition. Section 8.3 describes designs that address the problems of patient heterogeneity.

8.2.1 Comparing Two Groups

At the planning stage, we assumed a known subject-level variance τ^2 and in (8.2) derived the critical value c based on it. At the conclusion of the study we may revise this position and admit that τ^2 is in fact not known and use its estimator instead. The obvious estimators are

$$\hat{\tau}_T^2 = \frac{1}{n_T - 1} \sum_{j \in T} (y_{jT} - \bar{y}_T)^2,$$

for the variances within treatments $T = A$ or B, and

$$\hat{\tau}^2 = \frac{(n_A - 1)\,\hat{\tau}_A^2 + (n_B - 1)\,\hat{\tau}_B^2}{n_A + n_B - 2} \tag{8.6}$$

for their common value. When the outcomes Y are normally distributed (conditionally on the treatment applied), this estimator has a scaled χ^2 distribution:

$$(n_A + n_B - 2)\,\frac{\hat{\tau}^2}{\tau^2} \sim \chi^2_{n_A + n_B - 2}.$$

If τ^2 were known we would refer to the statistic

$$\frac{\widehat{\Delta\mu}_{AB}}{\tau} \sqrt{\frac{n_A n_B}{n_A + n_B}};$$

under the null-hypothesis it has the standard normal distribution. When τ is not known we replace τ by its estimator given by (8.6). The resulting statistic

$$T_{AB} = \frac{\widehat{\Delta\mu}_{AB}}{\hat{\tau}} \sqrt{\frac{n_A n_B}{n_A + n_B}} \tag{8.7}$$

is bound to be more dispersed as a consequence or replacing the constant denominator by a random variable. Note an ambiguity in the notation: by $\hat{\tau}$

we mean $\sqrt{\hat{\tau}^2}$. Although $\hat{\tau}^2$ is unbiased for τ^2, $\hat{\tau}$ is biased τ. Similarly, $1/\hat{\tau}$ and $1/\hat{\tau}^2$ are biased for the respective targets $1/\tau$ and $1/\tau^2$.

The statistic defined by (8.7) is an example of a t-statistic, named after *Student's t-distribution*. The t-distribution with m degrees of freedom, denoted by t_m, is defined as the distribution of the ratio

$$ t = \frac{X}{\sqrt{U}}\sqrt{m}, $$

where variable X has the standard normal distribution and U has the χ^2 distribution with m degrees of freedom, and X and U are independent. The t-distribution is continuous, unimodal, and symmetric around zero. The density of the t_m distribution is

$$ f(x) = \frac{\Gamma\left(\frac{m+1}{2}\right)}{\sqrt{m\pi}\,\Gamma\left(\frac{m}{2}\right)}\left(1 + \frac{x^2}{m}\right)^{-\frac{m+1}{2}}. $$

As its number of degrees of freedom m approaches $+\infty$, t_m converges to the standard normal distribution. This follows immediately from the limit identity $(1+y/n)^n \to \exp(y)$; we need not be concerned with working out the limit of the fraction involving the constants, because the limiting function, a density, has to integrate up to unity. For orientation, the densities of a few t-distributions are plotted in Figure 8.1. The distribution t_m does not have a mean or variance for $m = 1$. For $m > 1$, its mean is equal to zero, as implied by symmetry. The variance of t_m is defined only for $m > 2$.

To prove that T_{AB} has the $t_{n_{\mathrm{A}}+n_{\mathrm{B}}-2}$ distribution when $\mu_{\mathrm{A}} = \mu_{\mathrm{B}}$, we set $X = \widehat{\Delta}\mu_{\mathrm{AB}}/\tau\sqrt{n_{\mathrm{A}}\,n_{\mathrm{B}}/(n_{\mathrm{A}}+n_{\mathrm{B}})}$ and $U = (n_{\mathrm{A}}+n_{\mathrm{B}}-2)\,\hat{\tau}^2/\tau^2$. It remains to show that, with these definitions, X and U are independent. We show first that the within-treatment mean $\bar{y}_{\mathrm{T}} = \mathbf{y}_{\mathrm{T}}^\top \mathbf{1}$ and centred sum of squares $S_{\mathrm{T}} = (\mathbf{y}_{\mathrm{T}} - \bar{y}_{\mathrm{T}}\mathbf{1})^\top(\mathbf{y}_{\mathrm{T}} - \bar{y}_{\mathrm{T}}\mathbf{1})$ are independent. The latter can be expressed as $S_{\mathrm{T}} = \mathbf{y}_{\mathrm{T}}^\top(\mathbf{I}-\mathbf{P}_{\mathrm{T}})\mathbf{y}_{\mathrm{T}}$, where $\mathbf{P}_{\mathrm{T}}$ is the projection matrix, $\mathbf{P}_{\mathrm{T}} = n_{\mathrm{T}}^{-1}\mathbf{1}\mathbf{1}^\top$. Since $\mathbf{I}-\mathbf{P}_{\mathrm{T}}$ is idempotent, $\mathbf{I}-\mathbf{P}_{\mathrm{T}} = (\mathbf{I}-\mathbf{P}_{\mathrm{T}})^2$, and so $S_{\mathrm{T}} = \mathbf{y}_{\mathrm{T}}^\top(\mathbf{I}-\mathbf{P}_{\mathrm{T}})(\mathbf{I}-\mathbf{P}_{\mathrm{T}})\mathbf{y}_{\mathrm{T}}$. Now

$$ \mathrm{cov}\left\{(\mathbf{I}-\mathbf{P}_{\mathrm{T}})\mathbf{y}_{\mathrm{T}},\, \mathbf{1}^\top\mathbf{y}_{\mathrm{T}}\right\} = \tau_{\mathrm{T}}^2(\mathbf{I}-\mathbf{P}_{\mathrm{T}})\mathbf{1} = \mathbf{0}, $$

and no correlation of normally distributed variables implies their independence. Hence $\bar{y}_{\mathrm{T}}$ is also independent of a function of $\mathbf{y}_{\mathrm{T}} - \bar{y}_{\mathrm{T}}\mathbf{1}$, namely, of S_{T}. Finally, $(\bar{y}_{\mathrm{A}}, \bar{y}_{\mathrm{B}})$ is independent of $(S_{\mathrm{A}}, S_{\mathrm{B}})$, and so are their linear combinations. This concludes the proof that T_{AB} has the $t_{n_{\mathrm{A}}+n_{\mathrm{B}}-2}$ distribution.

The hypothesis that $\mu_{\mathrm{A}} \geq \mu_{\mathrm{B}}$ against the alternative $\mu_{\mathrm{B}} > \mu_{\mathrm{A}}$ is rejected when $T_{\mathrm{AB}} > c$, where c is the $(1-\alpha)$-quantile of the $t_{n_{\mathrm{A}}+n_{\mathrm{B}}-2}$ distribution. For $\alpha < 0.5$, this quantile is a decreasing function of the number of degrees of freedom and it converges to the corresponding quantile of the standard normal distribution as both sample sizes n_{A} and n_{B} increase above all bounds. The decrease is rapid for few degrees of freedom, and then it levels off. For example, the 0.95-quantile of t_1 is 6.31, of t_{10} is 1.81, and of t_{100} is 1.66, very close to

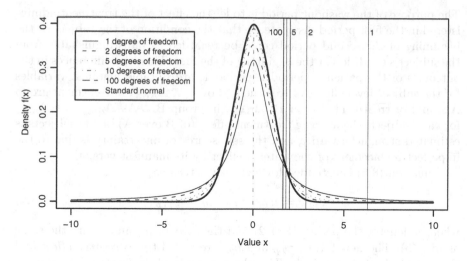

Fig. 8.1. The densities of the t-distributions with the indicated numbers of degrees of freedom and the normal distribution (highlighted). The vertical lines mark the 95th percentiles of the distributions; these cannot be distinguished for t_{100} (1.660) and the standard normal (1.645).

the 0.95-quantile of $t_{+\infty}$ or $\mathcal{N}(0,1)$, 1.645; see Figure 8.1. So, when estimating τ^2 with 100 or more degrees of freedom, we can ignore the uncertainty about it and compare the two groups (with normally distributed outcomes) as if the value of τ^2 were known and equal to $\hat{\tau}^2$.

8.3 Crossover Design

For a given pair of sample sizes n_A and n_B, the between-subject variance τ^2 governs the precision of the estimator $\widehat{\Delta}\mu_{AB}$. If the subject-level treatment effects $\Delta_{AB,j} = Y_j^{(B)} - Y_j^{(A)}$ vary much less than τ^2 or are constant, $\Delta\mu_{AB}$ could be estimated much more precisely if these treatment effects were observed, after administering both treatments to some or all of the subjects. This is a powerful rationale for the *crossover design*.

In a crossover trial, each subject is administered a sequence of treatments with the administrations separated by a *washout period*. In the simplest crossover design, n_{AB} subjects are administered treatment A in the first and treatment B in the second period. Another group, comprising n_{BA} subjects, are administered treatment B in the first and treatment A in the second period; usually $n_{AB} = n_{BA} = \frac{1}{2}n$, although the equality is not necessary and, in principle, some subjects could be administered the same treatment in both periods. The sequence of treatments administered, AB and BA in this example, is called a *regimen*. We refer to the treatment groups by their regimens.

The purpose of the washout period is to let the effect of the treatment administered in the first period dissipate, so that the condition of the subject at the beginning of the second period could be regarded as indistinguishable from the subject's condition at the beginning of the first. Then the differences in the outcomes of the patients, period 2–period 1, are suitable manifest variables for the subject-level effects of treatment B over A, $\Delta_{AB,i}$, in treatment group AB, and of treatment A over B, $\Delta_{BA,i}$, in group BA. As $\Delta_{BA,j} = -\Delta_{AB,j}$ for each subject, the average treatment effect (of B over A) of the subjects is estimated straightforwardly, and the sole source of uncertainty is due to the imperfect replacement of the (latent) effect by its manifest version.

Equation (8.5) is extended for a crossover trial as

$$Y_{jTp} = \mu_T + \gamma_{Tp} + \eta_p + \varepsilon_{jTp}, \qquad (8.8)$$

where p denotes the period (1 or 2) and the roles of μ_T and ε_j are the same as in (8.5). The new terms, γ_{Tp} and η_p, are called the *carryover effect* and the *period effect*, respectively. The observation-level deviations ε_{jTp} may be correlated within subjects. They could be decomposed into sums of subject- and observation-level terms, $\varepsilon_{jTp} = \delta_j + \nu_{jTp}$; these components are independent and their respective variances are denoted by τ^2 and σ^2. The latter variance can be estimated from within-subject contrasts, such as $Y_{jB2} - Y_{jA1}$ for subject j in treatment group AB, in which the subject-level terms δ_j cancel out.

Note that the term *effect* is used here differently from Chapter 7, even though the treatment order and period are controlled by design. They are more closely related to average effects (in the sample), but even that only under some assumptions that are unlikely to be satisfied. Foremost among them is the assumption that the subjects are a good representation of the relevant population. Section 8.4 addresses this issue in more detail. In (8.8), all pairs of indices jT are realised, as well as all pairs jp, but not all triplets jTp, because each subject receives any given treatment in only one period.

The values of γ_{A1} and γ_{B1} in (8.8) are constrained to zero because there is no treatment preceding the first period. Only the difference $\gamma_{B2} - \gamma_{A2}$ can be identified, so γ_{A2} is also constrained to zero. Therefore, $\gamma = \gamma_{B2}$ is the only parameter related to carryover. It can be described as an adjustment of the mean outcome of treatment B when it is administered in the second period, following treatment A in the first period. The period effect η_p is also identified only for one period, so we set, by convention, $\eta_1 = 0$. Then $\eta = \eta_2$ is the sole model parameter associated with the two periods.

The model in (8.8) presents a perspective different from that of Chapter 7. Here an infinite (very large) population is considered and its outcomes in response to the treatments are random. The model parameters can be interpreted as either applicable to every member of the population (including a common treatment effect) or as population averages. A clinical trial is sometimes referred to as a *group trial*, suggesting that inferences are sought only for the group of patients who participate in the trial, and the extrapolation to the relevant population is deferred to a separate analysis. Then the interpretation of the deviations ε is crucial. For example, if they are specific to each participant-treatment combination, then the treatment effect in a crossover trial is established with precision, because so is each subject's treatment effect.

8.3.1 Estimation

The model in (8.8), with the assumptions of normality, independence, and homoscedasticity, is an ordinary regression model. If the treatment, carryover, and period are represented by binary variables, equal to unity for treatment B, the treatment-period pair B2, and period 2, respectively, then the regression design matrix is

$$\mathbf{X} = \begin{pmatrix} 1 & 0 & 0 & 0 \\ 1 & 1 & 1 & 1 \\ 1 & 1 & 0 & 0 \\ 1 & 0 & 0 & 1 \end{pmatrix},$$

where the first two row-blocks contain n_{AB} rows each, and the next two n_{BA} each. Let the vector of outcomes be $\mathbf{y}$, with the corresponding partitioning

$$\mathbf{y} = \left(\mathbf{y}_{AB1}^\top, \mathbf{y}_{AB2}^\top, \mathbf{y}_{BA1}^\top, \mathbf{y}_{BA2}^\top \right)^\top,$$

in which the subscripts indicate the regimen and period. Then the least squares estimator of the vector $\boldsymbol{\theta} = (\mu_A, \Delta\mu_{AB}, \gamma, \eta)^\top$ is

$$\hat{\boldsymbol{\theta}} = \left(\mathbf{X}^\top \mathbf{X} \right)^{-1} \mathbf{X}^\top \mathbf{y}.$$

We have

$$\mathbf{X}^\top \mathbf{X} = \begin{pmatrix} 2n & n & n_{AB} & n \\ n & n & n_{AB} & n_{AB} \\ n_{AB} & n_{AB} & n_{AB} & n_{AB} \\ n & n_{AB} & n_{AB} & n \end{pmatrix}$$

and

$$\left(\mathbf{X}^\top \mathbf{X} \right)^{-1} = \begin{pmatrix} a & -a & a & -a \\ -a & b & -b & a \\ a & -b & 2b & -b \\ -a & a & -b & b \end{pmatrix},$$

where $a = 1/n_{AB}$ and $b = n/(n_{AB} n_{BA})$. This can be checked directly by multiplying the two matrices or derived by elementary operations. Note that $b - a = 1/n_{BA}$. Further,

$$\mathbf{X}^\top \mathbf{y} = \left(\mathbf{y}^\top \mathbf{1}, \mathbf{y}_{AB2}^\top \mathbf{1} + \mathbf{y}_{BA1}^\top \mathbf{1}, \mathbf{y}_{AB2}^\top \mathbf{1}, \mathbf{y}_{AB2}^\top \mathbf{1} + \mathbf{y}_{BA2}^\top \mathbf{1} \right),$$

so the estimator of the treatment effect (the second element of $\hat{\boldsymbol{\theta}}$) is

$$\widehat{\Delta \mu}_{AB} = -a\mathbf{y}^\top \mathbf{1} + b\mathbf{y}_{AB2}^\top \mathbf{1} + b\mathbf{y}_{BA1}^\top \mathbf{1} - b\mathbf{y}_{AB2}^\top \mathbf{1} + a\mathbf{y}_{AB2}^\top \mathbf{1} + a\mathbf{y}_{BA2}^\top \mathbf{1}$$

$$= -a\mathbf{y}_{AB1}^\top \mathbf{1} + (b-a)\mathbf{y}_{BA1}^\top \mathbf{1} \quad = \bar{y}_{AB1} - \bar{y}_{BA1}, \tag{8.9}$$

where the bar denotes the sample mean within the indicated period-treatment combination. Thus, the treatment effect is estimated solely based on the outcomes recorded in the first period. If the outcomes from the second period are not used at all, conducting it could not be justified; the anticipated advantages of the crossover design would not be realised. The sampling variance of the estimator in (8.9) is

$$(V =) \quad \mathrm{var}\left(\widehat{\Delta \mu}_{AB}\right) = (\tau^2 + \sigma^2)\left(\frac{1}{n_{AB}} + \frac{1}{n_{BA}}\right), \tag{8.10}$$

where τ^2 is the variance of the subjects' treatment effects and σ^2 is the inconsistency variance; in (8.8), $\mathrm{var}(\varepsilon) = \sigma^2 + \tau^2$.

The explanation of why the second period is redundant in (8.9) is that the model in (8.8) and the estimation based on it fail to take into account the purpose of the washout, to remove the carryover. We could either (optimistically) assume that the washout is effective and it removes the carryover or expose the subjects to only one treatment each. A compromise of these two solutions is based on the assumption that the carryover is small. Then the crossover design is useful, and the analysis is not tainted by the inappropriate assumption that $\gamma = 0$.

As an aside, note that the estimator $\widehat{\Delta \mu}_{AB}$ can be derived without evaluating the inverse of $\mathbf{X}^\top \mathbf{X}$. The means of the outcomes within the treatment-period combinations are a set of (minimal) linear sufficient statistics, and the four equations that match these statistics with their expectations are equivalent to least squares and maximum likelihood estimation. There are four statistics and four parameters, μ_A, μ_B, γ, and η, so there is at most one solution. Details are left for an exercise.

If the carryover is assumed to be absent, then the ordinary least squares estimator is

$$\widehat{\Delta \mu}_{AB}^{(0)} = \frac{1}{2}\left(\bar{y}_{AB2} - \bar{y}_{AB1}\right) + \frac{1}{2}\left(\bar{y}_{BA1} - \bar{y}_{BA2}\right);$$

outcomes from both periods contribute to estimating the treatment effect. Its sampling variance is

$$(V_0 =) \quad \mathrm{var}\left(\widehat{\Delta \mu}_{AB}^{(0)}\right) = \frac{\sigma^2}{2}\left(\frac{1}{n_{AB}} + \frac{1}{n_{BA}}\right), \tag{8.11}$$

substantially smaller than (8.10), especially when τ^2 is greater than σ^2. In the estimator $\widehat{\Delta \mu}_{AB}^{(0)}$, the periods contribute with equal weights, $\frac{1}{2}$ each, whereas with carryover as a nuisance parameter, only the first period contributes, so that the periods associated with the weights are 1 and 0. This motivates a compromise estimator in which the first period is assigned weight w greater than $\frac{1}{2}$ and the second is assigned its complement to unity, $1-w$. The difference of the weights, and therefore the information value of the observations from the two periods, would reflect our reduced confidence in the outcomes from the second period because they are tainted by a possibly imperfect but not totally ineffective washout.

8.3.2 Minimax Estimation

The MSEs of alternative estimators of the same target often depend on (unknown) parameters, and so finding the most efficient of them is not trivial. Some estimators have their *niches*, narrow regions of the parameter space where they are efficient or nearly so, and *weaknesses*, where their MSEs are much greater than for some other estimators. *Minimax* is a criterion for a class of estimators. We compare the maxima of their MSEs over the parameter space and select the one with the smallest maximum. Such an estimator, qualified by the class and the parameter space, is called minimax. It is the estimator of choice when we do not care about the niches or strengths of an estimator and seek the one with the least pronounced weaknesses. For an expensive experiment, such as a clinical trial, we would like to state in advance and with some level of certainty that the MSE of the selected estimator of the treatment effect, the key target, will not exceed a given level. With a minimax estimator, this level can be the smallest possible. In addition to the class of estimators and the parameter space, this has to be qualified by adherence to the plan (design) and validity of the assumptions made.

Suppose we are satisfied that the carryover effect does not exceed a certain limit Γ; we are confident that $|\gamma| < \Gamma$. We derive an estimator of $\Delta\mu_{AB}$ well suited for this threshold value of γ and explore its properties when $|\gamma| < \Gamma$. The problem is symmetric around $\gamma = 0$, so no generality is lost by assuming that $\gamma > 0$.

We have two estimators, $\widehat{\Delta}\mu_{AB}$ and $\widehat{\Delta}\mu_{AB}^{(0)}$. The former is unbiased but has a large variance, while the latter, although biased if $\gamma \neq 0$, is more efficient when $|\gamma|$ is small. We combine the two estimators so as to minimise the MSE of the combination when $\gamma = \Gamma$. The constituent estimators $\widehat{\Delta}\mu_{AB}$ and $\widehat{\Delta}\mu_{AB}^{(0)}$ have respective biases 0 and $\frac{1}{2}\Gamma$ and their sampling variances V and V_0 are given by (8.10) and (8.11), respectively. The covariance of the two estimators is V_0. This follows from independence of the two groups' observations and the identities

$$\text{cov}\left(\bar{y}_{BA,1}, \bar{y}_{BA,1} - \bar{y}_{BA,2}\right) = \text{cov}\left(\bar{\delta}_{BA} + \bar{\nu}_{BA,1}, \bar{\nu}_{BA,1} - \bar{\nu}_{BA,2}\right)$$

$$= \text{var}\left(\bar{\nu}_{BA,1}\right)$$

$$= \frac{\sigma^2}{n_{BA}},$$

and similarly

$$\mathrm{cov}\left(-\bar{y}_{\mathrm{AB},1}\,,\,\bar{y}_{\mathrm{AB},2}-\bar{y}_{\mathrm{AB},1}\right)=\frac{\sigma^2}{n_{\mathrm{AB}}}\,,$$

where bar denotes sample means within the indicated regimen-by-period combination and $\delta_j+\nu_{jGp}$ is the decomposition of ε_{jGp} in (8.8) to independent components for subject j in group (regimen) G and period $p=1,2$. Hence

$$\mathrm{cov}\left(\widehat{\Delta}\mu_{\mathrm{AB}}\,,\,\widehat{\Delta}\mu_{\mathrm{AB}}^{(0)}\right)=\frac{\sigma^2}{2}\left(\frac{1}{n_{\mathrm{AB}}}+\frac{1}{n_{\mathrm{BA}}}\right)=V_0\,.$$

A convex combination of the two estimators,

$$\widetilde{\Delta}\mu_{\mathrm{AB}}=(1-d)\widehat{\Delta}\mu_{\mathrm{AB}}+d\widehat{\Delta}\mu_{\mathrm{AB}}^{(0)}\,,$$

has the MSE

$$\mathrm{MSE}\left(\widetilde{\Delta}\mu_{\mathrm{AB}}\,;\,\Delta\mu_{\mathrm{AB}}\right)=(1-d)^2V+\left\{d^2+2d(1-d)\right\}V_0+\frac{d^2\gamma^2}{4}$$

$$=d^2\left(V-V_0+\frac{\gamma^2}{4}\right)-2d\left(V-V_0\right)+V\,.$$

This quadratic function of d attains its minimum for

$$d^*=\frac{4(V-V_0)}{4(V-V_0)+\gamma^2}\,,\qquad(8.12)$$

with

$$V-V_0=\left(\tau^2+\frac{\sigma^2}{2}\right)\left(\frac{1}{n_{\mathrm{AB}}}+\frac{1}{n_{\mathrm{BA}}}\right)\,.$$

As $0<d^*<1$, the estimator $\widetilde{\Delta}\mu_{\mathrm{AB}}$ has the anticipated interpretation. For $\gamma=0$, $d^*=1$ and we use only $\widehat{\Delta}\mu_{\mathrm{AB}}^{(0)}$. For very large γ, $d^*\doteq 0$, and we make little use of the second period; $\widetilde{\Delta}\mu_{\mathrm{AB}}\doteq\widehat{\Delta}\mu_{\mathrm{AB}}$. This concurs with intuition.

If γ were known to be equal to $\varGamma$ the minimum MSE would be

$$\mathrm{MSE}\left(\widetilde{\Delta}\mu_{\mathrm{AB}}\,;\,\Delta\mu_{\mathrm{AB}}\right)=V-\frac{4(V-V_0)^2}{4(V-V_0)+\varGamma^2}$$

$$=V_0+\frac{1}{4}\varGamma^2\,\frac{4(V-V_0)}{4(V-V_0)+\varGamma^2}\,;$$

the compromise estimator $\widetilde{\Delta}\mu_{\mathrm{AB}}$ would be more efficient than either of its constituents.

Let $\widetilde{\Delta}\mu_{\mathrm{AB}}^{(\varGamma)}$ be the estimator $\widetilde{\Delta}\mu_{\mathrm{AB}}$ with the coefficient d^* evaluated at $\gamma=\varGamma$. When γ has an arbitrary feasible value, $|\gamma|\leq\varGamma$, its MSE is

$$\mathrm{MSE}\left(\widetilde{\Delta}\mu_{\mathrm{AB}}^{(\varGamma)}\,;\,\Delta\mu_{\mathrm{AB}}\right)=\frac{(V-V_0)^2}{\left(V-V_0+\frac{1}{4}\varGamma^2\right)^2}\left(V-V_0+\frac{\gamma^2}{4}\right)$$

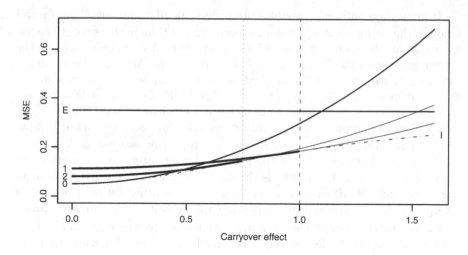

Fig. 8.2. The MSEs of estimators of the treatment effect $\Delta\mu_{AB}$ in a crossover trial with $n_{AB} = n_{BA} = 20$, $\sigma^2 = 1$, $\tau = 2.5$. The estimators are: E—$\widehat{\Delta}\mu_{AB}$, with the carryover estimated; 0—$\widehat{\Delta}\mu_{AB}^{(0)}$, with the carryover assumed absent; 1—$\widetilde{\Delta}\mu_{AB}^{(\Gamma)}$, minimax for $\Gamma = 1.0$; and 2—$\widetilde{\Delta}\mu_{AB}^{(\Gamma)}$, minimax for $\Gamma = 0.75$. The MSE of the optimal combination of estimators 'E' and '0', marked by 'I', is drawn by dots and dashes, obscured in most of the range $(0, 1)$.

$$-\frac{2(V - V_0)^2}{V - V_0 + \frac{1}{4}\Gamma^2} + V$$

$$= V - \frac{(V - V_0)^2}{\left(V - V_0 + \frac{1}{4}\Gamma^2\right)^2}\left\{V - V_0 + \frac{1}{4}\left(2\Gamma^2 - \gamma^2\right)\right\}.$$

$$(8.13)$$

This is an increasing linear function of γ^2, with slope smaller than $\frac{1}{4}$. By construction, it is efficient among the convex combinations $\widetilde{\Delta}\mu_{AB}$ when $\gamma = \Gamma$. Therefore, the MSE of any other convex combination $\widetilde{\Delta}\mu_{AB}$ exceeds the MSE in (8.13) when $\gamma = \Gamma$. Thus, $\widetilde{\Delta}\mu_{AB}^{(\Gamma)}$ is minimax among the convex combinations $\widetilde{\Delta}\mu_{AB}$ for $|\gamma| \leq \Gamma$.

Figure 8.2 gives an illustration. The MSE of the estimator $\widehat{\Delta}\mu_{AB}$, marked as E in the diagram, does not depend on the carryover effect γ. The estimator $\widehat{\Delta}\mu_{AB}^{(0)}$, marked as '0', is efficient when the carryover is absent or small but inefficient otherwise; it has a niche but also a weakness. For the setting $\Gamma = 1$, the estimator $\widehat{\Delta}\mu_{AB}^{(\Gamma)}$, marked as '1', is uniformly more efficient than $\widehat{\Delta}\mu_{AB}$ and is more efficient than $\widehat{\Delta}\mu_{AB}^{(0)}$ when the carryover is in the range 0.6–1.0. The MSE of $\widehat{\Delta}\mu_{AB}^{(0)}$ increases very steeply with carryover.

If we are too optimistic about Γ and the value of γ exceeds Γ by a small amount, the estimator $\widehat{\Delta}\mu_{AB}^{(\Gamma)}$ remains more efficient than both its constituents. If we can justify a smaller value of Γ, we are rewarded by uniformly higher efficiency in the plausible range of values of γ. The MSE of the minimax estimator based on $\Gamma = 0.75$, marked in the diagram by '2', is more efficient than estimator '1', so long as $|\gamma| < 0.75$. The MSE of estimator '2' increases with carryover at a faster rate, so that it is less efficient than estimator '1' for values of γ from about $\gamma = 0.85$ on. The penalty for using too small a value of Γ is quite harsh, especially with regard to the weaknesses of $\widehat{\Delta}\mu_{AB}^{(\Gamma)}$.

The optimal combination of the two constituent estimators, based on the value of γ as if it were known, is drawn by dots and dashes. It represents the lower limit of MSE, and its comparison with other estimators can be interpreted as the loss due to combining the constituent estimators $\widehat{\Delta}\mu_{AB}$ and $\widehat{\Delta}\mu_{AB}^{(0)}$ suboptimally. The minimax estimators give some ground against it for small Γ, but the loss is very small for large values of γ when they are plausible.

We have assumed that the values of σ^2 and τ^2 are known. In practice, they have to be estimated. This does not pose any substantial difficulties because for set sample sizes n_{AB} and n_{BA} the coefficient d^* in (8.12) depends only on the ratio $\gamma^2/(\tau^2 + \frac{1}{2}\sigma^2)$. In effect, we have to declare an upper bound on this ratio instead of on γ^2. It pays to be conservative, to protect our inferences against the possibility of high MSE.

8.4 Treatment Heterogeneity

The model in (8.8) and its submodels assume that a common treatment effect applies to every member of the population. In this section, we explore the consequences when this assumption is not satisfied. Suppose we can coarsely describe the effect of treatment B over A in a planned clinical trial as beneficial when $\mu_{AB} > \mu_1^*$, as innocuous (clinically unimportant) when $\mu_0^* \leq \mu_{AB} \leq \mu_1^*$, and as harmful when $\mu_{AB} < \mu_0^*$. The constants μ_0^* and μ_1^* depend on the scale defined for the outcomes, but they apply to any treatment that is or might be included in the clinical trial. When the treatment effect is constant (*homogeneous*), the treatment is beneficial, innocuous, or harmful to every member of the population equally.

When the treatment effect is not constant (is *heterogeneous*) we have to consider the three subpopulations defined by the classification of the treatment effect to beneficial, innocuous, and harmful or, in general, the distribution of the treatment effect. The patient selection process (by recruitment, screening, and informed consent) is not controlled by any sampling design, so it cannot ensure a good representation of the treatment effects among the recruited patients. By way of an example, suppose treatment B is beneficial (in comparison with A) for 50% of the population and innocuous for the remaining 50%.

In an analysis that assumes that the treatment effect is constant, we have no means of discovering this because heterogeneity has been ruled out. The only feasible conclusions are that we have or do not have sufficient evidence that the treatment is beneficial. The latter outcome should be interpreted as a state of ignorance ('we do not know'); this is different from evidence against a beneficial effect of the treatment, which is not sought by the trial.

If most subjects are recruited from the subpopulation for whom the treatment is beneficial, the estimator applied will be biased for the population mean treatment effect. This problem cannot be resolved by randomisation. Randomisation ensures that the treatment effect is estimated without bias for the target equal to the sample average of the treatment effects, not the population average. The problem is that, without any control over the recruitment process, the expectation of the sample average (over the sampling mechanism) may differ from the expectation of the treatment effects in the population. In brief, a clinical trial is both a survey and an experiment. The aspects of the experiment can be adhered to closely, at least in the plan (protocol), but the survey imperatives (good representation) cannot be satisfied.

Treatment heterogeneity leaves no trace in the outcomes, because it is confounded with the lack of constancy of the effects in the model and with the residual term. Replicate measurement of the outcomes may offer some insights into heterogeneity, enabling us to decompose the residual variance to its contribution due to heterogeneity and measurement error. However, population heterogeneity is not well represented in the sample, so the corresponding variance of the treatment effects is estimated with bias.

A solution might be to ignore the problem until the studied treatment has been distributed and used by patients who were prescribed it after an appropriate diagnosis. A survey may then establish the extent of treatment heterogeneity. However, in this setting, randomisation is no longer feasible, so any population inference remains problematic. In fact, now it appears that we should aim for inference not about the population of sufferers, but of those who (would) end up being prescribed the treatment. They may be a selected subpopulation, and the selection mechanism evolves as the reputation of the treatment develops over time. So the target of inference is not readily identified and is far from fixed at the time of the study, making a straightforward assessment of an estimator impossible. One might argue that treatment heterogeneity cannot be extreme, referring to the extensive successful experience with using drugs in medical practice. However, treatment homogeneity may be regarded as an equally extreme assumption.

8.5 Bioequivalence

Clinical trials described in Sections 8.2 and 8.3 are concerned with assessing evidence of *superiority* of one treatment over another. The pharmaceutical research and development sometimes require one to provide evidence that the effect of one treatment is very similar to the effect of another treatment over the same comparator; that is, the two treatments are *bioequivalent*. For example, if a company develops a much cheaper or reliable manufacturing process for a drug it already distributes commercially, it has to provide evidence to the regulatory authority that the product of the new process is, in effect, the same as the product of the old process. A company may have an exclusive licence to produce a drug for a limited period of time. When its licence runs out competitors may produce generic versions of the drug but may distribute it commercially only after they have provided evidence that their product has a very similar effect.

Clinical trials in which evidence of similarity of treatment effects is sought are called *bioequivalence* trials. Two treatments A and B are said to be bioequivalent if the treatment effect of B over A is equal to zero for every member of the population. This definition represents an absolute standard. A lower but much more constructive standard is based on the value of the *mean squared treatment effect*, defined as

$$\text{MSD}\,(Y; A, B) = \text{E}\left\{ \left(Y^{(B)} - Y^{(A)} \right)^2 \right\}$$

for outcomes Y in response to treatments A and B. The standard is that

$$\text{MSD}\,(Y; A, B) \leq D, \tag{8.14}$$

where D is a constant. The absolute standard corresponds to $D = 0$. The condition in (8.14) can be interpreted as a form of rationing for the deviations of the treatment effects from zero. There may be an average treatment effect $\sqrt{D}$ or $-\sqrt{D}$ if the treatment effect is homogeneous, or the standard deviation of the treatment effect may be up to $\sqrt{D}$ if the average treatment effect vanishes. And D can be split to the two components, the squared mean treatment effect and the treatment heterogeneity:

$$\text{MSD}\,(Y; A, B) = \left\{ \text{E}\left(Y^{(B)} - Y^{(A)} \right) \right\}^2 + \text{var}\left(Y^{(B)} - Y^{(A)} \right).$$

Every measurement of $Y^{(T)}$ is tainted with a composite of the measurement error and the everyday influences on the patient; instead of $Y^{(T)}$ we observe $Y_\dagger^{(T)} = Y^{(T)} + \varepsilon^{(T)}$. We have to distinguish between this manifest outcome and its latent version $Y^{(T)}$. The values of $Y_\dagger^{(T)}$ are inconsistent—the patient would respond differently to the same (identical) treatment on a different occasion, and it would not be solely because of a consistent change in the state of health. The latent outcome is consistent across replications of the treatment—it is the consistent component in replications of the same treatment. Therefore, the 'manifest' difference $Y_\dagger^{(B)} - Y_\dagger^{(A)}$ between the outcomes of two treatments comprises the (consistent) difference $Y^{(B)} - Y^{(A)}$ of the underlying latent values and the inconsistencies that accompany every administration of a treatment. The standard formulated by (8.14) refers to the latent values.

By definition, any treatment is bioequivalent with itself and satisfies the absolute standard, with $D = 0$ in (8.14), when compared with itself: $MSD(Y; A, A) = 0$. Bioequivalence trials use several periods, so that the 'manifest' differences between administrations of the same treatment can be pitted against the differences between administrations of alternative treatments. The former contain only the inconsistency in the responses, whereas the latter combine inconsistency with the treatment effects. The standard of bioequivalence with small positive D corresponds to the two sets of dispersions differing very little.

On the one hand, by administering treatments in more periods we obtain more information about inconsistency and treatment effects; on the other hand, we want to expose subjects to as little experimentation as possible. The minimal design that has some within- and between-treatment comparisons within subjects is the design with three periods in which one treatment group, denoted by ABB, is treated by A in the first period and by B in the second and third periods. Another group, with regimen BAA, is treated by B in the first and by A in the second and third periods. Patients are assigned to these regimens by randomisation. As an alternative, the regimens AAB and BBA may be applied. A more extensive design has four periods, with regimens ABAB and BABA, or ABBA and BAAB, or with all these four regimens. Symmetry in the design entails two aspects: equal within-regimen sample sizes and symmetry of regimens, as in (ABBA, BAAB); by swapping the labels A and B of the treatments we obtain the same set of regimens. Such symmetry simplifies the inference by eliminating some nuisance parameters.

The periods are separated by washouts, and we assume that they are perfect, so that there is no carryover. This assumption is somewhat more realistic with established treatments that have been studied extensively in the past, both in clinical trials (development) and observational studies (in operation, after approval). We also assume that the period effects vanish. This is mainly to keep the notation simple and to keep the focus on inference about bioequivalence, although it is often a reasonable assumption.

We assume that the outcomes (both manifest and latent) are jointly normally distributed. Denote by σ_A^2 and σ_B^2 the inconsistency variances associated with respective treatments A and B, by σ_{AB}^2 the variance of the treatment effects, and by $\Delta\mu_{AB}$ the mean treatment effect. That is, the manifest version of the within-subject differences of the outcomes in response to treatments B and A is

$$Y_\dagger^{(B)} - Y_\dagger^{(A)} \sim \mathcal{N}\left(\Delta\mu_{AB}, \sigma_{AB}^2 + \sigma_A^2 + \sigma_B^2\right),$$

whereas its latent version is $Y^{(B)} - Y^{(A)} \sim \mathcal{N}\left(\Delta\mu_{AB}, \sigma_{AB}^2\right)$. Suppose n_r subjects are assigned to regimen $r = \text{ABB}$ and BAA by randomisation and the protocol is adhered to throughout.

Let $\mathbf{y}_{r,t}$ be the vector of outcomes for the subjects in regimen $r = \mathrm{ABB}$, BAA in period $t = 1, 2, 3$ and denote the between-period within-subject sums of squares

$$s^2_{r,t_1,t_2} = \frac{1}{n_r} \left(\mathbf{y}_{r,t_2} - \mathbf{y}_{r,t_1}\right)^\top \left(\mathbf{y}_{r,t_2} - \mathbf{y}_{r,t_1}\right).$$

In regimen ABB, the comparisons of the outcomes in the second and third period have variance $2\sigma_B^2$, and both comparisons of first with second and first with third period have variance $\sigma_{AB}^2 + \sigma_A^2 + \sigma_B^2$; for $t = 2$ and 3,

$$\mathrm{E}\left(s^2_{\mathrm{ABB},1t}\right) = \sigma_{AB}^2 + \sigma_A^2 + \sigma_B^2 + \Delta\mu_{AB}^2,$$

$$\mathrm{E}\left(s^2_{\mathrm{ABB},23}\right) = 2\sigma_B^2. \tag{8.15}$$

The variances of the between-period comparisons in regimen BAA are derived by exchanging the roles of A and B:

$$\mathrm{E}\left(s^2_{\mathrm{BAA},1t}\right) = \sigma_{AB}^2 + \sigma_A^2 + \sigma_B^2 + \Delta\mu_{AB}^2,$$

$$\mathrm{E}\left(s^2_{\mathrm{BAA},23}\right) = 2\sigma_A^2.$$

The mean squared treatment effect is equal to $\sigma_{AB}^2 + \Delta\mu_{AB}^2$. We can estimate it without bias by

$$\widehat{\mathrm{MSD}}(Y; A, B) = \frac{s^2_{\mathrm{ABB},12} + s^2_{\mathrm{ABB},13} + s^2_{\mathrm{BAA},12} + s^2_{\mathrm{BAA},13}}{4} - \frac{s^2_{\mathrm{ABB},23} + s^2_{\mathrm{BAA},23}}{2}.$$

This is an example of a moment-matching estimator. We derived it by matching a (linear) combination of some suitably selected statistics with its expectation. Often there is no unique moment-matching estimator for a target. That is also the case here—there are many ways to combine the estimators s^2_{r,t_1,t_2}. We chose a formula in which all the statistics appear and do so symmetrically. Linear moment-matching estimators imply unbiasedness, but no claims about efficiency can be made. Note that $s^2_{\mathrm{ABB},12}$ and $s^2_{\mathrm{ABB},13}$ are correlated, because both involve outcomes for regimen ABB from period 1. This makes deriving the sampling distribution of $\widehat{\mathrm{MSD}}(Y; A, B)$ difficult.

An alternative moment-matching estimator is constructed from the vectors $\boldsymbol{\xi}_{r,\mathrm{X}} = \mathbf{y}_{r,1} - (\mathbf{y}_{r,2} + \mathbf{y}_{r,3})/2$ and $\boldsymbol{\xi}_{r,\mathrm{W}} = \mathbf{y}_{r,3} - \mathbf{y}_{r,2}$. Here X and W are symbols for 'across' (between) and 'within' treatment contrasts. The covariance of these two variables vanishes:

$$\mathrm{cov}\left(\xi_{r,\mathrm{X}}, \xi_{r,\mathrm{W}}\right) = \mathrm{cov}\left(Y_{r,1} - \frac{Y_{r,2} + Y_{r,3}}{2}, Y_{r,3} - Y_{r,2}\right)$$

$$= \mathrm{cov}\left(Y_{r,1}, Y_{r,3}\right) - \mathrm{cov}\left(Y_{r,1}, Y_{r,2}\right) + \frac{\mathrm{var}\left(Y_{r,3}\right) - \mathrm{var}\left(Y_{r,2}\right)}{2}$$

$$= 0,$$

where $\xi_{r,\mathrm{X}}$ denotes the component of $\boldsymbol{\xi}_{r,\mathrm{X}}$ for a subject. As $\xi_{r,\mathrm{X}}$ and $\xi_{r,\mathrm{W}}$ are uncorrelated and normally distributed, they are also independent. For moment matching with $\boldsymbol{\xi}_{r,\mathrm{W}}$ and $\boldsymbol{\xi}_{r,\mathrm{X}}$, we require the identities

$$\frac{1}{n_r} \mathrm{E}\left(\boldsymbol{\xi}_{r,\mathrm{X}}^{\top} \boldsymbol{\xi}_{r,\mathrm{X}}\right) = \sigma_{\mathrm{AB}}^2 + \sigma_{r_1}^2 + \frac{1}{2}\sigma_{r_2}^2 + \Delta\mu_{\mathrm{AB}}^2,$$

$$\frac{1}{n_r} \mathrm{E}\left(\boldsymbol{\xi}_{r,\mathrm{W}}^{\top} \boldsymbol{\xi}_{r,\mathrm{W}}\right) = 2\sigma_{r_2}^2,$$

where r_1 and r_2 are the treatments (A or B) administered in the respective periods 1 and 2 of regimen r. Hence the moment-matching estimator

$$\widetilde{\mathrm{MSD}}\,(Y;\mathrm{A},\mathrm{B}) = \frac{1}{2}\sum_r \frac{1}{n_r}\boldsymbol{\xi}_{r,\mathrm{X}}^{\top}\boldsymbol{\xi}_{r,\mathrm{X}} - \frac{3}{8}\sum_r \frac{1}{n_r}\boldsymbol{\xi}_{r,\mathrm{W}}^{\top}\boldsymbol{\xi}_{r,\mathrm{W}}, \qquad (8.16)$$

with summations over the regimens $r = \mathrm{ABB}$ and BAA. We relate the distribution of this estimator to χ^2 distributions. First, $\boldsymbol{\xi}_{r,\mathrm{W}}^{\top}\boldsymbol{\xi}_{r,\mathrm{W}}$ has a scaled χ^2 distribution with n_r degrees of freedom. The expectation of $\boldsymbol{\xi}_{r,\mathrm{X}}$ differs from zero, so we decompose $\boldsymbol{\xi}_{r,\mathrm{X}}^{\top}\boldsymbol{\xi}_{r,\mathrm{X}}$ to

$$\boldsymbol{\xi}_{r,\mathrm{X}}^{\top}\boldsymbol{\xi}_{r,\mathrm{X}} = \left(\boldsymbol{\xi}_{r,\mathrm{X}} - \bar{\xi}_{r,\mathrm{X}}\mathbf{1}\right)^{\top}\left(\boldsymbol{\xi}_{r,\mathrm{X}} - \bar{\xi}_{r,\mathrm{X}}\mathbf{1}\right) + n_r\,\bar{\xi}_{r,\mathrm{X}}^2,$$

where $\bar{\xi}_{r,\mathrm{X}}$ is the sample mean $\bar{\xi}_{r,\mathrm{X}} = \boldsymbol{\xi}_{r,\mathrm{X}}^{\top}\mathbf{1}/n_r$. The corrected sum of squares in this identity has χ^2 distribution with $n_r - 1$ degrees of freedom, one being lost because of estimating the mean treatment effect, the population version of $\bar{\xi}_{r,\mathrm{X}}$.

The squared sample mean $\bar{\xi}_{r,\mathrm{X}}^2$ has a scaled *noncentral* χ^2 distribution with one degree of freedom. The noncentral χ^2 distribution with one degree of freedom is defined as the square of a variable with distribution $\mathcal{N}(\mu, 1)$. The squared mean μ^2 is referred to as the *noncentrality parameter*. The distribution is denoted by χ_{1,μ^2}^2. Its mean is μ^2+1 and variance $\mu^4+6\mu^2+3$. The noncentral χ^2 distribution with $m > 1$ degrees of freedom is defined by the sum of two independent variables, one with χ_{1,μ^2}^2 and the other with χ_{m-1}^2 distribution. Its noncentrality parameter is defined as μ^2 and the distribution is denoted by χ_{m,μ^2}^2.

We can now describe the distribution of $\widetilde{\mathrm{MSD}}$ in (8.16) as a linear combination of six independent χ^2 distributions:

$$\widetilde{\mathrm{MSD}}(Y;\mathrm{A},\mathrm{B}) = \frac{1}{2}\frac{\sigma_{\mathrm{AB}}^2 + \sigma_{\mathrm{A}}^2 + \frac{1}{2}\sigma_{\mathrm{B}}^2}{n_{\mathrm{ABB}}}X_1 + \frac{1}{2}\frac{\sigma_{\mathrm{AB}}^2 + \frac{1}{2}\sigma_{\mathrm{A}}^2 + \sigma_{\mathrm{B}}^2}{n_{\mathrm{BAA}}}X_2$$

$$-\frac{3\sigma_{\mathrm{B}}^2}{8n_{\mathrm{BAA}}}X_3 - \frac{3\sigma_{\mathrm{B}}^2}{8n_{\mathrm{BAA}}}X_4$$

$$+\frac{1}{2}\left(\sigma_{\mathrm{AB}}^2 + \sigma_{\mathrm{A}}^2 + \frac{1}{2}\sigma_{\mathrm{B}}^2\right)X_5 + \frac{1}{2}\left(\sigma_{\mathrm{AB}}^2 + \frac{1}{2}\sigma_{\mathrm{A}}^2 + \sigma_{\mathrm{B}}^2\right)X_6,$$

where X_1, X_2, X_3, and X_4 are mutually independent random variables with χ^2 distributions with $n_{\mathrm{ABB}}-1$, $n_{\mathrm{BAA}}-1$, n_{ABB}, and n_{BAA} degrees of freedom, and X_5 and X_6 have noncentral χ^2 distributions with one degree of freedom each and respective noncentrality parameters

$$\frac{n_{\mathrm{ABB}}\,\Delta\mu_{\mathrm{ABB}}^2}{\sigma_{\mathrm{AB}}^2+\sigma_{\mathrm{A}}^2+\frac{1}{2}\sigma_{\mathrm{B}}^2}\quad\text{and}\quad\frac{n_{\mathrm{BAA}}\,\Delta\mu_{\mathrm{BAA}}^2}{\sigma_{\mathrm{AB}}^2+\frac{1}{2}\sigma_{\mathrm{A}}^2+\sigma_{\mathrm{B}}^2}\,.$$

The variance of this distribution is the sum of the variances of the six (independent) components. It is a formidable and unwieldy expression; it depends on the population variance σ_{AB}^2 as well as on the two inconsistency variances. Substituting estimates for the unknown variances is not appropriate, because the error committed in estimation is then committed again in estimating the sampling variance of the estimator. This highlights the difficulties of making inferences about variances in general. However, even with moderate sample sizes n_{ABB} and n_{BAA}, we have approximate normality, and a quantile of the estimator's distribution can be approximated using its (approximate) sampling variance.

Evidence of bioequivalence corresponds to small values of $\widetilde{\mathrm{MSD}}$. This corresponds to testing the hypothesis that the underlying value (population quantity) MSD is small. In practice, testing the hypothesis that MSD = 0 would require too great a sample size, and given that the original treatment has been proven to be beneficial, some deviation of MSD from zero can be allowed. The critical value is difficult to set without being too conservative because the variances σ_{AB}^2, σ_{A}^2, and σ_{B}^2 are not known. Their estimation can be improved by incorporating the (prior) information that these variances, and the latter two in particular, are not large. If such thresholds can be set for all three variances, the sampling variance of the test statistic could be evaluated for the least favourable setting. At the extreme, $\sigma_{\mathrm{AB}}^2=0$ may be adopted as prior information. Then we are concerned only with the common (mean) treatment effect $\Delta\mu_{\mathrm{AB}}$ and could base our inference on its estimator $\widehat{\Delta\mu}_{\mathrm{AB}}$. However, unlike in an assessment of superiority, we now seek evidence against large values of $|\Delta\mu_{\mathrm{AB}}|$, and so evidence of bioequivalence corresponds to $|\widehat{\Delta\mu}_{\mathrm{AB}}|<c$ for a suitable positive constant c.

To select the critical value c, we set first the largest value of Δ_{AB} that is still compatible with bioequivalence. That is, the mean treatment effect of B over A would just about be regarded as unimportant. Let this value of the mean effect be Δ_{AB}^*. The critical value c is then set so that the probability of rejecting the hypothesis of no bioequivalence, $|\Delta_{\mathrm{AB}}|>\Delta_{\mathrm{AB}}^*$, would not exceed the size of the test α (usually 0.05), whenever the hypothesis is valid. When the residual variance σ^2 is known and the outcomes are normally distributed, this probability is

$$\mathrm{P}(|\widehat{\Delta}_{\mathrm{AB}}|>c\,|\,\Delta_{\mathrm{AB}}^*)=\varPhi^{-1}\left(\frac{c-\Delta\mu_{\mathrm{AB}}^*}{2\sigma}\sqrt{n}\right)+\varPhi^{-1}\left(\frac{-c-\Delta\mu_{\mathrm{AB}}^*}{2\sigma}\sqrt{n}\right),$$

when $\Delta_{\mathrm{AB}}=\pm\Delta_{\mathrm{AB}}^*$, and it can be shown that the probability is smaller when $|\Delta_{\mathrm{AB}}|>\Delta_{\mathrm{AB}}^*$.

8.6 Incorporating Utilities

An outstanding weakness of hypothesis testing as a tool for making a binary (Yes/No) decision is that it is oblivious to the consequences of an erroneous choice. Instead of limiting the probabilities of the two kinds of error, whichever way we balance the probability of one kind against the probability of the other, we should evaluate the consequences of making an incorrect decision and make the choice for which the expected loss is minimised. Implementing this scheme is not elementary because we have to operate with several elements of uncertainty. Further, we have to evaluate what the losses would be in each particular circumstance.

We consider a clinical trial for superiority of treatment B over treatment A. In the trial, the mean treatment effect of B over A is estimated, assuming that the treatment effect is constant in the studied population. For a given class of designs, such as the two-period crossover design with balance ($n_{AB} = n_{BA}$), there is an obvious estimator of the treatment effect θ, denoted by $\hat{\theta}$, and its MSE is a function of the sample size:

$$v(n) = \mathrm{MSE}(\hat{\theta}; \theta \mid n);$$

we omit from the notation any other parameters on which the variance may depend. As a simple example, $v(n) = 4\sigma^2/n$ for the single-period randomised trial with $n/2$ subjects in either of the two treatment groups.

The consequences of a decision are governed by the cost of development and experimentation, possibly offset over time by income from sales (with the costs of production and distribution subtracted), and the risk of failure due to distributing a drug that turns out to be ineffective, or even harmful, compounded by the loss of good reputation. Experimentation costs depend on the sample size, and we assume that this is a linear function. There is a setup cost and a constant per-subject cost. Of course, the development of a drug involves several experiments, but we assume that these have been concluded successfully and subsume their cost in that of the development.

The utility of a drug is zero if the decision is not to distribute it commercially. Otherwise, as a simplification, we assume that the utility is a monotone function of θ, independent of all other parameters. It may be smooth, or smooth except for one or two 'jumps' at some critical values of θ. Establishing this utility function $U(\theta)$ is essential, because it has a profound impact on the (commercial) decision. For example, if the utility is extremely high throughout the range of feasible values of θ, experimentation is unnecessary. If the losses are modest even in the worst plausible scenario and the utility is positive and very large for a range of values of θ, the decision should be formed differently from when the losses may be catastrophic and the gains modest even in the most optimistic scenario.

The details of the utility function, its exact shape, are difficult to set. The regulatory authority might impose one, representing the population that will be affected in the future, or more generally the general public's interest in health care. The setting would reflect the society's priorities—to be sure that any treatment available for prescription is effective and to quantify the harm done by using an ineffective treatment. The developer, a pharmaceutical company, may have different priorities. They consider the profit that a successful drug might bring in the future and balance it with the risks of a possibly catastrophic failure if a drug turned out to be ineffective or even harmful after its appearance on the market. Possible loss of good reputation and of the public's confidence in the company's products are important considerations.

Let (θ_L, θ_H) be the range of plausible values within which the treatment effect θ is bound to lie. We simplify the task of setting the utility function by agreeing with the developer (or the regulatory agency) on the utilities for θ_L and θ_H, the extreme values of θ. Let them be $U_L = U(\theta_L)$ and $U_H = U(\theta_H)$. Usually, $U_L < 0$, $U_H > 0$, and $-U_L \gg U_H$; the risks greatly outweigh the possible profits. Further, let θ_0 be such that $U(\theta_0) = 0$; this is the break-even point; distribution of the product is beneficial (profitable) if $\theta > \theta_0$.

We now overlay a smooth function over the points (θ_L, U_L), $(\theta_0, 0)$, and (θ_H, U_H). The form of the function should be informed by the circumstances. For example, if the utility increases slowly for large θ and reaches a plateau at around θ_H and drops precipitously for large negative values of θ, a suitable function is

$$U(\theta) = c - \exp(a - b\theta), \tag{8.17}$$

with the constants a, $b > 0$ and $c > 0$ set so as to satisfy the conditions at θ_L, θ_0, and θ_H. A singular 'penalty' can be subtracted from the utility in (8.17) for negative θ. The utility function is then discontinuous at $\theta = 0$ but is monotone throughout.

We set the cost of experimentation to $C(n) = d_0 + d_1 n$, with positive constants d_0 and d_1. The cost may be a more complex function. In particular, it may have some discontinuities, related to the capacity to conduct trials. For example, the cost may increase by a singular quantity when additional staff have to be engaged for recruitment or the conduct of the trial.

Suppose θ will be estimated from the mean of the outcomes of the two treatment groups as $\hat{\theta} = \bar{y}_B - \bar{y}_A$, and the decision rule for marketing and distribution will have the form $\hat{\theta} > \theta^*$ for a sample-size-dependent value θ^*. For a given value of θ, the gain is defined as the expected utility adjusted for the cost of experimentation:

$$G(\theta^*, \theta; n) = U(\theta)\, P\left(\hat{\theta} > \theta^*\right) - C(n).$$

The gain is easy to calculate for any combination of θ and θ^*, assuming a known distribution of $\hat{\theta}$. The difficulty is that θ is not known. We want to set θ^* and n so as to maximise the gain G.

With increasing sample size, the cost $C(n)$ increases, so we have an incentive to keep the trial small. In contrast, disastrous decisions would have an appreciable probability if the sample size were very small, because the estimate $\hat{\theta}$ may exceed a high threshold θ^* even when θ is much smaller than θ_0.

8.7 Example

Suppose the feasible range of mean treatment effects of a novel drug against its established competitor is from $\theta_L = -2$ to $\theta_H = 6$, and the manifest variance, which can be interpreted as the amalgam of the measurement (assessment) error, temporal inconsistency, and subject-level heterogeneity, is $\sigma^2 = 2$. Further, suppose the break-even value is $\theta_0 = 0.5$, the utility at θ_H is $U_H = 10$, and the utility at θ_L is $U_L = -100$, with a singular penalty of 10 units applied when $\theta < 0$. We fit a utility function of the form (8.17) by the *Newton method*.

The univariate Newton method for solving the equation $f(x) = d$, for a differentiable function f, comprises iterations

$$x_{\text{new}} = x_{\text{old}} + \frac{d - f(x_{\text{old}})}{f'(x_{\text{old}})}, \tag{8.18}$$

where f' is the derivative of f regarded as a function of the same argument as f. This formula is derived by the Taylor expansion applied to the function f at the solution x_{new}:

$$f(x_{\text{new}}) \doteq f(x_{\text{old}}) + f'(x_{\text{old}})\,(x - x_{\text{old}}),$$

from which (8.18) follows immediately. The multivariate version of (8.18), with a vector of functions F and the search for the vector $\mathbf{x}^*$ for which $F(\mathbf{x}^*) = \mathbf{d}$, is

$$\mathbf{x}_{\text{new}} = \mathbf{x}_{\text{old}} + \left(\frac{\partial F}{\partial \mathbf{x}} \bigg|_{\mathbf{x} = \mathbf{x}_{\text{old}}} \right)^{-1} \{ \mathbf{d} - F(\mathbf{x}_{\text{old}}) \}.$$

In our case, F comprises three functions of (a, b, c), equal to $c - \exp(a - b\theta)$ for $\theta = \theta_L$, θ_0, and θ_H, and $\mathbf{x} = (a, b, c)$. The partial differentials of these functions are

$$\frac{\partial f}{\partial a} = -\exp(a - b\theta),$$

$$\frac{\partial f}{\partial b} = \theta \exp(a - b\theta),$$

$$\frac{\partial f}{\partial c} = 1,$$

and $\partial F / \partial \mathbf{x}$ comprises these values as three columns, evaluated at θ_L, θ_0, and θ_H. The penalty introduces a discontinuity. It can be dealt with by first removing it, finding a solution for the penalty-free problem with U_H adjusted accordingly (from -100 to -90), and then incorporating the penalty to the solution. An initial guess is required for x_{old} in the first iteration.

Table 8.1 gives details of the iterations. The distance in the right-most column is defined as the total of the squared deviations of $F(x_{old})$ from $\mathbf{U} = (U_L, U_0, U_H)$. The values of utility given in the table are already adjusted for the penalty. We see that the convergence is quite fast, despite a very poor starting solution. The fitted utility function is plotted in Figure 8.3.

Table 8.1. Iterations of the Newton method to find a suitable utility function.

| | Utility parameters | | | Values of utility | | | |
Iteration	a	b	c	$\theta_L = -2$	$\theta_0 = 0.5$	$\theta_H = 6$	Distance
Start	1.000	1.000	1.000	-29.09	-0.65	0.99	—
1	5.877	0.553	10.058	-1076.56	-260.45	-2.90	$\sim 10^6$
2	4.921	0.576	8.723	-435.38	-94.05	4.41	$\sim 10^5$
3	4.037	0.632	9.049	-201.58	-32.24	7.77	$\sim 10^4$
4	3.321	0.738	9.552	-121.67	-9.59	9.22	562.32
5	2.902	0.860	9.950	-101.76	-1.89	9.85	6.71
6	2.778	0.914	10.058	-100.01	-0.13	9.99	0.02
7	2.768	0.919	10.064	-100.00	0.00	10.00	$< 10^{-5}$
8	2.768	0.919	10.064	-100.00	0.00	10.00	$< 10^{-6}$

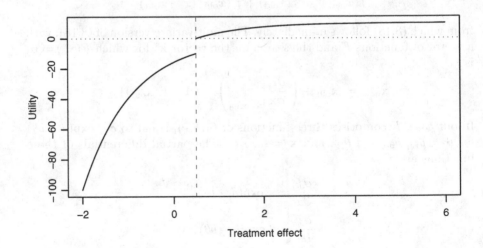

Fig. 8.3. The utility as a function of the treatment effect, with a penalty of 10 units at $\theta = 0.5$. Details of this function are given in the bottom row of Table 8.1.

Table 8.2. The expected gains for $n = 20$. The penalty of 10 units for $\theta < 0$ is not subtracted.

θ^*				θ					
	−2	−1	0	1	2	3	4	5	6
0.0	−0.537	−2.868	−3.566	3.149	7.207	8.686	9.250	9.466	9.549
0.2	−0.478	−1.677	−2.792	2.973	7.196	8.686	9.250	9.466	9.549
0.4	−0.458	−1.020	−2.092	2.712	7.169	8.686	9.250	9.466	9.549
0.6	−0.452	−0.692	−1.518	2.360	7.110	8.685	9.250	9.466	9.549
0.8	−0.451	−0.544	−1.091	1.932	6.992	8.684	9.250	9.466	9.549
1.0	−0.450	−0.483	−0.805	1.458	6.777	8.679	9.250	9.466	9.549
1.2	−0.450	−0.461	−0.630	0.985	6.424	8.666	9.250	9.466	9.549
1.4	−0.450	−0.453	−0.534	0.556	5.900	8.634	9.250	9.466	9.549
1.6	−0.450	−0.451	−0.486	0.204	5.194	8.563	9.249	9.466	9.549
1.8	−0.450	−0.450	−0.464	−0.057	4.332	8.422	9.248	9.466	9.549
2.0	−0.450	−0.450	−0.455	−0.233	3.382	8.166	9.242	9.466	9.549
2.2	−0.450	−0.450	−0.452	−0.340	2.431	7.745	9.229	9.466	9.549
2.4	−0.450	−0.450	−0.450	−0.399	1.570	7.120	9.195	9.466	9.549
2.6	−0.450	−0.450	−0.450	−0.428	0.863	6.278	9.120	9.465	9.549
2.8	−0.450	−0.450	−0.450	−0.442	0.339	5.252	8.970	9.464	9.549
3.0	−0.450	−0.450	−0.450	−0.447	−0.014	4.118	8.698	9.458	9.549

Suppose the cost of the trial is $C(n) = 0.25 + 0.01n$. The initial costs, $d_0 = 0.25$, are 2.5% of the gains from sales in the most optimistic scenario of $\theta = \theta_H$. We search for the best combination of critical value θ^* and sample size n by evaluating the function G over a rectangular grid of values of θ^* and θ for a range of sample sizes n. As an example, Table 8.2 presents the results for $n = 20$. For instance, if the critical value is set to $\theta^* = 1.0$ and the treatment effect is $\theta = 0$, the gain is -0.805, that is, the expected loss is much greater than $C(20) = 0.45$. This is because the decision to market the novel treatment, and therefore incur losses, has a large probability $P(\hat{\theta} > \theta^* \mid \theta = 0)$.

If the decision at the end of the trial is not to proceed with distribution, the gain is -0.45, the cost of the trial. For $\theta^* = 3.0$ and $\theta < 1$, the gain is -0.45 or only slightly higher, because $P(\hat{\theta} > \theta^* \mid \theta)$ is very small. In contrast, when $\theta = 6.0$, any setting of θ^* in the range $(0, 3)$ will lead to realising most of the possible gains.

The critical value θ^* and the sample size n are set by design, when θ is not known. Therefore, we cannot place our bets regarding the gains on any particular value of θ but have to average over its feasible values. We average over all the feasible values of θ, that is, evaluate

$$E\{G(\theta^*; n)\} = \int_{\theta_L}^{\theta_H} G(\theta^*, \theta; n) \, d\theta \qquad (8.19)$$

for a range of sample sizes n. We can approximate this integral by the summation

$$\sum_{\theta=\theta_{\mathrm{L}}}^{\theta_{\mathrm{H}}} G(\theta^*, \theta; n)\, \Delta\theta\,,$$

over a grid of feasible values of θ with gaps of $\Delta\theta$. We could use a finer grid, but that is not necessary, because first we hone in on the combinations of θ^* and n and evaluate the expected gains over a finer grid later.

We can also calculate the average gain, by integration or its approximation by summation with *weights*, describing our beliefs about the relative plausibility of each value of θ. The integral in (8.19) corresponds to equal weights, or *indifference* (no preference) among the values of θ in $(-2, 6)$. It can be motivated as a noninformative Bayes prior (Chapter 4). A more optimistic scenario corresponds to weights increasing with θ and a more pessimistic scenario to weights decreasing with θ.

The weights, as a function of θ, represent a distribution—they are nonnegative and, after scaling if necessary, their integral is equal to unity. The discrete version of the weights, when only a finite number or countably many values of θ are feasible, also represents a (discrete) distribution. The expected loss with a continuous prior distribution w is

$$\mathrm{E}\{G(\theta^*; n)\,|\,w\} = \int_{\theta_{\mathrm{L}}}^{\theta_{\mathrm{H}}} G(\theta^*, \theta; n)\; w(\theta)\,\mathrm{d}\theta\,. \tag{8.20}$$

Figure 8.4 displays the indifference, an optimistic, a pessimistic, and a focussed prior. The indifference prior is unique—it corresponds to the uniform distribution. However, there are priors more pessimistic than the one depicted in panel B. More probability can be concentrated on the negative values of θ; in principle, a prior could even rule out any positive values of θ. By symmetry, there are priors more optimistic than that in panel C. By a focussed prior (panel D), we incorporate in the analysis our belief about the location of the value of θ. More concentrated density corresponds to greater confidence and stronger commitment; at the same time, it presents a greater threat to the validity of the analysis, if its choice is not well founded. The qualifier 'focussed' is also relative. The knowledge that the value of θ is in a very narrow range represents a more focussed prior than the one in panel D. On the other hand, even the indifferent prior is 'slightly' focussed, since it rules out values of θ below -2.0 and above 6.0.

With the indifference (uniform) prior on $(-2, 6)$, the expected gains are approximated by the within-row averages of the gains in Table 8.2. These averages are listed in Table 8.3. The expected gain increases up to about 0.8 and then decreases at a somewhat faster rate. For example, the expected gain for $\theta^* = 3$ and $n = 20$ is 3.34. Thus, if $n = 20$ were chosen, the optimal critical value would be $\theta^* \doteq 0.8$.

Since we can also set the sample size n, we find the maximum expected gains for a range of sample sizes. These values are given in Table 8.4 in the

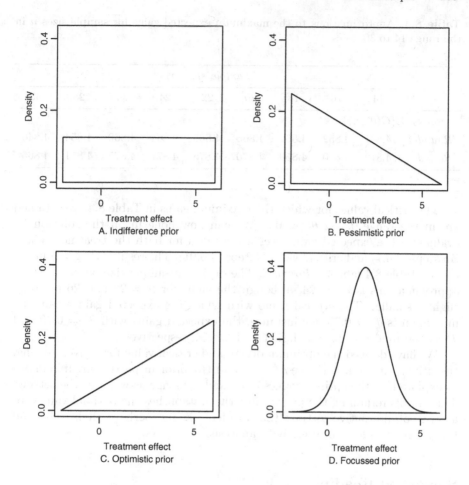

Fig. 8.4. Examples of prior distributions for the mean treatment effect θ.

Table 8.3. Approximate expected gains in the clinical trial with $n = 20$.

θ^*	0.0	0.2	0.4	0.6	0.8	1.0	1.2	1.4	...
$E\{G(\theta^*; 20)\}$	4.48	4.69	4.81	4.86	4.87	4.83	4.76	4.66	...

row with the heading *Round 1*. We see that the maximum gain is attained for $n = 20$ or 22. The maximum increases while $n < 20$ more steeply than it decreases when $n > 22$, so it is better to err on the side of setting a higher n, even when drop-out and other problems with the conduct of the trial are disregarded.

Table 8.4. Approximations to the maximum expected gains for sample sizes n in the range 14 to 30.

	Sample size (n)								
	14	16	18	20	22	24	26	28	30
$\max_{\theta^*} E\{G(\theta^*; n)\}$									
Round 1	4.831	4.852	4.862	4.865	4.865	4.864	4.860	4.854	4.846
Round 2	4.812	4.840	4.859	4.870	4.876	4.877	4.875	4.871	4.865

The critical values for which the maximum gains in Table 8.4 are attained are in the range $0.5 < \theta^* < 0.9$. We can now hone in on the solution by evaluating the expected gains over a finer grid for both the treatment effect (in steps of 0.1) and critical values (steps of 0.01). The results are given in the row of Table 8.4 labelled *Round 2*. The optimum sample size based on these approximations is $n^* = 24$, although the gains for $n = 22$ and 26 are only slightly smaller. The critical value with which the expected gain attains its maximum is $\theta^* = 0.75$; for instance, the expected gains with $\theta^* = 0.70$ and $\theta^* = 0.80$ (and $n = 24$) are 4.8751 and 4.8754, respectively.

We have derived the optimum design and critical value for a given setting, the utility function, variance $\sigma^2 = 2$, and the prior in particular. It remains to explore how the optimal values of θ^* and n change as we alter the setting. This entails rerunning the programme that establishes the optimal values for a range of alternative settings that are feasible and perhaps slightly beyond this range, as a form of sensitivity analysis.

Suggested Reading

There are several monographs on clinical trials, with a focus on testing a single hypothesis of equality of (mean) treatment effects, [4], [147], [51], [180], and [145]. Standard references to the design and analysis of crossover trials are [90] and [179]. The argument against including the carryover effect in the analysis is presented by [53]. The minimax estimator of the treatment effect in crossover trials is derived in [119]; the impact of treatment heterogeneity on the established methods of analysis is discussed in [117]. Several journals specialise in research on clinical trials; foremost among them are *Controlled Clinical Trials, Drug Information Journal,* and *Journal of Biopharmaceutical Statistics. Statistics in Medicine* also publishes many articles on statistical issues in clinical trials.

Bioequivalence is a relatively recent concern in clinical trials; see [18]. The method described in [174] is widely adopted in the pharmaceutical research and development, even though it assumes treatment homogeneity. An alternative proposal is developed by [171]; see [181] for a related discussion. The method presented in this chapter is described in greater detail in [118]. A critique of using hypothesis testing for decisions about bioequivalence is presented in [103]; the points it makes are applicable to clinical trials in general.

Two advanced topics related to clinical trials are not addressed in this chapter: testing several hypotheses (multiplicity), [78] and [6], and sequential trials (trials with interim decisions as to stop or continue, based on summaries of intermediate variables) [194].

Problems and Exercises

8.1. Verify that the assumption of normality is essential for the sample mean $\bar{X}$ and sample variance $\hat{U}$ to be independent. Generate random samples from different distributions (log-normal, beta, gamma, and the like) and estimate the correlation of $\bar{X}$ and $\hat{U}$. Repeat this exercise with some symmetric distributions, such as t and symmetric beta, $\mathcal{B}(b, b)$. Relate your findings to the definition of the t-distribution.

8.2. Empirically (by simulations) it is not possible to prove that a distribution, such as t_1 does not have an expectation. How could you get some indication by simulation that the expectation (or variance) of a t-distribution may not exist?

8.3. What kinds of treatments cannot be studied by trials with crossover design?

8.4. List the problems with estimation of the mean treatment effect that would arise in a crossover trial if all subjects were assigned to the same regimen, say, AB.

8.5. Derive the estimator of the treatment effect $\Delta\mu_{AB}$ by moment matching, as outlined in Section 8.3.1.

8.6. Repeat the derivation of the minimax estimator in Section 8.3.2 with the assumption that the absolute value of the carryover does not exceed a given fraction of the absolute value of the treatment effect; $|\gamma| \leq c\,|\Delta\mu_{AB}|$. Identify the problem(s) additional to those in the original derivation, and devise ways of circumventing them. Could a treatment have a zero effect and yet be associated with a nonzero carryover? Relate your answer to the appropriateness of the assumption about γ and $\Delta\mu_{AB}$.

8.7. Derive the value of the carryover effect γ for which the two minimax estimators, based on different maximum plausible carryover effects $\Gamma < \Gamma'$ have the same MSEs; that is, where their MSE curves (curves 1 and 2 in Figure 8.2) intersect.

8.8. Discuss the definitions of patient heterogeneity and treatment heterogeneity and which features of a clinical trial, if any, address either of them.

8.9. The definition of bioequivalence used in this chapter is called *individual* bioequivalence in much of the literature. In the definition of population bioequivalence, a constant treatment effect is assumed. That is, two treatments are declared bioequivalent if the absolute value of the average treatment effect of one in comparison with the other is smaller than a set threshold D. Define the corresponding mean squared deviation, MSD, and derive a moment-matching estimator for it. Compare your test of the hypothesis that $\mathrm{MSD} \leq D$ with the test derived by [174].

8.10. Discuss the rationale for regimens with more than one application of a treatment for studying population bioequivalence, and compare it with the rationale for studying individual bioequivalence.

8.11. Trace through the derivation of the distribution of $\widehat{\mathrm{MSD}}$ in Section 8.5 the importance of normality of the outcomes. For a contrast, consider the problem with binary outcomes. How could (individual) bioequivalence be assessed when, in essence, all that is recorded is whether the outcomes of each subject are in concordance (agreement) or discordance (disagreement)?
Hint: For one possible solution, recall the details of the permutation test.

8.12. Devise a graphical method for (informal) assessment of individual bioequivalence. Explore, for example, plots of the outcomes for one period against another, within regimens. Align such plots when they are for the same treatment and for different treatments. To make the exploration easier, generate (normally distributed) datasets from models that satisfy individual bioequivalence and that fail it by a wide margin.

8.13. Adopt the diagram from the previous exercise as a feature; see Section 1.3.1. Generate replicates of the dataset with the same sample sizes and model parameters as the fit for the realised dataset, but set the between-treatment variance σ_{AB}^2 to zero. Draw the diagram for each replicate and compare these simulated diagrams with the diagram for the realised dataset. If the latter stands out among them, then we declare evidence against individual bioequivalence. Summarise the advantages and drawbacks of this approach.

8.14. Implement the Newton method described in Section 8.6. For a particular set of treatment effects $(\theta_\mathrm{L}, \theta_0, \theta_H)$ and the associated utilities $(U_\mathrm{L}, U_0, Y_\mathrm{H})$, explore how poor the initial values (a, b, c) have to be for the Newton algorithm to fail.

8.15. For the setting of the example in Section 8.7, explore how the expected gains could be presented graphically. Explain why the results in the two rounds differ for a pair (θ, θ^*) for which the expected gains are evaluated on both occasions. Explore how different the expected gains and the optimum sample sizes are when the utility function or the unit expenditure in the trial are altered by a small amount. Similarly, explore the sensitivity of the optimum sample size with respect to the prior.

Hint: Replace the uniform prior by a beta prior with both parameters close to 1.0 or by a prior with a linear density.

8.16. Discuss how the formulation of the placebo incorporates the principle of blinding. In a typical clinical trial, none of the staff who are in contact with the subjects (patients) can identify the treatments they administer. That is, they are aware of the labels of the treatments, such as A and B, but do not know which is the novel and which is the established treatment. Explain why it is essential to maintain such blinding until all the outcomes are recorded.

9

Random Coefficients

Clustering is a common structure in populations. We belong to families, communities, educational institutions, places of employment, or, in general, *clusters*. Members of a cluster are often more similar to one another than members of the population in general. When the population comprises many clusters and studying each of them in isolation is not practical, it is meaningful to regard them as another population and study them as such. At the same time, each cluster on its own is a population, with its features that may be described by a model. Therefore, a clustered population may be described by a population of models, which can itself be regarded as a single model. The subject of this chapter are such models. We focus on populations of ordinary regression models, building on the familiar, and expand the horizons later in the chapter.

9.1 Introduction

In earlier chapters, we found linear regression an effective means of describing how two variables are associated. Originally, we considered designs in which the values of the stimuli X are set and done so with no regard for the anticipated values of Y. Such a setting enables inferences about the effect of X on Y, as defined in Chapter 7. More commonly, neither X nor Y entails any form of control, so any interpretation of the fitted regression coefficients as effects is highly problematic. Nevertheless, they are useful to describe how the two variables are associated in a particular context.

In a structured population, with members i within clusters d, we may consider a separate regression for each cluster:

$$y_{id} = \mathbf{x}_{id}\boldsymbol{\xi}_d + \varepsilon_{id},$$

where y_{id} is the outcome, $\mathbf{x}_{id}$ the corresponding row vector of the values of the covariates (with the intercept 1 as its first element), $\boldsymbol{\xi}_d$ the vector of regression coefficients for cluster d, and ε_{id} a random draw from $\mathcal{N}(0, \sigma_d^2)$. In a more compact notation,

$$(\mathbf{y}_d \mid \mathbf{T}_d, d) \sim \mathcal{N}\left(\mathbf{T}_d \boldsymbol{\xi}_d, \sigma_d^2 \mathbf{I}\right). \tag{9.1}$$

We refer to this as the *within-cluster model*. Such a model is well suited for one or a few clusters, but not for an entire population, especially when it comprises so many clusters that the listing of all sets of parameters $(\boldsymbol{\xi}_d, \sigma_d^2)$ would be impractical and would not inform us effectively without further analysis. We add d as a condition on the right-hand side of (9.1) to indicate that two clusters may have different regression coefficients $\boldsymbol{\xi}_d$ even when they have the same regression matrix $\mathbf{T}_d$.

We formulate a separate model for the population of clusters:

$$\boldsymbol{\xi}_d \sim \mathcal{N}(\mathbf{U}_d \boldsymbol{\eta}, \boldsymbol{\Sigma}_{\mathrm{B}}), \tag{9.2}$$

independently, that is,

$$\boldsymbol{\xi}_d = \mathbf{U}_d \boldsymbol{\eta} + \boldsymbol{\delta}_d,$$

with a known matrix $\mathbf{U}_d$, unknown vector of regression parameters $\boldsymbol{\eta}$, and a random sample $\boldsymbol{\delta}_d$ from $\mathcal{N}(\mathbf{0}, \boldsymbol{\Sigma}_{\mathrm{B}})$ with unknown variance matrix $\boldsymbol{\Sigma}_{\mathrm{B}}$. We refer to this as the *cluster-level* model. It is customary to assume a degenerate distribution for the residual variances σ_d^2, $\sigma_d^2 \equiv \sigma^2$, but this is by no means the only option. For instance, we can specify a linear model for $\log(\sigma_d^2)$ or add σ_d^2 as another component to the vector $\boldsymbol{\xi}_d$ in (9.2) and allow for σ_d^2 to be correlated with the components of $\boldsymbol{\xi}_d$. Model parsimony and relative computational simplicity are two reasons for preferring the assumption of homoscedasticity, $\sigma_d^2 \equiv \sigma^2$.

The models in (9.1) and (9.2), or the corresponding equations, can be combined to yield

$$\mathbf{y}_d = \mathbf{T}_d \mathbf{U}_d \boldsymbol{\eta} + \mathbf{T}_d \boldsymbol{\delta}_d + \boldsymbol{\varepsilon}_d, \tag{9.3}$$

so that

$$(\mathbf{y}_d \mid \mathbf{T}_d, \mathbf{U}_d, d) \sim \mathcal{N}\left(\mathbf{T}_d \mathbf{U}_d \boldsymbol{\eta} + \mathbf{T}_d \boldsymbol{\delta}_d, \sigma^2 \mathbf{I}\right). \tag{9.4}$$

As a convention, we assume that the first columns of $\mathbf{T}_d$ and $\mathbf{U}_d$ correspond to the intercept. The model in (9.4) is called *two-level*, to indicate that it combines models for members (elements or atoms) and clusters. It is a special case of the multilevel model in which models are combined for clusters at several levels. We discuss these in Section 9.6.

The regression matrix $\mathbf{T}_d \mathbf{U}_d$ can be interpreted as containing regression variables $\mathbf{T}$ defined for members, $\mathbf{U}$ defined for clusters, and all their interactions (products). Equation (9.3) states that the within-cluster regression coefficients are constant for all variables except for those in $\mathbf{T}$. The average (typical) regression is characterised by $\boldsymbol{\delta}_d = \mathbf{0}$, that is, by $\mathbf{T}\mathbf{U}\boldsymbol{\eta}$. The regression for cluster d deviates from the average regression by $\mathbf{T}\boldsymbol{\delta}$.

All the $\mathbf{T}$-by-$\mathbf{U}$ interactions are included in the model because the cluster-level model in (9.2) involves the same set of variables for each component of

$\boldsymbol{\xi}_d$. We can relax this substantially and simplify the model description at the same time. Instead of (9.3) we assume that

$$\mathbf{y}_d = \mathbf{X}_d \boldsymbol{\beta} + \mathbf{Z}_d \boldsymbol{\delta}_d + \boldsymbol{\varepsilon}_d, \tag{9.5}$$

where $\boldsymbol{\delta}_d$, $d = 1, \ldots, D$, is a random sample from a centred (multivariate) normal distribution, $\mathcal{N}(\mathbf{0}, \boldsymbol{\Sigma}_{\mathrm{B}})$, and $\boldsymbol{\varepsilon}_d$ are independent random vectors with distributions $\mathcal{N}(\mathbf{0}, \sigma^2 \mathbf{I}_{n_d})$; n_d is the subsample size within cluster d. The two sets of random vectors, $\boldsymbol{\delta}_d$ and $\boldsymbol{\varepsilon}_d$, are mutually independent. The variables in $\mathbf{X}$ contain the intercept, and the variables in $\mathbf{Z}$ are a selection from those in $\mathbf{X}$; $\mathbf{Z}$ always contains the intercept, unless $\mathbf{Z}$ is empty. The variables in $\mathbf{X}$ that are not included in $\mathbf{Z}$ form the *regression part* of the model; these variables are denoted by $\mathbf{R}$. The variables in $\mathbf{Z}$ form the (cluster-level) *variation part* of the model. The regression and variation parts are also referred to as *fixed* and *random*, respectively, but we reserve these two qualifiers for use solely in conjunction with replications (fixed — constant; random — varying). We denote the numbers of variables in $\mathbf{X}$ and $\mathbf{Z}$ by p and r, respectively.

The model in (9.5) can be interpreted as a collection of regressions:

$$\mathbf{y}_d = \mathbf{R}_d \boldsymbol{\beta}^{(\mathrm{R})} + \mathbf{Z}_d \left(\boldsymbol{\beta}^{(\mathrm{V})} + \boldsymbol{\delta}_d \right) + \boldsymbol{\varepsilon}_d,$$

where $\boldsymbol{\beta}_d^{(\mathrm{V})} = \boldsymbol{\beta}^{(\mathrm{V})} + \boldsymbol{\delta}_d$ is the vector of within-cluster regression coefficients on $\mathbf{Z}$ and $\boldsymbol{\beta}^{(\mathrm{R})}$ and $\boldsymbol{\beta}^{(\mathrm{V})}$ are the subvectors of $\boldsymbol{\beta}$ that correspond to the respective regression and variation parts of the model. The regressions share the same slopes for the variables in $\mathbf{R}$, while their slopes on $\mathbf{Z}$ differ. The differences among the slopes can be effectively described by their (cluster-level) variance matrix $\boldsymbol{\Sigma}_{\mathrm{B}}$. We this discuss in Section 9.2. A variable can be moved from $\mathbf{R}$ to $\mathbf{Z}$, but then the corresponding variance in $\boldsymbol{\Sigma}_{\mathrm{B}}$ is equal to zero. As a convention, we can rule out such moves, although $\boldsymbol{\Sigma}_{\mathrm{B}}$ may still contain some zero variances when we do not know that they are equal to zero.

The variance of an observation comprises two terms,

$$\mathrm{var}(y_{id}) = \sigma^2 + \mathbf{z}_{id} \boldsymbol{\Sigma}_{\mathrm{B}} \mathbf{z}_{id}^{\mathsf{T}},$$

which correspond to the two levels. They are referred to as *variance components*. When $\mathbf{z}$ is univariate, $z_{id} \equiv 1$, both components are constant. In the model with no covariates, $y_{id} = \mu + \delta_d + \varepsilon_{id}$, the relative sizes of the variances are sometimes of interest. They are related to the within-cluster correlation, $\mathrm{cor}(y_{id}, y_{i'd}) = \sigma_{\mathrm{B}}^2 / (\sigma^2 + \sigma_{\mathrm{B}}^2)$, for $i \neq i'$.

9.2 Patterns of Variation

For simplicity, we consider first a model with a single covariate X defined for members (elements):

$$\mathbf{y}_d = \mathbf{X}_d\boldsymbol{\beta} + \mathbf{X}_d\boldsymbol{\delta}_d + \boldsymbol{\varepsilon}_d,$$

where $\mathbf{X}$ comprises the intercept and the covariate. The within-cluster regressions are $\mathrm{E}(\mathbf{y}_d \mid \mathbf{X}_d, d) = \mathbf{X}_d(\boldsymbol{\beta}+\boldsymbol{\delta}_d)$, so the regression coefficients $\boldsymbol{\beta}_d = \boldsymbol{\beta}+\boldsymbol{\delta}_d$ have cluster-level distribution $\mathcal{N}(\boldsymbol{\beta}, \boldsymbol{\Sigma}_B)$.

When every cluster has the same regression, then $\boldsymbol{\Sigma}_B = \mathbf{0}$. When the regressions are parallel (they share the same slope but have different intercepts), $\boldsymbol{\Sigma}_B = \begin{pmatrix} \sigma_1^2 & 0 \\ 0 & 0 \end{pmatrix}$; σ_1^2 is the variance in $\boldsymbol{\Sigma}_B$ that corresponds to the intercept. We use the notation σ_{1x} and σ_x^2 for the other two independent elements of $\boldsymbol{\Sigma}_B$. When the regressions differ in both their intercepts and slopes they may cross at a single point. Let this point be x^*, and denote $\mathbf{x}^* = (1, x^*)$. Then $\mathrm{var}\,(\mathbf{x}^*\boldsymbol{\delta}_d) = \mathbf{x}^*\boldsymbol{\Sigma}_B\mathbf{x}^{*\top} = 0$. Since $\mathbf{x}^* \neq \mathbf{0}$, $\boldsymbol{\Sigma}_B$ is singular. Further, assuming that $\sigma_x^2 > 0$, the identity

$$\sigma_1^2 + 2\sigma_{1x}x^* + \sigma_x^2 x^{*2} = 0$$

implies that $x^* = -\sigma_{1x}/\sigma_x^2$.

Finally, when $\boldsymbol{\Sigma}_B$ is nonsingular, we can describe the differences among the regressions (that is, the cluster-level variation) by $\mathrm{var}(\mathbf{x}\boldsymbol{\delta}_d) = \mathbf{x}\boldsymbol{\Sigma}_B\mathbf{x}^\top$. This quadratic function of x has a unique minimum, equal to $\sigma_1^2 - \sigma_{1x}^2/\sigma_x^2$ and attained at $x^* = -\sigma_{1x}/\sigma_x^2$. The minimum-variance value x^* may be within the range of the values of X in the population; then the regression lines go through a knot at x^*, where the cluster-level variance $\mathbf{x}\boldsymbol{\Sigma}_B\mathbf{x}^\top$ is smallest. The tightness of the knot depends on $\mathrm{var}(\mathbf{x}^*\boldsymbol{\delta}) = \sigma_1^2 - \sigma_{1x}^2/\sigma_x^2$, that is, on the proximity of the matrix $\boldsymbol{\Sigma}_B$ to singularity. When $\boldsymbol{\Sigma}_B$ is singular and the slopes vary ($\sigma_x^2 > 0$), all the regressions go through a single point $(x^*, \mathbf{x}^*\boldsymbol{\beta})$. When x^* is smaller than all the values of X in the population, then the variance of the regressions increases throughout the range. When it exceeds all the values of X the variance decreases, and when it lies within the range the variance decreases up to x^* and then it increases. Figure 9.1 illustrates these patterns of variation. The within-cluster regressions are drawn in the left-hand panels and the variance as a function of X in the right-hand panels.

The patterns of variation with two or more variables associated with variation are more difficult to discuss or represent graphically, because variation occurs in more than two dimensions. We may reduce our attention to one variable at a time and to the corresponding 2×2 submatrix of $\boldsymbol{\Sigma}_B$, akin to conditioning on the regressions with respect to the other variables.

9.2.1 Invariance with Respect to Linear Transformations

In ordinary regression models we subscribe to the following hierarchy of covariates:

1. intercept is always included in the model;
2. with any interaction $X^{(1)}X^{(2)}$, both its constituent variables, $X^{(1)}$ and $X^{(2)}$, are included;

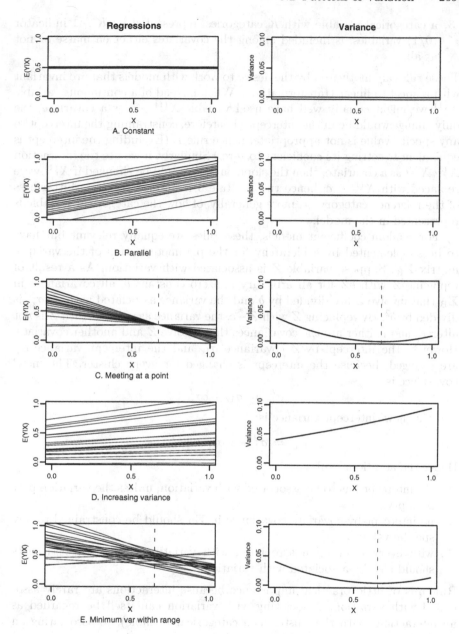

Fig. 9.1. Patterns of cluster-level variation. The within-cluster regressions $\mathbf{x}\beta_d$ are plotted in the left-hand panels and the corresponding variances $\mathbf{x}\boldsymbol{\Sigma}_B\mathbf{x}^\top$ in the right-hand panels. Vertical dashes mark the value of x for which the cluster-level variance attains its minimum.

3. a categorical variable with K categories, represented by $K - 1$ indicator (0/1) variables, is included among the covariates either en masse or not at all.

These rules are motivated by the desire to work with models that are invariant with respect to linear transformations. When instead of a continuous variable $X^{(1)}$ we might equally well have used variable $X^{(1)} - c$ as a covariate, the only change would be in the intercept. Therefore, constraining the intercept to any specific value is not appropriate; hence rule 1. (Excluding the intercept is equivalent to setting its coefficient to zero.) Similarly, if we use the interaction $X^{(1)} X^{(2)}$ as a covariate, then the slope on $X^{(2)}$ would be changed if $X^{(1)}$ were replaced with $X^{(1)} - c$; hence rule 2. Rule 3 is implied by the arbitrariness of the reference category or, more generally, of how the categorical variable is represented in the model.

For random coefficient models, these rules are equally relevant but have to be supplemented by a hierarchy for the parameterisation of the variance matrix Σ_B. Suppose variable Z is associated with variation. As a result of replacing Z with bZ for an arbitrary nonzero constant b, all covariances in Σ_B that involve Z are divided by b and the variance associated with Z, σ_z^2, is divided by b^2. By replacing Z with $Z - c$, the variance associated with Z is not altered, and neither are the covariances that involve Z and another covariate. However, the intercept-by-Z covariance σ_{1z} and the intercept variance σ_1^2 are changed, because the intercept is changed for every cluster. The 'new' covariance is

$$\sigma'_{1z} = \sigma_{1z} + c\sigma_z^2$$

and the 'new' intercept variance is

$$\sigma_1^{2'} = \sigma_1^2 + 2c\sigma_{1z} + c\sigma_z^2.$$

Hence the additional rules:

4. the intercept has to be associated with variation, unless the variation part is empty;
5. no intercept-by-covariate covariance in Σ_B should be constrained to any specific value;
6. with every interaction associated with variation both its constituents should also be associated with variation.

Rule 6 is of little practical importance because interactions are rarely associated with variation. Associating with variation can itself be regarded as an interaction (with the cluster as a categorical variable), so associating an interaction with variation is akin to a three-way interaction.

9.3 Maximum Likelihood Estimation

In this section, we describe a method for fitting the random coefficient model in (9.5) by maximum likelihood (ML). The starting point is an expression for the likelihood. As the vectors $\mathbf{y}_d$, $d = 1, \ldots, D$, are mutually independent (conditionally on $\mathbf{X}_d$) and normally distributed, the log-likelihood for $\mathbf{y} = (\mathbf{y}_1^\top, \ldots, \mathbf{y}_D^\top)^\top$ is

$$l = \sum_{d=1}^{D} l_d,$$

with the log-likelihoods (contributions) for each cluster d equal to

$$l_d = -\frac{1}{2} \left[n_d \log(2\pi) + \log\{\det(\mathbf{V}_d)\} + \mathbf{e}_d^\top \mathbf{V}_d^{-1} \mathbf{e}_d \right],$$

where $\mathbf{V}_d = \mathrm{var}\,(\mathbf{y}_d \,|\, \mathbf{X}_d)$ and $\mathbf{e}_d = \mathbf{y}_d - \mathbf{X}_d \boldsymbol{\beta}$. The overall sample size is denoted by n; $n = n_1 + \cdots + n_D$. For the variance matrices, we have

$$\mathbf{V}_d = \sigma^2 \mathbf{I}_{n_d} + \mathbf{Z}_d \boldsymbol{\Sigma}_\mathrm{B} \mathbf{Z}_d^\top.$$

When the sample size n_d is much greater than the number of variables in the variation part, r, the inverse and the determinant of this variance matrix can be evaluated with computational economy by the formulas

$$\det(\mathbf{V}_d) = \sigma^{2n_d} \det(\mathbf{G}_d),$$

$$\mathbf{V}_d^{-1} = \frac{1}{\sigma^2} \mathbf{I}_{n_d} - \frac{1}{\sigma^4} \mathbf{Z}_d \boldsymbol{\Sigma}_\mathrm{B} \mathbf{G}_d^{-1} \mathbf{Z}_d^\top,$$

(9.6)

where $\mathbf{G}_d = \mathbf{I}_r + \sigma^{-2} \mathbf{Z}_d^\top \mathbf{Z}_d \boldsymbol{\Sigma}_\mathrm{B}$. Note that $\mathbf{G}_d$ is an $r \times r$ matrix, irrespective of the value of n_d. The identity for the inverse can be proved by checking that the product of $\mathbf{V}_d$ and the expression for $\mathbf{V}_d^{-1}$ is equal to the identity matrix:

$$\left(\sigma^2 \mathbf{I}_{n_d} + \mathbf{Z}_d \boldsymbol{\Sigma}_\mathrm{B} \mathbf{Z}_d^\top \right) \left(\frac{1}{\sigma^2} \mathbf{I}_{n_d} - \frac{1}{\sigma^4} \mathbf{Z}_d \boldsymbol{\Sigma}_\mathrm{B} \mathbf{G}_d^{-1} \mathbf{Z}_d^\top \right)$$

$$= \mathbf{I}_{n_d} + \frac{1}{\sigma^2} \mathbf{Z}_d \boldsymbol{\Sigma}_\mathrm{B} \mathbf{Z}_d^\top - \frac{1}{\sigma^2} \mathbf{Z}_d \boldsymbol{\Sigma}_\mathrm{B} \left(\mathbf{G}_d - \mathbf{I}_r \right) \mathbf{G}_d^{-1} \mathbf{Z}_d^\top - \frac{1}{\sigma^2} \mathbf{Z}_d \boldsymbol{\Sigma}_\mathrm{B} \mathbf{G}_d^{-1} \mathbf{Z}_d^\top$$

$$= \mathbf{I}_{n_d}.$$

To prove the identity for $\det(\mathbf{V}_d)$, consider the matrix with the partitioning

$$\begin{pmatrix} \sigma^2 \mathbf{I}_{n_d} & -\mathbf{Z}_d \boldsymbol{\Sigma}_\mathrm{B} \\ \mathbf{Z}_d^\top & \mathbf{I}_r \end{pmatrix}.$$

(9.7)

The determinant of this matrix is not altered if we subtract the $\sigma^{-2} \mathbf{Z}_d^\top$ (or any other) premultiple of the blocks at the top from the blocks at the bottom. This results in the matrix

$$\begin{pmatrix} \sigma^2 \mathbf{I}_{n_d} & -\mathbf{Z}_d \boldsymbol{\Sigma}_\mathrm{B} \\ \mathbf{0} & \mathbf{G}_d \end{pmatrix},$$

and its determinant is $\sigma^{2n_d} \det(\mathbf{G}_d)$. Neither is the determinant of the matrix in (9.7) altered by subtracting from its left-hand blocks the $\mathbf{Z}_d^\top$ postmultiples of the right-hand blocks. This results in the matrix

$$\begin{pmatrix} \mathbf{V}_d & \mathbf{Z}_d\Sigma_{\mathrm{B}} \\ \mathbf{0} & \mathbf{I}_r \end{pmatrix},$$

so its determinant is equal to $\det(\mathbf{V}_d)$. Hence the determinant identity in (9.6).

We find the maximum of the likelihood using the *Fisher scoring algorithm*. The algorithm proceeds by iterations of the updating formula

$$\hat{\boldsymbol{\theta}}_{\mathrm{new}} = \hat{\boldsymbol{\theta}}_{\mathrm{old}} + \left\{ \mathcal{I}\left(\hat{\boldsymbol{\theta}}_{\mathrm{old}}\right)\right\}^{-1} \mathbf{s}\left(\hat{\boldsymbol{\theta}}_{\mathrm{old}}\right),$$

where $\boldsymbol{\theta}$ is the vector of all the parameters; $\hat{\boldsymbol{\theta}}_{\mathrm{old}}$ and $\hat{\boldsymbol{\theta}}_{\mathrm{new}}$ its current (provisional) and updated estimate, respectively; $\mathcal{I}$ the expected information matrix; and $\mathbf{s}$ the score vector; $\mathcal{I}$ and $\mathbf{s}$ are evaluated at $\hat{\boldsymbol{\theta}}_{\mathrm{old}}$. The vector of parameters $\boldsymbol{\theta}$ comprises σ^2, all the components of $\boldsymbol{\beta}$, and all the nonduplicated elements of Σ_{B}, that is, $1+p+r(r+1)/2$ elements in total. The difference $\Delta\hat{\boldsymbol{\theta}} = \hat{\boldsymbol{\theta}}_{\mathrm{new}} - \hat{\boldsymbol{\theta}}_{\mathrm{old}}$ is referred to as the *updating* vector.

We simplify the task of maximising l by introducing the scaled variance matrix $\Omega = \sigma^{-2}\Sigma_{\mathrm{B}}$ and the matrices $\mathbf{W}_d = \sigma^{-2}\mathbf{V}_d$, so that

$$l_d = -\frac{1}{2}\left[n_d \log(2\pi) + n_d \log\left(\sigma^2\right) + \log\{\det(\mathbf{W}_d)\} + \frac{1}{\sigma^2}\,\mathbf{e}_d^\top \mathbf{W}_d^{-1}\mathbf{e}_d\right]$$

and $\mathbf{W}_d = \mathbf{I}_{n_d} + \mathbf{Z}_d\Omega\mathbf{Z}_d^\top$. The advantage of this is that σ^2 can now be estimated separately from the remaining parameters. We have

$$2\frac{\partial l_d}{\partial \sigma^2} = -\frac{n_d}{\sigma^2} + \frac{1}{\sigma^4}\mathbf{e}_d^\top \mathbf{W}_d^{-1}\mathbf{e}_d,$$

since neither $\mathbf{e}_d$ nor $\mathbf{W}_d$ involves σ^2 (after introducing Ω). The score function for σ^2, $\partial l / \partial \sigma^2$, has the root

$$\hat{\sigma}_{\mathrm{new}}^2 = \frac{1}{n}\sum_{d=1}^{D} \hat{\mathbf{e}}_d^\top \hat{\mathbf{W}}_d^{-1}\hat{\mathbf{e}}_d \tag{9.8}$$

obtained after adding up the derivatives of l_d over the clusters d. By adding carets $\hat{}$ we indicate that $\mathbf{e}_d$ and $\mathbf{W}_d$ are not available, and expressions for them have to be evaluated using the current values of $\hat{\boldsymbol{\beta}}$ and $\hat{\Omega}$, respectively.

The score vector for the regression parameters $\boldsymbol{\beta}$ is derived from the identity

$$\frac{\partial l_d}{\partial \boldsymbol{\beta}} = \frac{1}{\sigma^2}\mathbf{X}_d^\top \mathbf{W}_d^{-1}\mathbf{e}_d,$$

so that

$$\frac{\partial l}{\partial \beta} = \frac{1}{\sigma^2} \sum_{d=1}^{D} \mathbf{X}_d^\top \mathbf{W}_d^{-1} \mathbf{e}_d = \frac{1}{\sigma^2} \mathbf{X}^\top \mathbf{W}^{-1} \mathbf{e},$$

where $\mathbf{W}$ is the block-diagonal matrix composed of $\mathbf{W}_1, \ldots, \mathbf{W}_D$ as its diagonal blocks, and $\mathbf{e} = \mathbf{y} - \mathbf{X}\beta$ is the vector of residuals; $\mathbf{e} = (\mathbf{e}_1^\top, \ldots, \mathbf{e}_D^\top)^\top$. The root of the score vector with respect to β is

$$\hat{\beta}_{\text{new}} = \left(\mathbf{X}^\top \hat{\mathbf{W}}^{-1} \mathbf{X} \right)^{-1} \mathbf{X}^\top \hat{\mathbf{W}}^{-1} \mathbf{y}. \tag{9.9}$$

This is equivalent to the updating formula

$$\hat{\beta}_{\text{new}} = \hat{\beta}_{\text{old}} + \left(\mathbf{X}^\top \hat{\mathbf{W}}^{-1} \mathbf{X} \right)^{-1} \mathbf{X}^\top \hat{\mathbf{W}}^{-1} \hat{\mathbf{e}},$$

which we would obtain using the Fisher scoring algorithm.

Finally, we deal with estimating the elements of $\mathbf{\Omega}$. It turns out that we need to apply Fisher scoring only for these parameters. Let ω be an arbitrary element of $\mathbf{\Omega}$. It can be expressed as $\omega = \mathbf{i}_1^\top \mathbf{\Omega} \mathbf{i}_2$, where $\mathbf{i}_1$ and $\mathbf{i}_2$ are the respective indicator vectors of the row and column of ω in $\mathbf{\Omega}$. An indicator vector comprises zeros, with one exception, unity, for the element it indicates. For example, suppose $\mathbf{\Omega}$ is 4×4. Then for the covariance $\Omega_{2,3}$, $\mathbf{i}_1 = (0, 1, 0, 0)^\top$ and $\mathbf{i}_2 = (0, 0, 1, 0)^\top$. As $\Omega_{2,3} = \Omega_{3,2}$, the values of $\mathbf{i}_1$ and $\mathbf{i}_2$ could be swapped. The element of the score vector for ω is

$$\frac{\partial l}{\partial \omega} = -\frac{1}{2} \frac{\partial \log\{\det(\mathbf{W})\}}{\partial \omega} + \frac{1}{2\sigma^2} \mathbf{e}^\top \mathbf{W}^{-1} \frac{\partial \mathbf{W}}{\partial \omega} \mathbf{W}^{-1} \mathbf{e}. \tag{9.10}$$

Here, a diagonal block of $\partial \mathbf{W}/\partial \omega$ is

$$\frac{\partial \mathbf{W}_d}{\partial \omega} = \mathbf{Z}_d \frac{\partial \mathbf{\Omega}}{\partial \omega} \mathbf{Z}_d^\top. \tag{9.11}$$

When $\omega = \mathbf{i}_1^\top \mathbf{\Omega} \mathbf{i}_2$ is a covariance,

$$\frac{\partial \mathbf{\Omega}}{\partial \omega} = \mathbf{i}_1 \mathbf{i}_2^\top + \mathbf{i}_2 \mathbf{i}_1^\top. \tag{9.12}$$

When ω is a variance in $\mathbf{\Omega}$, $\partial \mathbf{\Omega}/\partial \omega = \mathbf{i}\mathbf{i}^\top$, where $\mathbf{i}$ indicates the column and row of ω in $\mathbf{\Omega}$. When ω is half of a variance, $\omega = \frac{1}{2} \mathbf{i}^\top \mathbf{\Omega} \mathbf{i}$, the derivative matrix $\partial \mathbf{\Omega}/\partial \omega = 2\mathbf{i}\mathbf{i}^\top$ has the same form as for a covariance, with $\mathbf{i}_1 = \mathbf{i}_2 = \mathbf{i}$. Then (9.12) holds for every parameter in $\mathbf{\Omega}$, and we do not have to distinguish between the two types of parameters ω.

We derive an expression for the derivative of the log-determinant indirectly. The expectation of the score vanishes, $\mathrm{E}(\partial l/\partial \omega) = 0$, so (9.10) implies that

$$\frac{\partial \log\{\det(\mathbf{W})\}}{\partial \omega} = \frac{1}{\sigma^2} \mathrm{E}\left(\mathbf{e}^\top \mathbf{W}^{-1} \frac{\partial \mathbf{W}}{\partial \omega} \mathbf{W}^{-1} \mathbf{e} \right)$$

$$= \frac{1}{\sigma^2} \operatorname{tr} \left\{ \mathbf{W}^{-1} \frac{\partial \mathbf{W}}{\partial \omega} \mathbf{W}^{-1} \operatorname{E} \left(\mathbf{e} \mathbf{e}^{\top} \right) \right\}$$

$$= \operatorname{tr} \left(\mathbf{W}^{-1} \frac{\partial \mathbf{W}}{\partial \omega} \right),$$

as $\operatorname{E}(\mathbf{ee}) = \operatorname{var}(\mathbf{e}) = \mathbf{V} = \sigma^2 \mathbf{W}$. Therefore, (9.10) with (9.11) and (9.12) becomes

$$\frac{\partial l}{\partial \omega} = -\frac{1}{2} \sum_{d=1}^{D} \left\{ \operatorname{tr} \left(\mathbf{W}_d^{-1} \frac{\partial \mathbf{W}_d}{\partial \omega} \right) - \frac{1}{\sigma^2} \mathbf{e}_d^{\top} \mathbf{W}_d^{-1} \frac{\partial \mathbf{W}_d}{\partial \omega} \mathbf{W}_d^{-1} \mathbf{e}_d \right\}$$

$$= -\frac{1}{2} \sum_{d=1}^{D} \left\{ \operatorname{tr} \left(\mathbf{Z}_d^{\top} \mathbf{W}_d^{-1} \mathbf{Z}_d \frac{\partial \mathbf{\Omega}}{\partial \omega} \right) - \frac{1}{\sigma^2} \mathbf{e}_d^{\top} \mathbf{W}_d^{-1} \mathbf{Z}_d \frac{\partial \mathbf{\Omega}}{\partial \omega} \mathbf{Z}_d^{\top} \mathbf{W}_d^{-1} \mathbf{e}_d \right\}$$

$$= -\sum_{d=1}^{D} \left(\mathbf{i}_1^{\top} \mathbf{Z}_d^{\top} \mathbf{W}_d^{-1} \mathbf{Z}_d \mathbf{i}_2 - \frac{1}{\sigma^2} \mathbf{e}_d^{\top} \mathbf{W}_d^{-1} \mathbf{Z}_d \mathbf{i}_1 \, \mathbf{e}_d^{\top} \mathbf{W}_d^{-1} \mathbf{Z}_d \mathbf{i}_2 \right), \qquad (9.13)$$

exploiting the properties of the trace operator and the symmetry of the way ω is expressed in terms of $\mathbf{\Omega}$.

The result of premultiplying an arbitrary matrix $\mathbf{M}$ by an indicator vector $\mathbf{i}$ is a row of $\mathbf{M}$, so pre- and postmultiplying $\mathbf{M}$ by indicator vectors is equivalent to extracting an element of $\mathbf{M}$. Similarly, the product of a vector and an indicator vector is an element of the former. For the concluding expression in (9.13), we require the matrices $\mathbf{U}_d = \mathbf{Z}_d^{\top} \mathbf{W}_d^{-1} \mathbf{Z}_d$ and vectors $\mathbf{u}_d = \mathbf{Z}_d^{\top} \mathbf{W}_d^{-1} \mathbf{e}_d$. Note that $\mathbf{U}_d = \sigma^{-2} \operatorname{E} \left(\mathbf{u}_d \mathbf{u}_d^{\top} \right)$. Evaluation $\mathbf{U}_d$ and $\mathbf{u}_d$ is simplified by (9.6) adapted for $\mathbf{W}_d$. The inverse of $\mathbf{W}_d$ is $\mathbf{W}_d^{-1} = \mathbf{I}_{n_d} - \mathbf{Z}_d \mathbf{\Omega} \mathbf{G}_d^{-1} \mathbf{Z}_d^{\top}$, and so

$$\mathbf{Z}_d^{\top} \mathbf{W}_d^{-1} = \mathbf{Z}_d^{\top} - \mathbf{Z}_d^{\top} \mathbf{Z}_d \mathbf{\Omega} \mathbf{G}_d^{-1} \mathbf{Z}_d^{\top}$$

$$= \left\{ \mathbf{I}_r - (\mathbf{G}_d - \mathbf{I}_r) \mathbf{G}_d^{-1} \right\} \mathbf{Z}_d^{\top} \quad = \mathbf{G}_d^{-1} \mathbf{Z}_d^{\top}. \qquad (9.14)$$

Hence $\mathbf{U}_d = \mathbf{G}_d^{-1} \mathbf{Z}_d^{\top} \mathbf{Z}_d$ and $\mathbf{u}_d = \mathbf{G}_d^{-1} \mathbf{Z}_d^{\top} \mathbf{e}_d$. Denote by $U_{d,hk}$ the (h, k)-element of $\mathbf{U}_d$ and by $u_{d,h}$ the h-element of $\mathbf{u}_d$. Then for a covariance $\omega_{hk} = \Omega_{hk}$ or a half-variance $\omega_{kk} = \frac{1}{2} \Omega_k$, (9.13) becomes

$$\frac{\partial l}{\partial \omega_{hk}} = -\sum_{d=1}^{D} \left(U_{d,hk} - \frac{u_{d,h} \, u_{d,k}}{\sigma^2} \right).$$

In summary, the scoring vector for the elements of $\mathbf{\Omega}$ requires the summaries $\mathbf{Z}_d^{\top} \mathbf{X}_d$ and $\mathbf{Z}_d^{\top} \mathbf{y}_d$. It turns out that the former are sufficient also for evaluating the expected information matrix for $\mathbf{\Omega}$.

Let $\omega_1 = \mathbf{i}_1^{\top} \mathbf{\Omega} \mathbf{i}_2$ and $\omega_2 = \mathbf{i}_1'^{\top} \mathbf{\Omega} \mathbf{i}_2'$ be covariances or half-variances in $\mathbf{\Omega}$, expressed in terms of their indicator vectors. In terms of the elements of $\mathbf{\Omega}$ they represent, $\omega_1 = \Omega_{hk}$ and $\omega_2 = \Omega_{h'k'}$, or their respective halves if $h = k$ or $h' = k'$. Then by differentiating (9.13) we obtain

$$\frac{\partial^2 l}{\partial \omega_1 \partial \omega_2} = \sum_{d=1}^{D} \left\{ \text{tr} \left(\mathbf{U}_d \frac{\partial \Omega}{\partial \omega_1} \mathbf{U}_d \frac{\partial \Omega}{\partial \omega_2} \right) - \frac{2}{\sigma^2} \mathbf{u}_d^{\top} \frac{\partial \Omega}{\partial \omega_1} \mathbf{U}_d \frac{\partial \Omega}{\partial \omega_2} \mathbf{u}_d \right\}.$$

Note that $\text{E}(\mathbf{u}_d \mathbf{u}_d^{\top}) = \sigma^2 \mathbf{G}_d^{-1} \mathbf{Z}_d^{\top} \mathbf{W}_d \mathbf{Z}_d \mathbf{G}_d^{-1^{\top}} = \sigma^2 \mathbf{U}_d$. An element of the expected information matrix is

$$-\text{E} \left(\frac{\partial^2 l}{\partial \omega_1 \partial \omega_2} \right) = - \sum_{d=1}^{D} \text{tr} \left(\mathbf{U}_d \frac{\partial \Omega}{\partial \omega_1} \mathbf{U}_d \frac{\partial \Omega}{\partial \omega_2} \right)$$

$$+ \frac{2}{\sigma^2} \sum_{d=1}^{D} \text{tr} \left\{ \frac{\partial \Omega}{\partial \omega_1} \mathbf{U}_d \frac{\partial \Omega}{\partial \omega_2} \text{E} \left(\mathbf{u}_d \mathbf{u}_d^{\top} \right) \right\}$$

$$= \sum_{d=1}^{D} \text{tr} \left(\mathbf{U}_d \frac{\partial \Omega}{\partial \omega_1} \mathbf{U}_d \frac{\partial \Omega}{\partial \omega_2} \right)$$

$$= \sum_{d=1}^{D} \left(\mathbf{i}_1^{\top} \mathbf{U}_d \mathbf{i}_1' \; \mathbf{i}_2^{\top} \mathbf{U}_d \mathbf{i}_2' + \mathbf{i}_1^{\top} \mathbf{U}_d \mathbf{i}_2' \; \mathbf{i}_2^{\top} \mathbf{U}_d \mathbf{i}_1' \right)$$

$$= \sum_{d=1}^{D} \left(U_{d,hh'} U_{d,kk'} + U_{d,hk'} U_{d,kh'} \right). \tag{9.15}$$

Evaluation of this expression requires only the matrices $\mathbf{U}_d$.

The iterations of the Fisher scoring algorithm can avoid handling the original data $(\mathbf{X} \; \mathbf{y})$ altogether by evaluating and storing all the sufficient summaries before the first iteration. For estimating β, we require the quadratic forms $\mathbf{X}_d^{\top} \mathbf{W}_d^{-1} \mathbf{X}_d$ and $\mathbf{X}_d^{\top} \mathbf{W}_d^{-1} \mathbf{y}_d$, and these can be expressed as

$$\mathbf{X}_d^{\top} \mathbf{W}_d^{-1} \mathbf{t}_d = \mathbf{X}_d^{\top} \mathbf{t}_d - \mathbf{X}_d^{\top} \mathbf{Z}_d \Omega \mathbf{G}_d^{-1} \mathbf{Z}_d^{\top} \mathbf{t}_d,$$

where $\mathbf{t}_d$ is an arbitrary vector of length n_d. Therefore, we require the within-cluster totals of crossproducts $(\mathbf{X}_d \; \mathbf{y}_d)^{\top} (\mathbf{X}_d \; \mathbf{y}_d)$. In fact, it suffices to have $(\mathbf{X}_d \; \mathbf{y}_d)^{\top} \mathbf{Z}_d$. The remaining summaries can be replaced by the overall totals of crossproducts $(\mathbf{X} \; \mathbf{y})^{\top} (\mathbf{X} \; \mathbf{y})$. The quadratic form $\mathbf{e}^{\top} \mathbf{W}^{-1} \mathbf{e}$, used for updating $\hat{\sigma}^2$, is economically evaluated as

$$\mathbf{e}^{\top} \mathbf{W}^{-1} \mathbf{e} = \begin{pmatrix} -\beta \\ 1 \end{pmatrix}^{\top} (\mathbf{X} \; \mathbf{y})^{\top} \mathbf{W}^{-1} (\mathbf{X} \; \mathbf{y}) \begin{pmatrix} -\beta \\ 1 \end{pmatrix},$$

without having to access the elementary-level data.

For parallel regressions, when Ω comprises the variance ratio $\omega = \sigma_{\text{B}}^2 / \sigma^2$ as its sole parameter, the univariate versions of U_d and u_d are $U_d = n_d / (1 + n_d \omega)$ and $u_d = \bar{e}_d n_d / (1 + n_d \omega)$, where $\bar{e}_d = \mathbf{e}_d^{\top} \mathbf{1}_{n_d} / n_d$ is the mean of the residuals in cluster d. The equations for Fisher scoring collapse to

$$\frac{\partial l}{\partial \omega} = -\frac{1}{2} \sum_{d=1}^{D} U_d \left(1 - \frac{\bar{e}_d^2}{\sigma^2} U_d \right) ,$$

$$-\mathrm{E} \left(\frac{\partial^2 l}{\partial \omega^2} \right) = \frac{1}{2} \sum_{d=1}^{D} U_d^2 .$$

In this case, the sufficient data summaries are the within-cluster totals $(\mathbf{X}_d \ \mathbf{y}_d)^\top \mathbf{1}_{n_d}$ and the matrix $(\mathbf{X} \ \mathbf{y})^\top (\mathbf{X} \ \mathbf{y})$ of the overall totals of crossproducts.

9.3.1 Restricted Maximum Likelihood

Just like the ML estimator of the residual variance in ordinary regression, ML estimators of the variances and covariances in random coefficient models are biased. The estimator of the elementary-level variance σ^2 takes no account of the fact that the regression parameters $\boldsymbol{\beta}$ (as well as the between-cluster variance matrix $\boldsymbol{\Sigma}_\mathrm{B}$) are estimated; that is, the ML estimator $\hat{\sigma}^2$ coincides with the ML estimator that would be derived if $\boldsymbol{\beta}$ were known and happened to be equal to $\hat{\boldsymbol{\beta}}$. A sign of the problem is that $\hat{\sigma}^2 = \mathbf{e}^\top \mathbf{W}^{-1} \mathbf{e}/n$, whereas $n - p$, interpreted as the number of degrees of freedom, might be regarded as a more appropriate denominator; p degrees of freedom have been lost due to estimating $\boldsymbol{\beta}$.

This problem, if regarded as such, is resolved by maximising the likelihood for the so-called *error contrasts*. They are linear transformations of the outcome vector $\mathbf{y}$, $\mathbf{Py}$, where $\mathbf{P}$ is an $(n - p) \times n$ matrix of full rank $n - p$, such that $\mathbf{PX} = \mathbf{0}$. In effect, the transformation eliminates any dependence of the outcomes on $\boldsymbol{\beta}$, since $\mathrm{E}(\mathbf{Py}) = \mathbf{PX}\boldsymbol{\beta} = \mathbf{0}$, and isolates the estimation of σ^2 and $\boldsymbol{\Omega}$ to $\mathbf{Py}$. The choice for $\mathbf{P}$ turns out to be immaterial because the likelihoods for the choices differ only by a constant (multiplicative) factor which has no impact on likelihood maximisation. The likelihood for $\mathbf{Py}$ is called *restricted*, and its maximisation is referred to as restricted maximum likelihood (REML). Apart from a constant that depends on none of the parameters or on $\mathbf{y}$, the restricted likelihood is $l^{(\mathrm{re})} = l - \Delta l$, where the adjustment Δl is

$$\Delta l = \frac{1}{2} \log \left\{ \det \left(\mathbf{X}^\top \mathbf{V}^{-1} \mathbf{X} \right) \right\} . \qquad (9.16)$$

This adjustment does not depend on $\boldsymbol{\beta}$, so the expression for estimating $\boldsymbol{\beta}$ in (9.9) is unchanged. However, it now involves a different estimator of $\mathbf{W}$, and so the REML estimator of $\boldsymbol{\beta}$, $\hat{\boldsymbol{\beta}}^{(\mathrm{re})}$, differs from the ML estimator $\hat{\boldsymbol{\beta}}$. The difference (in their distributions) is usually inconsequential.

By extracting σ^2 as a factor in (9.16), using the identity $\mathbf{V} = \sigma^2 \mathbf{W}$, we obtain the REML counterpart of (9.8):

$$\hat{\sigma}^2_{\mathrm{re,new}} = \frac{1}{n - p} \sum_{d=1}^{D} \hat{\mathbf{e}}_d^\top \hat{\mathbf{W}}_d^{-1} \hat{\mathbf{e}}_d ;$$

the denominator for $\hat{\sigma}_{\mathrm{re}}^2$ is adjusted for the degrees of freedom used for estimating $\boldsymbol{\beta}$.

The adjustment for the parameters involved in $\boldsymbol{\Omega}$ is somewhat more involved; its starting point is the identity

$$\frac{\partial \Delta l}{\partial \omega} = -\frac{1}{\sigma^2} \mathrm{tr} \left\{ (\mathbf{X}^\top \mathbf{W}^{-1} \mathbf{X})^{-1} \sum_{d=1}^{D} \mathbf{X}_d^\top \mathbf{W}_d^{-1} \mathbf{Z}_d \frac{\partial \mathbf{W}_d}{\partial \omega} \mathbf{Z}_d^\top \mathbf{W}_d^{-1} \mathbf{X}_d \right\} .$$

REML would seem to be more essential for $\boldsymbol{\Omega}$ (or $\boldsymbol{\Sigma}_{\mathrm{B}}$) than for σ^2, because D (or a smaller number) is more appropriate than n for the role of degrees of freedom in estimating $\boldsymbol{\Omega}$. Usually $D \ll n$, so the relative change in the degrees of freedom from D to $D - p$ is much greater than from n to $n - p$. To see why estimation of $\boldsymbol{\Omega}$ should be associated with D or $D - p$ degrees of freedom, consider the setting in which each of the D clusters is represented in the data by so many elements (observations) that the uncertainty about the corresponding values of $\boldsymbol{\delta}_d$ can be ignored. Then $\boldsymbol{\Sigma}_{\mathrm{B}} = \mathrm{var}_D(\boldsymbol{\delta}_d)$ would be estimated by

$$\frac{1}{D} \sum_{d=1}^{D} \boldsymbol{\delta}_d \boldsymbol{\delta}_d^\top$$

or a similar expression with the denominator $D - p$; the distributions of the estimators of the variances in $\boldsymbol{\Sigma}_{\mathrm{B}}$ would then be related by scaling to χ^2_{D-p} distribution. In practice, we have much less information (every cluster has only finitely many elements in the data), so $\hat{\boldsymbol{\Sigma}}_{\mathrm{B}}$ and $\hat{\boldsymbol{\Omega}}$ are likely to be associated with fewer than $D - p$ degrees of freedom. As an extreme example, when each cluster is represented in the data by only one element, only the total $\sigma^2 + \sigma_{\mathrm{B}}^2$ can be estimated in a model with parallel regressions. In this case, there are no degrees of freedom available for estimating σ_{B}^2. We revisit this issue in Section 9.5.

Small MSE, not small bias, is the criterion for efficient estimation. Therefore, the adjustment by REML does not serve our purpose directly. When D is much greater than p, the adjustment is unimportant. When p is a large fraction of D or even of n, quantities of interest may be estimated more efficiently by ML (or REML) fitted to some submodels, for which the bias incurred is more than offset by variance reduction. In any case, the property of unbiasedness is lost by nonlinear transformations. Synthesis (Section 2.3) has a potential for estimation with even smaller MSE, but it is difficult to explore and implement. Model selection has limitations similar to those in ordinary regression.

9.3.2 Residuals

The model in (9.5) contains two kinds of random terms, $\boldsymbol{\delta}_d$ and ε_{id}. Their realisations can be estimated by their estimated conditional expectations. Such estimation refers to a very strange (conditional) replication scheme in which the target δ_d for a given d, or ε_{id} for a given pair (i, d), is fixed, while the remaining deviations are random, with the between-replication variation specified by the model. To emphasise that we consider a specific cluster d, we denote it by j. The conditional distribution of δ_j given all the model parameters and the data is derived from the joint distribution of $\mathbf{y}_j$ and δ_j; the rest of the vector $\mathbf{y}$, denoted by $\mathbf{y}_{-d}$, can be discarded because it is independent of δ_j. From the distributional identity

$$\begin{pmatrix} \mathbf{y}_j \\ \delta_j \end{pmatrix} \sim \mathcal{N}\left\{ \begin{pmatrix} \mathbf{X}_j \beta \\ \mathbf{0} \end{pmatrix}, \begin{pmatrix} \mathbf{V}_j & \mathbf{Z}_j \Sigma_{\mathrm{B}} \\ \Sigma_{\mathrm{B}} \mathbf{Z}_j^\top & \Sigma_{\mathrm{B}} \end{pmatrix} \right\},$$

we obtain the conditional distribution of δ_j given $\mathbf{y}_j$:

$$(\delta_j \mid \mathbf{y}_j; \mathbf{X}_j, \beta, \sigma^2, \Sigma_{\mathrm{B}}) \sim \mathcal{N}\left(\Sigma_{\mathrm{B}} \mathbf{Z}_j^\top \mathbf{V}_j^{-1} \mathbf{e}_j, \ \Sigma_{\mathrm{B}} - \Sigma_{\mathrm{B}} \mathbf{Z}_j^\top \mathbf{V}_j^{-1} \mathbf{Z}_j \Sigma_{\mathrm{B}} \right).$$

After applying the identity in (9.14), this simplifies to

$$(\delta_j \mid \mathbf{y}_j; \mathbf{X}_j, \beta, \sigma^2, \Sigma_{\mathrm{B}}) \sim \mathcal{N}\left(\Omega \mathbf{G}_j^{-1} \mathbf{Z}_j^\top \mathbf{e}_j, \ \Sigma_{\mathrm{B}} \mathbf{G}_j^{-1} \right). \tag{9.17}$$

For parallel regressions, when only the intercept is associated with cluster-level variation, this reduces to

$$(\delta_j \mid \mathbf{y}_j; \mathbf{X}_j, \beta, \sigma^2, \sigma_{\mathrm{B}}^2) \sim \mathcal{N}\left(\frac{n_j \omega}{1 + n_j \omega} \, \bar{e}_j, \ \frac{\sigma_{\mathrm{B}}^2}{1 + n_j \omega} \right).$$

By a similar process we derive the conditional distribution of ε_j from the joint distribution of $\mathbf{y}_j$ and ε_j. It is normal, with expectation $\mathbf{W}_j^{-1} \mathbf{e}_j$ and variance matrix $\sigma^2 \mathbf{Z}_j \Sigma_{\mathrm{B}} \mathbf{G}_j^{-1} \mathbf{Z}_j^\top$. Note that

$$\mathbf{Z}_j \, \mathrm{E}(\delta_j \mid \mathbf{y}_j) + \mathrm{E}(\varepsilon_j \mid \mathbf{y}_j) = \mathbf{e}_j; \tag{9.18}$$

the conditional expectations of δ_j and ε_j 'apportion' the overall residual $\mathbf{e}_j$ to its cluster-level (consistent) and elementary-level components.

9.3.3 Borrowing Strength

An alternative estimator of δ_j that might at first appear better motivated is

$$\hat{\delta}_j^\dagger = \left(\mathbf{Z}_j^\top \mathbf{Z}_j \right)^{-1} \mathbf{Z}_j^\top \mathbf{e}_j.$$

It is derived by ordinary least squares. If we regard cluster j as the universe, the estimator is conditionally unbiased and its sampling variance is

$$\mathrm{var}\left(\hat{\delta}_j^\dagger \mid \delta_j \right) = \sigma^2 \left(\mathbf{Z}_j^\top \mathbf{Z}_j \right)^{-1}.$$

The difference of this and the variance matrix in (9.17) is positive definite. We show it first for a positive definite $\boldsymbol{\Omega}$.

$$
\begin{aligned}
\sigma^2 \left(\mathbf{Z}_j^\top \mathbf{Z}_j\right)^{-1} - \boldsymbol{\Sigma}_B \mathbf{G}_j^{-1} &= \boldsymbol{\Sigma}_B \left\{ \left(\mathbf{Z}_j^\top \mathbf{Z}_j \boldsymbol{\Omega}\right)^{-1} - \mathbf{G}_j^{-1} \right\} \\
&= \boldsymbol{\Sigma}_B \left\{ \left(\mathbf{G}_j - \mathbf{I}\right)^{-1} \mathbf{G}_j - \mathbf{I} \right\} \mathbf{G}_j^{-1} \\
&= \boldsymbol{\Sigma}_B \left(\mathbf{G}_j - \mathbf{I}\right)^{-1} \mathbf{G}_j^{-1} \\
&= \sigma^2 \left(\mathbf{Z}_j^\top \mathbf{Z}_j\right)^{-1} \mathbf{G}_j^{-1} ,
\end{aligned} \tag{9.19}
$$

and both matrix-factors in the concluding expression are positive definite. A limiting argument, considering a sequence of positive definite matrices $\boldsymbol{\Omega}$ that converges to a singular variance matrix, can be applied to show that the difference is positive definite even when $\boldsymbol{\Sigma}_B$ is singular. The univariate version of the identity in (9.19) is

$$
\text{var}\left(\delta_j^\dagger \mid \delta_j\right) - \text{var}\left(\delta_j \mid \mathbf{y}_j\right) = \frac{\sigma^2}{n_j} \frac{1}{1 + n_j \omega} ; \tag{9.20}
$$

the difference is positive. These identities show that we can improve on unbiased estimation of the within-cluster regression coefficients, which is focussed on the data from the cluster concerned (j), by incorporating information from the rest of sample, in the form of the variance matrix $\boldsymbol{\Omega}$. This improvement is referred to as *borrowing strength* (across clusters). Alternatively, we can describe it as *exploiting the similarity* of the clusters. In (9.20), we can see that the gain (variance reduction) is greater for smaller $n_j \omega$ —for small clusters and when the clusters are more similar.

Borrowing strength has to be carefully qualified. First, some losses vis-à-vis (9.19) and (9.20) are incurred because $\boldsymbol{\beta}$ and $\boldsymbol{\Omega}$ are not known. Second, the improvement is only on average, after taking expectation over the (estimated) cluster-level distribution of $\boldsymbol{\delta}_d$. And finally, the gains are derived under the assumption that the model is appropriate. Although this condition applies equally to the ordinary regression model, the two-level model entails the variation part as a specification additional to that for the ordinary regression.

9.3.4 EM Algorithm—A Connection to Missing Data

Although the Fisher scoring algorithm for ML estimation, with some remaining details given in the next section, is satisfactory in most settings, we outline an alternative that is connected to incompleteness (Chapter 5). If we regard the deviations $\boldsymbol{\delta}_d$ as missing data the complete-data analysis amounts to fitting ordinary regression to the adjusted outcomes $\mathbf{y}_d' = \mathbf{y}_d - \mathbf{Z}_d \boldsymbol{\delta}_d$:

$$
\mathbf{y}_d' = \mathbf{X}_d \boldsymbol{\beta} + \boldsymbol{\varepsilon}_d . \tag{9.21}
$$

The EM algorithm (Section 5.4) can be applied to this setting. The data summaries required for fitting this model are $\mathbf{X}_d^\top \mathbf{X}_d$, $\mathbf{X}_d^\top \mathbf{y}_d'$, and $\mathbf{y}_d'^\top \mathbf{y}_d'$. They are linear and quadratic functions of $\boldsymbol{\delta}_d$. The E-step evaluates the conditional expectations of $\boldsymbol{\delta}_d$, involved in $\mathbf{X}_d^\top \mathbf{y}_d'$, and of $\boldsymbol{\delta}_d \boldsymbol{\delta}_d^\top$, involved in $\mathbf{y}_d'^\top \mathbf{y}_d'$. For evaluating the latter, the identity

$$\mathrm{E}\left(\boldsymbol{\delta}_d \boldsymbol{\delta}_d^\top \mid \mathbf{y}_d\right) = \mathrm{var}\left(\boldsymbol{\delta}_d \mid \mathbf{y}_d\right) + \mathrm{E}\left(\boldsymbol{\delta}_d \mid \mathbf{y}_d\right) \mathrm{E}\left(\boldsymbol{\delta}_d \mid \mathbf{y}_d\right)^\top$$

is useful. The equations for the conditional expectations and variances are given in (9.17).

In the M-step, the ordinary regression model in (9.21) is fitted, with the linear sufficient statistics $\mathbf{X}_d^\top \mathbf{y}_d'$ and $\mathbf{y}_d'^\top \mathbf{y}_d'$ replaced by their conditional expectations that were evaluated in the preceding E-step. The between-cluster variance matrix $\boldsymbol{\Sigma}_\mathrm{B}$ is estimated by moment matching:

$$\hat{\boldsymbol{\Sigma}}_\mathrm{B} = \frac{1}{D} \sum_{d=1}^{D} \mathrm{E}\left(\boldsymbol{\delta}_d \boldsymbol{\delta}_d^\top \mid \mathbf{y}_d\right).$$

With each updating of the estimates of β, σ^2, and $\boldsymbol{\Sigma}_\mathrm{B}$, the conditional expectations and variance matrices of $\boldsymbol{\delta}_d$ are altered, and so the pairs of E and M steps have to be iterated until convergence. The EM algorithm requires the same expressions as Fisher scoring, $\mathbf{U}_d = \mathbf{Z}_d^\top \mathbf{W}_d^{-1} \mathbf{Z}_d$ and $\mathbf{u}_d = \mathbf{Z}_d^\top \mathbf{W}^{-1} \mathbf{e}_d$, but uses them differently. The convergence with the Fisher scoring algorithm is in general much faster. In contrast, an advantage of the EM algorithm is that its convergence, together with an increased value of the log-likelihood at every iteration, is supported by theory. Also, each provisional estimate of $\boldsymbol{\Sigma}_\mathrm{B}$ or of $\boldsymbol{\Omega}$ in the EM algorithm is nonnegative definite; in the Fisher scoring algorithm, it may have a negative eigenvalue at any iteration. Iterations of the two methods can be combined to take advantage of their respective strengths.

9.3.5 Technical Details

The first iteration of Fisher scoring requires a set of provisional (initial) estimates of all the parameters. For the regression parameters, the ordinary least squares (OLS) fit $\hat{\beta}_0 = \left(\mathbf{X}^\top \mathbf{X}\right)^{-1} \mathbf{X}^\top \mathbf{y}$ is suitable. It is the ML estimator when $\hat{\boldsymbol{\Omega}} = \mathbf{0}$. For σ^2, the estimate of the residual variance in the OLS fit can be used. For $\boldsymbol{\Omega}$, there is no obvious initial estimator, although the estimates of all its covariances can be set to zero. The estimate of the cluster-level intercept variance can initially be set to a fraction of the OLS estimate $\hat{\sigma}_0^2$. The other variances may be set to zero or to a fraction of the corresponding initial values of $\hat{\beta}_x^2$. This can be motivated as follows. If a regression slope is equal to β_x, then the corresponding between-cluster variance is likely to be of the order β_x^2. Of course, this 'guess' is not always very good, but the first few iterations of the Fisher scoring algorithm are likely to make up for it.

An iteration of Fisher scoring may yield an estimated variance matrix $\hat{\Omega}$ that is not nonnegative definite. An updated estimate of a variance may be negative or an estimated covariance may be so large in absolute value that the corresponding correlation is outside the interval $[-1, 1]$. These examples do not exhaust all the possibilities. For instance, the matrix

$$\begin{pmatrix} 5 & 4 & 4 \\ 4 & 5 & 1 \\ 4 & 1 & 5 \end{pmatrix}$$

is not a variance matrix; its determinant is equal to -8. At the outset, the estimated variance matrix is positive definite. It will remain so if we halve the updating for each parameter ω in Ω sufficiently many times. This may slow the progress toward convergence, especially when the ML estimate of Ω is singular, but all the provisional estimates $\hat{\Omega}$ will be positive definite and will be allowed to converge to a singular variance matrix. In the EM algorithm described in the previous section, this problem is not encountered.

Another fail-safe solution is based on the parameterisation of Ω that uses the *Cholesky decomposition* $\Omega = \mathbf{L}\mathbf{L}^{\top}$, where $\mathbf{L}$ is a lower triangular matrix (a matrix with zeros above the diagonal) with positive entries on its diagonal. The Cholesky decomposition of a nonsingular variance matrix is unique. The score vector and information matrix with respect to the elements of $\mathbf{L}$ are evaluated similarly as for the elements of Ω. The equations are somewhat more complex because the elements of $\mathbf{L}$ are not linear in Ω. For elements θ, θ_1, and θ_2 of $\mathbf{L}$, we have

$$\frac{\partial \Omega}{\partial \theta} = \mathbf{L} \frac{\partial \mathbf{L}^{\top}}{\partial \theta} + \frac{\partial \mathbf{L}}{\partial \theta} \mathbf{L}^{\top},$$

$$\frac{\partial^2 \Omega}{\partial \theta_1 \partial \theta_2} = \frac{\partial \mathbf{L}}{\partial \theta_1} \frac{\partial \mathbf{L}^{\top}}{\partial \theta_2} + \frac{\partial \mathbf{L}}{\partial \theta_2} \frac{\partial \mathbf{L}^{\top}}{\partial \theta_1};$$

all the second-order partial derivatives $\partial^2 \mathbf{L}/(\partial \theta_1 \partial \theta_2)$ vanish. When a provisional (or the final) estimate of Ω is singular, the expected information matrix for the elements of $\mathbf{L}$ is also singular. Nonuniqueness of $\mathbf{L}$ in this case is resolved by setting the element in the bottom right-hand corner of $\mathbf{L}$ to zero and not estimating it any further. If that is not sufficient to get rid of the singularity of the information matrix, further elements of $\mathbf{L}$ have to be constrained to zero, starting with those in the next-to-last column.

The iterations are terminated when a convergence criterion is satisfied. Such a criterion can be that any element of the updating vector $\Delta\hat{\theta}$ is smaller than the precision of rounding, such as 10^{-4}, or that the mean squared updating $\Delta\hat{\theta}^{\top}\Delta\hat{\theta}/q$ is smaller than a set tolerance, such as 10^{-8}; q is the number of estimated parameters. The criterion may also include the change in the value of the log-likelihood between two consecutive iterations. In an orderly convergence, the log-likelihood increases at every iteration except the first, and the changes get smaller at a geometric rate. Slow and erratic convergence are signs of having too many covariates in the regression or variation part of the model or of having too little data.

9.4 Model Validity

The two-level model in (9.5) assumes that clusters are selected by a simple random sampling design from an infinite population of clusters. Each cluster, as a population, is assumed to contain infinitely many elements, and their representation in the realised sample is according to a simple random sampling design. Thus, a replication of the study would yield a different collection (sample) of clusters, and for a cluster that happens to be drawn in two replications their sets of subjects would be different.

In many settings, these assumptions are not satisfied, but the model in (9.4) is constructive nevertheless, because it provides a compact description of the population, by regression in a typical (average) cluster (β), variation of the within-cluster regressions (Σ_B), and the (conditional) within-cluster, or residual, variance σ^2. With such an application, we have to bear in mind that the description by the model fit then describes the compendium of the population and the sampling design. Good representation, for both elements and clusters, is very difficult to arrange, as the following examples show. Suppose the clusters in a finite population have unequal (finite) numbers N_d of elements and a simple random (not clustered) sampling design is applied. Then some clusters may not be represented in a sample at all. Clusters of small size N_d are less likely to be represented than large clusters. We have no means of adjusting the analysis for such a distortion. As a consequence, larger samples have a greater say in the model fit, without our intention to bring about such a disparity. The assumption about the deviations δ_d is that their expectation vanishes. In this assumption, each cluster is given equal weight. Therefore, good representation has to be arranged not for members, but for clusters *and* for members within each selected cluster.

When a clustered sampling design is applied, with sampling clusters coinciding with the clusters d in the model, and a simple random sample of a fixed and common size $n^{(1)} = n_1 = \ldots = n_D$ is drawn within each cluster, elements from small clusters have a greater probability of appearing in a sample. Sometimes most of the clusters are small, such as with individuals in human families. Then it is practical to include every member of a selected cluster in the sample. When included, a cluster is always represented in the sample by the same set of elements. The consequences of such departures from the model assumptions are difficult to assess and require detailed information about the sampling mechanism, because the problem cannot be detected by inspecting the data.

A replication of a study may end up with the same set of clusters. A case in point arises when the clusters are the districts of a country and the realised survey sample includes most of the districts. Then it is more appropriate to regard the districts as fixed. This may at first appear to be inconvenient because one of the rationales for declaring the deviations $\boldsymbol{\delta}_d$ as random is to facilitate their compact description by a variance matrix. However, a variance matrix is well defined also for a finite (and fixed) set of quantities, as

$$\mathbf{V}_\delta = \frac{1}{D} \sum_{d=1}^{D} \left(\boldsymbol{\delta}_d - \bar{\boldsymbol{\delta}}\right) \left(\boldsymbol{\delta}_d - \bar{\boldsymbol{\delta}}\right)^\top,$$

where $\bar{\boldsymbol{\delta}} = (\boldsymbol{\delta}_1 + \cdots + \boldsymbol{\delta}_D)/D$ is their population mean. When the deviations $\boldsymbol{\delta}_d$ are not known estimation of $\bar{\boldsymbol{\delta}}$ and $\mathbf{V}_\delta$ is subject to uncertainty, and further uncertainty arises when some $\boldsymbol{\delta}_d$ are not represented in the sample. Without some assumption that relates $\boldsymbol{\delta}_d$ for a cluster not represented in the data to $\boldsymbol{\delta}_d$ for the represented clusters, $\bar{\boldsymbol{\delta}}$ cannot be estimated without the threat of a substantial bias.

The model in (9.5) assumes that the within-cluster regression matrices $\mathbf{X}_d$, as well as the subsample sizes n_d, are given. This is rarely the case in practice, especially when data are collected by a survey. When the values of $\mathbf{X}_d$ are not assigned or may have been assigned nonignorably, no inferences about the coefficients $\boldsymbol{\beta}$ as (causal) effects are warranted. Without some assumptions external to the data, usually not verifiable, only an assignment of the values of $\mathbf{X}$ that is not informed by the values of the outcomes $\mathbf{y}$ enables us to make causal inferences.

Fixed or Random?

An estimate of the conditional expectation in (9.17) can be used as an estimate of the deviation $\boldsymbol{\delta}_j$, assuming that this deviation is fixed and the other deviations are random. If the uncertainty about $\boldsymbol{\beta}$ and $\boldsymbol{\Omega}$ is ignored, this estimator is unbiased on average:

$$\mathrm{E}_{\mathcal{D}} \left\{ \mathrm{E}\left(\hat{\boldsymbol{\delta}}_j \mid \boldsymbol{\delta}_j\right) \right\} = \boldsymbol{\Omega} \mathbf{G}_j^{-1} \mathbf{Z}_j^\top \mathbf{Z}_j \, \mathrm{E}_{\mathcal{D}}(\boldsymbol{\delta}_j) = \mathbf{0}.$$

We have unbiasedness only after averaging over the distribution of $\boldsymbol{\delta}_d$. If each realisation of cluster j entails a different value of $\boldsymbol{\delta}_j$, then the quantities $\boldsymbol{\delta}_j$ will be estimated without average bias in the long run.

In contrast, if we regard $\boldsymbol{\delta}_j$ as fixed (otherwise $\boldsymbol{\delta}_j$ is like a moving goalpost), its expectation is

$$\mathrm{E}\left(\hat{\boldsymbol{\delta}}_j \mid \boldsymbol{\delta}_j\right) = \boldsymbol{\Omega} \mathbf{G}_j^{-1} \mathbf{Z}_j^\top \mathbf{Z}_j \, \boldsymbol{\delta}_j,$$

so $\hat{\boldsymbol{\delta}}_j$ is biased. For parallel regressions,

$$\mathrm{E}\left(\hat{\boldsymbol{\delta}}_j \mid \boldsymbol{\delta}_j\right) = \frac{n_j \, \omega}{1 + n_j \omega} \, \boldsymbol{\delta}_j,$$

so its bias is $\delta_j/(1 + n_j\omega)$. Large values of δ_d are underestimated and small (large negative) values are overestimated. In their expectations, the estimators of the deviations δ_j are shrunk toward zero.

The interpretation of $\Sigma_B G_j^{-1}$ as a sampling variance or MSE is equally problematic, even when β, σ^2, and Ω are known. When δ_j is fixed,

$$\text{var}\left(\hat{\delta}_j \mid \delta_j\right) = \Omega G_j^{-1} Z_j^\top (\sigma^2 I_{n_j}) Z_j G_j^{-1^\top} \Omega$$
$$= \Sigma_B G_j^{-1} Z_j^\top Z_j G_j^{-1^\top} \Omega,$$

so that the MSE of $\hat{\delta}_j$ in estimating δ_j is

$$\text{MSE}\left(\hat{\delta}_j \mid \delta_j\right) = \Sigma_B G_j^{-1} Z_j^\top Z_j G_j^{-1^\top} \Omega$$
$$+ \left(\Omega G_j^{-1} Z_j^\top Z_j - I\right) \delta_j \delta_j^\top \left(\Omega G_j^{-1} Z_j^\top Z_j - I\right)^\top.$$

Only after taking the expectation over the distribution of δ_d, when $\delta_j\delta_j^\top$ is replaced by $\Sigma_B = \sigma^2\Omega$, we obtain the conditional variance in (9.17):

$$E_{\mathcal{D}}\left\{\text{MSE}\left(\hat{\delta}_j \mid \delta_j\right)\right\} = \Sigma_B G_j^{-1} Z_j^\top Z_j G_j^{-1^\top} \Omega + \Sigma_B - 2\Sigma_B G_j^{-1}\left(G_j - I\right)$$
$$+ \Sigma_B G_j^{-1}\left(G_j - I\right) Z_j^\top Z_j G_j^{-1^\top} \Omega$$
$$= \Sigma_B Z_j^\top Z_j G_j^{-1^\top} \Omega - \Sigma_B + 2\Sigma_B G_j^{-1}$$
$$= \Sigma_B G_j^{-1},$$

exploiting the fact that the evaluated expectation is a symmetric matrix. In summary, $\text{MSE}(\hat{\delta}_j \mid \delta_j) \neq \Sigma_B G_j^{-1}$, even when β, σ^2, and Ω are known; equality holds only after averaging over the clusters.

Assessing Normality

If we regard $\hat{\delta}_d$ as estimators of the deviations δ_d, we might use them to assess whether the assumptions associated with δ_d are satisfied. This is problematic first of all because each $\hat{\delta}_d$ is intended as an estimator of the individual value of δ_d (for fixed d); the collection $\{\hat{\delta}_d\}$ need not have any good properties even when each individual $\hat{\delta}_d$ has them all. Next, the cluster-level matrices Z_d are involved in $\hat{\delta}_d$ in such a way that when $Z_d^\top Z_d\Omega$ is small relative to I_r, the estimator $\hat{\delta}_d$ is shrunk a lot toward 0. At an extreme, when cluster d is not represented in the data, $\hat{\delta}_d = 0$ with certainty. Thus, the matrices Z_d and, when $Z_d = 1$, the within-cluster subsample sizes n_d, influence the pattern of the values of $\hat{\delta}_d$. Similar problems arise with the estimators $\hat{\varepsilon}_d = \hat{W}_d^{-1}\hat{e}_d$. And finally, note that univariate normality of each component of δ_d does not imply multivariate normality of the vector δ_d.

Any one of these undesirable features can be dealt with by a suitable transformation of $\hat{\boldsymbol{\delta}}_d$, but possibly at the price of exacerbating another. As an alternative, we propose the simulation-based method described in Section 1.3.1. We generate 19 (or 99) datasets from the model fitted to the collected data using the design for the study. Then we evaluate a feature (or multi-feature) on each dataset and shuffle the 20 (or 100) features, so that the realised feature could not be recognised solely by its location among them. If one of these features stands out, and after its identification it turns out to be the realised feature, we have evidence against the model assumptions.

A practical approach to choosing a feature for simulation reflects the concern we have about the values of $\boldsymbol{\delta}_d$. We define a summary of $\hat{\boldsymbol{\delta}}_d$ that is likely to detect the departure if the values of $\boldsymbol{\delta}_d$ were available. For example, if the skewnesses of the components of $\boldsymbol{\delta}_d$, denoted by $\kappa(\boldsymbol{\delta}_{\mathcal{D}})$, are a concern we evaluate $\kappa(\hat{\boldsymbol{\delta}}_{\mathcal{D}})$ for the fit based on the collected data and on 19 datasets simulated according to the model fit with the same set of matrices $\mathbf{X}_d$.

9.5 Inference About Variation

The variance matrix $\boldsymbol{\Sigma}_{\mathrm{B}}$, or its scaled version $\boldsymbol{\Omega}$, is a very convenient descriptor of the pattern of variation of the within-cluster regressions. However, inference about their elements is much more difficult than about the regression parameters. To see this, consider a simple version of the problem. Suppose the univariate cluster-level deviations δ_d are known. Then their variance σ_{B}^2 is estimated straightforwardly by

$$\hat{\sigma}_{\mathrm{B}}^2 = \frac{1}{D} \sum_{d=1}^{D} \delta_d^2.$$

The distribution of $D\hat{\sigma}_{\mathrm{B}}^2/\sigma_{\mathrm{B}}^2$ is χ_D^2, so $\hat{\sigma}_{\mathrm{B}}^2$ is unbiased for σ_{B}^2, and its sampling variance is $2\sigma_{\mathrm{B}}^4/D$. The standard error of $\hat{\sigma}_{\mathrm{B}}^2$ is estimated by $\hat{s} = \hat{\sigma}_{\mathrm{B}}^2 \sqrt{2/D}$ without bias, but $\hat{\sigma}_{\mathrm{B}}^2$ and $\hat{s}$ are perfectly correlated. So, an error in estimating σ_{B}^2 is duplicated as an error in estimating $s = \sqrt{\mathrm{var}\,(\hat{\sigma}_{\mathrm{B}}^2)}$.

In more realistic settings, with finite within-cluster sample sizes, this problem is equally pressing, although its diagnosis is more difficult. For example, the expected information about ω in a model with parallel regressions is

$$\mathcal{I}(\omega, \omega) = \frac{1}{2} \sum_{d=1}^{D} \frac{n_d^2}{(1 + n_d \omega)^2},$$

so it also depends on ω, but in a way that is more difficult to analyse. When each cluster has the same sample size $n_\bullet$, the asymptotic variance of the ML estimator $\hat{\omega}$, equal to $1/\mathcal{I}(\omega, \omega)$, is $2(1/n_\bullet + \omega)^2/D$. Knowing the values of δ_d corresponds to $n_\bullet = +\infty$. The estimated asymptotic standard error $(1/n_\bullet + \hat{\omega})\sqrt{2/D}$ is also perfectly correlated with the estimator $\hat{\omega}$.

As an aside, we derive an approximation for the number of degrees of freedom associated with the ML estimator $\hat{\omega}$. We match the asymptotic (approximate) sampling variance of $\hat{\omega}$ with the variance of a χ^2 distribution. Let this χ^2 distribution have m degrees of freedom; then we solve the equation

$$\frac{2\omega^2}{m} = \frac{2(1/n_\bullet + \omega)^2}{D}.$$

The solution is $m = D/\{1 + 1/(n_\bullet \omega)\}^2$; naturally, it involves ω. When the within-cluster sample sizes are unequal, a good approximation to m is obtained by replacing $n_\bullet$ with the harmonic mean of the sample sizes,

$$n_\bullet^* = \frac{D}{\displaystyle\sum_{d=1}^{D} \frac{1}{n_d}}. \tag{9.22}$$

Thus, for a fixed value of ω, information about ω increases with $n_\bullet^*$ but does not do so linearly. The increments get smaller with increasing $n_\bullet^*$. This is an indirect consequence of borrowing strength across clusters; the borrowing is greater for clusters with sparser representation. Of course, another reason for incomplete information is that only a finite number of clusters is represented in the overall sample.

9.5.1 Confounding in Cluster-Level Variation

For ordinary regression, we have powerful algebraic equipment for understanding the correlation structure and estimability of the OLS estimator $\hat{\beta}$. For example, estimability is equivalent to full rank $p \leq n$ of the $n \times p$ regression matrix $\mathbf{X}$. With a modicum of approximation, it can be applied also to its counterpart in a random coefficient model.

For the parameters in $\boldsymbol{\Omega}$, a similar diagnosis is much more difficult to make. The number of parameters to be estimated, $\frac{1}{2}r(r+1)$, proliferates with increasing number r of variables in the variation part of the model and a connection to linear algebra is much more difficult to establish. In (9.15) we expressed the elements of the information matrix for the parameters in $\boldsymbol{\Omega}$ in terms of the elements of the matrices $\mathbf{U}_d = \mathbf{Z}_d^\top \mathbf{W}_d^{-1} \mathbf{Z}_d = \mathbf{G}_d^{-1} \mathbf{Z}_d^\top \mathbf{Z}_d$. We form the cluster-level variables $\mathbf{H}_{hk} = (U_{1,hk}, U_{2,hk}, \ldots, U_{D,hk})^\top$ from the (h, k) elements of the matrices $\mathbf{U}_d$. These variables depend on the variation matrix $\mathbf{Z}$ as well as on $\boldsymbol{\Omega}$.

For simplicity, we discuss the case of one variable in the variation part, when $\boldsymbol{\Omega}$ involves three parameters, two half-variances and a covariance. The information matrix for these parameters is

$$\mathcal{U} = \begin{pmatrix} 2\mathbf{H}_{11}^\top \mathbf{H}_{11} & 2\mathbf{H}_{12}^\top \mathbf{H}_{12} & 2\mathbf{H}_{11}^\top \mathbf{H}_{12} \\ 2\mathbf{H}_{12}^\top \mathbf{H}_{12} & 2\mathbf{H}_{22}^\top \mathbf{H}_{22} & 2\mathbf{H}_{12}^\top \mathbf{H}_{22} \\ 2\mathbf{H}_{11}^\top \mathbf{H}_{12} & 2\mathbf{H}_{12}^\top \mathbf{H}_{22} & \mathbf{H}_{11}^\top \mathbf{H}_{22} + \mathbf{H}_{12}^\top \mathbf{H}_{12} \end{pmatrix}.$$

Each matrix $\mathbf{U}_d$ is nonnegative definite and is positive definite whenever $\mathbf{Z}_d$ is of full rank 2, that is, when the values of the covariate in the variation part are not constant. Therefore

$$\mathbf{H}_{12}^\top \mathbf{H}_{12} \leq \mathbf{H}_{11}^\top \mathbf{H}_{22} \,,$$

with equality when all matrices $\mathbf{Z}_d$ are of rank 1. Further, by the Cauchy-Schwartz inequality,

$$\left(\mathbf{H}_{11}^\top \mathbf{H}_{22}\right)^2 \leq \mathbf{H}_{11}^\top \mathbf{H}_{11} \, \mathbf{H}_{22}^\top \mathbf{H}_{22} \,.$$

Equality in both these relations occurs only when all matrices $\mathbf{U}_d$ are singular, that is, when all matrices $\mathbf{Z}_d^\top \mathbf{Z}_d$ are singular. Apart from this trivial case, the submatrix of $\mathcal{U}$ for the two half-variances (the first two rows and columns) is always positive definite. A similar discussion applies to any other pair of parameters (a covariance and a half-variance), but it is much more difficult to extend to the entire 3×3 matrix $\mathcal{U}$.

9.6 Multilevel Models and Other Extensions

The clusters can themselves be clustered, in several layers, or *levels of nesting*. Then we have elements within clusters of level 2, these within clusters of level 3, and so on. Each cluster is associated with its own (conditional) regression, and the vectors of coefficients in these regressions at a given level of nesting vary according to a multivariate normal distribution. This description corresponds to the three-level model

$$\mathbf{y}_{ad} = \mathbf{X}_{ad}\boldsymbol{\beta} + \mathbf{Z}_a^{(3)}\boldsymbol{\delta}_a^{(3)} + \mathbf{Z}_{ad}^{(2)}\boldsymbol{\delta}_{ad}^{(2)} + \boldsymbol{\varepsilon}_{ad} \,, \tag{9.23}$$

in which $\boldsymbol{\delta}_a^{(3)}$ and $\boldsymbol{\delta}_{ad}^{(2)}$, $d = 1, \ldots, D_a$ and $a = 1, \ldots, A$, are mutually independent random samples from respective multivariate normal distributions $\mathcal{N}(\mathbf{0}_{r_3}, \boldsymbol{\Sigma}_3)$ and $\mathcal{N}(\mathbf{0}_{r_2}, \boldsymbol{\Sigma}_2)$, both independent of $\boldsymbol{\varepsilon}_{ad} \sim \mathcal{N}(\mathbf{0}_{n_{ad}}, \sigma^2 \mathbf{I}_{n_{ad}})$, which are themselves mutually independent. Extensions to more than three levels are obvious, although a neater notation for them is necessary. We say that the data have three levels; the term *multilevel* is used for data (analysis, model, and the like) with an unspecified number of levels.

Figure 9.2 gives an illustration of varying regressions. The average regression $\mathbf{x}\boldsymbol{\beta}$, with a single covariate, $\mathbf{x} = (1, x)$, is drawn by a thick line and the within level-3 cluster regressions $\mathbf{x}\boldsymbol{\beta} + \delta_a^{(3)}$ by lines of medium thickness. These lines are indented and marked by asterisks. The level-2 regressions $\mathbf{x}\boldsymbol{\beta} + \delta_a^{(3)} + \mathbf{x}\boldsymbol{\delta}_{ad}^{(2)}$ are drawn by thin lines, except for those belonging to one level-3 cluster, which are drawn by dashes, so they stand out. In the model used for generating this example, the level-3 regressions are parallel, with variance $\sigma_3^2 = 0.08$, and the level-2 regressions within each level-3 cluster have

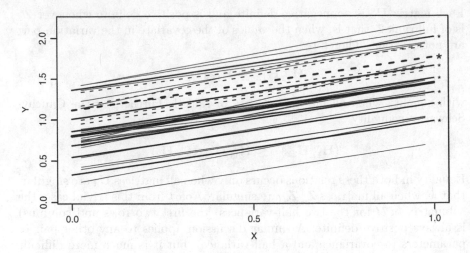

Fig. 9.2. Illustration of a three-level model. The average regression is drawn by a thick solid line. The regressions of the level-2 clusters are indented, and those within one level-3 super-cluster are drawn by dashes. The level-3 regressions are marked in the right-hand margin by asterisks; the asterisk for the highlighted super-cluster is enlarged.

the normal distribution with mean vector $\boldsymbol{\beta} = (0.8, 0.65)$ and variance matrix $\boldsymbol{\Sigma}_2 = \begin{pmatrix} 0.0100 & 0.0025 \\ 0.0025 & 0.0100 \end{pmatrix}$. The highlighted level-2 regressions indicate that they are much more similar within a level-3 cluster than in general. This is a consequence of the relatively large variance σ_3^2.

The random vector $\boldsymbol{\delta}_{ad}^{(2)}$ describes the deviation of the regression within level-2 cluster ad from the regression in its level-3 cluster (or super-cluster) a, and $\boldsymbol{\delta}_a^{(3)}$ describes the deviation of the regression in level-3 cluster a from the average (typical) cluster or from the overall regression $\mathbf{X}\boldsymbol{\beta}$. The variables in $\mathbf{Z}^{(h)}$, $h = 2, 3$, are said to be associated with variation at level h; $\mathbf{Z}^{(h)}$ contains a subset of the variables in $\mathbf{X}$ with the intercept as its first column, unless $\mathbf{Z}^{(h)}$ is empty.

The model in (9.23) can be fitted by ML. We relate it to ML estimation with a two-level model. For a cluster a at level 3, form $\mathbf{y}_a$ by vertical stacking of the vectors of outcomes $\mathbf{y}_{ad}$, $d = 1, \ldots, D_a$. Define similarly $\mathbf{X}_a$ and $\mathbf{e}_a = \mathbf{y}_a - \mathbf{X}_a\boldsymbol{\beta}$. Let $\boldsymbol{\Omega}_h = \sigma^{-2}\boldsymbol{\Sigma}_h$, $h = 2, 3$, and $\mathbf{W}_{a,3} = \sigma^{-2}\mathrm{var}(\mathbf{y}_a)$. The log-likelihood is $l = l_1 + \cdots + l_A$, where

$$l_a = -\frac{1}{2}\left[n_a \log(2\pi) + n_a \log(\sigma^2) + \log\{\det(\mathbf{W}_{a,3})\} + \frac{1}{\sigma^2}\mathbf{e}_a^\top \mathbf{W}_{a,3}^{-1}\mathbf{e}_a\right].$$

Each matrix $\mathbf{W}_{a,3}$ can be expressed as

$$\mathbf{W}_{a,3} = \mathbf{W}_{a,2} + \mathbf{Z}_a^{(3)}\boldsymbol{\Omega}_3\mathbf{Z}_a^{(3)^\top},$$

where $\mathbf{W}_{a,2} = \mathrm{diag}_d (\mathbf{W}_{ad,2})$ is the block-diagonal matrix comprising the blocks $\mathbf{W}_{ad,2} = \mathbf{I} + \mathbf{Z}_{ad}^{(2)} \boldsymbol{\Omega}_2 \mathbf{Z}_{ad}^{(2)}{}^{\top}$, $d = 1, \ldots, D_a$, on the diagonal. For the determinant and inverse of $\mathbf{W}_{a,3}$ we have expressions similar to those in (9.6):

$$\det (\mathbf{W}_{a,3}) = \det (\mathbf{W}_{a,2}) \det (\mathbf{G}_{a,3}) ,$$

$$\mathbf{W}_{a,3}^{-1} = \mathbf{W}_{a,2}^{-1} - \mathbf{W}_{a,2}^{-1} \mathbf{Z}_a^{(3)} \boldsymbol{\Omega}_3 \, \mathbf{G}_{a,3}^{-1} \mathbf{Z}_a^{(3)}{}^{\top} \mathbf{W}_{a,2}^{-1} ,$$

(9.24)

and

$$\mathbf{G}_{a,3} = \mathbf{I}_{r_3} + \mathbf{Z}_a^{(3)}{}^{\top} \mathbf{W}_{a,2}^{-1} \mathbf{Z}_a^{(3)} \boldsymbol{\Omega}_3 ,$$

$$= \mathbf{I}_{r_3} + \sum_{d=1}^{D_a} \mathbf{Z}_{ad}^{(3)}{}^{\top} \mathbf{W}_{ad,2}^{-1} \mathbf{Z}_{ad}^{(3)} \boldsymbol{\Omega}_3 .$$

These identities reduce the problem of dealing with $\mathbf{W}_{a,3}$ to the problem of dealing with matrices $\mathbf{W}_{ad,2}$, which have the form of scaled variance matrices for two-level data. Equations for maximising the likelihood carry over from Section 9.3, using the identities in (9.24) instead of those in (9.6). They require various expressions that involve $\mathbf{W}_{ad,2}$, and these are evaluated using (9.6).

The identities in (9.24) can be generalised substantially. They state that if a matrix $\mathbf{W}$ has a decomposition $\mathbf{W} = \mathbf{W}_0 + \mathbf{Z}_1 \mathbf{Z}_2^{\top}$ in which both $\mathbf{Z}_1$ and $\mathbf{Z}_2$ have only a few columns and $\mathbf{W}_0$ is much easier to invert than $\mathbf{W}$ directly, then the determinant and inverse of $\mathbf{W}$ can be expressed in terms of their counterparts for $\mathbf{W}_0$ and $\mathbf{I} + \mathbf{Z}_2^{\top} \mathbf{W}_0^{-1} \mathbf{Z}_1$. An application of this expresses the likelihood for an M-level model in terms of several quadratic forms and determinants for $(M-1)$-level likelihood and, by recursive application of the identities in (9.24), eventually in terms of quadratic forms and determinants for only two levels.

At the end of such a recursion, the matrix $\mathbf{W}_0$ need not be the identity matrix; it merely has to be a matrix that is relatively easy to invert and its determinant easy to evaluate. In particular, $\mathbf{W}_0$ may be a diagonal matrix. This is useful when the observations are associated with unequal elementary-level variances σ^2. The variances may depend on some covariates, such as $\sigma_{adi}^2 = \exp \left(\mathbf{Z}_{adi}^{(1)} \boldsymbol{\alpha} \right)$ or $\sigma_{adi}^2 = \left(\mathbf{Z}_{adi}^{(1)} \boldsymbol{\alpha} \right)^2$ for a vector of parameters $\boldsymbol{\alpha}$. In both cases, we assure that every elementary-level variance σ^2 is non-negative. The latter parameterisation is more natural because the variables in the cluster-level variation part of the model also contribute to the overall variance by a quadratic function, so we can refer to $\mathbf{Z}^{(1)}$ as variables associated with elementary-level variation. Such models can also be developed as generalisations of the single-level model with heteroscedasticity,

$$y_j = \mathbf{x}_j \boldsymbol{\beta} + \mathbf{z}_j \varepsilon_j ,$$

where ε_j is a random sample from a centred multivariate normal distribution and $\mathbf{Z}$ is formed as a selection of variables in $\mathbf{X}$.

A consequence of associating variables with variation, at any level, is that the variance of an observation depends on the values of these variables. We can take advantage of this by associating variables with variation not for the original purpose, but for describing the heteroscedasticity (varying variance) of the outcomes. This has to be done with care, to avoid confounding because, compared to the regression, data usually contain very sparse information about the *shape of the variance*, defined as a function of some variables.

Random coefficients can be considered for models other than regression, so long as they involve parameters that describe them. In a general setting, each cluster d is associated with a vector of quantities $\boldsymbol{\theta}_d$, which would be regarded as parameters if we focussed solely on cluster d as the population. A cluster-level distribution is specified for $\boldsymbol{\theta}_d$. Multivariate normal distributions are advantageous for this purpose because their class is complete (for any variance matrix there is a distribution), self-contained (closed with respect to taking margins, conditioning, and linear operations), and easy to handle (their densities, expectations, and variance matrices are simple expressions). In principle, any other class of distributions can take over this role, but not without introducing considerable analytical complexity. When the parameters $\boldsymbol{\theta}_d$ differ in only one component, this problem is tractable in some settings. Some of them are discussed in Chapter 10.

9.7 Estimating Many Quantities

Multilevel models involve many quantities of several kinds that may be of interest. It is often tempting to list as a default all the inferential statements, such as the (ML or REML) estimate and the associated estimated root-MSE $(\hat{\theta}, \hat{s}_\theta)$ for every quantity (parameter or deviation) θ, inspect them, and focus the report on the findings that we regard as interesting or believe that our client would find them so. The alternative is to state in advance of any data inspection and analysis what would be reported and how (in what context) and to declare in advance how each possible configuration of estimates (and associated estimated root-MSEs) would be interpreted. This might appear to be an unnecessary straitjacket, imposing a lot of abstract work in advance of what is often regarded as the most interesting activity—evaluating estimators (computing) and improvising the discussion of the results. One might argue that after learning from the data we are in a better position to state what the important findings are and to document them appropriately.

The principal argument for preparing a protocol for analysis and its report, that is, for imposing a straitjacket on them, is that the properties of an estimator used, such as its (estimated) MSE, are quoted appropriately only when they are reported unconditionally. For example, reporting the estimate $\hat{\beta}_x = 1.17$ with the associated estimated root-MSE $\hat{s}(\hat{\beta}_x) = 0.22$ would invite the interpretation that β_x is almost certainly greater than, say, 0.5. We should downgrade our confidence in this statement if its reporting is a result of sifting through the estimates of many other quantities. Given that $\hat{\beta}_x$ is reported, the distribution of the estimator $\hat{\beta}_x$ differs from its unconditional distribution, that is, the distribution conditional only on the model that was selected a priori.

The problem is most acute for inferences about the clusters, especially if we regard them before the analysis as anonymous, without any preconceptions that some of them may be exceptional in any particular way—their deviations δ_d are assumed to have an unknown (normal) distribution. After inspecting the results that list the clusters and their estimates $\hat{\delta}_d$, we may promote a cluster to the status of being of interest and worthy of a (mention in the) report. The act of *promotion*, denoted by $\mathcal{R}$, is random (data dependent); in a replication of the data-generating process followed by the process of inspecting the results, a different cluster d may be promoted to the status of being of interest. The problem is that the unconditional distribution of $\hat{\delta}_d$ differs from the conditional distribution of $(\hat{\delta}_d \mid \mathcal{R})$, and they both differ from the distribution of $\hat{\delta}_{d^{\mathcal{R}}}$, which attempts to identify the cluster that would be selected for promotion if the values of δ_d were known. These distributions, $(\hat{\delta}_d \mid \mathcal{R})$ and $(\hat{\delta}_{d^{\mathcal{R}}})$, depend on the promotion process. In general, they are difficult to derive or estimate and without a rigorous definition of the promotion process, even their approximation is next to impossible. The confusion of the realised index $d^{\mathcal{R}}$ (an integer) with the index $d^{\mathcal{R}}$ as an integer random variable is called *personalisation*.

The most common example of a promotion process is reporting the cluster with the largest (or smallest) value of $\hat{\delta}_d$ in the fit of a model with parallel regressions. Having observed that the maximum occurs for a cluster d^*, an analyst may declare that this cluster is of interest. However, the distributions of $\hat{\delta}_{d^*}$ and $\max_d \hat{\delta}_d$ differ, as can easily be established by simulations, and neither is a good estimator of $\max_d \delta_d$. The core of the problem is that by promoting d^* we have committed personalisation—we confused inference about an a priori declared cluster with inference about the (unknown) cluster that has a particular attribute, such as the largest value of δ_d. If we 'trust' the model we have applied, we may estimate the largest value of δ_d directly by sampling from the fitted cluster-level distribution $\mathcal{N}(\mathbf{0}, \hat{\sigma}_B^2)$ and improve on this by acknowledging the uncertainty about σ_B^2. This entails generating several plausible values (replicate imputations) of σ_B^2 as random draws from the estimated sampling distribution of $\hat{\sigma}_B^2$ and then simulating the extreme value of δ_d based on each of these plausible variances $\tilde{\sigma}_B^2$.

The promotion of a cluster is appropriate when we can, with integrity, defend the position that not declaring the cluster in the protocol for the analysis was an oversight. That is, if we could roll the clock back to the state prior to data inspection and prepare the protocol with greater care, the cluster would have been declared of interest, for a particular reason, without having gained any information about the values of the outcomes in the dataset.

9.8 Some Applications

Multilevel models are well suited for data collected in populations that have a hierarchical structure. In this section, we discuss four such applications. For each we point out that the setting of the application is not perfectly matched by multilevel models.

9.8.1 Small-Area Estimation

Small-area statistics is concerned with estimating population means and proportions or, more generally, regressions in a division of the domain, such as in the districts of a country. When there are many districts, it is attractive to associate them with random terms, referring to a superpopulation which would yield a 'different country' in every replication. This is usually in conflict with the inferential goal of estimation for a *specific set* of districts into which a country is divided—the same districts would appear in replications of the survey because the country is regarded as fixed at the time point for which inferences are sought.

The problem can be resolved by applying models with random coefficients representing the districts but followed up by an analysis of the consequences of using an invalid model. For example, the standard errors derived by the assumption of randomness of the districts may be unbiased for this replication scheme but are biased under the more realistic scheme in which the deviations δ_d are fixed.

Setting these issues aside, a two-level model is formulated with the purpose of reducing the variation at both levels as much as possible. If the between-district variance were reduced to zero, the same regression formula would apply in every district. Any prediction for the district would then, in effect, be based on the data from the entire survey. Caution has to be applied in following this plan, because if we use sufficiently many covariates the *estimated* between-district variation may indeed be reduced substantially, but this may be achieved at the cost of substantial inflation of the sampling variation of the regression parameter estimator $\hat{\beta}$. If the between-district variation were reduced to zero the district-level means would be estimated by $\hat{x}_d \hat{\beta}$, where $\hat{x}_d$ is an estimator of the vector of means of the covariates for district d. The estimator may combine information from the analysed survey with other surveys, or some components of x_d may even be known precisely. The uncertainty about $\hat{x}_d$ is a factor additional to $\text{MSE}(\hat{\beta}; \beta)$ and the magnitude of Σ_B. As a consequence, a better-fitting model need not result in more efficient small-area estimation.

An alternative approach to small-area estimation was described in Section 3.8.

9.8.2 Performance Assessment of Institutions

We dealt with this topic in Section 7.5, regarding it as an application of causal analysis. Setting aside the issue of whether institutions should be regarded as a fixed set or as a random draw from a superpopulation, institutions with their clients (students, patients, customers, and the like) have a hierarchical structure, as assumed in two-level models. Assessing the performance of institutions can then be regarded as inference about the deviations of the institution-specific regressions from the typical (average) regression. The covariates in these regressions have the role of *adjustment* for the differing distributions (*profiles*) of their clientele or caseload; institutions with clients who require more attention, are more difficult to treat, and so on, should not be handicapped in the assessment. In other words, the covariates are meant to take account of the (self-)selection process that results in the assignment of the particular clients (cases) to institutions (treatments).

In variance with the approach in Chapter 7, in which the potential outcomes of a client are fixed, the outcomes in two-level models are regarded as random. The attribution of a value of ε_{id} for case i in institution d to the deviation from the regression part of the model ($\mathbf{X}\beta$) or to variation across replications is ambiguous. (Would the case have the same outcome in every replication, or is its value of ε_{id} due mainly to its consistent idiosyncrasy?) Some of this ambiguity can be resolved by studying the measurement process involved in establishing the values of the outcomes. Several arguments presented in Section 7.5 are against the application of random coefficient or other linear models. Foremost among them is that regression is too smooth and inflexible, especially when fitted over a wide range of values, and inferences for an institution at one end of the scale should not be influenced in any way by institutions at the other end or even near the centre of the scale. In this respect, treating the problem as that of missing data for the unrealised potential outcomes is more principled and does not rely so heavily on the optimistic assumption that the model applied is good enough. Validity of the model cannot be established by model diagnostics, that is, solely by inspecting the visible features of the data.

9.8.3 Progression over Time

Studies in which subjects are observed several times, at a sequence of time points, are called *longitudinal*. We can regard an observation (on a subject at a time point) as an element and the set of observations on a subject as a cluster. The time is an obvious covariate, and it is meaningful to associate it with subject-level variation to allow for subjects to have different speeds of change or, more generally, different patterns of change over time.

When the time points are set by design, the same set for every subject, multivariate analysis can be applied, regarding the subjects' responses at the T time points as a single outcome. When the subjects' time points differ we may have to resort to models with random coefficients. However, the process of how the time points are set should be carefully considered. When subjects choose their time points purposefully, with some agenda or purpose in mind, such as to record an exceptional value of the outcome variable, we observe a distorted version of what we believe the data represent. Values of the outcome variable at time points are selected *nonignorably*, related to or influenced by the value to be recorded.

Variables used in longitudinal analysis may be defined for observations (elements) and subjects (clusters). If treatment effects are the targets, intermediate variables, recorded after the treatment has been assigned, should not be included among the covariates. Observation-level covariates should be scrutinised for this in particular, except for time and its transformations, when time is set by design and the scheduled treatment that is applied in a crossover trial.

The subject of longitudinal analysis is treated in greater detail in Chapter 11.

9.8.4 Studying Families

Families and their members are studied with a wide range of inferential agenda that includes the inheritance of physical, mental, and intellectual traits and diseases and the effect of upbringing (nurture). In such studies, the family-level variation is of interest, being interpreted as a descriptor of how much families differ and in what way. Such an interpretation has a strong 'causal' flavour, inviting highly speculative judgments of how different certain offspring would be if he or she had different parents. These are poorly supported because, in the terminology of Chapter 7, they refer to an assignment that could not possibly have been realised. It would be meaningful to discuss the 'effect of parents' only if parents could be regarded as assignable treatments.

Associated with this is the problem that the values of most covariates in **X** could not possibly have been assigned either. Nor can the number of children and the timing of their births. If we regard parents as the treatment applied to their children, then essentially all the variables defined for children are intermediate and their presence in the model is problematic, because they bear the stamp of the treatment. But parents make conscious choices not only about their children's environment and context in which they would be or are growing up, but also about their own, even prior to the births of their children. Thus, variables defined for parents, at a time preceding the birth of their children, should also be regarded as intermediate, and so their role as covariates is therefore problematic.

While all these comments are negative, models fitted to data about families can reveal how variables are associated and how their associations vary. As a typical family has only a few children, if any, and the children tend to be similar in most characteristics and attributes, there is little scope for complex modelling of between-family variation. Studies of twins might be regarded as an application of random coefficient models, but most of the inferences can be based on summaries defined for the pairs. An essential assumption is that twins do not differ from single-birth children in any systematic way related to the outcome variables.

Suggested Reading

Early developments of random coefficient models were stimulated by applications in agriculture, and animal breeding in particular; [76] is a pioneering contribution; see also [77]. Maximum likelihood estimators for the setting with the standard normality assumptions were derived first by [67]. A series of papers [42]–[45] discussed the advantages of random coefficient models for estimating the quantities associated with each cluster. Key papers on REML are [142] and [69]. The Fisher scoring algorithm for data with arbitrarily many layers of nesting is described in [112]. Prominent early applications using the EM algorithm are presented in [159] and [34]; the method is treated in detail by [13]. There is a rich literature on the Bayesian versions of random coefficient models; a good entry point to it is [93].

Applications connected to computational algorithms are discussed in detail by [113] and [60], the latter motivated mainly by educational research and associated with the software MLwin; see www.cmm.bristol.ac.uk/MLwin/ based on the method of iteratively reweighted least squares. A comprehensive library of Splus functions and the theory supporting them is documented in [146]. A detailed account of models for variance components is given by [177]; it also contains a detailed historical review.

Prominent applications of random coefficient models to performance assessment are [2] and [62]. Small-area estimation with random coefficient models is treated in detail by [154]; Part II of [121] gives details and applications of an alternative approach outlined in Section 3.8.

Problems and Exercises

9.1. Work through all the details of the random coefficient model given by the equations for its two levels:

$$\mathbf{y}_d = \mathbf{X}_d \boldsymbol{\beta}_d + \boldsymbol{\varepsilon}_d,$$

$$\boldsymbol{\beta}_d = \mathbf{Z}_d \boldsymbol{\gamma} + \boldsymbol{\delta}_d,$$

with the standard assumptions of independence and normality of $\boldsymbol{\delta}_d$ and $\boldsymbol{\varepsilon}_d$, when both $\mathbf{X}$ and $\mathbf{Z}$ comprise a continuous and a categorical variable.

9.2. Covariates in two-level models can be defined for elements or clusters. Cluster-level covariates can be constructed as summaries of the values of elementary-level covariates; for instance, the within-cluster sample mean $\bar{x}_d$ of a continuous variable X is such a covariate. Relate to the material in Chapter 6 the problems with using such a covariate, especially when the within-cluster sample sizes n_d are small.

Hint: Study the correlation of X and the variable constructed by expanding $\bar{x}_d$ to the subjects in such a way that each subject in cluster d has the value $\bar{x}_d$. Compare this correlation with its population counterpart, $\mathrm{cor}(X, X_{[d]})$, where $X_{[d]}$ is formed by expanding the within-cluster population means. Why should a cluster-level covariate not be associated with variation?

9.3. Describe some patterns of variation with a singular 3×3 variance matrix Σ_B. Devise a way of presenting these patterns graphically.

9.4. List the rules related to invariance with respect to linear transformations when the within-cluster regressions are polynomial. As an example, consider the setting with cubic average regression and the within-cluster regressions differing from it by quadratic functions.

9.5. Prove the identity

$$(\mathbf{I}_n + \rho \mathbf{J}_n)^{-k} = \mathbf{I}_n - \frac{1}{n} \frac{g_n^k - 1}{g_n^k} \mathbf{J}_n \tag{9.25}$$

for $k = \pm 1, \pm 2, \ldots$, where $g_n = 1 + n\rho$.

Hint: Prove it first for $k = -1$, and then apply mathematical induction.

Suppose $\mathbf{Z}$ is an $n \times r$ matrix of full rank $r < n$ and $\boldsymbol{\Omega}$ is a variance matrix, not necessarily nonsingular. Prove the identity

$$(\mathbf{I}_n + \mathbf{Z}\boldsymbol{\Omega}\mathbf{Z}^\top)^k = \mathbf{I}_n - \mathbf{Z}(\mathbf{Z}^\top \mathbf{Z})^{-1}(\mathbf{I}_n - \mathbf{G}^k)\mathbf{Z}^\top$$

where $\mathbf{G} = \mathbf{I} + \mathbf{Z}^\top \mathbf{Z}\boldsymbol{\Omega}$ and $k = \pm 1, \pm 2, \ldots$. This identity generalises (9.25) and the second identity in (9.6).

9.6. This exercise relates to the setting of Section 9.3. Show that when the sample size n_d exceeds the number of variables associated with variation, r, the variance matrix $\mathbf{V}_d = \mathrm{var}(\mathbf{y}_d)$ has eigenvalue σ^2 with multiplicity $n_d - r$.

9.7. Derive the part of the Fisher scoring algorithm in Section 9.3 for σ^2 with the original parameterisation, using $\mathbf{V}_d$ and Σ_B. Can you avoid having to derive the diagonal element of the information matrix for σ^2?

9.8. A two-level dataset is called *balanced* if each cluster has the same matrix $\mathbf{Z}_d$. A slightly more general definition of balance requires only that $\mathbf{Z}_d^\top \mathbf{Z}_d$ is the same for every cluster d. Derive the ML estimator of $\boldsymbol{\beta}$ for a balanced dataset and the equations for the ML estimates of σ^2 and $\boldsymbol{\Omega}$.

9.9. Derive the conditional distribution of $\boldsymbol{\varepsilon}_d$ given in the text leading up to (9.18).

9.10. A two-level model can be associated with the ANCOVA model that differs from it only by the status of the cluster-level deviations δ_d. Two such models are called *paired*. For a simple model, say with a single covariate X and parallel regressions (no group-by-X interactions), derive the estimators of the deviation δ_1 for the first cluster in the two models. Make the necessary assumptions, e.g., that the variance ratio ω is known, under which the MSEs of two estimators can be compared analytically. Discuss how the comparison should be made empirically.

9.11. A two-level model $y_{id} = \mathbf{x}_{id}\beta + \delta_d + \varepsilon_{id}$ can be 'collapsed' to the cluster level by defining a similar model for the cluster-level averages as

$$\bar{y}_d = \bar{\mathbf{x}}_d\gamma + \delta'_d,$$

where the bar $^-$ denotes the averaging and $\delta'_d = \delta_d + \bar{\varepsilon}_d$. Give an example or a reason why the parameters β and γ may have very different values, even when the within-cluster sample sizes n_d are identical. This phenomenon is known as *ecological fallacy*.
Hint: Consider a setting in which the values of δ_d are associated with the means $\bar{\mathbf{x}}_d$.

9.12. Two-level models are sometimes called *empirical Bayes*; [42]. That is, the model would be Bayes if the cluster-level variance (matrix) were known; the corresponding distribution $\mathcal{N}(\mathbf{0}, \boldsymbol{\Sigma}_B)$ would then play the role of the prior for the deviations δ_d. Give a complete Bayes specification of the two-level model, with priors for all the model parameters. Discuss or resolve the ambiguity about the role of δ_d. Are they on par with ε_d, or are they model parameters? Is the distinction essential?

9.13. Work out all the details of the EM algorithm for fitting a two-level model.

9.14. If the assumption of normality of δ_d in a two-level model is problematic, a more general assumption, that their distribution is a mixture of two unrelated centred normal distributions, may be adopted. Describe how the EM algorithm could be combined with the Fisher scoring to fit such a model.

9.15. Verify empirically the approximation given by (9.22).

9.16. Show that the regression matrix $\mathbf{X}$ is of full rank $p < n$ if and only if $\mathbf{X}^\top\mathbf{V}^{-1}\mathbf{X}$ is of full rank. Relate this equivalence to the relationship between estimability of the vector of regression parameters in the ordinary regression model ($\mathbf{y} = \mathbf{X}\beta + \varepsilon$) and in the two-level model with the same regression matrix $\mathbf{X}$ and a nonsingular variance matrix $\mathbf{V} = \text{var}(\mathbf{y})$. Does the presence of some clusters d for which the regression matrix $\mathbf{X}_d$ is singular affect the estimability of β in any way? Can δ_d be estimated for such clusters? Could the $p \times 1$ vector β be estimated even when every cluster has a sample size smaller than p?

9.17. For a finite structured population, the population mean of a variable Y may differ substantially from the mean of the within-cluster means, $(\bar{Y}_1 + \cdots + \bar{Y}_D)/D$. Construct such an example. Explain why the sample mean $\bar{y}$ may differ substantially from the ML estimator of the parameter μ in the two-level model $y_{id} = \mu + \delta_d + \varepsilon_{id}$. Generalise this conclusion to the comparison of the OLS estimator $\hat{\beta} = (\mathbf{X}^\top \mathbf{X})^{-1} \mathbf{X}^\top \mathbf{y}$ and the ML estimator $\tilde{\beta} = (\mathbf{X}^\top \hat{\mathbf{W}}^{-1} \mathbf{X})^{-1} \mathbf{X}^\top \hat{\mathbf{W}}^{-1} \mathbf{y}$ for a suitable regression matrix $\mathbf{X}$ and nonsingular estimate of the scaled variance matrix $\mathbf{W}$.

9.18. In the software of your choice, write a programme for fitting the two-level model with parallel regressions. Include in the output the estimates of the deviations δ_d and the elementary-level residuals $\hat{\varepsilon}_{id}$. The dataset in file EXMa.dat on www.sntl.co.uk/BookA/Data contains log-values of the assets and liabilities of the 1965 French companies listed on the stock exchange in 1980. The companies are classified to 71 industrial sectors. Regard these sectors as clusters, and fit the two-level model of the log-liabilities as the outcomes. Explore the results for exceptional sectors.

9.19. Using the dataset from the previous exercise and the software developed, devise a method for checking the assumption of parallel within-cluster regressions.
Hint: Fit the ordinary regressions within each cluster of sufficient size or in the clusters in which the regression can be fitted. Compare the variation of the regression slope estimates with the variation that one would expect if all the regression slopes were identical. The latter can be established either analytically, from the matrices of crossproducts $\mathbf{X}_d^\top \mathbf{X}_d$, or by simulations. Consider also the compromise in which only replicate sets of estimates are generated, without any replicate outcomes.

9.20. Extend the programme you compiled earlier to fit two-level models with a covariate associated with variation and reanalyse the dataset in EXMa.dat. Try out several ways of forcing the provisional (and final) estimates of the scaled variance matrix $\mathbf{\Omega}$ to be nonnegative definite. Describe the pattern of cluster-level variation implied by $\hat{\mathbf{\Omega}}$. Draw the fitted deviations $\mathbf{z}\hat{\delta}_d$ for $\mathbf{z}$ in the same range as the values in the dataset, and discuss whether these lines agree with the pattern implied by $\hat{\mathbf{\Omega}}$. Compare the sample variance of the estimates of the slope with the estimated variance, $\hat{\sigma}^2 \hat{\Omega}_\mathrm{x}$, and explain the discrepancy.

9.21. Prepare a complete list of the assumptions for a causal interpretation of the setting of a two-level model. Carefully define the various average effects. Discuss the advantages and drawbacks of regression and matching and why matching should be done within clusters.

9.22. Suppose a two-level model with parallel regressions is appropriate for a particular setting, and this is confirmed when the model is fitted (and compared with some alternatives). What is likely to happen to the property of parallelness when the outcome or a covariate is subjected to a nonlinear transformation? Check your conjectures or conclusions by experimenting with the dataset in EXMa.dat.

9.23. Suppose a very large population comprises many clusters, each of them of substantial size. The population also comprises two types, such as men and women, who are present in each cluster with abundance. The within-cluster differences of the means of a key variable for these two types are constant; $\Delta_{AB} = \mu_{A,d} - \mu_{B,d}$ for every cluster d. A survey is to be conducted with the purpose of estimating Δ_{AB}. Its sample size is fixed at n. Suppose the variance ratio σ_B^2/σ^2 is known to be in the range 0.07–0.12. Discuss the design of the survey. Advise about the number of clusters and the composition of the types within the clusters.

Hint: Study the information matrix for the target.

9.24. Consider the two-level model with parallel regressions,

$$y_{id} = \beta_0 + \beta_x x_d + \beta_u u_{id} + \delta_d + \varepsilon_{id},$$

in which X is a cluster-level variable ($x_{id} = x_d$) and U is such that $u_{1d} + u_{2d} + \cdots + u_{n_d d} = $ const. For example, for the setting of classrooms and students, X may be an attribute of the classroom and U gender of the student, and each classroom has the same number of boys as girls in the sample. Show that the maximum likelihood estimators of $\hat{\beta}_x$ and $\hat{\beta}_u$ are uncorrelated. Further, show that $\hat{\beta}_x$ and the estimate of the cluster-level variance, $\hat{\sigma}_B^2$, are not altered when U is dropped from the model.

10

Generalised Linear Models

Normality of the conditional distributions in ordinary regression and in other models is a very constraining assumption because outcomes in a wide range of settings have distributions that are distinctly not normal. This section presents a generalisation of the ordinary regression beyond normality, which retains several features of the ordinary regression. In Section 10.5 we extend multilevel models similarly.

10.1 Introduction

For motivation, we consider the setting with conditionally independent binary outcomes Y given a continuous covariate X. The plot of the realised values $\mathbf{y}$ against the values of $\mathbf{x}$ is not very informative because Y is supported by only two points, 0 and 1. An illustration is given in Figure 10.1. The outcomes, equal to zero or unity, are marked by circles ∘. The figures printed in the diagram are the proportions of positive outcomes within the $\frac{1}{2}$-point bands of values of X. For example, in the band on the extreme left, 3.0–3.5, all seven outcomes are negative. The conditional probability of a positive outcome, $p(x) = \mathrm{P}(Y = 1 \,|\, X = x)$, is related to x; greater values of X are associated with higher probabilities $p(x)$. The curve drawn in the diagram is the function $p(x)$ and the vertical ticks on it mark its values for the realised values of X. More details about this curve (function), called *logistic*, are given later.

The function $p(x)$ could not be nonconstant linear and at the same time bounded by zero and unity, just like the outcomes and probabilities are. Yet, relating $p(x)$ to a linear function would be very convenient, for the same reasons that underlie our preference for linear regression with normally distributed outcomes—analytical simplicity and easy interpretation. Transformations of $p(x)$ provide a solution; we assume that

$$g\{p(x)\} = \beta_0 + \beta_1 x \tag{10.1}$$

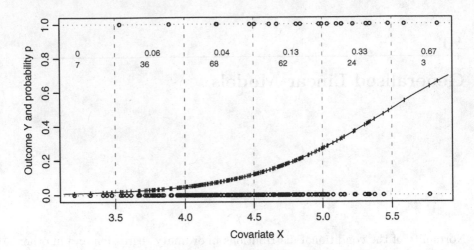

Fig. 10.1. Example of a logistic regression with a single covariate. The outcomes are marked by circles and the underlying probabilities $p(x)$ by short vertical ticks on the logistic curve. The numbers at the height of 0.8 give the proportions of positive outcomes and the numbers of observations within the bands 0.5 wide.

for some (unknown) coefficients $\boldsymbol{\beta} = (\beta_0, \beta_1)^\top$. More generally, $g\{p(\mathbf{x})\} = \mathbf{x}\boldsymbol{\beta}$ for a vector of covariates $\mathbf{x}$ and a regression parameter vector $\boldsymbol{\beta}$. As a convention, the first components of $\mathbf{x}$ and $\boldsymbol{\beta}$ represent the intercept. By $\mathbf{X}$ we denote the regression matrix formed by vertical stacking of the rows $\mathbf{x}$ for the observed units, and by $\mathbf{y}$ the corresponding vector of outcomes. The function $\mathbf{x}\boldsymbol{\beta}$ is referred to as the *linear predictor*.

The function g is called the *link* function. Practical choices for g are monotone functions that map the interval $(0, 1)$ to the entire real axis. These include the *logit*,

$$g(p) = \log\left(\frac{p}{1-p}\right),\qquad(10.2)$$

complementary log-log,

$$g(p) = -\log\{-\log(p)\},$$

and *probit*,

$$g(p) = \Phi^{-1}(p),$$

where Φ^{-1} is the inverse of the distribution function of the standard normal distribution $\mathcal{N}(0, 1)$. Instead of Φ, we could use the distribution function of any continuous distribution supported on $(-\infty, +\infty)$.

The logit link stands out among these options because it is connected to the likelihood in a special way. The log-likelihood for $\boldsymbol{\beta}$ given by (10.1) and g by (10.2) is

$$l(\boldsymbol{\beta}; \mathbf{y}; \mathbf{x}) = \sum_{j=1}^{n} y_j \log \left\{ \frac{p(x_j)}{1 - p(x_j)} \right\} + \sum_{j=1}^{n} \log \left\{ 1 - p(x_j) \right\}$$

$$= \mathbf{y}^{\top} \mathbf{X} \boldsymbol{\beta} - \sum_{j=1}^{n} \log \left\{ 1 + \exp (\mathbf{x}_j \boldsymbol{\beta}) \right\},$$

so $\mathbf{X}^{\top} \mathbf{y}$ is a set of minimal linear sufficient statistics for $\boldsymbol{\beta}$. Maximisation of this log-likelihood corresponds to moment matching, as

$$\frac{\partial l}{\partial \boldsymbol{\beta}} = \mathbf{X}^{\top} \mathbf{y} - \sum_{j=1}^{n} p(x_j) \mathbf{x}_j,$$

and $\mathrm{E}(y_j \,|\, X = x_j) = p(x_j)$. Further,

$$-\frac{\partial l^2}{\partial \boldsymbol{\beta} \, \partial \boldsymbol{\beta}^{\top}} = \sum_{j=1}^{n} p(x_j) \left\{ 1 - p(x_j) \right\} \mathbf{x}_j \mathbf{x}_j^{\top}.$$

This does not depend on the outcomes $\mathbf{y}$, so the observed and expected information matrices for $\boldsymbol{\beta}$ coincide.

We refer to the model implied by (10.1) as a regression and to the model with the logit link as *logistic regression*. The connection with ordinary regression is made more obvious by the equivalent expression

$$\mathrm{E}(Y \,|\, X = x) = g^{-1} (\beta_0 + \beta_1 x), \qquad (10.3)$$

so that the regression is linear, but for the application of the inverse of the link function. Ordinary regression is subsumed in these models by setting the link to identity; $g(x) = x$.

The three link functions for binary outcomes are compared in the left-hand panel of Figure 10.2. A link function g can be regarded as identical with any of its nontrivial linear transformations $a + bg$, with $b \neq 0$, because such a transformation can be compensated for in the linear regression by using $\beta_0' = (\beta_0 - a)/b$ and $\beta_1' = \beta_1/b$. In the right-hand panel, the complementary log-log and probit are linearly transformed to match the logit link as closely as possible in the range $p \in (0.25, 0.75)$. The graph shows that the three link functions differ very little in the mid-range of probabilities, and probit and logit differ only slighly even in the tails. Probit and logit links are symmetric around $\frac{1}{2}$, that is, $g(p) = -g(1 - p)$, unlike the complementary log-log. The functions $-\log\{-\log(1-p)\}$ and $-\log\{-\log(p)\}$ represent substantially different links.

The generalisation of the model in (10.3) to multiple regression is straightforward—we replace $\beta_0 + \beta_1 x$ by $\mathbf{x}\boldsymbol{\beta}$ for a row vector $\mathbf{x}$ of values of the covariates preceded by the intercept 1. For the conditional distribution of Y, assumed to be binary thus far, we can specify other classes of distributions, to match the information we have about Y prior to data collection as closely

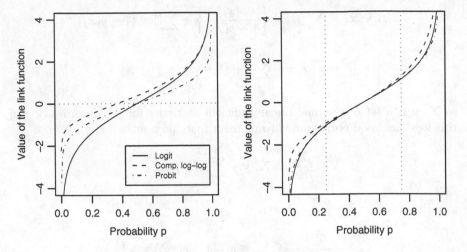

Fig. 10.2. The logit, complementary log-log, and probit link functions for binary outcomes, as defined (left-hand panel) and after linear transformations (right-hand panel).

as possible. With these two generalisations, we obtain the class of *generalised linear models* (GLMs). They are specified by

- linear regression $\mathbf{X}\boldsymbol{\beta}$;
- link function g; and
- a class conditional distributions of Y given $\mathbf{x}$.

The link operates for classes of equivalence; links within a class are linearly related. A link function is monotone and one-to-one. We lose no generality by considering only links that are increasing functions.

Maximisation of the log-likelihood for GLM is, in general, a nontrivial computational task involving iterative procedures. The pairing of binary distribution and logit link is an example in which the problem is simpler because the likelihood for the regression parameters $\boldsymbol{\beta}$ depends on the outcomes $\mathbf{y}$ through a short list of sufficient statistics, $\mathbf{X}^\top\mathbf{y}$. Such a link function, associated with a specified class of conditional distributions $(Y \mid \mathbf{X} = \mathbf{x})$, is called *canonical*; logit is the canonical link for binary outcomes.

A very wide class of distributions suitable for GLMs is given by the *exponential family of distributions*. It is specified by the densities or probabilities

$$f(y; \mathbf{x}, a, b, c, \theta) = \exp\left\{ \frac{y\theta - b(\theta)}{a} + c(y, a) \right\}, \qquad (10.4)$$

where a is a positive constant, called the *scale*, b and c are functions, and θ is a value underlying the conditional expectation of y given $\mathbf{x}$; $\theta = \nu(\mathbf{x}\boldsymbol{\beta})$.

We derive a connection between a and b in (10.4) and the expectation and variance of the distribution. For any parametric class of densities $f(y; \theta)$,

$$\frac{\partial}{\partial \theta} \int f(y; \theta) \, dy = 0,$$

because the integral is equal to unity for every θ. If $f(y; \theta)$ is a smoothly differentiable function of θ for every value of y,

$$\frac{\partial}{\partial \theta} \int f(y; \theta) \, dy = \int \frac{\partial f(y; \theta)}{\partial \theta} \, dy$$

$$= E\left[\frac{\partial \log \{f(y; \theta)\}}{\partial \theta}\right] = 0,$$

so long as the order of differentiation and integration can be exchanged. For distributions in the exponential family, this identity yields

$$\frac{\partial}{\partial \theta} \int f(y; \mathbf{x}, a, b, \theta) \, dy = \frac{y - b'}{a}.$$

As the expectation of this derivative vanishes,

$$E\left[\frac{\partial \log \{f(y; \mathbf{x}, a, b, \theta)\}}{\partial \theta}\right] = \frac{E(Y) - b'(\theta)}{a} = 0,$$

$E(Y) = b'(\theta)$. In the following, we suppress the arguments $\mathbf{x}$, a, and b of a density f.

If the density f is twice continuously differentiable in θ for every y, its further differentiation yields the identity

$$\frac{\partial}{\partial \theta} E\left[\frac{\partial \log \{f(y; \theta)\}}{\partial \theta}\right] = \int \frac{\partial^2 \log \{f(y; \theta)\}}{\partial \theta^2} f(y; \theta) \, dy$$

$$+ \int \left[\frac{\partial \log \{f(y; \theta)\}}{\partial \theta}\right]^2 f(y; \theta) \, dy$$

$$= E\left[\frac{\partial^2 \log \{f(y; \theta)\}}{\partial \theta^2}\right] + E\left[\frac{\partial \log \{f(y; \theta)\}}{\partial \theta}\right]^2.$$

For an exponential family of distributions, this yields

$$-E\left[\frac{\partial^2 \log \{f(y; \theta)\}}{\partial \theta^2}\right] = \frac{1}{a^2} \mathrm{var}(Y),$$

and hence

$$\mathrm{var}(Y) = a b''(\theta).$$

In a GLM, the observations are associated with a common pair of functions b and c and scale a, and θ is related to the covariates by the identity

$$\theta_j = \nu(\mathbf{x}_j \boldsymbol{\beta}).$$

The canonical link corresponds to the identity function ν. The expectation $b'(\theta)$ is equal to the inverse of the canonical link.

In some settings, it is difficult to identify a suitable distribution for y, and it is much easier to specify how the conditional variance and expectation are related. The *variance function* is defined as $\text{var}(y \mid \mathbf{x}) = V(\mu)$, where $\mu = \text{E}(y \mid \mathbf{x})$, that is, as a function of the expectation. It provides an alternative to specifying the conditional distribution in a GLM. Some combinations of variance and link functions do not correspond to a distribution, but that is in general no hindrance to their application.

10.2 Examples of GLMs

The ordinary regression is a special case of GLM. It is defined by the identity link, $g(\theta) = \theta$, and the normal distributions or the constant variance function $V(\mu) = a$. The normal distributions are a member of the exponential family, defined by $a = \sigma^2$, $b(\theta) = \frac{1}{2}\mu^2$, and

$$c(y, \sigma^2) = -\tfrac{1}{2} \log\left(2\pi\sigma^2\right) - \frac{y^2}{2\sigma^2}.$$

The Poisson distributions are given by the sets of probabilities

$$P(Y = k; \lambda) = e^{-\lambda} \frac{\lambda^k}{k!}$$

for $k = 0, 1, \ldots$, and parameter $\lambda > 0$. The Poisson distributions belong to the exponential family, with $a = 1$, $\theta = \log(\lambda)$, and $c(k, a) = \log(k!)$. The mean and variance of Y are both equal to λ, so $V(\lambda) = \lambda$. The canonical link for the Poisson distribution is the log function. Poisson is often selected as the class of distributions for modelling count data. A Poisson distribution can be derived as the limit of a sequence of binomial distributions $\mathcal{B}(n, p_n)$ such that n diverges to infinity and np_n converges to a positive constant. It can also be derived as the number of random draws from an exponential distribution before their total exceeds a given threshold. These derivations and the simple form of their probabilities motivate the use of the Poisson distributions. However, the assumption that the mean and variance coincide may be unrealistic. It can be relaxed by adopting the variance function $V(\mu) = a\mu$ and estimating the constant a by moment matching; see later. This may be useful even if a distribution with such a variance function does not exist.

The Gamma distributions are given by the densities

$$f(y; \theta, \xi) = \frac{\theta^\xi y^{\xi-1} \exp(-\theta y)}{\Gamma(\xi)}$$

for $y > 0$ and positive values of the parameters θ and ξ. These distributions are members of the exponential family, with $a = -1$, $b(\theta) = \xi \log(\theta)$, and

$c(y, a) = (\xi - 1) \log(y) - \log\{\Gamma(\xi)\}$, when the value of ξ is known. The mean and variance of the Gamma distributions are ξ/θ and ξ/θ^2, respectively.

The family of exponential distributions can be expanded further by monotone transformations. If the distribution of a continuous variable Y is in the exponential family, then its differentiable increasing transformation $h(Y)$ has the density

$$\exp\left\{\frac{h^{-1}(u)\theta - b(\theta)}{a} + c^{\dagger}(u, a)\right\}, \tag{10.5}$$

where $c^{\dagger}(u, a) = c\{h(y), a\} + h'\{h^{-1}(u)\}$. Transformations of the parameters (reparameterisation) offer further extensions.

10.3 Maximum Likelihood Estimation

The special form of the exponential family of distributions enables us to maximise the log-likelihood by the Newton–Raphson or Fisher scoring algorithms. For a vector of outcomes $\mathbf{y}$, mutually conditionally independent given the matrix of covariates $\mathbf{X}$, the log-likelihood is

$$l(\beta; \mathbf{y}, \mathbf{X}) = \frac{1}{a}\sum_{j=1}^{n} y_j \theta_j - \frac{1}{a}\sum_{j=1}^{n} b(\theta_j) + \sum_{j=1}^{n} c(y_j, a),$$

where $\theta_j = \eta(\mathbf{x}_j \beta)$ is a transformation of the linear predictor $\mathbf{x}_j \beta$. The score vector for β is

$$\frac{\partial l}{\partial \beta} = \frac{1}{a}\sum_{j=1}^{n} \{y_j - b'(\theta_j)\}\frac{\partial \theta_j}{\partial \eta_j}\mathbf{x}_j, \tag{10.6}$$

where the differential is of θ_j as a function of $\eta_j = \mathbf{x}_j \beta$. For the canonical link, $\theta_j = \mathbf{x}_j \beta$, and so $\partial \theta_j / \partial \eta_j = 1$. The score vector can be thought of as a weighted total of crossproducts of the residuals $y_j - b'(\mathbf{x}_j \beta)$ and the covariates $\mathbf{x}_j$, with the weights $\partial \theta_j / \partial \eta_j$. The observed information matrix for β is

$$-\frac{\partial l^2}{\partial \beta \, \partial \beta^{\top}} = \frac{1}{a}\sum_{j=1}^{n} b''(\theta_j)\left(\frac{\partial \theta_j}{\partial \eta_j}\right)^2 \mathbf{x}_j \mathbf{x}_j^{\top} + \sum_{j=1}^{n} \{y_j - b'(\theta_j)\}\frac{\partial \theta_j^2}{\partial^2 \eta_j}\mathbf{x}_j \mathbf{x}_j^{\top}.$$

Its expectation, the expected information matrix, is equal to the first summation on the right-hand side:

$$-\mathrm{E}\left(\frac{\partial l^2}{\partial \beta \, \partial \beta^{\top}}\right) = \frac{1}{a}\sum_{j=1}^{n} b''(\theta_j)\left(\frac{\partial \theta_j}{\partial \eta_j}\right)^2 \mathbf{x}_j \mathbf{x}_j^{\top}. \tag{10.7}$$

For the canonical link, the observed and expected information matrices coincide and are equal to $a^{-1}\sum_j b''(\theta_j)\mathbf{x}_j \mathbf{x}_j^{\top}$.

The maximum likelihood estimates are found by iterative updating

$$\hat{\beta}_{\text{new}} = \hat{\beta}_{\text{old}} + \mathcal{I}_{\beta,\beta}^{-1}\left(\hat{\beta}_{\text{old}}, \hat{\beta}_{\text{old}}\right) \mathbf{s}_{\beta}\left(\hat{\beta}_{\text{old}}\right),$$

where $\mathbf{s}_{\beta}$ and $\mathcal{I}_{\beta,\beta}$, given by (10.6) and (10.7), respectively, are evaluated at the current solution $\hat{\beta}_{\text{old}}$. A provisional solution is required for the first iteration. The ordinary least squares fit, $(\mathbf{X}^{\top}\mathbf{X})^{-1}\mathbf{X}^{\top}\mathbf{y}$, suitably scaled for the (approximated) variances $b''(\theta_j)/a$, can be used. An alternative is based on the fit with all the slopes in $\hat{\beta}$ set to zero. For a canonical link, this is obtained by transforming the mean $\bar{y} = \mathbf{y}^{\top}\mathbf{1}_n/n$ to the scale of the linear predictor, that is, solving the equation $b'(\hat{\beta}_0) = \bar{y}$.

There is no guarantee that the Fisher scoring algorithm would converge, and a general discussion of the problems entailed is not possible. Some but not all of the problems can be related to the ill-conditioning of the regression matrix $\mathbf{X}$. In general, the convergence is faster for simpler models and when the factors $w_j = b''(\theta_j)(\partial\theta_j/\partial\eta_j)^2$ in (10.7) are smooth functions of the linear predictor $\mathbf{x}\beta$ and, evaluated at $\hat{\beta}$ or $\hat{\beta}_{\text{old}}$, are distant from both zero and $+\infty$.

The factors w_j can be interpreted as weights, ascribing relative importance to the observations as compared to ordinary regression, in which every weight is equal to unity. For example, with binary outcomes and logit link, $w_j = \hat{p}_j(1-\hat{p}_j)$, where $\hat{p}_j = 1/\{1+\exp(-\mathbf{x}_j\hat{\beta})\}$ is the fitted probability. Therefore, observations with fitted probabilities $\hat{p}_j$ distant from zero and unity are relatively less important than observations with $\hat{p}_j$ close to $\frac{1}{2}$, for which w_j is close to $\frac{1}{4}$. This agrees with intuition: observations with their values of the covariates $\mathbf{x}$ in a region where $\hat{p}_j$ is small contain little information because almost all the corresponding outcomes are the same (equal to zero).

We emphasize that w_j represents *relative* importance, because the values of $\mathbf{x}_j$ have an impact on how useful an observation is even when w_j are constant. Further, importance cannot be assigned to each observation in isolation from the rest, because, for instance, dispersion of the values of $\mathbf{x}_j$ is associated with information about the regression parameters.

The formulae for the Fisher scoring algorithm can be expressed in terms of the weights w_j. Define the generalised residuals as

$$e_j^* = \frac{y_j - b'(\theta_j)}{b''(\theta_j)\,\partial\theta_j/\partial\eta_j}$$

and their vector as $\mathbf{e}^* = (e_1^*, \ldots, e_n^*)^{\top}$. Further, let $\mathbf{W}$ be the diagonal matrix with the weights w_j on its diagonal. Then the score vector and expected information matrix are

$$\frac{\partial l}{\partial \beta} = \frac{1}{a}\mathbf{X}^{\top}\mathbf{W}\mathbf{e}^*,$$

$$-\mathrm{E}\left(\frac{\partial^2 l}{\partial\beta\,\partial\beta^{\top}}\right) = \frac{1}{a}\mathbf{X}^{\top}\mathbf{W}\mathbf{X}. \tag{10.8}$$

The weights depend on the linear predictor $\mathbf{x}_j\boldsymbol{\beta}$, so their estimated version $\hat{w}_j$ as a function of $\hat{\boldsymbol{\beta}}$ has to be updated at each iteration. Thus, fitting a GLM can be described as *iteratively reweighted least squares*.

10.3.1 Overdispersion

In the terminology of GLM, the normal-identity model involves a scale (σ^2) that is estimated. In models for binary and Poisson-distributed outcomes, the scale is implied by the distributional assumption and is equal to unity in both cases. The scale may be set to a different value, and for the Poisson distributions it can even be estimated. The assumption that the mean λ is associated with the variance $c\lambda$ for a particular value of c, whether known or not, may in some settings be appropriate. With $c \neq 1$, we seek a match of the association of the mean and variance, $V = c\mu$, without reference to any particular class of distributions. A distribution with the posited association need not even exist.

For binary outcomes, the mean (probability) and variance can be connected only by the variance function $V(p) = p(1 - p)$. However, even for counts in a given number of trials, for which the binomial would be the distributions of choice, the variance function may be greater than for the binomial. When the set of m trials from which an outcome is derived are conditionally independent, given the values of the covariates, the variance function is $V(p) = mp(1 - p)$. When the trials yield conditionally positively correlated outcomes, the variance function is $V(p; m) = cmp(1 - p)$ for a constant $c > 1$. This phenomenon is referred to as *overdispersion*. If the conditional correlation of outcomes within a set of trials is equal to ρ, then $c = 1 + (m - 1)\rho$.

Conditionally correlated outcomes may arise when the list of covariates is not complete. That is, if one or several further variables were included among the covariates, the outcomes would be independent after conditioning on all of them, but with an incomplete list of covariates they are conditionally correlated. This is easy to demonstrate on a simple example. Suppose $n = 1280$ binomially distributed outcomes with denominator $m = 6$ are generated according to a logistic regression model $\text{logit}(p_j) = -0.5 + 0.2x_j$, where x_j have integer values in the range 1–10. Figure 10.3 summarises such a (simulated) dataset by the distribution of the covariate and the conditional probabilities of 'success' for each value of the covariate. If the covariate is ignored, the fitted model is derived directly by transforming the overall sample mean proportion. For a particular realisation, we have $\hat{p} = 0.64$, so $\hat{\beta}_0 = 0.576$. The sample variance of the outcomes is 1.489, higher than $m\hat{p}(1 - \hat{p}) = 1.382$, derived by assuming that the $m = 6$ trials that constitute a unit are independent and ignoring the uncertainty about $\hat{p}$. The difference between these two estimated variances is substantial and does not arise solely by chance. To verify this, we replicate the simulation 1000 times. The realised proportions of success are in the range $(0.626, 0.660)$, with mean 0.643; the corresponding (estimated) binomial variances, $m\hat{p}(1 - \hat{p})$ are in the range $(1.346, 1.405)$.

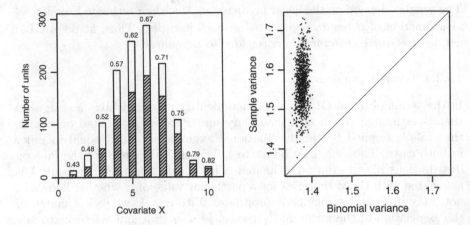

Fig. 10.3. The sample and binomial variances in a simulation of simple logistic regression (right-hand panel). In the left-hand panel, the distribution of the covariate is plotted, with the conditional probability of success given above each bar and indicated by shading. The right-hand panel summarises the sample variances.

However, the simulated sample variances $\sum_{j=1}^{n}(Y_j - \bar{Y})^2/(n-1)$ are 1.011–1.254 times greater, in the range $(1.378, 1.731)$. The right-hand panel of Figure 10.3 plots the sample and binomial variances. So, although not dramatic, the overdispersion is persistent.

The example highlights the importance of the *conditional* as a qualifier for independence of the outcomes in regression models in general. For a given dataset, overdispersion in this example has no impact on the estimates because the multiplicative inflation of the variances and weights in $\mathbf{X}^\top \mathbf{W} \mathbf{e}^*$ and $\mathbf{X}^\top \mathbf{W} \mathbf{X}$ in (10.8) cancels out. However, the information matrix is reciprocally proportional to the inflation factor, so the standard errors are affected.

Overdispersion need not be multiplicative. We are at liberty to specify any variance function V, so it can be related to the variance function V^* for a known distribution in essentially any way that maintains positivity of V. One such example arises by assuming that the outcomes as counts contain an excess of zeros. That is, conditionally on the values of the covariates, the distribution of the outcomes is a mixture of a Poisson (binomial or some other discrete) distribution and the identical zero. In a setting with no covariates, let the (mixture) probability of identical zero be ρ and the mean of the other, say, Poisson-distributed, component λ. Note that the probability of a zero outcome is greater than ρ because zero may also be generated by the Poisson component. The expectation of the mixture is $\lambda(1-\rho)$ and its variance is $\lambda(1-\rho)(1+\lambda\rho)$. Thus, in relation to the expectation of the mixture, $\lambda(1-\rho)$, an excess of zeros always amounts to overdispersion. In contrast, when related to the original Poisson-distributed variable, overdispersion arises only when $(1-\rho)(1+\lambda\rho) > 1$, that is, when $\lambda > 1/(1-\rho)$.

Suppose the mean λ depends on the values of some covariates, but the proportion ρ is independent of them. Then the extent of overdispersion, measured on the multiplicative scale, depends on λ. The overdispersion is greater for greater values of λ, when zero is a more extreme value in the conditional mixture distribution. When there are fewer zeros than the Poisson (or another discrete) reference distribution would have, we have a case of *underdispersion*.

Models for under- and overdispersion can be fitted by specifying an appropriate variance function, although difficulties may be encountered when the probability associated with the mixture components has to be estimated and when it depends on some covariates. The EM algorithm, in which the identity of the mixture component for each observation is regarded as the missing data, addresses this problem. In the E-step, the outcomes equal to zero are apportioned to the two components according to the probability of zero outcome given the nondegenerate (Poisson, binomial, or some other specified) distribution. In the M-step, which itself involves iterations, this distribution is updated, based on the apportionment from the preceding E-step, and the iterations of E- and M-steps are repeated until convergence.

10.3.2 Model Selection

Often a range of alternative models is considered and one of them is selected as the most suitable description of the data-generating process. The elemental part of this is a choice between two models, based on how well they fit the data. The fit of two models, A and B, such that A is a submodel of B, can be compared by the *likelihood ratio*. Suppose these models involve p_A and $p_B > p_A$ unconstrained regression parameters. Denote by D_A and D_B the -2-multiple of the log-likelihood evaluated at the fit of the respective models A and B. Then, if model A is valid and the values of the model parameters are not on the boundary of the parameter space (for A), $D_A - D_B$ has asymptotically χ^2 distribution with $p_B - p_A$ degrees of freedom. This provides a prescription for selecting between the two models. We choose A if the realised value of $D_A - D_B$ does not exceed the a priori set quantile of the χ^2 distribution; otherwise we choose B. Such a model selection can be related to hypothesis testing in which we adopt model A as the default and choose B only when there is evidence against A, in the form of a value of $D_A - D_B$ that would be exceptional if model A were valid.

This procedure has all the drawbacks of its counterpart for ordinary regression. First, it is not informed by the target of estimation, the purpose for which the model is to be employed. Second, the procedure is concerned with probabilities of correct choice, not with minimising the undesirable consequences of the two kinds of incorrect choices. And third, we have no means of estimating the sampling distribution (or the MSE) of the selected-model-based estimator given the model-selection process. Any (estimated) summary of the conditional sampling distribution, given the selected model, such as the standard error of a model parameter, is misleading because the corresponding summary of the unconditional distribution, which is a mixture of the selected-model-based estimators, should be quoted.

Let C be the selected model; C = A or C = B. Suppose a quantity θ would be estimated by $\hat{\theta}_A$ or $\hat{\theta}_B$, depending on which model is selected. With the model selection, the estimator is

$$\hat{\theta}_C = I_A \hat{\theta}_A + I_B \hat{\theta}_B,$$

where $I_A = 1 - I_B$ indicates the selection of model A. This estimator is not efficient even if $\hat{\theta}_A$ and $\hat{\theta}_B$ would be efficient if the respective model A or B were selected unconditionally. Further, if $\hat{s}_A^2$ and $\hat{s}_B^2$ are unbiased estimators of the MSEs of the respective estimators $\hat{\theta}_A$ and $\hat{\theta}_B$, then $\mathrm{MSE}(\hat{\theta}_C; \theta)$ is estimated by $\hat{s}_C^2 = I_A \hat{s}_A^2 + I_B \hat{s}_B^2$ with bias. In fact,

$$\mathrm{MSE}\left(\hat{\theta}_C; \theta\right) = p_A \operatorname{var}\left(\hat{\theta}_A \mid I_A = 1\right) + p_B \operatorname{var}\left(\hat{\theta}_B \mid I_B = 1\right)$$
$$+ p_A \left\{ \mathrm{E}(\hat{\theta}_A \mid I_A = 1) - \theta \right\}^2 + p_B \left\{ \mathrm{E}(\hat{\theta}_B \mid I_B = 1) - \theta \right\}^2,$$

where $p_A = \mathrm{P}(I_A = 1)$ and $p_B = \mathrm{P}(I_B = 1)$. The bottom line in this formula can be interpreted as the inflation of the MSE due to model uncertainty.

In Section 2.3, we applied synthesis as an alternative to model selection. Synthesis estimates θ by

$$\tilde{\theta} = \left(1 - \hat{b}_\theta\right) \hat{\theta}_A + \hat{b}_\theta \hat{\theta}_B,$$

with $\hat{b}_\theta$ estimating the coefficient b_θ that would minimise the MSE of $\tilde{\theta}$ for θ. Estimation of $\operatorname{var}(\hat{\theta}_A)$ and $\operatorname{var}(\hat{\theta}_B)$, involved in b_θ, is more complex because of the dependence of $\operatorname{var}(Y)$ on $\mathrm{E}(Y)$ and because the sampling variance is usually only approximated, from the inverse of the expected information matrix. The targets are often on the scale of the outcomes, such as probabilities in logistic regression, and so the sampling variances $\operatorname{var}(\hat{\theta}_A)$ and $\operatorname{var}(\hat{\theta}_B)$ involve further approximations. The MSE of neither $\hat{\theta}_C$ nor $\tilde{\theta}$ can be evaluated or estimated without bias, except by simulations.

Example 15. The dataset analysed in this example was generated by an experiment in which the stimulus x was set to one of the integers 1, 2, ..., 10, and the outcome y was binary. The values of x are distributed approximately uniformly on 1–10; the frequencies of the values are in the range 81–114. One thousand observations were made in total.

The logistic regression yields the fit $-0.112 + 0.071x$ with the standard error of the slope estimated by 0.023. We are interested in estimating the probability of positive outcome for each integer value $x = 1, 2, \ldots, 10$ of the stimulus, perhaps with some mild extrapolation to $x = 0$ and $x = 11$ and $x = 12$. These probabilities are estimated straightforwardly, by transforming the fitted value of the linear predictor to the probability scale. For example, for $x = 10$ we obtain the prediction by transforming the linear fit $-0.112 + 10 \times 0.071 = 0.598$ to the probability scale; we obtain $\hat{p}_{10} = 0.645$. An alternative estimator is the frequency of positive outcomes, based on all 1000 observations. It ignores the values of the stimulus, so this estimator is biased for prediction at all values of x, except perhaps one near the mean $\bar{x}$. At the same time, its variance is smaller than for the regression-based estimator because we have 'saved' one degree of freedom. The estimate is $\hat{p} = 0.566$ and the associated sampling variance is estimated by 2.456×10^{-4}. The latter is unbiased only when the probabilities p_x do not depend on x. However, it differs only slightly from its counterpart based on the logistic regression,

$$\widehat{\mathrm{var}}(\hat{p}\,|\,\hat{\beta}) = \frac{1}{n^2} \sum_{j=1}^{n} \hat{p}_{x_j} \left(1 - \hat{p}_{x_j}\right), \tag{10.9}$$

equal to 2.433×10^{-4}.

Using the logistic regression, we estimate first the standard error of the prediction on the logit scale. For $x = 10$, this is

$$10^{-4} \begin{pmatrix} 1 \\ 10 \end{pmatrix}^{\mathsf{T}} \begin{pmatrix} 189 & -28 \\ -28 & 5 \end{pmatrix} \begin{pmatrix} 1 \\ 10 \end{pmatrix} = 0.01589, \tag{10.10}$$

where the 2×2 matrix is the 10^4-multiple of the estimated sampling variance matrix of $\hat{\beta}$. Since all the probabilities involved are in the range $(0.45, 0.70)$, far away from zero or unity, we can approximate the logit and its inverse by linear functions, with slopes equal to 4 and $\frac{1}{4}$, respectively. Thus, $\hat{p}_{10}$ is approximately unbiased, with estimated standard error $\frac{1}{4}\sqrt{0.01589} = 0.0315$, or about 3%.

We combine the two estimators of the conditional probability of positive outcome p_x; $\hat{p}_x$ derived from logistic regression fit and the sample proportion $\hat{p}$. The former is nearly unbiased and its sampling variance is approximately equal to

$$\mathrm{var}\,(\hat{p}_x) \doteq \{p_x(1 - p_x)\}^2 \, \mathbf{x} \left(\mathbf{X}^{\mathsf{T}}\mathbf{W}\mathbf{X}\right)^{-1} \mathbf{x}^{\mathsf{T}},$$

where $\mathbf{x} = (1, x)$ is the regression vector for the target. The covariance of the two estimators is approximated by

$$C_x = \frac{1}{n} p_x(1 - p_x) \mathbf{x} \left(\mathbf{X}^{\mathsf{T}}\mathbf{W}\mathbf{X}\right)^{-1} \mathbf{X}^{\mathsf{T}}\mathbf{W}\mathbf{1}.$$

These two quantities are estimated naively, as is the bias of $\hat{p}$, by $\hat{B}_x = \hat{p} - \hat{p}_x$, and $\mathrm{var}(\hat{p}_x)$ is estimated by (10.9).

The optimal combination of the estimators $\hat{p}_x$ and $\hat{p}$ is $\tilde{p}_x = (1 - b_x)\hat{p}_x + b_x\hat{p}$, with

$$b_x = \frac{\mathrm{var}(\hat{p}_x) - C_x}{\mathrm{var}(\hat{p}_x) + \mathrm{var}(\hat{p}) - 2C_x + B_x^2}, \tag{10.11}$$

Table 10.1. Synthetic estimation of the probabilities by logistic regression.

	Regression/Selection		Synthesis		
x	$\hat{p}_x$	$\sqrt{\widehat{\mathrm{var}}(\hat{p}_x)}$	$\tilde{p}_x$	$\sqrt{\widehat{\mathrm{MSE}}(\tilde{p}_x\,;p_x)}$	$\hat{b}_x$
0	0.4718	0.0343	0.4807	0.0330	0.0945
1	0.4896	0.0294	0.4968	0.0284	0.0951
2	0.5073	0.0248	0.5129	0.0240	0.0956
3	0.5251	0.0207	0.5290	0.0202	0.0960
4	0.5428	0.0175	0.5450	0.0173	0.0976
5	0.5603	0.0159	0.5611	0.0158	0.1443
6	0.5777	0.0161	0.5765	0.0161	0.1051
7	0.5950	0.0181	0.5922	0.0179	0.0944
8	0.6120	0.0213	0.6077	0.0208	0.0918
9	0.6287	0.0249	0.6231	0.0242	0.0898
10	0.6451	0.0289	0.6382	0.0279	0.0878
11	0.6612	0.0328	0.6531	0.0317	0.0856
12	0.6769	0.0366	0.6677	0.0353	0.0833

where B_x is the bias of $\hat{p}$ in estimating p_x. The coefficient b_x is estimated naively, using the naive estimators of the quantities required in (10.11). The estimates and associated standard errors for $x = 0, 1, \ldots, 12$ are given in Table 10.1.

The table shows that the regression estimates $\hat{p}_x$ are altered by synthesis only slightly; the sample proportion $\hat{p}$ is assigned small weight $\hat{b}_x$, around 0.1, for all values of x. The coefficients are nearly identical because the problem is very similar to synthesis in simple regression, where the coefficient is common to all values of x. The small differences arise because of slight heteroscedasticity, weak dependence of $\mathrm{var}(Y \mid X = x)$ on x, and nonlinearity of the logit function in the range of the fitted probabilities. Figure 10.4 summarises the results graphically. Although the differences between the pairs of maximum likelihood and synthetic estimators are small, they are perceptible.

The estimated standard errors require a careful qualification. First, we did not state up front whether we would have contemplated the logistic model with no covariates, which would yield the common estimator $\hat{p}$ for all values of x. If so, we would have to declare the selection criterion. In some replications, this 'empty' model might be accepted by the model-selection criterion. For the synthetic estimator, the uncertainty about $\hat{b}_x$ is ignored in estimating its MSE. Thus, a fair comparison can be made only by simulations, as done in Section 2.3 for a different example. The simulations confirm that the synthetic estimator is slightly more efficient than $\hat{p}_x$ or its model-selection counterpart, and that model selection can be counterproductive, resulting in inflated MSE

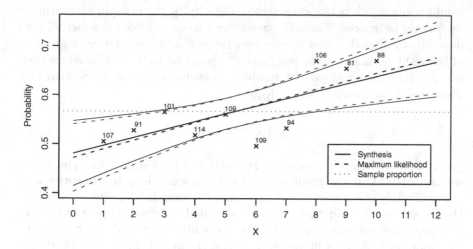

Fig. 10.4. The synthetic and maximum likelihood estimates of the probabilities p_x (thicker lines) and the associated pointwise 95% confidence limits (thinner lines). The subsample proportions for the values of x are marked by crosses and are accompanied by the number of observations.

of prediction. Details are omitted because the conclusions are similar to those based on simple regression.

10.4 Residuals

In ordinary regression, each deviation ε_j can be regarded as a target and estimated by $e_j = y_j - \mathbf{x}_j\hat{\boldsymbol{\beta}}$ or its standardisation $e_j^\dagger$ that arranges $\mathrm{var}(e_j^\dagger)$ to be constant. In GLM, there is no direct analogue of ε_j, but we can adopt the deviation $y_j - \mathrm{E}(y_j \mid \mathbf{x}_j) = y_j - b'(\theta_j)$, or its naive estimator, $y_j - b'(\hat{\theta}_j)$, as a generalisation of the residual. In ordinary regression we would study the patterns among the residuals; in GLM this is not always useful. Residuals for binary outcomes represent an extreme example. For each value of $\mathbf{x}_j\hat{\boldsymbol{\beta}}$ there are only two possible values of the residual, $1 - b'(\mathbf{x}_j\hat{\boldsymbol{\beta}})$ and $-b'(\mathbf{x}_j\hat{\boldsymbol{\beta}})$, so the pattern of the residuals is strongly influenced by the pattern of the values of the covariates.

In other cases, even with continuous outcomes, the expectation is associated with the variance of the outcomes, so a particular pattern of the residuals can be expected when fitting valid models. The so-called Pearson residuals,

$$e_j^{(\mathrm{P})} = \frac{y_j - b'(\mathbf{x}_j\hat{\boldsymbol{\beta}})}{\sqrt{b''(\mathbf{x}_j\hat{\boldsymbol{\beta}})}},$$

would remove such patterns (heteroscedasticity) if the error in estimating β by $\hat{\beta}$ could be ignored. The scale parameter a could be added as a factor in the denominator, but that is of no relevance because only the relative magnitudes of the residuals matter. The residuals $e_j^{(P)}$ could be further adjusted for their unequal influence, as done with residuals in ordinary regression (Section 1.3). These residuals are $e_j^{(P)}/\sqrt{h_j}$, where

$$h_j = \mathbf{x}_j \left(\mathbf{X}^{*\top} \mathbf{W} \mathbf{X}^* \right)^{-1} \mathbf{x}_j^\top.$$

A simple diagnostic procedure is motivated by Figure 10.1. The values of the estimated linear predictor $\mathbf{x}_j\hat{\beta}$ are coarsened into K categories with approximately equal numbers of units, and the sample proportions $\hat{p}_k$ within the categories are compared with the estimated expected proportions $p_k(\hat{\beta})$. The latter are evaluated as the means of the fitted probabilities. Substantial deviations indicate poor fit and suggest that the model should be revised. The categories should be defined so that each would have a sufficient number of units. However, if there are too few categories the assessment of the model may be too crude and some consistent deviations from the model may be missed by averaging over too many subjects.

The simulation-based version of this procedure, introduced in Section 1.3.1, in which the vector of the within-category deviations is the feature, avoids the need for a judgment as to whether a deviation is unusual. The procedure requires a definition for the coarsening that can be implemented on the computer after fitting the model to a replicate (simulated) dataset.

For outcomes other than binary, a similar procedure compares the within-category means or other summaries of the outcomes with their expected counterparts. In principle, the within-category empirical distributions can be compared with their expected versions, but this is practical only for very large datasets.

Deviance Residuals

The deviance is defined as the -2-multiple of the log-likelihood. The log-likelihood is used only for comparisons of its values and for differentiation, so it can be defined subject to an arbitrary constant additive term. For example, the constant $n\log(2\pi)$ in a log-likelihood for normally distributed outcomes, or $n\log(m!)$ in a log-likelihood involving binomial outcomes (x successes in m trials), can always be dropped without any impact on ML estimation.

Deviance is sometimes preferred to the log-likelihood because of its connection with the likelihood ratio test, which is a comparison of the deviances, but also because it represents a summary of the failure to fit the outcomes perfectly. In this context, perfect fit corresponds to $y_j = g^{-1}(\mathbf{x}_j\hat{\beta})$ for every subject j. Thus, a well-motivated definition of the deviance uses the version that attains the value of zero when a perfect fit is attained. Let a particular version of the deviance be D. Its arguments are $\mathbf{y}$, the vector of outcomes, and $\boldsymbol{\mu}$, the conditional expectation given $\mathbf{X}$. Then

$$D^*(\mathbf{y}; \boldsymbol{\mu}) = D(\mathbf{y}; \boldsymbol{\mu}) - D(\mathbf{y}; \mathbf{y})$$

is the version of the deviance for which $D^* = 0$ when $\boldsymbol{\mu} = \mathbf{y}$. For some GLMs, D^* is not defined. For example, for binary outcomes with logit link perfect fit corresponds to a singularity, with all fitted probabilities equal to either zero or unity. But then the corresponding linear predictors are all equal to $+\infty$ or $-\infty$. In ordinary regression, D^* is well defined only when the variance σ^2 is fixed. The estimate of σ^2 with the perfect fit would be zero, also resulting in a singularity.

As a nontrivial example, consider outcomes with exponential distributions and reciprocal link to the linear predictor. The density of the exponential distribution is $\mu^{-1} \exp(-y/\mu)$, where μ is its expectation, so each observation y_j contributes to the log-likelihood with $l_j = -\log(\mu_j) - y_j/\mu_j$, where the linear predictor is $\mathbf{x}_j \boldsymbol{\beta} = 1/\mu_j$. The deviance D^* is equal to $D_1^* + \cdots + D_n^*$, where the contribution $D_j^* = D^*(y_j, \mu_j)$ of subject j is

$$D_j^* = -2\left\{-\frac{y}{\mu_j} - \log(\mu_j)\right\} + 2\left\{-1 - \log(y)\right\}$$

$$= 2\left(\frac{y_j}{\mu_j} - 1\right) - 2\log\left(\frac{y_j}{\mu_j}\right). \tag{10.12}$$

It is left for an exercise to show that D_j^* is nonnegative and when μ_j is fixed its minimum of zero is attained for $y_j = \mu_j$.

The *deviance residuals* $e_j^{(\mathrm{D})}$ are defined as $\mathrm{sign}(y_j - \mu_j)\sqrt{D_j}$, where sign is the function with values $+1$ for positive, -1 for negative arguments, and zero when its argument is equal to zero. When one or a small number of the observations make disproportionately large contributions to the deviance, they deserve scrutiny—the analyst should explore whether they are outliers due to errors in the data-collection process or due to some exceptional circumstances in the data-generating process. The difficulty in this proposal is that 'disproportional' requires a judgment that may not be straightforward to make. If computing power is not a limiting factor, simulation-based diagnostics are an alternative. We define a feature, possibly based on the deviance residuals, generate 19 (or 99) simulated versions of this feature, and inspect the anonymised set of 20 (or 100) features to see whether any of them stands out. If one of them is identified and it turns out to be the realised feature, we have evidence against validity of the model we have applied, and the model should be revised.

10.4.1 Overall Assessment of Fit

The fit of a model can be assessed by defining a feature, evaluating it on the realised data, and comparing it with its version generated by simulations from the fitted model. The feature can be based on the residuals, but these are not very useful for binary outcomes. An alternative approach defines a coarsening of the linear predictor $\mathbf{x}\hat{\boldsymbol{\beta}}$ to a suitable (finite) set of categories and compares the means of the outcomes with the means of the fitted values $g(\mathbf{x}\hat{\boldsymbol{\beta}})$ within these categories. As g is a monotone function, coarsening based on the values of $\mathbf{x}\hat{\boldsymbol{\beta}}$ is equivalent to a coarsening based on $g(\mathbf{x}\hat{\boldsymbol{\beta}})$. Good fit corresponds to close agreement of the two sets of the means, although this has to be qualified by the subsample sizes involved. This method is particularly useful for binary outcomes, for which there are few effective alternatives.

For a particular coarsening of $\mathbf{x}\hat{\boldsymbol{\beta}}$ or $g(\mathbf{x}\hat{\boldsymbol{\beta}})$, denote the subsample sizes within the coarse categories by n_h, $h = 1, \ldots, H$. We refer to these categories as bins, to help draw parallels with the diagnostic method used in Example 14 in Section 6.7. For a binary outcome variable and a model fit to its values, let $\hat{p}_h$ be the proportion of positive outcomes among the observations that fell into bin h, and let $\hat{r}_h$ be the average of the fitted probabilities $g(\mathbf{x}_j\hat{\boldsymbol{\beta}})$ for these outcomes. The statistic

$$S = \sum_{h=1}^{H} n_h \frac{(\hat{p}_h - \hat{r}_h)^2}{\hat{r}_h}$$

assesses the proximity of the proportions $\hat{p}_h$ to the estimated proportions $\hat{r}_h$. It is motivated by the test of the hypothesis that a set of sample proportions is compatible with a set of (underlying) probabilities. If we ignore the uncertainty about each $\hat{r}_h$, then under the null hypothesis that $\hat{p}_h$ are compatible with $\hat{r}_h$, the statistic S has asymptotic χ^2 distribution with $H - 1$ degrees of freedom. The qualifier *asymptotic* refers to many observations in each bin. It suggests that the number of bins should not be excessive, and each of them should contain many observations. Details can be explored by a simple simulation study, but defining too many bins, several of them sparsely occupied, is not practical anyway. The uncertainty about $\hat{r}_h$ can also be addressed by simulation, declaring the statistic S as a feature and evaluating it on replicate datasets generated according to the fitted model.

10.5 Random Coefficients

In this section, we adapt GLMs for structured populations, with elements in clusters. GLMs involve linear regression:

$$E(y \mid \mathbf{x}; \boldsymbol{\beta}) = g^{-1}(\mathbf{x}\boldsymbol{\beta}),$$

where g is the link function. A constraining assumption of GLM is that the outcomes are conditionally independent. It is easily challenged with structured observations, such as with units within clusters. The model formulation in terms of varying regressions (Chapter 9) carries over from the setting with normally distributed outcomes, although the nonlinearity of the link function as well as the departure from normality bring about a host of analytical complexities. We explore these later in this section.

Suppose observations are made on subjects within clusters and each cluster is associated with a different regression. The regressions have a common link function and the conditional (within-cluster) distributions of the outcomes belong to the same class. It is practical to introduce the notation

$$\mathrm{GLM}(\mathcal{F}, g, \mathbf{X}\boldsymbol{\beta})$$

for the GLM with the class of distributions $\mathcal{F}$ (e.g., binary), link function g (e.g., probit), regression matrix $\mathbf{X}$, and vector of regression parameters $\boldsymbol{\beta}$. Then a general model for the setting with elements $i = 1, \ldots, n_d$ within clusters $d = 1, \ldots, D$ can be concisely specified as

$$(\mathbf{y}_d \mid \boldsymbol{\delta}_d; \mathbf{X}_d, \mathbf{Z}_d) \sim \mathrm{GLM}(\mathcal{F}, g, \mathbf{X}_d\boldsymbol{\beta} + \mathbf{Z}_d\boldsymbol{\delta}_d) ,$$

$$\boldsymbol{\delta}_d \sim \mathcal{N}(\mathbf{0}, \boldsymbol{\Sigma}_{\mathrm{B}}) . \tag{10.13}$$

Here the vector of regression parameters $\boldsymbol{\beta}$ represents the typical regression and the vector of cluster-level deviations $\boldsymbol{\delta}_d$, or the corresponding term $\mathbf{z}\boldsymbol{\delta}_d$ that is specific to cluster d, is the deviation of the regression in cluster d from the typical regression. The matrices $\mathbf{X}_d$ and $\mathbf{Z}_d$ are the segments of the respective matrices $\mathbf{X}$ and $\mathbf{Z}$ that correspond to cluster $d = 1, \ldots, D$. The variation (design) matrix $\mathbf{Z}$ is usually formed by a selection from the columns of $\mathbf{X}$. The regression slopes with respect to the variables in $\mathbf{Z}$ vary across the clusters, and with respect to the other variables in $\mathbf{X}$ they are constant. These models, GLM with random coefficients (GLMrc), are also known as generalised linear mixed models (GLMM); the qualifier *mixed* refers to the combination of within-cluster regression slopes constant for some and varying for other covariates.

The 'rules' for model specification listed in Section 9.2.1 apply also to GLMM, irrespective of the link function used. However, nonlinearity of the link function brings about a lot of complexity that requires a careful discussion. With identity link $g(\mu) = \mu$, we can refer to $\mathbf{x}\boldsymbol{\beta}$ as the average regression, because the expectation over the clusters and the link function can be interchanged:

$$\mathrm{E}_{\mathcal{D}}\{g(\mathbf{x}\boldsymbol{\beta} + \mathbf{z}\boldsymbol{\delta}_d)\} = g\{\mathrm{E}_{\mathcal{D}}(\mathbf{x}\boldsymbol{\beta} + \mathbf{z}\boldsymbol{\delta}_d)\} = \mathbf{x}\boldsymbol{\beta}$$

for any fixed vectors $\mathbf{x}$ and $\mathbf{z}$. For nonlinear link functions we have this identity only in some special cases, such as when $\mathbf{x}\boldsymbol{\beta} = 0$ and g is symmetric around zero, since the multivariate normal distribution is symmetric around zero. Therefore it is misleading to refer to $\mathbf{x}\boldsymbol{\beta}$ as the average regression. We use the qualifier *typical*, since $\boldsymbol{\beta}$ does not stand out among the within-cluster regression coefficients $\boldsymbol{\beta} + \Delta\boldsymbol{\beta}_d$ in any way. (The vector $\Delta\boldsymbol{\beta}_d$ is formed by supplementing $\boldsymbol{\delta}_d$ with zeros for the variables not associated with variation.) By way of a simple example, suppose $\beta_0 = -3$ in a logit model for binary data with no covariates, and the between-cluster regression is very large, say $\sigma^2 = 4$. The typical within-cluster probability is equal to $\exp(-3)/\{1 + \exp(-3)\} = 0.0474$; it is the median of the within-cluster probabilities. However, these probabilities are highly skewed; on the one hand, they can be smaller than the median by no more than 0.0474 because they are all positive, and on the other hand, within-cluster probabilities in excess of 0.50 are not exceptional, as their probability is equal to $1 - \Phi(1.5) = 0.067$. The marginal probability is equal to

$$\frac{1}{\sqrt{2\pi}} \int \frac{\exp(\beta + \sigma\delta)}{1 + \exp(\beta + \sigma\delta)} \exp\left(-\frac{\delta^2}{2}\right) d\delta.$$

It can be approximated by quadrature methods described in Section 10.5.1. As an alternative that is easier to programme, the marginal probability can be approximated as the mean of the transformation of a random sample of logits, in our case as $E[\exp(U)/\{1 + \exp(U)\}]$, where $U \sim \mathcal{N}(-3, 4)$. The probability is equal to approximately 0.1295, way in excess of the typical probability 0.0474.

In a GLMM with univariate cluster-level deviations δ_d, when only the intercept is associated with variation, the within-cluster regressions are not parallel. The lines $\mathbf{x}\beta + \delta_d$, $d = 1, \ldots, D$, are parallel, but after the nonlinear transformation, $g(\mathbf{x}\beta + \delta_d)$, they are not, even though they do not intersect. The within-cluster regressions are linear only on the scale of the linear predictor. This is illustrated in Figure 10.5 by examples of logistic regression with several patterns of variation. In the left-hand panels, the within-cluster regressions are plotted on the logit (linear) scale, so they are linear functions. In the right-hand panels, these regressions are plotted on the probability scale, after the inverse-logit transformation, so they are not linear. However, the departure from linearity is not dramatic and is perceptible only outside the interval $(-1, 1)$. Thus, we can exchange averaging and the application of the logit link function, so long as all the logits involved are within this range, that is, the probabilities are in the range $(0.25, 0.75)$.

The marginal regression in a GLM is defined as the expectation of an outcome with a set vector of covariates $\mathbf{x}$, $E(Y \mid \mathbf{x})$, after averaging over the clusters. It can be derived from the within-cluster regressions as

$$E(Y \mid \mathbf{x}) = \int \ldots \int E(Y \mid \boldsymbol{\delta}, \mathbf{x}) \, \phi(\boldsymbol{\delta}; \mathbf{0}, \boldsymbol{\Sigma}_B) \, d\boldsymbol{\delta},$$

where ϕ denotes the density of the multivariate normal distribution with the mean vector and variance matrix given as its arguments. For multivariate $\boldsymbol{\delta}$ this integral is multiple. Unlike for random coefficient models with identity link, the marginal distribution need not belong to the same class of regressions as the within-cluster regressions. For example, the marginal regression in a logistic GLMM is not logit, and its approximation by a logit is good only in a region that involves no probabilities outside the range $(0.25, 0.75)$. That is, the approximation is good only when the link function is very close to being linear.

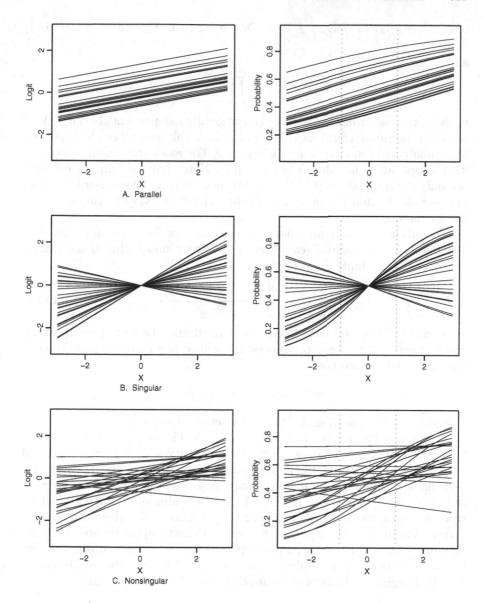

Fig. 10.5. Examples of varying logistic regressions, drawn on the logit and probability scales. In the right-hand panels, the vertical dots delineate the interval $(-1, 1)$, within which the logit is very close to linearity.

10.5.1 Fitting GLMM

The log-likelihood for a GLMM is equal to the total of the log-likelihoods for the observations within clusters: $l = l_1 + \cdots + l_D$, where

$$\exp(l_d) = \int \dots \int f^{(c)} \left(\mathbf{y}_d \, | \, \mathbf{X}_d, \boldsymbol{\delta}_d \right) \phi \left(\boldsymbol{\delta}; \mathbf{0}, \boldsymbol{\Sigma}_{\mathrm{B}} \right) \mathrm{d}\boldsymbol{\delta} \tag{10.14}$$

and

$$f^{(c)} \left(\mathbf{y}_d \, | \, \mathbf{X}_d, \boldsymbol{\delta}_d \right) = \prod_{j=1}^{n_d} f \left(y_{jd} \, | \, \mathbf{x}_{jd}, \boldsymbol{\delta}_d \right),$$

as the outcomes within a cluster are conditionally independent given $\boldsymbol{\delta}_d$. With normally distributed outcomes and identity link, this integral can be expressed in an analytical form, as done is Chapter 9. For most other combinations of distribution and link, this is not possible. Note that we want to evaluate not only the integrals in (10.14) but also their first- and second-order partial differentials, to find the maximum likelihood by the Newton–Raphson or a similar method.

We outline several approaches to maximising the likelihood for a GLMM. The first-order partial differentials of an arbitrary smooth function q can be approximated by finite differences as

$$q'(x) \doteq \frac{q(x+h) - q(x-h)}{2h} \tag{10.15}$$

for a small h. This approximation can be derived from the mean value theorem, which states that for a smooth function q defined in an interval (a,b) there is a point $c \in (a,b)$ such that

$$q(b) - q(a) = (b-a) \, q'(c).$$

The sought approximation is obtained by setting $b = x + h$ and $a = x - h$; the error of approximation is equal to $q'(c) - q'(x)$. The step h in (10.15) has to be small, so that the values of the derivative q' vary very little in the interval $(x - h, x + h)$; otherwise the approximation is not very good. However, for very small h, numerical imprecision may arise when evaluating the ratio of two very small numbers in (10.15). A suitable value of h can be found by trial and error, using functions similar to q, but for which their derivative is known. The second-order partial differentials can be approximated by finite differences of the first-order partial differentials. So, at least in principle, we require only a method for evaluating the contributions l_d to the log-likelihood.

The integral in (10.14) can be approximated by the finite sum

$$\frac{1}{M} \sum_{m=1}^{M} f^{(c)} \left(\mathbf{y}_d \, | \, \mathbf{X}_d; \boldsymbol{\delta}_m \right)$$

for the vectors $\boldsymbol{\delta}_m$, $m = 1, \dots, M$, selected so that they represent well the distribution $\mathcal{N}(\mathbf{0}, \boldsymbol{\Sigma}_{\mathrm{B}})$. For example, $\boldsymbol{\delta}_m$ could be a random draw from the distribution. Although simple to implement, this approach requires very extensive computing and is affordable only in some simple problems. An alternative is to choose the values $\boldsymbol{\delta}_m$ deliberately, aiming to achieve a set precision with a small number M. This problem is solved for univariate (and normally distributed) δ by the so-called *Gaussian quadrature*. The requisite values can be found in statistical tables or software.

For multivariate δ, we can express the integral in terms of $\delta^* = \Sigma^{-\frac{1}{2}}\delta$, the components of which are independent and have unit variances; $\mathrm{var}(\delta^*) = \mathbf{I}$. For δ^*, Gaussian quadrature can be applied to each component separately. Even for a moderate number of points M in the quadrature for each dimension, the number of summands with three or more dimensions is very large; for example, for $M = 10$ and three-dimensional δ, the approximation has 1000 terms for one cluster and $1000D$ for a dataset with D clusters in a single iteration. In most settings, Gaussian quadrature is practical to implement only for one- or two-dimensional random terms δ.

10.5.2 Exact Derivatives of the Log-Likelihood

The log-likelihood can be differentiated analytically, by exchanging integration and differentiation, leaving us with the task of integrating a function similar to the joint density, although somewhat more complex. We assume that the conditional density f belongs to the exponential family given by (10.4) and that the canonical link is used. Then

$$\frac{\partial l_d}{\partial \beta} = \frac{1}{L_d} \int f^{(c)} \left(\mathbf{y}_d \,|\, \mathbf{X}_d, \delta\right) \mathbf{s}_{\mathrm{x},d}(\delta)\, \phi\left(\delta; 0, \Sigma_{\mathrm{B}}\right) \mathrm{d}\delta\,,$$

where $L_d = \exp(l_d)$ and

$$\mathbf{s}_{\mathrm{x},d}(\delta) = \frac{1}{a} \sum_{j=1}^{n_d} \left\{y_{jd} - b'(\mathbf{x}_{jd}\beta + \mathbf{z}_{jd}\delta)\right\} \mathbf{x}_{jd}\,.$$

The second-order partial differentials with respect to β are expressed similarly. In general, they involve $\partial^2 \theta_{jd} / \left(\partial\beta\,\partial\beta^{\top}\right)$, but for canonical link this vanishes. We have

$$\frac{\partial^2 l_d}{\partial\beta\,\partial\beta^{\top}} = -\frac{\partial l_d}{\partial\beta}\frac{\partial l_d}{\partial\beta^{\top}} + \frac{1}{L_d} \int f^{(c)}\left(\mathbf{y}_d \,|\, \mathbf{X}_d, \delta\right) \mathbf{S}_{\mathrm{xx},d}(\delta)\, \phi\left(\delta; 0, \Sigma_{\mathrm{B}}\right) \mathrm{d}\delta\,,$$

where

$$\mathbf{S}_{\mathrm{xx},d}(\delta) = \mathbf{s}_{\mathrm{x},d}(\delta)\left\{\mathbf{s}_{\mathrm{x},d}(\delta)\right\}^{\top} - \frac{1}{a}\sum_{j=1}^{n_d} b''(\mathbf{x}_{jd}\beta + \mathbf{z}_{jd}\delta)\,\mathbf{x}_{jd}\mathbf{x}_{jd}^{\top}\,.$$

For differentiating with respect to parameters involved in Σ_{B}, it is advantageous to extract Σ_{B} from ϕ and compensate for it in the terms that involve $\mathbf{z}_{jd}\delta$. Then similar expressions to those for $\partial l_d/\partial\beta$ are obtained:

$$\frac{\partial l_d}{\partial\omega} = \frac{1}{L_d} \int f^{(c)}\left(\mathbf{y}_d \,|\, \mathbf{x}_d, \Sigma_{\mathrm{B}}^{\frac{1}{2}}\gamma\right) \mathbf{s}_{\mathrm{z},d}\left(\Sigma_{\mathrm{B}}^{\frac{1}{2}}\gamma\right) \frac{\partial\Sigma_{\mathrm{B}}^{\frac{1}{2}}}{\partial\gamma}\,\gamma\,\phi\left(\gamma; 0, \mathbf{I}\right) \mathrm{d}\gamma\,,$$

where ω is a parameter involved in $\boldsymbol{\Sigma}_B$ (but not in $\boldsymbol{\beta}$), $\boldsymbol{\gamma}$ represents $\boldsymbol{\Sigma}_B^{-\frac{1}{2}}\boldsymbol{\delta}$, and

$$\mathbf{s}_{z,d}(\boldsymbol{\delta}) = \frac{1}{a}\sum_{j=1}^{n_d}\left[\{y_{jd} - b'(\mathbf{x}_{jd}\boldsymbol{\beta} + \mathbf{z}_{jd}\boldsymbol{\delta})\}\,\mathbf{z}_{jd}\right].$$

Further, for parameters ω_1 and ω_2, both involved in $\boldsymbol{\Sigma}_B$ but neither in $\boldsymbol{\beta}$,

$$\frac{\partial^2 l_d}{\partial\omega_1\,\partial\omega_2} = -\frac{\partial l_d}{\partial\omega_1}\frac{\partial l_d}{\partial\omega_2}$$

$$+ \frac{1}{L_d}\int f^{(c)}(\mathbf{y}_d;\mathbf{x}_d,\boldsymbol{\Sigma}_B)\,\boldsymbol{\gamma}^\top\mathbf{S}_{zz,d}\left(\boldsymbol{\Sigma}^{\frac{1}{2}}\boldsymbol{\gamma}\right)\boldsymbol{\gamma}\frac{\partial\boldsymbol{\Sigma}_B^{\frac{1}{2}}}{\partial\omega_1}\frac{\partial\boldsymbol{\Sigma}_B^{\frac{1}{2}}}{\partial\omega_2}\,\phi\left(\boldsymbol{\gamma};\mathbf{0},\mathbf{I}\right)\,\mathrm{d}\boldsymbol{\gamma}$$

$$+ \frac{1}{L_d}\int f^{(c)}\left(\mathbf{y}_d;\mathbf{x}_d,\boldsymbol{\Sigma}_B^{\frac{1}{2}}\boldsymbol{\gamma}\right)\mathbf{s}_{z,d}\left(\boldsymbol{\Sigma}_B^{\frac{1}{2}}\boldsymbol{\gamma}\right)\boldsymbol{\gamma}\frac{\partial^2\boldsymbol{\Sigma}_B^{\frac{1}{2}}}{\partial\omega_1\,\partial\omega_2}, \qquad (10.16)$$

where

$$\mathbf{S}_{zz,d}(\boldsymbol{\delta}) = \mathbf{s}_{z,d}(\boldsymbol{\delta})\,\mathbf{s}_{z,d}(\boldsymbol{\delta})^\top - \frac{1}{a}\sum_{j=1}^{n_d}b''(\mathbf{x}_{jd}\boldsymbol{\beta} + \mathbf{z}_{jd}\boldsymbol{\delta})\,\mathbf{z}_{jd}\,\mathbf{z}_{jd}^\top.$$

Note that the concluding term in (10.16) vanishes when ω_1 and ω_2 are linear functions of $\boldsymbol{\Sigma}_B^{\frac{1}{2}}$. Thus, some computational advantage is conferred by such a parameterisation, together with the canonical link. Instead of the square-root matrix $\boldsymbol{\Sigma}_B^{\frac{1}{2}}$, the Cholesky decomposition, $\boldsymbol{\Sigma}_B = \mathbf{L}\mathbf{L}^\top$ with a lower tridiagonal matrix $\mathbf{L}$ can be used as a basis for parameterisation of the between-cluster variation.

10.5.3 Laplace Approximation

Although the expressions derived in the previous section are all of the same type as for evaluating the log-likelihood, their evaluation is nevertheless not always feasible. A computationally simpler method is based on approximating the log-likelihood by an expression that involves no integrals.

For this, we apply the Taylor expansion to the conditional log-likelihood $\log\{f^{(c)}(\mathbf{y}_d;\mathbf{x}_d,\boldsymbol{\delta}_d)\}$ around $\log\{f^{(c)}(\mathbf{y}_d;\mathbf{x}_d,\mathbf{0})\}$:

$$\log\left\{f^{(c)}(\mathbf{y}_d;\mathbf{x}_d,\boldsymbol{\delta}_d)\right\} = \log\left\{f^{(c)}(\mathbf{y}_d;\mathbf{x}_d,\mathbf{0})\right\} + \frac{1}{a}\boldsymbol{\delta}_d^\top\mathbf{s}_{z,d}(\mathbf{0})$$

$$-\sum_{k=2}^{\infty}\sum_{j=1}^{n_d}\frac{1}{a\,k!}\left(\mathbf{z}_{jd}\boldsymbol{\delta}_d\right)^k\frac{\partial^{k-2}w_{jd}}{\{\partial(\mathbf{z}_{jd}\boldsymbol{\delta})\}^{k-2}}\Bigg|_{\boldsymbol{\delta}=0},$$

where $w_{jd} = b''(\mathbf{x}_{jd}\boldsymbol{\beta} + \mathbf{z}_{jd}\boldsymbol{\delta})$. We approximate the contribution l_d by the integral of the sum of the first three terms in this expansion:

$$l_d \doteq \log\left\{f^{(c)}(\mathbf{y}_d\,;\mathbf{x}_d\,,\mathbf{0})\right\} - \tfrac{1}{2}r\log(2\pi) - \tfrac{1}{2}\log\left\{\det(\boldsymbol{\Sigma}_{\mathrm{B}})\right\}$$

$$- \log\left[\textstyle\int \exp\left\{\tfrac{1}{a}\boldsymbol{\delta}^{\top}\mathbf{s}_{z,d}(\mathbf{0}) - \tfrac{1}{2}\boldsymbol{\delta}^{\top}\left(\boldsymbol{\Sigma}_{\mathrm{B}}^{-1} + \tfrac{1}{a}\mathbf{Z}_d^{\top}\mathbf{W}_d\mathbf{Z}_d\right)\boldsymbol{\delta}\right\}\,\mathrm{d}\boldsymbol{\delta}\right], \qquad (10.17)$$

where $\mathbf{W}_d$ is the diagonal matrix with its diagonal elements equal to w_{jd}, $j = 1,\ldots,n_d$. The integrand is the exponential of a quadratic function of $\boldsymbol{\delta}$, so it can be matched with the density of an r-variate normal distribution. For brevity, we denote $\mathbf{H}_d = \boldsymbol{\Sigma}_{\mathrm{B}}^{-1} + a^{-1}\mathbf{Z}_d^{\top}\mathbf{W}_d\mathbf{Z}_d$. The integrand is equal to

$$\exp\left[-\frac{1}{2}(\boldsymbol{\delta} - \mathbf{A}_d)^{\top}\mathbf{H}_d(\boldsymbol{\delta} - \mathbf{A}_d) - \frac{1}{2}\left\{\mathbf{s}_{z,d}(\mathbf{0})\right\}^{\top}\mathbf{H}_d^{-1}\mathbf{s}_{z,d}(\mathbf{0})\right],$$

for $\mathbf{A}_d = a^{-1}\mathbf{H}_d^{-1}\mathbf{s}_{z,d}(\mathbf{0})$. In evaluating the integral in (10.17), we make use of the fact that any multivariate normal density integrates to unity. Thus,

$$l_d \doteq \log\left\{f^{(c)}(\mathbf{y}_d\,;\mathbf{x}_d\,,\mathbf{0})\right\} - \frac{1}{2}r\log(2\pi) - \frac{1}{2}\log\left\{\det(\boldsymbol{\Sigma}_{\mathrm{B}})\right\}$$

$$- \frac{1}{2}\log\left\{\det(\mathbf{H}_d)\right\} - \frac{1}{2}\mathbf{A}_d^{\top}\mathbf{H}_d\mathbf{A}_d$$

$$= C + \log\left\{f^{(c)}(\mathbf{y}_d\,;\mathbf{x}_d\,,\mathbf{0})\right\} - \frac{1}{2}\log\left\{\det(\mathbf{G}_d)\right\} - \frac{1}{2a^2}\mathbf{s}_{z,d}^{\top}\boldsymbol{\Sigma}_{\mathrm{B}}^{\frac{1}{2}}\mathbf{G}_d^{-1}\boldsymbol{\Sigma}_{\mathrm{B}}^{\frac{1}{2}}\mathbf{s}_{z,d},$$

where $\mathbf{G}_d = \mathbf{I} + a^{-1}\mathbf{Z}_d^{\top}\mathbf{W}\mathbf{Z}_d\boldsymbol{\Sigma}_{\mathrm{B}}$ and C is a constant. This expression has the form of a log-likelihood for normally distributed outcomes, with deviations $\mathbf{e}_d = \boldsymbol{\Sigma}_{\mathrm{B}}^{\frac{1}{2}}\mathbf{s}_{z,d}(\mathbf{0})$ and variance matrix $a^{-1}\mathbf{W} + \mathbf{Z}_d\boldsymbol{\Sigma}_{\mathrm{B}}\mathbf{Z}_d^{\top}$. If we ignore that $\mathbf{G}_d$ depends on $\boldsymbol{\Sigma}_{\mathrm{B}}$, we could maximise it by the Fisher scoring algorithm applied to the 'normal' version of the likelihood. The estimates of the matrices $\mathbf{G}_d$ have to be updated in every iteration, as $\hat{\boldsymbol{\Sigma}}_{\mathrm{B}}$ and $\hat{\mathbf{W}}_d$ are altered by the iterations.

In the derivations we assumed that $\boldsymbol{\Sigma}_{\mathrm{B}}$ is nonsingular. These methods work also for singular $\boldsymbol{\Sigma}_{\mathrm{B}}$ without needing any adjustments because inversion of $\boldsymbol{\Sigma}_{\mathrm{B}}$ is avoided throughout; only the matrices $\hat{\mathbf{G}}_d$ have to be inverted.

10.5.4 Some Generalisations and Alternatives

We pointed out earlier that the principal rationale for using normally distributed cluster-level deviations is expediency—the multivariate normal distributions have several very convenient properties, foremost among them an analytical form of the density. With GLMs we have to numerically evaluate integrals involved in the likelihood or use some approximations for them, even with normally distributed cluster-level deviations, so the appeal of the normal distributions is not as strong. Instead of the normal densities we might as well use any other class. Nevertheless, it is advantageous to retain some connection with normality. Two devices for this are using transformations of the normal distribution and mixtures of GLMMs.

If we replace normality of the cluster-level deviations by the assumption that they have a class of distributions formed by one or a class of transformations of the normal, the log-likelihood has a similar form, so its maximisation does not introduce any new difficulties. Some classes of transformations retain some features of the normal, such as symmetry and unimodality. It is also advantageous for the transformed distribution to have zero mean, but that can be arranged by subtracting the mean.

As an alternative, we may choose a class of distributions for the coefficients associated with the clusters for which the integrals involved in the marginal distribution can be evaluated analytically. As an example, suppose the outcomes are binary, with no covariates,

$$P(Y_{jd} = 1 \mid p_d) = p_d,$$

so that the marginal distribution is

$$P(Y_{jd} = y) = \int p^y (1 - p)^{1-y} f(p)\, dp,$$

$y = 0, 1$. This integral is easy to evaluate for the density of the beta distribution,

$$f(p) = \frac{\Gamma(a+b)}{\Gamma(a)\,\Gamma(b)} p^{a-1}(1 - p)^{b-1},$$

which has the same form as the probability for the binary distributions, but with the roles of parameters and values of the outcomes interchanged. The beta and binomial distributions are said to be *conjugate*. The marginal probability of positive outcomes in a cluster of m trials is

$$
\begin{aligned}
P(Y_d = y) &= \binom{m}{y} \frac{\Gamma(a+b)}{\Gamma(a)\,\Gamma(b)} \int_0^1 p^{a+y-1}(1-p)^{b+m-y-1}\, dp \\
&= \frac{\Gamma(m+1)\,\Gamma(a+b)}{\Gamma(a)\,\Gamma(b)\,\Gamma(a+b+m)} \frac{\Gamma(a+y)\,\Gamma(b+m-y)}{\Gamma(1+y)\,\Gamma(1+m-y)},
\end{aligned} \tag{10.18}
$$

exploiting the fact that the density of the beta distribution integrates to unity.

The impact of the parameters a and b can be explored on distributions with small m. For $m = 2$, the simplest nontrivial case, the probabilities in (10.18) are $(b^2 + b)/B$, $2ab/B$, and $(a^2 + a)/B$ for $y = 0, 1, 2$, where $B = (a + b)(a + b + 1)$. Compared to the binomial distribution with probabilities $b^2/(a+b)^2$, $2ab/(a+b)^2$, and $a^2/(a+b)^2$ for $y = 0, 1, 2$, the probabilities for $y = 0$ and 2 are increased, $(1+1/b)/\{1+1/(a+b)\}$ and $(1+1/a)/\{1+1/(a+b)\}$ times, respectively, whereas for $y = 1$ they are reduced $1 + 1/(a + b)$ times.

Although the probabilities in (10.18) involve no integrals, ML estimation based on them is far from simple. Moment matching is an alternative. It can be interpreted as finding parameter values $\hat{a}$ and $\hat{b}$ for which the level of overdispersion agrees with its sample (data-based) version. The mean and variance of the beta distribution are $a/(a+b)$ and $ab/(a+b)/(a+b+1)$, respectively. Hence the mean and variance of the marginal distributions are

$$E(Y) = \frac{ma}{a+b}$$

and

$$\text{var}(Y) = \text{var}_{\mathcal{B}}(mp) + E_{\mathcal{B}}\{mp(1-p)\}$$
$$= \frac{m^2ab}{(a+b)^2(a+b+1)} + \frac{ma}{a+b} - \frac{ma(a+1)}{(a+b)(a+b+1)}$$
$$= \frac{mab}{(a+b)(a+b+1)}\left(1 + \frac{m}{a+b}\right),$$

where the subscript $\mathcal{B}$ indicates expectation or variance with respect to the beta distribution. In relation to the binomial distribution with expectation $ma/(a+b)$, $\text{var}(Y)$ is $\{1 - 1/(a+b+1)\}\{1 + m/(a+b)\}$ times greater.

Conjugate cluster-level distributions cannot be defined with elementary-level covariates, when the value of a covariate is defined for every trial within the binomial sequence. Even with cluster-level covariates only categorical variables can be dealt with easily, in essence regarding each category as a separate dataset.

In earlier sections we considered only additive cluster-level deviations. When the multiplicative scale is natural, multiplicative cluster-level deviations are well motivated and give us the advantage of working on the original scale, without any transformations. Models with multiplicative deviations are an alternative to GLM with log link. For instance, with the class of Poisson distributions, the log link converts multiplication to addition on the scale of the linear predictor.

Suppose the outcomes are positive and satisfy the model

$$y_{jd} = y_{jd}^{\circ}\delta_d, \tag{10.19}$$

where y_{jd}° is the outcome that would be realised if the unit were in a 'typical' cluster, for which $\delta_d = 1$. The deviations δ_d are a random sample from a distribution supported on $(0, +\infty)$, with unit mean; $E(\delta_d) = 1$. It is independent of y_{jd}. This distribution is usually skewed, so that its median differs from unity. For y_{jd}° we specify a GLM, so that $E(y_{jd}^{\circ})$ is linked to a linear predictor $\mathbf{x}_{jd}\boldsymbol{\beta}$ and y_{jd}° are mutually independent. To make the problem tractable, we assume that all the covariates are defined for the clusters d, so that within each cluster d, y_{jd}° have identical distributions.

The joint distribution of the outcomes within a cluster cannot be established (the relevant distributions are not specified), so we apply moment matching. Its starting point is evaluation of the means, variances, and covariances of the outcomes. We denote by μ_d the common expectation of y_{jd}°, $j = 1, \ldots, n_d$, and by $V_d = V(\mu_d)$ their common variance. We have

$$E(y_{jd}) = E(y_{jd}^o) E(\delta_d) = \mu_d,$$

$$\text{var}(y_{jd}) = E_{\mathcal{D}}\left(\delta_d^2 V_d\right) + \text{var}_{\mathcal{D}}\left(\delta_d \mu_d\right),$$

$$= \left(1 + \sigma_B^2\right) V_d + \sigma_B^2 \mu_d^2$$

$$\text{cov}\left(y_{j_1 d}, y_{j_2 d}\right) = E_{\mathcal{D}}\left\{\delta_d^2 \text{cov}(y_{j_1 d}, y_{j_2 d})\right\} + \text{cov}_{\mathcal{D}}\left(\delta_d \mu_d, \delta_d \mu_d\right)$$

$$= \sigma_B^2 \mu_d^2,$$

where the subscript $\mathcal{D}$ indicates expectation, variance, or covariance with respect to the distribution of δ_d and $\sigma_B^2 = \text{var}_{\mathcal{D}}(\delta_d)$.

The variance matrix for the set of outcomes in cluster d, $\mathbf{y}_d$, can be expressed compactly as

$$\text{var}(\mathbf{y}_d) = \left(1 + \sigma_B^2\right) V_d \mathbf{I}_{n_d} + \sigma_B^2 \mu_d^2 \mathbf{J}_{n_d}.$$

The within-cluster sample mean $\bar{y}_d = (y_{1d} + \cdots + y_{n_d d})/n_d$ has expectation μ_d and variance

$$U_d = \text{var}(\bar{y}_d) = \frac{1 + \sigma_B^2}{n_d} V_d + \sigma_B^2 \mu_d^2.$$

If the variance σ_B^2 were known we would estimate the regression parameters by fitting a regression to the sample means $\bar{y}_d$. This entails solving the system of nonlinear equations

$$\sum_{d=1}^{D} n_d \frac{\partial \mu_d}{\partial \beta} \hat{U}_d (\bar{y}_d - \hat{\mu}_d) = 0. \tag{10.20}$$

To estimate the variance σ_B^2, we match the expectation of the sum-of-squares statistic $S = \sum_{d=1}^{D} \sum_{j=1}^{n_d} (y_{jd} - \bar{y}_d)^2$ with its expectation. We have

$$E(S) = \sum_{d=1}^{D} E_{\mathcal{D}} \left\{ \sum_{j=1}^{n_d} E\left(y_{jd}^o \delta_{jd} - \frac{1}{n_d} \sum_{j'=1}^{n_d} y_{j'd}^o \delta_{j'd} \right)^2 \right\}$$

$$= \sum_{d=1}^{D} \sum_{j=1}^{n_d} E_{\mathcal{D}} \left\{ \text{var}\left(y_{jd}^o \delta_{jd} - \frac{1}{n_d} \sum_{j'=1}^{n_d} y_{j'd}^o \delta_{j'd} \right) + \mu_d^2 \left(\delta_{jd} - \bar{\delta}_d \right)^2 \right\}$$

$$= \sum_{d=1}^{D} (n_d - 1) \left(V_d + \mu_d^2 \right) \sigma_B^2,$$

where $\bar{\delta}_d = (\delta_{1d} + \cdots + \delta_{n_d d})/n_d$ is the within-cluster sample mean of the δs. Hence the moment-matching estimator

$$\hat{\sigma}_B^2 = \frac{S}{\sum_{d=1}^{D} \left(\hat{V}_d + \hat{\mu}_d^2 \right) (n_d - 1)}. \tag{10.21}$$

This estimator can be motivated as gauging the excess within-cluster variation, on the multiplicative scale. It may seem strange that σ_B^2, a characteristic related to between-cluster variation, is estimated from a within-cluster sum-of-squares statistic. There are alternatives to the statistic S, such as the between-cluster sum of squares $\sum_d n_d (\bar{y}_d - \bar{y})^2$. This statistic is derived from the D sample means $\bar{y}_d$ and can be loosely associated with $D - 1$ degrees of freedom. The heteroscedasticity induced by multiplicative random terms leaves an imprint also on the within-cluster statistic S. We prefer to use S because it is associated with many more degrees of freedom, about $n - D$.

Equations (10.20) and (10.21) have to be iterated because after updating the regression parameter estimates $\hat{\boldsymbol{\beta}}$ we have to recalculate the value of S, and after updating $\hat{\sigma}_B^2$ the values of $\hat{U}_d$ and $\hat{\mu}_d$ are altered and (10.20) has to be solved (iteratively) again. There is no guarantee that this algorithm converges. For starting values of $\hat{\boldsymbol{\beta}}$, we may set $\hat{\sigma}_B^2 = 0$ and solve (10.20). Statistics alternative to S can be used for diagnostics. For the fitted model we evaluate such a statistic T and generate its values for datasets simulated according to the fitted model. Evidence against validity of the model corresponds to the value of T for the realised dataset being at the extreme or outside the range of the simulated values of T.

Suggested Reading

The original paper on GLM is [138], and [132] is without dispute the principal reference on GLM. The GLM methods were implemented in the software GLIM (web site

www.nottingham.ac.uk/is/services/software/is-machines/appls/glim.phtml),

which had a near monopoly on model fitting until the advent in the early 1990s of the new generation of statistical software and Splus in particular. Textbooks on GLM with a practical orientation include [1], [38] and [84], the last focussing on the logistic regression. Concise descriptions of methods for overdispersion are found in [195] and [11].

Some analytical difficulties with GLM can be overcome by defining suitable approximations to the densities or probabilities or to the log-likelihood. The term *quasi-likelihood* is often used in this context; see [193] for the original contribution and [137] for an extension. Approximate maximum likelihood for GLMM using the Laplace transformation is derived in [12], and the Gaussian quadrature is described in [114]. More recent developments in statistical computing, motivated mainly by problems in Bayesian analysis and supported by greatly enhanced computational power, have made these methods somewhat obsolete; see [133]. Inference with models with multiplicative random deviations is discussed in [49]. A likelihood-related theory that bypasses all the difficulties with integration is developed in [99] and extended in [100].

Problems and Exercises

10.1. Generalised ANOVA. A set of D independent binomial outcomes, with y_d successes out of m_d independent trials with probabilities p_d, $d = 1, \ldots, D$, differs from the ANOVA setting only by the distributional assumption. Derive the maximum likelihood estimators of the probabilities p_d and verify that they coincide with the estimators derived from the fit of the logistic regression model

$$\text{logit} \{P(y_{jd} = 1)\} = \beta_0 + \beta_d,$$

where y_{jd} is the ith (binary) outcome in set d. Generalise this to other link functions for binomial outcomes. Can this equivalence be extended to outcomes with other distributions?

10.2. Compile a programme (function) for fitting GLM to conditionally independent binary outcomes. In the programme, the link function should be an argument. In the output, include information about the speed of convergence and an assessment of the fit of the model.

10.3. Generate the values of a variable X on a sample of subjects of size $n = 250$ as a random sample from the uniform distribution, and for these values generate a set of binary outcomes Y according to the logistic regression model

$$\text{logit} \{P(y_j = 1)\} = \beta_0 + x_j \beta_x,$$

with $\beta_0 = -0.5$ and $\beta_x = 0.75$. Fit the logistic regression by maximum likelihood and compare the estimates $\hat{\beta}_0$ and $\hat{\beta}_x$ with the fit of the ordinary regression of Y on X (disregarding the obvious nonnormality of Y). Describe how and explain why the two pairs of estimates are related. Repeat the exercise with the probit link function.

10.4. For a binary outcome Y with probability p, $\text{var}(Y) = p(1 - p)$. Suppose $\hat{p}$ is the proportion of successes in a sequence of n independent trials, each with probability p. Is $\hat{p}(1 - \hat{p})/n$ an unbiased estimator of $\text{var}(\hat{p})$? If not, adjust this estimator for its bias. Explain the problem that arises when $\hat{p} = 0$, and devise some remedies.

10.5. Describe all the circumstances in which the logistic regression with a single covariate cannot be fitted because the provisional information matrix for the regression parameters is singular. Do your conclusions carry over to other link functions?

10.6. Derive the score and information matrix for the linear regression for binary outcomes with the complementary log-log link.

10.7. Explore GLMs for outcomes with conditional beta distribution, and discuss their connection to GLMs for binary outcomes.

10.8. *Binomial outcomes with excess zeros.* Suppose outcomes are generated as random samples from a distribution that is a mixture of a binomial with denominator $n = 12$ and identical zero. The binomial is realised with probability $r = 0.7$ and the (excess) zero with probability 0.3. Derive the mean and variance of this mixture distribution and work out when the mixture amounts to overdispersion. Devise a method for estimating the proportion of extra zeros.

10.9. Show that a mixture of two Poisson distributions, with expectations λ_1 and λ_2 and respective probabilities p and $1 - p$, can be used for modelling overdispersion of counts. (Derive the expectation and variance of the mixture, and show that the variance exceeds the expectation.) Describe the impact the probability p and the absolute difference $|\lambda_1 - \lambda_2|$ have on the extent of overdispersion. Generalise this description to mixtures with several components.

10.10. Generate random samples from binomial distributions and assess their proximity to a Poisson distribution by comparing the sample proportions of the values of the outcomes with the probabilities of the Poisson distribution that fits to them best. Define a rule of thumb that arbitrates whether the distribution for a probability p and number of trials m is close to a Poisson distribution. Relate this rule to the condition that np^2 is smaller than a set threshold.

10.11. Adapt the programme compiled in Exercise 10.2 to a limited set of other distributions and the associated canonical links. The dataset in file EX9a.dat on www.sntl.co.uk/BookA/Data contains the numbers of homicides in the cities with population greater than 50 000 in a country in 2001. The population of each city and the proportion of substandard residential housing is also given. Relate the number of homicides to these two covariates and assess the quality of the fit and presence of outliers. Can it be concluded that poor housing is a cause of high homicide rate?

10.12. Suppose the survival to the age of one month of a young of a species of mammal is independent of the survival of the siblings in the litter given the litter's probability of survival. Marginally, the litters' probabilities of survival have a beta distribution, $\mathcal{B}(a, b)$ with $a = 0.2$ and $b = 0.8$. Try to guess the probability that the whole litter of five survives one month after birth and the probability that none of the litter survives, and then compare your guesses with the results obtained by simulations. Compare the marginal probability of survival with the probability of survival in a typical litter, in which the probability of survival is $a/(a + b)$.

10.13. Explore how importance sampling (Section 4.2) can be applied to evaluate the integral in (10.14) and its partial differentials, first for the case of parallel regressions (univariate integration). Describe the difficulties that arise when a distribution different from the normal is used for δ_d.

10.14. A binary outcome can be regarded as a coarse version of a normally distributed outcome. This motivates an application of the missing data methods in which incompleteness is brought about by coarsening. Develop this idea and discuss its (computational) advantages in the setting of random coefficient models.

10.15. A national employment agency applies the policy of finding three vacant posts for each client (job seeker) in the first round of their engagement. The headquarters produces quarterly summaries of its nationwide business with first-time clients by tabulating the numbers of offers made to them within four weeks of the date of application. For example, the table for the third quarter of 2005 (27 161 clients) is

	Number of offers			
	0	1	2	3
Number of applicants	8035	10 770	6191	2165

As a refinement, they intend to fit a logistic regression to such data in the future, assuming that the conditional distribution of the outcomes is binomial (with denominator $m = 3$), given suitable covariates, such as qualifications, experience, age, flexibility and the like, suitably coded. Give advice on the potential value of such an analysis.

Hint: If a suitable set of covariates is used, then the conditional variance of the outcome for client j is equal to $mp_j(1 - p_j)$, where p_j is the probability implied by the model. Therefore, a diagnostic procedure may be based on an assessment of whether the estimates of such variances agree with the sample variances within narrow bands (bins) of the predictions $\hat{p}_j$. If one or several important covariates are dropped, overdispersion can be expected. Hence, the usefulness of any covariates can be assessed by the extent of overdispersion in the 'unadjusted' data in the table.

10.16. Adapt the programme you compiled in Exercise 9.19 or 9.21 for random coefficient models with the normality assumptions to their counterpart for logistic regression using Laplace approximation.

10.17. Derive the marginal distribution, that is, the probabilities $P(X = k)$, $k = 0, 1, \ldots$, for the model with conditional Poisson distributions,

$$P(X = k \mid \lambda_d, d) = \frac{e^{-\lambda_d} \lambda_d^k}{k!}$$

within clusters d, and gamma distribution of their conditional expectations λ_d, with the density

$$f(\lambda; \theta, c) = \frac{1}{\Gamma(c)} \theta^c \lambda^{c-1} \exp(-\lambda\theta)$$

for parameters $c > 0$ and $\theta > 0$.

Longitudinal and Time-Series Analysis

Longitudinal analysis is concerned with studying the progression of the values of a variable over time for the members of a population. If time is defined as a categorical variable, longitudinal analysis is closely related to multivariate analysis, studying vectors of outcomes. When time is a continuous variable, longitudinal analysis studies the subjects' curves (trajectories), and random coefficient models are well suited for this purpose. We can associate each time point with a separate variable, in the spirit of the original definition of the term *variable*. Then longitudinal analysis is the study of collections of variables; in most applications the variables are strongly associated. Features of this association are frequently the targets of inference.

11.1 Introduction

In longitudinal studies we work with populations and variables that are well defined at specified time points. For example, all those obliged to make annual declarations of income to the tax authority of a country are a population and the income of each of them is well defined by the rules of the authority in every year. Figure 11.1 summarises the income of a small random sample of taxpayers aged 25 in 1995 (year 0) in a country over the period of seven years, 1996–2002, coded as 1–7. The left-hand panel plots the values of income on the original scale and the right-hand panel on the logarithmic scale. The seven values of a subject are connected by straight lines. In the diagram, we can identify and describe certain features, such as the extent to which the lines criss-cross, how much they fan out over the seven years, and for how many subjects there are substantial changes from one year to the next. As an alternative, the values of the income may be described by a seven-variate distribution. The normal distribution would be convenient for this purpose because we are familiar with it. By applying the log-transformation to each component, the assumption of normality becomes much more palatable, so a

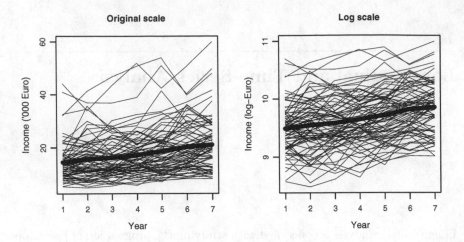

Fig. 11.1. Income (in Euros) of a simple random sample of 80 taxpayers who were 25 years old in 1995, in a country over the seven following years (1996–2002). The thick line represents their average on the original and log scales in the respective panels.

suitable description is provided in the form $\log(\mathbf{Y}) \sim \mathcal{N}(\boldsymbol{\mu}, \boldsymbol{\Sigma})$ for the vector of incomes $\mathbf{Y}$.

On the original scale, in Euros, there appear to be a few subjects whose income is exceptionally high throughout the seven years. The distribution of incomes is skewed in every year. The annual distributions of log-income are much closer to symmetry, and the annual maxima of log-income are much less exceptional than they are on the original scale. For most subjects, income does not change a great deal from one year to the next, so few of those with high income in year 1 have low income in year 7 or vice versa.

We can complement the plots in Fig. 11.1 by the within-year univariate summaries, such as the sample means and variances:

$$\hat{\mu} = 10^3 \times (14.45, \ 15.64, \ 16.12, \ 17.13, \ 18.55, \ 20.20, \ 20.93) \,,$$

$$\operatorname{diag}\left(\hat{\boldsymbol{\Sigma}}\right) = 10^6 \times (49.37, \ 61.18, \ 63.95, \ 73.59, \ 89.60, \ 80.13, \ 97.71)$$

on the original scale and

$$\hat{\mu} = (9.49, \ 9.55, \ 9.58, \ 9.65, \ 9.72, \ 9.82, \ 9.85) \,,$$

$$\operatorname{diag}\left(\hat{\boldsymbol{\Sigma}}\right) = (0.17, \ 0.23, \ 0.20, \ 0.20, \ 0.21, \ 0.18, \ 0.20) \tag{11.1}$$

on the log scale. These summaries confirm that the average income increases over the years and becomes more dispersed on the original scale, but they do not inform us about the year-to-year changes in the income of individual

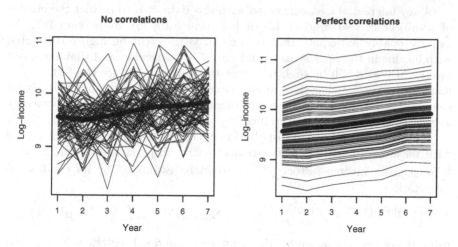

Fig. 11.2. Examples of extreme patterns of changes of income, based on the summaries in (11.1).

subjects. At one extreme, annual income varying wildly from one year to the next, and at another, income increasing in an orderly manner, are compatible with the description in (11.1). Figure 11.2 gives corresponding examples. In the left-hand panel, the incomes in any pair of distinct years are independent, whereas in the right-hand panel they are perfectly correlated. The two scenarios are equally unrealistic, but they both conform with the summaries in (11.1).

These summaries are incomplete because they convey no information about the associations of income across time. This is remedied by the sample correlation matrix (for log-income), equal to

$$\widehat{\text{cor}}(\mathbf{Y}) = \frac{1}{100} \begin{pmatrix} 100 & 84 & 83 & 78 & 75 & 74 & 77 \\ 84 & 100 & 90 & 85 & 81 & 78 & 74 \\ 83 & 90 & 100 & 89 & 87 & 81 & 80 \\ 78 & 85 & 89 & 100 & 90 & 91 & 88 \\ 74 & 78 & 81 & 85 & 91 & 100 & 91 \\ 77 & 74 & 80 & 84 & 88 & 91 & 100 \end{pmatrix} .$$

In the right-hand panel of Figure 11.2, $\text{cor}(\mathbf{Y}) = \mathbf{I}$, and in the left-hand panel $\text{cor}(\mathbf{Y}) = \mathbf{1}\mathbf{1}^{\top}$. Our data are closer to the latter case. The annual incomes of a subject are highly correlated, especially for consecutive years.

Working with log-income is advantageous because the data conform much more closely to multivariate normality. A small difference Δ on the log-scale is easily converted to relative change as $\exp(\Delta) - 1 \doteq \Delta$, that is, an increase by approximately $100\Delta\%$. For example, $\Delta = 0.03$ corresponds to $\exp(0.03) - 1 = 1.0305$, or an increase by 3.05%.

A key inferential task connected with this dataset is to predict the income of a subject in year 8, given his or her income history from years 1–7. We can reasonably anticipate that income in year 8 will be highly correlated with income in the earlier years, and year 7 in particular, and that the mean income in year 8 will be slightly higher than in year 7, since the (estimated) mean annual income has risen in every one of the seven years for the analysed sample. The estimated variances, the diagonal of $\hat{\Sigma}$, show no trend, so we may assume that the population variance in year 8 will be in the range $(0.17, 0.23)$.

If we knew that the joint distribution of the incomes in years 1–8 is normal with mean vector $\mu^{(1-8)}$ and variance matrix $\Sigma_{(1-8)}$, the income in year 8 for a given income history $y^{(1-7)}$ could be estimated by its conditional expectation

$$\mathrm{E}\left(Y^{(8)} \mid \mathbf{Y}^{(1-7)} = \mathbf{y}^{(1-7)}\right) = \mu^{(8)} + \Sigma_{(8,1-7)}\Sigma_{(1-7)}^{-1}\left(\mathbf{y}^{(1-7)} - \mu^{(1-7)}\right),$$

using the obvious notation for the submatrices and subvectors of $\Sigma_{(1-8)}$ and $\mu^{(1-8)}$, and with all population quantities replaced by their estimates. The conditional variance,

$$\Sigma_{(8\mid 1-7)} = \Sigma_{8,8} - \Sigma_{(8,1-7)}\Sigma_{(1-7)}^{-1}\Sigma_{(1-7,8)},$$

or its estimator, indicates the uncertainty about the (future) value of $Y^{(8)}$, assuming that $\mu^{(1-8)}$ and $\Sigma_{(1-8)}$ are known. We refer to $\sqrt{\Sigma_{(8\mid 1-7)}}$ as the conditional standard deviation.

Without information external to the data, inferences about the mean and variance of the incomes in year 8 are difficult to make, because they are based, in effect, on only seven observations, the corresponding summaries for years 1–7. They would be based on only seven observations (degrees of freedom) even if the entire population were observed in years 1–7 and the values of $\mu^{(1-7)}$ were known. Although no radical changes may have been observed in years 1–7, the seven years of observations are not sufficient to rule out a sudden shock that would have an effect on the employment and income of the studied population. Such shocks happen infrequently and without any recognisable signals announcing their arrival in the near future.

We face an apparently similar problem when studying a small population that contains a small fraction of exceptional members. A random sample of small size might contain no such members as its subjects. In studying the years 1–7, we may also consider a population of years, e.g., dating back to a notable year, such as the end of World War II, but the years 1–7 cannot be regarded as a random sample from them. Nevertheless, income in years 1–7 is the most relevant for information about income in year 8.

We could condition our inferences about $(Y^{(8)} \mid \mathbf{Y}^{(1-7)} = \mathbf{y})$ on particular scenarios, described by the mean vector $\mu^{(1-8)}$ and variance matrix $\Sigma_{(1-8)}$, and carefully qualify them by these assumptions. By way of an example, we consider the three income histories given in Table 11.1 and assume two scenarios:

Table 11.1. Prediction for log-income histories with scenarios 1 and 2 (see text). For the scenarios, predictions and the associated standard errors (in parentheses) are given for three income histories.

| Subject | Income history (year) | | | | | | | Scenario | |
	1	2	3	4	5	6	7	1	2
A	9.24	9.01	9.18	9.45	9.14	9.21	9.01	9.26 (0.18)	9.27 (0.28)
B	9.20	9.18	9.24	9.25	9.24	9.27	9.27	9.34 (0.18)	9.43 (0.28)
C	9.10	9.20	9.35	9.45	9.52	9.60	9.71	9.74 (0.18)	9.76 (0.28)

1. $\mu^{(8)} = 9.89$, $\Sigma_8 = 0.20$ and $\mathbf{R}_{(8,1-7)} = \frac{1}{100}(91, 88, 84, 80, 77, 74, 70)$;

2. $\mu^{(8)} = 9.94$, $\Sigma_8 = 0.25$ and $\mathbf{R}_{(8,1-7)} = \frac{1}{100}(81, 78, 76, 74, 72, 70, 68)$,

where $\mathbf{R}_{(1-8)}$ is the correlation matrix that corresponds to $\Sigma_{(1-8)}$. The first scenario can be regarded as more settled, with smaller variance and higher correlations, and the second as more volatile, with greater variance and smaller correlations. The three subjects for whom predictions are sought are represented by their income histories. Subject A has a relatively volatile history of income, with substantial drops and increases from one year to the next, subject B has nearly constant income over the seven years, and subject C has above-average increases in most years.

The predictions differ somewhat under the two scenarios, but by far less than the conditional standard deviations. Uncertainty within a scenario is much greater than the uncertainty about the scenario, although the latter is not trivial either. Within a scenario, the subjects' conditional standard deviations are the same, equal to 0.18 and 0.28. This is a consequence of the normality assumptions. Although analytically very convenient, it may not be realistic. For example, we would expect a greater standard error of prediction for subject A because his or her history suggests less predictability than for subjects B and C. Also, the predictions have the following translation property. For any vector of constants $\mathbf{c}$,

$$E\left(Y^{(8)} \mid \mathbf{Y}^{(1-7)} = \mathbf{y} + \mathbf{c}\right) = d + E\left(Y^{(8)} \mid \mathbf{Y}^{(1-7)} = \mathbf{y}\right),$$

where d is a constant that does not depend on $\mathbf{y}$. In fact, $d = \Sigma_{(8,1-7)} \Sigma_{(1-7)}^{-1} \mathbf{c}$.

The importance of the distant past for prediction can be assessed by comparing the predictions in Table 11.1 with their counterparts obtained after discarding the data for the first few years. Judging by the conditional standard deviations, the years 1, 2, and 3 are not important; the estimated standard deviations $\sqrt{\hat{\Sigma}_{(8|4-7)}}$ are greater than $\sqrt{\hat{\Sigma}_{(8|1-7)}}$ by only 0.0023 and 0.0039 for the respective scenarios 1 and 2. However, the predictions are altered out of proportion with these figures for subject A; they are increased by 0.030

(scenario 1) and 0.051 (scenarios 2). The corresponding changes for the other two subjects are much smaller, 0.018 and -0.017 for scenario 1 and -0.009 and 0.024 for scenario 2 for the respective subjects B and C.

11.2 Markov Property

In the example analysed in the previous section, we could have used for prediction only data from year 7 and the conditional standard deviations would not have been much greater than if data from all years 1–7 were used (0.185 and 0.293, compared to 0.176 and 0.283, respectively). In both scenarios, the annual incomes are close to having the property that $\left(Y^{(8)} \mid \mathbf{Y}^{(1-7)}\right) \sim \left(Y^{(8)} \mid Y^{(7)}\right)$ or, more generally, that two observations in time are conditionally independent given any intermediate observation:

$$\left(Y^{(k)} \mid Y^{(h_1)}, Y^{(h_2)}\right) \sim \left(Y^{(k)} \mid Y^{(h_1)}\right),$$

when $k > h_1 > h_2$. This is called the *Markov property*. The Markov property can be detected in the variance matrix of the sequence $\mathbf{Y}$ or, more precisely, in its inverse. The inverse of the variance matrix is called the *concentration matrix*. We use the notation 'con' for concentration matrices; for example, $\text{con}(\mathbf{Y}) = \boldsymbol{\Sigma}^{-1}$. For submatrices of a concentration matrix, we have to indicate the original matrix because, in general, the concentration matrix of a subvector $\mathbf{Y}^{(1)}$ of $\mathbf{Y}$ is not equal to the corresponding submatrix of $\text{con}(\mathbf{Y})$. An unambiguous notation is $\text{con}\left(\mathbf{Y}^{(1)}, \mathbf{Y}^{(2)} \mid \mathbf{Y}\right)$ for the submatrix of $\text{con}(\mathbf{Y})$ that corresponds to $\mathbf{Y}^{(1)}$ (rows) and $\mathbf{Y}^{(2)}$ (columns).

A sequence of variables $Y^{(1)}, \ldots, Y^{(K)}$ has the Markov property when the inverse of their variance matrix is tridiagonal; that is, the only nonzero elements of the inverse are on the diagonal and immediately below and above it. To prove this for vectors with multivariate normal distribution, we derive first a seemingly more general result. Let $\mathbf{Y}^{(1)}$, $\mathbf{Y}^{(2)}$, and $\mathbf{Y}^{(3)}$ be three vectors such that $\mathbf{Y}^{(1)}$ and $\mathbf{Y}^{(3)}$ are conditionally independent given the value of $\mathbf{Y}^{(2)}$. Let their variance matrix be

$$\boldsymbol{\Sigma} = \begin{pmatrix} \boldsymbol{\Sigma}_{11} & \boldsymbol{\Sigma}_{12} & \boldsymbol{\Sigma}_{13} \\ \boldsymbol{\Sigma}_{21} & \boldsymbol{\Sigma}_{22} & \boldsymbol{\Sigma}_{23} \\ \boldsymbol{\Sigma}_{31} & \boldsymbol{\Sigma}_{32} & \boldsymbol{\Sigma}_{33} \end{pmatrix},$$

partitioned compatibly with $\mathbf{Y}_1$, $\mathbf{Y}_2$, and $\mathbf{Y}_3$, and denote its inverse similarly, with indices in the superscript; for example, $\boldsymbol{\Sigma}^{(12)} = \text{con}\left(\mathbf{Y}^{(1)}, \mathbf{Y}^{(2)} \mid \mathbf{Y}\right)$. Then $\boldsymbol{\Sigma}^{(13)} = \mathbf{0}$. That is, conditional independence of $\mathbf{A}$ and $\mathbf{C}$ given condition $\mathbf{B} = \mathbf{b}$ corresponds to zeros in the concentration submatrix

$$\text{con}\left(\mathbf{A}, \mathbf{C} \mid \mathbf{A}, \mathbf{B}, \mathbf{C}\right).$$

(We could omit $\mathbf{A}$ and $\mathbf{C}$ from the condition.)

We derive first an alternative characterisation of conditional independence. Conditional independence of $\mathbf{Y}^{(1)}$ and $\mathbf{Y}^{(3)}$ given a value of $\mathbf{Y}^{(2)}$ is equivalent to the equality of the distributions

$$\left(\mathbf{Y}^{(1)} \mid \mathbf{Y}^{(2)} = \mathbf{y}^{(2)}\right) \sim \left(\mathbf{Y}^{(1)} \mid \mathbf{Y}^{(2)} = \mathbf{y}^{(2)}, \mathbf{Y}^{(3)} = \mathbf{y}^{(3)}\right),$$

for any vectors $\mathbf{y}^{(2)}$ and $\mathbf{y}^{(3)}$. For the corresponding conditional variance matrices, this means that

$$\boldsymbol{\Sigma}_{11} - \boldsymbol{\Sigma}_{12}\boldsymbol{\Sigma}_{22}^{-1}\boldsymbol{\Sigma}_{21} = \boldsymbol{\Sigma}_{11} - \begin{pmatrix} \boldsymbol{\Sigma}_{21} \\ \boldsymbol{\Sigma}_{31} \end{pmatrix}^{\top} \begin{pmatrix} \boldsymbol{\Sigma}_{22} & \boldsymbol{\Sigma}_{23} \\ \boldsymbol{\Sigma}_{32} & \boldsymbol{\Sigma}_{33} \end{pmatrix}^{-1} \begin{pmatrix} \boldsymbol{\Sigma}_{21} \\ \boldsymbol{\Sigma}_{31} \end{pmatrix}. \tag{11.2}$$

For the inverse on the right-hand side, we have the expression

$$\begin{pmatrix} \boldsymbol{\Sigma}_{22} & \boldsymbol{\Sigma}_{23} \\ \boldsymbol{\Sigma}_{32} & \boldsymbol{\Sigma}_{33} \end{pmatrix}^{-1} = \begin{pmatrix} \boldsymbol{\Sigma}_{22}^{-1} + \mathbf{E}\mathbf{F}^{-1}\mathbf{E}^{\top} & -\mathbf{E}\mathbf{F}^{-1} \\ -\mathbf{F}^{-1}\mathbf{E}^{\top} & \mathbf{F}^{-1} \end{pmatrix}, \tag{11.3}$$

where $\mathbf{E} = \boldsymbol{\Sigma}_{22}^{-1}\boldsymbol{\Sigma}_{23}$ and $\mathbf{F} = \boldsymbol{\Sigma}_{33} - \boldsymbol{\Sigma}_{32}\boldsymbol{\Sigma}_{22}^{-1}\boldsymbol{\Sigma}_{23}$. The formula for the inverse can be verified by multiplication with the original matrix. With this formula, the identity in (11.2) is equivalent to

$$\mathbf{0} = \begin{pmatrix} \boldsymbol{\Sigma}_{21} \\ \boldsymbol{\Sigma}_{31} \end{pmatrix}^{\top} \begin{pmatrix} \mathbf{E}\mathbf{F}^{-1}\mathbf{E}^{\top} & -\mathbf{E}\mathbf{F}^{-1} \\ -\mathbf{F}^{-1}\mathbf{E}^{\top} & \mathbf{F}^{-1} \end{pmatrix} \begin{pmatrix} \boldsymbol{\Sigma}_{21} \\ \boldsymbol{\Sigma}_{31} \end{pmatrix}$$

$$= \left(\boldsymbol{\Sigma}_{12}\mathbf{E} - \boldsymbol{\Sigma}_{13}\right)\mathbf{F}^{-1}\left(\boldsymbol{\Sigma}_{12}\mathbf{E} - \boldsymbol{\Sigma}_{13}\right)^{\top},$$

that is,

$$\boldsymbol{\Sigma}_{13} = \boldsymbol{\Sigma}_{12}\boldsymbol{\Sigma}_{22}^{-1}\boldsymbol{\Sigma}_{23}, \tag{11.4}$$

since $\mathbf{F}$ is positive definite. We obtained the univariate version of this identity in Chapter 6 in connection with impartiality, interpreting it as absence of the partial correlation of $\mathbf{Y}^{(1)}$ and $\mathbf{Y}^{(3)}$ given the value of $\mathbf{Y}^{(2)}$. Finally, we relate this identity to the submatrices of $\boldsymbol{\Sigma}^{-1}$. We have

$$\boldsymbol{\Sigma}_{21}\boldsymbol{\Sigma}^{(11)} + \boldsymbol{\Sigma}_{22}\boldsymbol{\Sigma}^{(21)} + \boldsymbol{\Sigma}_{23}\boldsymbol{\Sigma}^{(31)} = \mathbf{0},$$

$$\boldsymbol{\Sigma}_{31}\boldsymbol{\Sigma}^{(11)} + \boldsymbol{\Sigma}_{32}\boldsymbol{\Sigma}^{(21)} + \boldsymbol{\Sigma}_{33}\boldsymbol{\Sigma}^{(31)} = \mathbf{0},$$

since these are off-diagonal blocks in the product $\boldsymbol{\Sigma}^{-1}\boldsymbol{\Sigma} = \mathbf{I}$. By subtracting the $\boldsymbol{\Sigma}_{32}\boldsymbol{\Sigma}_{22}^{-1}$ premultiple of the first equation from the second and exploiting the identity in (11.4), we obtain the identity

$$\left(\boldsymbol{\Sigma}_{33} - \boldsymbol{\Sigma}_{32}\boldsymbol{\Sigma}_{22}^{-1}\boldsymbol{\Sigma}_{23}\right)\boldsymbol{\Sigma}^{(31)} = \mathbf{0},$$

which, since $\mathbf{F} = \boldsymbol{\Sigma}_{33} - \boldsymbol{\Sigma}_{32}\boldsymbol{\Sigma}_{22}^{-1}\boldsymbol{\Sigma}_{23}$ is positive definite, is satisfied only when $\boldsymbol{\Sigma}^{(13)} = \mathbf{0}$. Although we proved this characterisation only for multivariate normally distributed vectors, it holds generally, for all vectors with finite variance matrices.

For a vector $\mathbf{Y}$ with the Markov property, Y_{k-1} and Y_{k+1} are conditionally independent given the value of Y_k for $k = 2, \ldots, K - 1$. Then $(Y_1, \ldots, Y_{k-1})$ and $(Y_{k+1}, \ldots, Y_K)$ are conditionally independent given the value of Y_k, and so the elements $C_{h,m}$ of $\mathbf{C} = \mathrm{con}(\mathbf{Y})$ vanish whenever $0 < h < k < m \leq K$. This is the case for each $k = 2, \ldots, K - 1$, so $\mathbf{C}$ is tridiagonal.

The joint density of a vector $\mathbf{Y}$ with the Markov property can be factorized as

$$f(y_1)\, f(y_2 \mid y_1)\, f(y_3 \mid y_2)\, \cdots\, f(y_K \mid y_{K-1}) \tag{11.5}$$

into a product of univariate conditional densities. Thus, any likelihood-related analysis, such as maximum likelihood, comprises K univariate analyses, although estimation of parameters shared by these K distributions would involve all the outcomes. Further, when we can rely on some structural symmetry in how Y_k are related to the preceding outcomes, the same model can be posited for each conditional distribution in (11.5). Of course, the model parameters are likely to be time-dependent. Then the model specification is reduced to the model for Y_1 and for the 'one-step' conditional distributions $(Y_{k+1} \mid Y_k = y)$. Regression models are prime candidates for the latter, for normally distributed outcomes and, more generally, for distributions in the exponential family. We can take advantage of the full flexibility of GLM by specifying models by a variance function instead of a class of distributions.

The joint density of $\mathbf{Y}$ can be expressed in terms of univariate conditional densities even without the Markov property, but these densities involve progressively more extensive conditioning:

$$f(y_1)\, f(y_2 \mid y_1)\, f(y_3 \mid y_1, y_2)\, \cdots\, f(y_K \mid y_1, y_2, \ldots, y_{K-1}).$$

We can check how close the annual incomes are to the Markov property. The sample concentration matrix in scenario 1 (see Table 11.1) is

$$
\begin{pmatrix}
26.3 & -11.9 & 6.7 & 0.6 & 4.2 & 1.0 & -13.8 & 11.8 \\
-11.9 & 31.0 & -16.1 & -7.0 & 0.6 & -5.9 & 12.5 & -13.5 \\
-6.7 & -16.1 & 43.4 & -10.4 & -12.3 & 4.9 & -1.3 & -0.8 \\
0.6 & -7.0 & -10.4 & 38.1 & -13.9 & -0.8 & -6.3 & 2.3 \\
4.2 & 0.6 & -12.3 & -13.9 & 46.9 & -20.2 & -7.2 & 1.1 \\
1.0 & -5.9 & 4.9 & -0.8 & -20.2 & 50.7 & -17.2 & -18.8 \\
-13.8 & 12.5 & -1.3 & -6.3 & -7.2 & -17.2 & 54.0 & -52.5 \\
11.8 & -13.5 & -0.8 & 2.3 & 1.1 & -18.8 & -52.5 & 168.9
\end{pmatrix} ;
$$

although the elements outside the diagonal strip do not vanish, many of them are quite small. The concentration matrix for scenario 2 has similar features.

11.3 Time Series

Among multivariate normal vectors with the Markov property, a special case is defined by the same model for each one-step conditional distribution $(Y_{k+1} \mid Y_k)$, $k = 1, \ldots, K - 1$:

$$Y_{k+1} = \beta_0 + \beta_1 Y_k + \varepsilon^{(k)}, \tag{11.6}$$

where $\varepsilon^{(k)} \sim \mathcal{N}(0, \sigma^2)$. The realisations of $\varepsilon^{(k)}$ are independent both within a time point k (for different subjects) and across time points $k = 1, \ldots, K - 1$. A separate model has to be specified for time point 1, such as $Y_1 \sim \mathcal{N}(\mu, \tau^2)$. To avoid any trivial cases, we assume that $\sigma^2 > 0$ and $K > 2$.

We may consider an infinite sequence $\mathbf{Y} = (Y_1, Y_2, \ldots)$; it is called a *time series*. A time series $\mathbf{Y}$ is said to be *stationary* if its components have identical distributions. The model given by (11.6) is stationary only when $\beta_0 = 0$, $\beta_1 = 1$ and $\tau^2 = 0$. A condition weaker than stationarity is that the components of $\mathbf{Y}$ have a limiting distribution. This condition is satisfied when $|\beta_1| < 1$, and the limiting distribution is then $\mathcal{N}\{\beta_0/(1 - \beta_1), \sigma^2/(1 - \beta_1^2)\}$. Note that the parameters of the initial distribution, μ and τ^2, play no role in the limiting distribution, when it exists.

A sequence defined by (11.6) is called *autoregressive* (AR). The assumption of normality may be dropped and replaced by that of a centred distribution for ε with a finite variance. The AR time series can be generalised by replacing the simple (one-step) regression with regression on the preceding m outcomes:

$$Y_{k+m} = \beta_0 + \beta_1 Y_{k+m-1} + \beta_2 Y_{k+m-2} + \cdots + \beta_m Y_k + \varepsilon^{(k+m)}.$$

The corresponding series $\mathbf{Y}$ is called AR or order m, denoted by AR(m), so that the sequence defined by (11.6) is AR(1). In an AR(m) series, components Y_k and Y_{k+h} ($k > 0$ and $h > 0$) are conditionally independent given the intermediate history, the values $(Y_{k+1}, \ldots, Y_{k+h-1})$, so long as $h \geq m$. Therefore the concentration matrix $\mathbf{C}$ of a segment $\mathbf{Y}^{(1-K)}$ has nonzero entries only up to the distance m from the diagonal: $C_{k_1 k_2} = 0$ if $|k_1 - k_2| > h$.

We can regard longitudinal data as replicates of a segment of time series. The replication is invaluable for efficient estimation of the parameters that govern the underlying process. Autoregressive time series motivates the model in which the concentration matrix has zeros in entries distant from the diagonal. The corresponding log-likelihood is $l = l_1 + \cdots + l_K$, where observations $\mathbf{y}_j$ of subject j contribute with

$$l_j = \frac{1}{2} \log\{\det(\mathbf{C})\} - \frac{1}{2}(\mathbf{y}_j - \boldsymbol{\mu})^\top \mathbf{C}(\mathbf{y}_j - \boldsymbol{\mu}), \tag{11.7}$$

and $\mathbf{Y} \sim \mathcal{N}(\boldsymbol{\mu}, \mathbf{C}^{-1})$. The log-likelihood can be maximised by the Fisher scoring algorithm, making use of the formulae for differentiation of matrices, as done in Chapter 9.

11.3.1 Moving Average

Let $\xi_1, \xi_2, \ldots$ be a sequence of random draws from a centred distribution, such as $\mathcal{N}(0, \kappa^2)$. The sequence defined by the identity

$$Y_{k+1} = \gamma_0 + \gamma_1 \xi_{k+1} + \gamma_2 \xi_k, \tag{11.8}$$

with Y_1 defined arbitrarily (as a constant or a variable) is called a *moving average*; γ_0, γ_1, and γ_2 are parameters (constants). Outcomes more than one time point apart are independent. A generalisation, MA of order m, MA(m), is defined by the identity

$$Y_{k+1} = \gamma_0 + \gamma_1 \xi_{k+1} + \gamma_2 \xi_k + \cdots + \gamma_{m+1} \xi_{k-m+1}.$$

In MA(m), observations $m + 1$ time points apart are independent. Thus, MA(m) can be recognised in the variance matrix $\boldsymbol{\Sigma} = \text{var}(\mathbf{Y})$ by zeros for every element $\Sigma_{hh'}$ of $\boldsymbol{\Sigma}$ such that $|h - h'| > m$. The log-likelihood for an MA sequence $\mathbf{y}$ is given by

$$l = -\frac{1}{2} \log \{\det(\boldsymbol{\Sigma})\} - (\mathbf{y} - \boldsymbol{\mu})\boldsymbol{\Sigma}^{-1}(\mathbf{y} - \boldsymbol{\mu})^\top,$$

similar to (11.7), except that it is preferable to use a parameterisation for the variance matrix instead of one for the concentration matrix.

Autoregressive moving average (ARMA) models combine the features of AR and MA. They are specified by the orders of the AR and MA parts of the model; thus, ARMA(m_A, m_M) is defined by the equation

$$Y_{k+1} = \gamma_0 + \sum_{j=1}^{m_A} \beta_j Y_{k-j+1} + \sum_{j=1}^{m_M+1} \gamma_j \xi_{k-j+2} + \varepsilon^{(k+1)}.$$

(The AR constant β_0 is absorbed in the MA constant γ_0; only their total can be identified.) In principle, the outcomes of an ARMA process can be decomposed into their AR and MA components, linear combinations of Y and ξ, respectively, and their log-likelihood maximised. A difficulty in this is that for AR and MA we prefer different parameterisations ($\mathbf{C}$ vs. $\boldsymbol{\Sigma}$), and these cannot be reconciled. In practice, the order of either the AR or the MA part is small; then the parameterisation better suited for the other part makes the likelihood maximisation simpler.

11.4 Targets, Designs, and Models

The setting of the example in Section 11.1 is rather artificial because it is concerned with the subpopulation of a country who were born in a particular year. We refer to them as an *age cohort*, implying a division of the country into cohorts according to age or year of birth. Cohorts can be defined similarly according to entry into the labour force, the beginning or completion of a course of studies, and the like.

Why would one be interested in a particular age cohort, those aged 25 in 1995, but not those who are a bit younger or older? The cohort of 1970 (the year of birth) may be regarded as a good representation of those who are a few years younger or older, so that, although the targets relate to this cohort, the inferences about it can be interpreted as applying also to the neighbouring cohorts.

It is important to distinguish between changes in a subpopulation over time and comparisons of subpopulations at a given time. For inferences about changes, a sample of such changes has to be observed, so subjects have to be observed at the relevant time points. In contrast, for comparisons of cohorts at a time, samples from the cohorts at the time point have to be observed. The two kinds of inferences—longitudinal and cohort—in general differ. For example, the statement that an age cohort of men is taller than their fathers on average by, say 10 cm, is a comparison of subpopulations (sons and fathers). It is unreasonable to deduce from this the longitudinal comparison that in the next 25 years or so, when they reach their fathers' ages, the sons will lose about 10 cm of their height on average.

A study may combine the two goals, for example, by comparing the changes made over a given period of time by two or several cohorts. If only a few cohorts are to be compared, the study can be regarded as a union of related longitudinal studies, one for each cohort. It is often more practical to regard the cohorts on a continuum and represent them by a continuous variable, such as age or calendar year. The principles of good representation of each cohort are then still relevant, but it may not be necessary for each cohort to be represented in the survey by a sufficiently large subsample.

The cohort can be incorporated in the analysis by specifying a separate model for each cohort; the samples for the cohorts are usually mutually independent. With the assumptions of multivariate normality, we may posit the general model

$$(\mathbf{Y} \mid k) \sim \mathcal{N}\left(\boldsymbol{\mu}^{(k)}; \boldsymbol{\Sigma}^{(k)}\right) . \tag{11.9}$$

The cohort-specific models may have some parameters in common. For example, they may have a common variance matrix; $\boldsymbol{\Sigma}^{(k)} \equiv \boldsymbol{\Sigma}$. The vectors $\boldsymbol{\mu}^{(k)}$ may have a pattern, such as constant differences, $\boldsymbol{\mu}^{(k)} - \boldsymbol{\mu}^{(h)} = \Delta \mu_{kh} \mathbf{1}$, or fanning out, $\boldsymbol{\mu}^{(k)} = \boldsymbol{\mu}^{(0)} + a_k \mathbf{d}$ for a nondecreasing sequence $\mathbf{d}$ and some constants a_k.

These models can be expressed in the form of a single equation as

$$\mathbf{Y} = \mathbf{X}\mathbf{B} + \boldsymbol{\varepsilon}, \tag{11.10}$$

where $\mathbf{Y}$ is the matrix of outcomes $(n \times K)$, $\mathbf{B}$ the $(p \times K)$ matrix of regression parameters, $\boldsymbol{\varepsilon}$ the $(n \times K)$ matrix of model deviations, and $\mathbf{X}$ the regression (design) matrix. Note that $\mathbf{Y}$ in (11.10) is a matrix of values, whereas in (11.9) it is a random vector; we cannot avoid the clash of notation. The model in (11.10), with its various generalisations, is for a *multivariate regression*. From now on, we use the term *univariate* as a qualifier for the regression models with univariate outcomes.

The matrix $\mathbf{X}$ is formed just like for univariate regression, with a column representing the intercept and further columns identifying the cohort. For example, if the rows of $\mathbf{Y}$ are sorted by the cohort and there are four cohorts, then

$$\mathbf{X} = \begin{pmatrix} 1 & 0 & 0 & 0 \\ 1 & 1 & 0 & 0 \\ 1 & 0 & 1 & 0 \\ 1 & 0 & 1 & 0 \end{pmatrix},$$

where the vertical partitioning corresponds to the observations from the four cohorts. In the parameter matrix $\mathbf{B}$, the first row is the population mean vector for the reference cohort 1, $\boldsymbol{\mu}^{(1)}$, and the second to fourth rows are the respective differences between cohorts 2–4 and 1, $\boldsymbol{\mu}^{(k)} - \boldsymbol{\mu}^{(1)}$, $k = 2, 3, 4$; that is, the cohort is treated like any other categorical covariate. Alternative parameterisations use a different reference cohort, omit the intercept but represent each cohort by an indicator, or linearly transform each column, perhaps except the first, so that the column total is equal to zero.

The matrix $\mathbf{X}$ can include further covariates (columns). Each column of $\mathbf{X}$, denoted by $\mathbf{X}^{(k)}$ corresponds to a row $\mathbf{B}^{(k)}$ of $\mathbf{B}$. Their matrix product, $\mathbf{X}^{(k)}\mathbf{B}^{(k)}$, is a contribution to the expectation of the matrix of outcomes $\mathbf{Y}$. For a covariate other than an indicator of the cohort, it does not depend on the cohort; the association of the outcomes with the covariate is the same in each cohort. By introducing interactions of covariates with the cohort, we allow the within-cohort regressions to differ. When there are K cohorts, the interaction of a (continuous) covariate with the cohorts is represented by $K-1$ variables, each of them equal to the product of the covariate with an indicator variable that represents the cohort. Interactions of other covariates are defined similarly, although, unlike in univariate regression where they are represented in the regression parameter vector $\boldsymbol{\beta}$ by one or several parameters, each of them is represented in $\mathbf{B}$ by one or several rows. The greater flexibility in modelling the association of $\mathbf{Y}$ and $\mathbf{X}$ that is attained by interactions has to be carefully weighed against the proliferation of the parameters involved.

Each column of $\mathbf{B}$ can be interpreted as the vector of parameters in the regression for the corresponding column of the (random) vector $\mathbf{Y}$. Therefore, if no constraints that span several columns are imposed on the elements of $\mathbf{B}$, then multivariate regression yields the same estimates as the collection of univariate regressions conducted separately for each column of the matrix $\mathbf{Y}$. The multivariate regression adds to this a description of the covariance structure across the time points. This is a valuable addition in many settings. By the univariate regressions we can estimate the variances in the matrix $\boldsymbol{\Sigma}$ but none of the covariances.

Covariates can be defined for subjects (vectors—rows of the matrix $\mathbf{Y}$) or for the elementary observations (on a subject at a time point). They are called subject- and elementary-level covariates, respectively. The former can be incorporated in $\mathbf{X}$ straightforwardly. The latter, also called *time-dependent*, can be accommodated only in more general models discussed in Section 11.5. The principles regarding causal analysis carry over from univariate regression.

We can refer to the elements or rows of $\mathbf{B}$ as (multivariate) effects only when the designer can assign the values of the covariates in $\mathbf{X}$ and does so without any regard for the values of $\mathbf{Y}$. Randomisation is one way of arranging this. Of course, in many settings it is not possible to assign subjects to cohorts. Then it is not meaningful to talk about cohort effects, and effects (of other covariates) cannot be estimated without bias.

When one of a set of alternative treatments is assigned to subjects by randomisation, causal inferences can be made. Care has to be exercised when including any covariates to accompany the treatment indicators in the model; inclusion of any intermediate variables is particularly problematic, just like in univariate models. With longitudinal outcomes, the effects are vectors, so it is much more difficult to specify what amounts to a substantial treatment effect. For example, we cannot expect the effect to be present at the first time point if it immediately follows the administration of the treatment. A favourable outcome may be that the expected differences increase over time and, perhaps, they settle at a particular level that is regarded as being of substantive importance. The pattern in which the differences first increase and are then reduced to a small value or even reverse their sign is more difficult to interpret. Although an effect is present it is of little relevance when a persistent effect, present over a long period of time (such as a permanent cure), is sought.

The elements of $\boldsymbol{\Sigma}$ can be constrained to have a particular pattern, such as conditional independence (tridiagonal $\boldsymbol{\Sigma}^{-1}$), compound symmetry ($\boldsymbol{\Sigma} = \sigma_W^2 \mathbf{I} + \sigma_B^2 \mathbf{J}$, where $\mathbf{J}$ is a matrix of unities), compound symmetry with changing dispersion ($\boldsymbol{\Sigma} = \sigma_W^2 \operatorname{diag}(\mathbf{c})^2 + \sigma_B^2 \mathbf{c}\mathbf{c}^\top$ for a vector $\mathbf{c}$), or the like. Without any such constraint, the multivariate regression model in (11.10) is fitted by the multivariate version of the ordinary least squares:

$$\hat{\mathbf{B}} = \left(\mathbf{X}^\top\mathbf{X}\right)^{-1}\mathbf{X}^\top\mathbf{Y},$$

$$\hat{\boldsymbol{\Sigma}} = \frac{1}{n-p}\mathbf{Y}^\top\left\{\mathbf{I} - \mathbf{X}\left(\mathbf{X}^\top\mathbf{X}\right)^{-1}\mathbf{X}^\top\right\}\mathbf{Y}.$$

The maximum likelihood estimator of $\boldsymbol{\Sigma}$ is the $(n-p)/n$-multiple of $\hat{\boldsymbol{\Sigma}}$; it has the denominator n instead of $n-p$.

The assumption that the variance matrix $\boldsymbol{\Sigma}$ is common to all the observations can be relaxed substantially, just like in univariate regression. Each cohort k can be associated with a separate variance matrix $\boldsymbol{\Sigma}^{(k)}$, and these matrices may have some features in common. For example, they may be proportional, $\boldsymbol{\Sigma}^{(k)} = c_k\boldsymbol{\Sigma}^{(1)}$, or have the same correlation matrix $\mathbf{R}$: $\boldsymbol{\Sigma}^{(k)} = \mathbf{D}^{(k)}\mathbf{R}\mathbf{D}^{(k)}$, where $\mathbf{D}^{(k)}$ are diagonal matrices. More generally, the (residual) variance matrix $\boldsymbol{\Sigma}$ can be specified as a function of some (categorical or continuous) covariates. Of course, this has to be done in such a way that $\boldsymbol{\Sigma}(\mathbf{x})$ is positive definite for every configuration of covariates $\mathbf{x}$. It may be difficult to define this function in such a way that its values would be realistic for all plausible values of $\mathbf{x}$.

11.4.1 Panels

Some inferential agenda remains relevant over a long period of time. For example, basic economic and demographic indicators, such as per capita income, retail price index, rate of unemployment, birth rate, and prevalence of some diseases, are estimated annually, quarterly, or even more frequently. Regularly conducted surveys in which a different sample is drawn on each occasion are suitable for estimating the state of the population at each time point (year). But they can offer no insight into the changes made by the individual members. For example, if the rate of unemployment is not changed between two quarters, we can only speculate whether the subpopulations of unemployed at the two time points are the same or how large their overlap is. More generally, if subjects' recall cannot be relied on, information about long-term unemployment can be collected only in surveys in which subjects are interviewed repeatedly.

However, only a limited response burden can be imposed on a subject, so he or she can be retained as a respondent only for a few rounds (waves) of a survey. For example, the UK Labour Force Survey (LFS) is conducted every quarter, that is, in January–March 2006, April–June 2006, and so on. Each subject is retained in the sample for five quarters, such as from January–March 2006 until January–March 2007. In this setting, a sample has several meanings. According to our definition, it is the set of all subjects in a wave, such as in January–March 2007. This sample comprises five subsamples defined by the wave in which the subject concerned was included for the first time; see Figure 11.3 for illustration. These subsamples are cohorts, and their union, the sample, is referred to as the *panel*. After each survey, the cohort that was just interviewed for the fifth time is retired and replaced by a new cohort. This design is called a *rotating panel* design; this term refers to the sequence of surveys. The panel for each wave (quarter) of the survey comprises five cohorts, one 'new' and one about to be retired and replaced in the next quarter.

In fact, LFS is conducted continually; a subsample of the panel is interviewed every week, so that the division of the data-collection effort into waves is almost entirely administrative. Even the subsamples of subjects interviewed during a week are representative of the population, at least in some aspects, so that a 'survey' could be defined for each week.

Panel designs respond to the need for information about the population at several time points and about changes made by their members. An unrelated advantage of panel designs is that a subject whose cooperation has been gained and who has been located will provide more information than if he or she were interviewed only once. The second and subsequent interviews could be made by phone or email, eliminating the costs of travel, arranging an appointment, and the like. On the other hand, however, the second and subsequent responses of a subject may be highly correlated with the first, so less information is gained than from a subject responding for the first (and

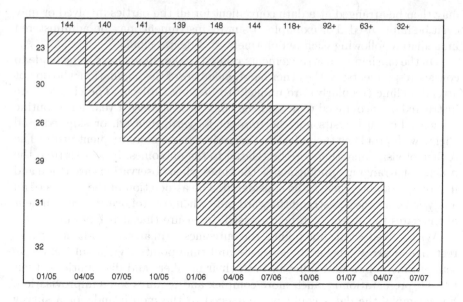

Fig. 11.3. Illustration of a rotating panel design. The numbers at the top are the sizes (in thousands, rounded) of the panels between the dates given at the bottom (e.g., 144 000 in January–March 2005), and the sizes of the cohorts are given at the left-hand margin (e.g., 23 000 interviewed for the first time in January–March 2005). The present time is July 2006; for the panels in the future only the totals over the cohorts already drawn are given and indicated by '+'.

Note: The diagram is motivated by the design of the UK LFS but the sizes of cohorts and panels are not equal to their counterparts in the design or realisation of LFS.

only) time. This highlights the importance of choosing an appropriate time-span between consecutive interviews, to ensure that changes in the recorded categories (statuses) of outcome variables occur with appreciable probability, while the probability of more than one change within the time-span is small. If several changes take place between two interviews, some may not be recorded because only information about current status is collected. Of course, administrative convenience should also be taken into account.

11.5 Irregular Time Points and Time-Specific Covariates

In previous sections we considered sequences of outcomes over discrete sets of time points that were fixed by design, although the example of LFS could be interpreted as having continuous time, coarsened for the purposes of reporting and management. The time is often meaningfully defined on a continuum and an observation of the outcome variable could conceivably be made at any point in time. An interview in which the current status of the subject is established may then be arranged at a date convenient for all the parties involved or may even be improvised. For example, a survey instrument may be administered immediately following each appointment at a dental clinic.

On the one hand, no arrangements related to the survey have to be made to contact respondents; on the other hand, members of the population who do not attend a clinic (regularly) are unlikely to become subjects. The clientele are instructed or encouraged to attend the clinic at least once a year for a routine checkup, but such visits may be brought forward, delayed, or skipped, and clients with problems they identify themselves make more frequent visits. The regime of visits may therefore be related to the outcomes. In this setting, the process of arranging appointments, the times when observations are made and its nonignorability, have to be considered. The association of the results of an analysis with causes is straightforward only when control over the assignment of the dates to subjects can be exercised, to ensure that it is ignorable.

With a fixed set of time points, the outcomes form an easy-to-handle $n \times K$ rectangular array labelled by subjects and time points. When subjects have sets of time points that differ in both their numbers and distributions, their tabular presentation is much more complex and requires some improvisation. For example, the dates could be coarsened to the month and, for a survey conducted over one year, the data could be presented in an $n \times 12$ array, with missing values for subject-by-month entries when no observation was made. For a subject-by-month with several observations, only a summary, such as the mean, would be given, accompanied by a special symbol. An illustration is given in Table 11.2 for the first few subjects of a larger dataset comprising 90 subjects with a total of 514 observations. For example, the record for subject 1, with exact dates, is:

Date (2005)	7/7	28/9	9/10	4/11	7/12
Outcome	135.5	125.7	132.6	163.6	204.8

and the entry for subject 3 in April is the mean of the outcomes 105.8 and 130.9, recorded on the 9th and 26th of April, respectively.

In Table 11.2 or a similar display, we should draw a distinction between cells that are empty because no appointment was made and those where an appointment was arranged but not kept. A symbol could be used for the latter to indicate that an observation was planned. However, even without such absences, the time points of a subject may be selected nonignorably, if appointments are arranged shortly before the visit, prompted by an event or change in status that are related to the outcome planned to be observed. The (causal) dependence of the date (appointment) on the outcome is a profound complication. It could not be resolved without modelling the process that generates the appointments. In the presence of a multitude of incentives,

Table 11.2. Illustration of a longitudinal dataset (part) with coarsened irregular time points. Asterisk * marks entries for two (or more) observations in a month; for them, their mean is given.

Id.	Jan	Feb	Mar	Apr	May	June	July	Aug	Sept	Oct	Nov	Dec
						Month (year 2005)						
1							135.5		125.7	132.6	163.6	204.8
2				125.6			122.1		176.2			120.8
3			118.3*			132.1	162.2			128.0	185.6	
4						158.7	131.5		178.9			
5					142.9		148.8*		157.1	128.1		
6	105.7	123.7	110.7				115.0		142.8		186.8	231.7
7							123.9	154.6		168.6	145.7	125.0
8	105.0		129.3*				129.5*			168.8		
9	100.1	114.5		129.2			125.5		140.1*		145.1	121.9

habits, and attitudes to one's health care and to the services available, this is a nontrivial undertaking.

The dates of all the observations are concisely summarised in Figure 11.4. Each subject is represented by a horizontal line interrupted by dots that mark the dates of the observations. A similar display of the outcomes, by a plot of the dates on the horizontal axis and the values of the outcomes on the vertical, may be misleading because the diagram would be dominated by the segments connecting the consecutive observations of a subject. Segments connecting distant observations are prominent, yet they are associated with less information than segments connecting observations made more frequently. Figure 11.5 gives an example based on the nine subjects whose observations are listed in Table 11.2.

Covariates may be defined for the subjects. A categorical subject-level variable can be represented in Figure 11.5 by ordering the subjects according to their values and inserting gaps to separate the subsamples from the categories. The values of a categorical outcome variable can also be represented in a diagram like Figure 11.5 by distinct symbols, such as circles and crosses for binary outcomes, instead of the dots that mark the appointments. A coarsened version of a continuous outcome variable may be indicated similarly. The size of the symbol may reflect the value of the outcome.

Covariates may also be defined for the elementary observations. Such elementary-level covariates may be functions of the time (day) but may also be specific to the observations. In most settings, the values of such variables are observed without the designer of the study exercising any control over them, and we can only speculate about the mechanism that assigns its value

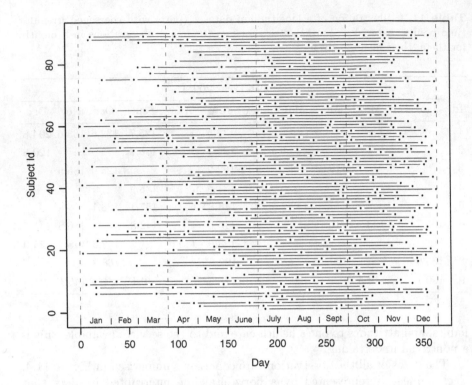

Fig. 11.4. The dates of the observations in a longitudinal study. Each subject is represented by a horizontal segment joining the dates of the first and last appointments and interrupted at the intermediate appointments. The vertical dashes mark the quarters of the year 2005 in which the study was conducted.

to a subject at a time point. The presumption or hypothesis that it is an intermediate variable, affected by the values of the variables with controlled assignment, is often well founded. The inclusion of such a variable as a covariate in a regression model is therefore problematic even if it would result in a substantially better fit as judged by data-based criteria.

11.6 Analysis

The observations from a longitudinal study have the structure of elements within clusters, so they are well suited for analysis with random coefficient models (Chapter 9). One model is posited for the outcomes of each subject (member of the population) and another describes the variation of the parameters in these models. Regression on time and its transformations is the natural choice for the former, leading to the model

$$y_{jt} = \mathbf{x}_{jt}\boldsymbol{\beta} + \mathbf{z}_{jt}\boldsymbol{\delta}_j + \varepsilon_{jt},$$

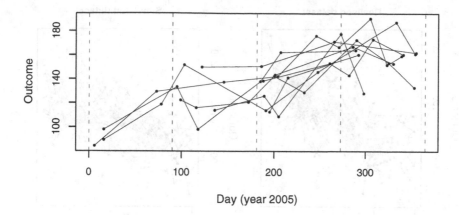

Fig. 11.5. The dates and outcomes for the subjects listed in Table 11.2. The vertical dashes delineate the quarters of the year.

with a random sample $\boldsymbol{\delta}_j$, $i = 1, \ldots, n$, from $\mathcal{N}(\mathbf{0}, \boldsymbol{\Sigma})$ and ε_{jt} an independent random sample from $\mathcal{N}(0, \sigma^2)$. Time is the obvious candidate for a covariate in both the regression and variation parts of the model. Greater flexibility is achieved by including a quadratic and higher powers of time. In general, we should include fewer such terms in the variation than in the regression part, while adhering to the rules that ensure invariance of the model with respect to linear transformations. The regression part, $\mathbf{x}$, may contain variables defined for subjects or elements (appointments). Subject-level variables should not be included in the variation part because they are constant for the observations of each subject, and so regressions on them could not be identified even if many observations were made on the subject. However, the variance matrix $\boldsymbol{\Sigma}$ may itself depend on one or several subject-level variables; for example, it may be specified as $c_h \boldsymbol{\Sigma}$ for subjects in category h of a variable. The constants c_h would usually be estimated, except for $c_1 = 1$, set for the sake of identifiability.

We can interpret the estimated conditional expectation $\mathbf{x}\hat{\boldsymbol{\beta}} + \mathbf{z}\hat{\boldsymbol{\delta}}_j$ as the fit to the observations for subject j. The values of some components of $\mathbf{x}$ and $\mathbf{z}$ are given, but for time and its transformations we can, in principle, substitute any values. This is appropriate within the range of time points of the subject, and possibly slightly beyond (both earlier and later), but the further we attempt to extrapolate, the more heavily the fit depends on the details of the model specification.

For the dataset partly summarised in Table 11.2 and Figure 11.5, we obtained the fit

$$E(y) = 101.478 + 0.187t$$

with estimated residual variance $\hat{\sigma}^2 = 430.80$ and estimated variance ratio $\hat{\omega} = -0.0033$. Instead of this negative value, zero can be quoted as the estimate and the ordinary regression fit adopted. It differs very little from the

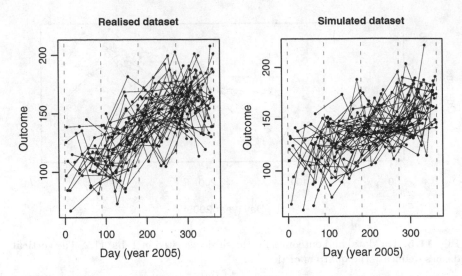

Fig. 11.6. The realised and a simulated longitudinal dataset. To avoid congestion, the progressions are plotted only for subjects with odd order numbers.

maximum likelihood fit with negative $\hat{\omega}$: $101.465 + 0.187t$, with estimated residual variance 429.37. The difference of the deviances for the two models is only 0.015. The estimated standard error of the slope on time t is 0.0094. The estimated standard error of $\hat{\omega}$ is 0.024, so the standard error of the between-subject variance estimator is about 10.0. Therefore, although the fit indicates that the subjects' curves do not differ, the uncertainty about the estimated parameters is such that even substantial between-subject variance is plausible. Quadratic regression and varying within-subject regression do not improve the model fit either. Appropriateness of the model with linear time and identical regressions can be assessed by generating datasets from the model fit and comparing their features with the realised dataset. A pair of such graphs is displayed in Figure 11.6. We may identify some features in which the two panels, for the realised and a simulated dataset, differ. However, we are interested only in features that would be replicated on most simulated datasets. In practice, the realised dataset is compared with several simulated datasets, but the corresponding features (graphs) cannot be printed in the limited space of a publication.

11.6.1 Missing Values

When an outcome is not recorded, because the appointment is not kept or some problems in the measurement process arise, it is tempting to disregard the anticipated data record in the subsequent analysis. A more principled approach regards the record as missing, considers the planned data as the complete dataset, and formulates a model for imputation; see Chapter 5. The obvious candidates that inform about the missing value are the observations from the recent past and near future, relying on the continuity of the outcome as a variable defined in time.

Common nonresponse patterns are those of dropping out, when a subject cooperates perfectly up to a time point and from then on provides no observations. Imputations for records with such patterns are simpler because they can be converted to sequences of univariate imputation problems. A drop-out is usually associated with a single cause of nonresponse, triggered at the first time point with nonresponse, when the subject makes a conscious decision to withdraw from the study, or some other circumstance makes continuation impossible. A difficulty with irregular time points is that for a drop-out we may have to impute an (irregular) schedule of appointments and outcomes based on them.

11.6.2 Multivariate and Cluster-Longitudinal Data

Multivariate outcomes can be motivated as longitudinal outcomes in which the time is a discrete variable represented by the components of the vector of outcomes. Although in such a setting multivariate analysis is usually simpler than an analysis with random coefficients, there are some exceptions. When there are many components and most subjects have incomplete records (by design), the imputation task to complete them (multiply) may be too complex, even when the nonresponse mechanism is MCAR. In a random coefficient model, the K components of the outcome vector are represented by $K-1$ indicator variables. Assuming multivariate normality of the outcomes, in the most general model these indicator variables are included in both regression and variation parts. Submodels can be specified by imposing constraints on the pattern of variation and the differences among the categories, while maintaining model invariance with respect to linear transformations. It is advantageous to avoid specifications in which the variance matrix is singular.

In some settings, the subjects are observed at a time point indirectly. For example, a summary of the prices of the residential properties in a district is observed only through the properties sold, which may be recorded in a register of sales. The resulting data can be regarded as having three levels, with transactions within district-years within districts. Within each district-year we have a different set of properties (houses or flats) that were sold during the year. If they are a random sample of the housing stock their prices represent well the market values of the entire stock. In ideal circumstances, we would analyse the underlying means, which are a set of time series over the years of the study; for them longitudinal analysis would be appropriate.

We regard the properties sold during a year in a district as a cluster and refer to the study (the dataset) of such clusters for several years as a *cluster-longitudinal* study (dataset). Missing-data methods can be applied for their analysis. It is natural to declare the district-year means (or other summaries that are relevant) as the missing data and apply the EM algorithm, when feasible, and multiple imputation otherwise, with a method for longitudinal analysis used for the complete data.

Functional data analysis is concerned with longitudinal data in which observations on a variable continuous in time are made so frequently that the association of the outcome with time is observed for the subjects completely. For example, the movement of a fixed point of the human body can be recorded at the speed of 100 records (locations) per second. Treating such data by longitudinal analysis is not practical. Alternatives include representing the motion as a function, in some applications multivariate, in a suitably defined system of coordinates using a basis of functions, $\mathbf{b} = (b_0, b_1, \ldots)$. For example, they may be the polynomials, with b_0 the constant function; there are obvious advantages to using an orthonormal basis. Thus, the observed function f for a subject is projected onto this basis, expressing it as

$$f(u) = \sum_{h=0}^{\infty} c_h b_h(u),$$

and approximating it by the summation of the first H terms. The analysis then proceeds by studying the vectors of coefficients $\mathbf{c} = (c_0, c_1, \ldots, c_H)$, that is, the coordinates with respect to the basis, as the outcomes. Using more terms yields a better approximation to f but is associated with greater complexity.

11.6.3 Mixture Models

When continuous outcomes are not (conditionally) normally distributed but we do not have a suitable class of (conditional) multivariate distributions for their description, mixture models can be applied with advantage. With them, we assume that the population comprises a small number of subpopulations, each with a description in terms of a multivariate normal distribution, either unconditionally or given some covariates; a different regression applies in each subpopulation. The membership of a subpopulation (category) is not known for any subject. In practice, the number of categories is not known either.

Let I_m be the variable that indicates whether a member belongs to category m, and let $\mathcal{M}$ be the categorical variable that states to which category a member belongs. That is, $I_{\mathcal{M}} \equiv 1$. Assuming that the values of all the covariates are fixed, we can define (latent) outcomes $\mathbf{Y}^{(m)}$, so that the observed outcome is

$$\mathbf{Y}^{(\mathcal{M})} = \sum_{m=1}^{M} I_m \mathbf{Y}^{(m)}. \tag{11.11}$$

Since $\mathbf{Y}^{(m)}$ can be defined without any restrictions other than agreement with $\mathbf{Y}^{(\mathcal{M})}$, no generality is lost by assuming that the indicators I_m and outcomes $\mathbf{Y}^{(m)}$ are independent for every category m.

We came across an expression similar to (11.11) in Chapter 7 when considering M potential outcomes of a subject, corresponding to M distinct treatments. There we denoted by W the indicator of the treatment applied; the indicator of the category, I, has a similar role here. Thus, mixture models can be motivated by the setting in which the treatment applied is not known. The targets of inference are the conditional distributions $\left(\mathbf{Y}^{(m)} \mid I_m = 1\right)$, $m = 1, \ldots, M$. By construction, the indicators I_m are independent of the (potential) outcomes $\mathbf{Y}^{(m)}$. However, the realised outcomes $\mathbf{Y}^{(\mathcal{M})}$ contain information about $\mathcal{M}$, the identity of the category.

Mixture models can be fitted by the EM algorithm in which the indicators I_m are the missing values. The E-step of this algorithm evaluates the conditional expectations $p_{j,m}$ of I_m for each subject j, and the subsequent M-step executes separate analyses for each category, with I_m (and I_m^2) replaced by $p_{j,m}$. The E-step expectations are

$$\hat{p}_{j,m}^{(\text{new})} = \frac{\hat{r}_m^{(\text{old})} L_{j,m}^{(\text{old})}}{\hat{r}_1^{(\text{old})} L_{j,1}^{(\text{old})} + \cdots + \hat{r}_M^{(\text{old})} L_{j,M}^{(\text{old})}},$$

where $L_{j,m}^{(\text{old})}$ is the contribution to the likelihood made by subject j, evaluated assuming that its category is m and with the current estimates of the model parameters substituted for the parameter values; $\hat{r}_m$ is the estimated (marginal) probability of belonging to category m. The superscripts 'old' and 'new' indicate the current and updated values, and carets $\hat{\ }$ are added to indicate that the quantities involved are estimates. In the M-step, the analysis for category m maximises the log-likelihood

$$\sum_{j=1}^{n} \hat{p}_{j,m}^{(\text{new})} \log\left(L_{j,m}^{(\text{old})}\right).$$

The marginal probabilities of the category m are estimated by the means of the subject-specific probabilities:

$$\hat{r}_m^{(\text{new})} = \frac{1}{n} \sum_{j=1}^{n} \hat{p}_{j,m}^{(\text{new})}.$$

The outcome of an analysis is a fitted distribution for each category and the estimated marginal probabilities $\hat{r}_m$. The categories need not have an interpretation in terms of distinct subpopulations. They are simply the best division of the sample in terms of minimising the likelihood with a normal distribution within each category. For instance, if we adopted another class of multivariate models, such as a class of multivariate gamma distributions, the division of the subjects to categories would be different. In fact, any continuous distribution can be approximated, with arbitrary precision, by a mixture of multivariate normal distributions. This property is not specific to the multivariate normals. For example, the multivariate uniform distribution, defined by the constant density on a rectangle, also has this property of forming, together with the operation of mixing, a basis for the space of continuous multivariate distributions.

The division, as indicated by the estimated conditional probabilities $\hat{p}_{j,m}$, is usually subject to uncertainty. Not only are these probabilities estimated, but they are also distant from zero and unity. This is easy to illustrate on a mixture of univariate normal distributions. For the density $f_m(x)$ of category m, we define the scaled density as $r_m f_m(x)$. When $M = 2$, the uncertainty about the mixture category is greatest at the intersection of the scaled densities, where $r_1 f_1(x) = r_2 f_2(x)$; for an observation j at that point; $p_{j,1} = p_{j,2} = \frac{1}{2}$.

Mixtures of normal distributions may be multimodal, asymmetric, and have long tails. In a multivariate setting, a variety of shapes of the density can be generated by mixtures of even very few distributions. Greater generality is achieved by considering mixtures of models, not only mixtures of joint (data) distributions from the same model. For example, different sets of covariates may be included in the models for the subpopulations. In principle, a category may comprise outliers; they are characterised by large variance, small marginal probability, and few or no covariates.

Settings in which the number of the mixture components (categories) is known are rare and unusual. More commonly, mixtures of some known (classes of) distributions are used as an approximation for an unknown distribution. It is then practical to proceed by fitting mixtures of two, three, and more distributions, stopping when the model fit with M components is very similar to the fit with $M - 1$ components. Similarity can be assessed by the likelihood ratio test, although for very large datasets this would invite us to fit exceedingly complex models with very small fractions of the population belonging to each component. A more practical rule is to stop when one of the fitted components has a small probability. At an extreme, an attempt to fit M components may result in a singularity, when the estimated probability $\hat{r}_m$ for a category approaches zero after a few iterations. Then the most complex mixture model we can fit is with $M - 1$ components.

The EM algorithm requires an initial solution. When fitting a sequence of models with increasing numbers of components, it is practical to make use of the previous solution. For instance, the initial solution for the three-component mixture can be the two-component fit supplemented by the parameterwise averages as the third component. The properties of the likelihood for a mixture model are difficult to explore, and multiple local maxima cannot be ruled out. Therefore it is prudent to fit a mixture model several times, with a range of starting values, especially when the number of components M is large. Slow convergence is often a reliable indication of such problems.

11.7 Example: House Prices in New Zealand

In this section, we describe a study of the residential property prices in the districts of New Zealand in the period 1996–2002. We are concerned with the house-price inflation—the increase of prices over the studied period. In the established approach, the mean or median price is calculated over each year, and these summaries are compared straightforwardly. Medians are preferred because they reduce the influence of the few very expensive properties. We prefer to work with the means of the log-prices because the property prices are much closer to normality, and symmetry in particular, on the log scale.

A problem with comparing any summaries of the house prices is that they refer to the properties sold, whereas inferences are desired for the housing stock in general or for a given property (a typical or 'standard' house or flat). Otherwise the comparison of prices may reflect the amalgam of improvements of, additions to, and removals from the housing stock, the selection of properties (by sellers and buyers), together with genuine inflation—change in the prices that can be attributed solely to time. For example, relatively more large properties may be sold in one period than in another, complicating the comparisons intended for a set of unchanging properties that are sold in both periods or for a set of properties sold in one period matched for all relevant characteristics by a set of properties sold in the other.

New Zealand comprises 74 districts (local authorities); 49 of them are on the North Island, 24 on the South Island, and one district, Chatham Islands, is several hundreds of miles east of either island in the Pacific Ocean. It is sparsely populated and there are only a few transactions in any year; we omit these from our study. Rounded to hundreds, there are records of 485 400 transactions in the study, 93 500, 83 600, 64 600, 60 500, 53 700, 59 200, and 70 200 in the respective years 1996–2002 (years 1–7).

New Zealand has about 4.0 million inhabitants and about 1.5 million single-household residential units. These are very unevenly distributed across the districts. The four districts that comprise the Auckland Metropolitan Area (Auckland City, Manukau, Waitakere, and North Shore) account for about a quarter of the population and a somewhat greater proportion of the transactions. In general, properties tend to be more expensive in urban areas and their prices are believed to have risen in the studied period at a higher rate than in towns and rural areas. A graphical summary of the annual log-mean prices in the districts is given in Figure 11.7. The lines connect the log-means of the prices for a district over the seven years. We refer to them as *inflation trajectories*. For orientation, the log-price of 11.0 corresponds to NZ$59 875 and 12.0 to NZ$162 750; in 2006, the exchange rate was about NZ$2.75 to UK£1.00.

The diagram shows that the districts tend to maintain their ranking of log-mean prices, but the log-means have gotten more dispersed over the years; the inflation trajectories are close to forming a right-facing megaphone. The trajectory highlighted in the right-hand panel, marked as Q in both margins,

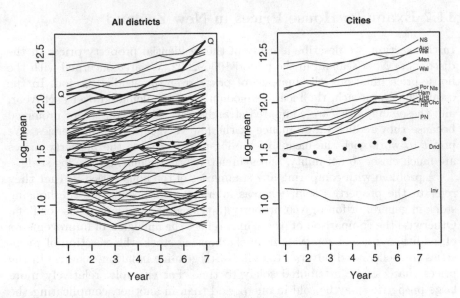

Fig. 11.7. The inflation trajectories for the districts of New Zealand from 1996 (year 1) to 2002 (year 7). The mean of the district-level log-means is indicated by dots. The right-hand panel is an extract for the fifteen city districts: North Shore (NS), Auckland City (Auc), Wellington (Wel), Manukau (Man), Waitakere (Wai), Porirua (Por), Nelson (Nel), Hamilton (Ham), Upper Hut (UHt), Napier (Nap), Christchurch (Chc), Hutt (Htt), Palmerston North (PN), Dunedin (Dnd), and Invercargill (Inv). Nelson, Christchurch, Dunedin, and Invercargill are on the South Island.

Adapted from [126], with permission of L. Erlbaum Associates.

is for Queenstown Lakes, a district in the South Island, parts of which have undergone substantial development as a holiday and adventure resort.

The pattern of the inflation trajectories can be summarised by the means of the district-level vectors of annual log-means:

$$\hat{\boldsymbol{\mu}} = (11.466, \ 11.505, \ 11.504, \ 11.555, \ 11.600, \ 11.615, \ 11.677)^\top,$$
$$(11.12)$$

marked in Figure 11.7 by large dots, variances

$$\frac{1}{1000} \ (140, \ 171, \ 188, \ 198, \ 214, \ 224, \ 243) \ ,$$

and the correlation matrix

$$\frac{1}{1000} \begin{pmatrix} 1000 & 990 & 979 & 966 & 966 & 965 & 958 \\ 990 & 1000 & 990 & 979 & 976 & 973 & 964 \\ 979 & 990 & 1000 & 993 & 988 & 983 & 971 \\ 966 & 979 & 993 & 1000 & 991 & 988 & 978 \\ 966 & 976 & 988 & 991 & 1000 & 995 & 986 \\ 965 & 973 & 983 & 988 & 995 & 1000 & 993 \\ 958 & 964 & 971 & 978 & 986 & 993 & 1000 \end{pmatrix}.$$

These confirm our observations from Figure 11.7: the variances increase over the years and the correlations are very high. The correlations decrease with distance in time, but they are very high even six years apart. The districts' trajectories cross one another very little.

The means in (11.12) differ substantially from the national means of log-prices, which are

$$(11.840,\ 11.887,\ 11.851,\ 11.887,\ 11.914,\ 11.932,\ 11.983)^\top. \qquad (11.13)$$

In the vector $\hat{\mu}$ in (11.12), the districts' means are of equal importance, ir-respective of the numbers of their transactions. In contrast, in (11.13) each transaction is of equal importance, so districts with fewer transactions have less influence on the mean.

Our analysis is based on an enumeration of the transactions, so no sampling issues arise. However, some of the districts are very sparsely populated and have fewer than one hundred transactions in a year. We might consider a replication of the year's real-estate business in each district, in which some other properties would be sold, and those that happen to be sold in both replications would be sold at different prices. Such within-district variation is accounted for by the two-level model

$$y_{tda} = \mu_a + \gamma_{da} + \varepsilon_{tda}, \qquad (11.14)$$

for log-price y in transaction t of district d in year a; the vectors $\gamma_d = (\gamma_{d1}, \ldots, \gamma_{d7})^\top$, $d = 1, \ldots, D = 73$, are a random sample from a centred seven-variate normal distribution (one component for each year), and ε_{tda} are independent random samples from centred (univariate) normal distributions. The samples $\{\gamma_d\}$ and $\{\varepsilon_a\}$, $a = 1, \ldots, 7$, are mutually independent. Denote $\text{var}_{\mathcal{D}}(\gamma_d) = \Sigma_{\mathrm{D}}$ and $\text{var}(\varepsilon_{tda}) = \sigma_a^2$. We allow the within-district variances σ_a^2 to differ from year to year; we have ample data for estimating each of them with high precision.

The fit of the model in (11.14), obtained by pooling the within-district variances, closely resembles the summaries of the district-level means, but we have an additional description in terms of the estimated within-district variances:

$$\sigma_{\mathrm{A}}^2 = \frac{1}{1000} (201,\ 200,\ 220,\ 232,\ 244,\ 249,\ 249) .$$

Table 11.3. Summary of the three-component mixture model fit to the log-sale prices.

Comp.	1	2	3	4	5	6	7	
				Year				
	log-mean							*Probability*
1	11.256	11.256	11.223	11.270	11.307	11.312	11.366	0.42
2	11.558	11.603	11.621	11.681	11.733	11.757	11.822	0.34
3	11.760	11.823	11.841	11.885	11.946	11.965	12.032	0.23
	District-level variances							
1	0.097	0.120	0.138	0.157	0.180	0.177	0.193	
2	0.112	0.133	0.136	0.137	0.154	0.169	0.187	
3	0.078	0.080	0.070	0.066	0.059	0.058	0.066	
	Transaction-level (within-district) variances							*Correlations*
1	0.259	0.261	0.295	0.313	0.341	0.351	0.345	0.942–0.996
2	0.205	0.197	0.209	0.215	0.224	0.218	0.228	0.958–0.997
3	0.144	0.144	0.158	0.167	0.164	0.168	0.169	0.962–0.998

Adapted from [126], with permission of L. Erlbaum Associates.

Thus, the within-district variances also increase over the period of the study.

Mixture models provide a more detailed description. For brevity, we give only the three-component mixture fit (see Table 11.3) and condense the correlation matrices into the ranges of the correlations. In all three fitted correlation matrices, the correlations decrease with distance in time, with very few exceptions, all of which are minor.

The first component has the lowest and the third the highest mean throughout the seven years. Although these differences appear to be substantial, they are only moderate when compared to the district-level standard deviations. A district-level variance of, say 0.09, corresponds to standard deviation of 0.30, and the distances between the pairs of means are of the same order of magnitude. Therefore, the district-level means in one mixture component have a substantial overlap with the means in another.

The district-level variances are estimated with little precision, because the 73 or slightly fewer degrees of freedom are split among the three components. However, we can discern that these variances increase in categories 1 and 2 and in category 3 remain small and are close to being constant. The transaction-level variances also increase over the seven years and are well separated; category 1 has the highest and category 3 the lowest variances. The correlations are very high for each component and the small differences among them are of no importance.

The marginal probabilities are 0.42, 0.34, and 0.23; they correspond to 31, 25, and 17 districts in the respective categories 1, 2, and 3. In fact, each

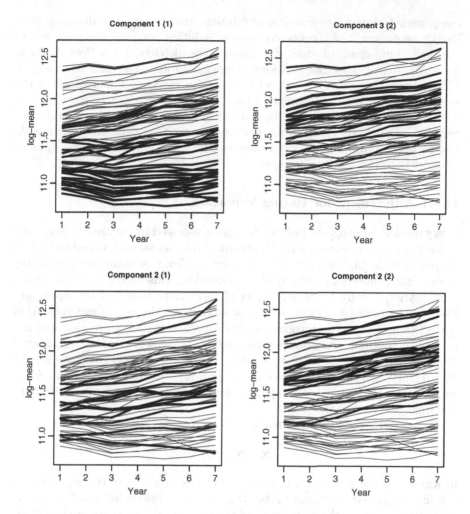

Fig. 11.8. The assignments of the districts' inflation trajectories to mixture categories according two- and three-component mixture model fits. The category in the two-component fit is given in the titles in parentheses.

Adapted from [126], with permission of L. Erlbaum Associates.

district is assigned to a category with probability in excess of 0.99. It seems that the three fitted distributions are well separated in the seven dimensions. There are no regions in which more than one distribution has an appreciable density. Figure 11.8 displays the assignment of the districts to mixture categories. For completeness, it includes the assignment of districts according to the two-component fit. The three-component fit can be described as forming a new component by taking some districts from either category of the two-component fit. Component 1 of the two-component solution becomes component 1 of the three-component solution, after losing some districts. Similarly, component 2 of the two-component solution becomes component 3 of the three-component solution, after losing some districts. These 'lost' districts form component 2 of the three-component solution. The panels of Figure 11.8 confirm that the district-level variances in category 1 increase over the seven years, while in component 3 the trajectories are nearly parallel, and component 2 (bottom two panels, split according to the category of the two-component solution) represents a halfway house. Note that the diagrams do not display the transaction-level variances which also influence the assignment of districts to the mixture categories.

11.7.1 Adjustment for Rating Valuation

Every residential property in New Zealand is assessed by its district authority annually or once in three years. The result of this assessment, called the *rating valuation*, is the capital value (CV), a figure in NZ\$, that estimates the market value of the property on the day of the valuation. This date is common within each district, usually 1st of September of every third year, but the dates vary from district to district. Being a large-scale exercise, the assessment is far from perfect as it is bound to involve subjective judgment and convention and has to rely on faithful and timely reporting by homeowners of all substantial alterations to the property. Nevertheless, CV is a very good covariate for the size, quality, and other attributes of the property, so that by adjusting for it we get closer to the ideal of comparing the sale prices in a district as like with like from one year to the next.

We consider the two-level model

$$y_{td} = \mathbf{x}_{td}(\boldsymbol{\beta} + \boldsymbol{\delta}_d) + \varepsilon_{td}, \tag{11.15}$$

in which $\mathbf{x}$ is the row vector of covariate values, comprising the logarithm of CV in force on 1st of January 2003, denoted by v, the scaled number of days (day/1000) between the valuation and the date of sale, u, its squared distance from $\frac{1}{2}$, $\left(u - \frac{1}{2}\right)^2$, and the intercept. Each of these variables is included in the variation part of the model. We divide the number of days by 1000, so that the corresponding estimates are not very small; a period between two rating valuations (three years) corresponds to about 1.1 on this scale. In the computational algorithm, the log-values v and y are replaced by $v - 11.5$ and $y - 11.5$, respectively, to reduce any numerical problems due to adding a large number of values. The adjustment of the computer output, so that it refers to v and y is straightforward.

The single-component model fit is

$$\hat{\mathrm{E}}(y) = 0.936v - 0.883u - 0.0570\left(u - \tfrac{1}{2}\right)^2 + 0.7053,$$
$$\hat{\sigma}^2 = 0.0705,$$

Table 11.4. The two-component mixture model fit for regression on capital value and time elapsed since valuation. All the figures are multiplied by 10 000.

	Component 1 (29 districts)				Component 2 (44 districts)			
	CV	u	$\left(u-\frac{1}{2}\right)^2$	1	CV	u	$\left(u-\frac{1}{2}\right)^2$	1
$\hat{\beta}$	9429	847	−746	6311	9312	908	−449	7456
$\hat{\sigma}^2$				590				843
$\hat{\Omega}_D$	1053 −502 201 −604				855 −424 −29 −452			
	−502 967 160 21				−424 1164 −91 22			
	−201 160 2632 −380				−29 −91 3953 −618			
	−604 21 −580 697				−452 22 −618 860			

$$\hat{\Omega}_D = \frac{1}{10\,000} \begin{pmatrix} 983 & -476 & 39 & -509 \\ -476 & 1164 & -6 & 14 \\ 39 & -6 & 3778 & -686 \\ -509 & 14 & -686 & 915 \end{pmatrix},$$

where $\Omega_D = \sigma^{-2}\Sigma_D$ is the scaled district-level variance matrix and $\hat{\Omega}_D$ is its estimate. This fit can be interpreted only by calculating the fitted values and variances for a range of values of v and u. This we do for the two-component solution given in Table 11.4.

The average regression slope on CV is close to unity and is smaller than 1.0 for both components, but the fitted variation of the district-level slopes is large (estimated standard deviation $\sqrt{0.0590 \times 0.1053} = 0.079$ for component 1 and 0.085 for component 2). This indicates that a large fraction of the districts have slopes greater than unity. However, the deviations of the slopes on v, u, and $\left(u - \frac{1}{2}\right)^2$ are correlated, so the district-level variation is explored more adequately by examples.

Figure 11.9 plots the fitted expectations and standard deviations for properties with capital values of NZ\$100 000, NZ\$160 000, and NZ\$250 000 over a period of three years since the rating valuation, for the solution given in Table 11.4. These three cases are marked as A, B, and C, respectively, and the two components as 1 and 2, so that, for instance, B1 stands for the expected log-price of a property with CV of NZ\$160 000 using the first (left-hand) component in Table 11.4. The horizontal dots indicate the CV.

The left-hand panel shows that the first components have uniformly higher values, although the differences get smaller toward year 3, and shows how much, on average they differ from the associated CVs, the values intended at time $u = 0$. The right-hand panel displays the fitted district-level standard deviations. These generally increase. The small reductions at the beginning of the period could be due to the inflexibility of the fitted curve for the variance,

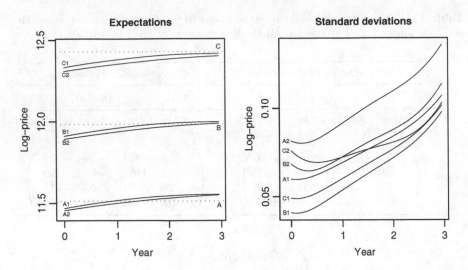

Fig. 11.9. The fitted expectations and district-level standard deviations for properties with capital values of NZ$100 000 (A), NZ$160 000 (B), and NZ$250 000 (C) for mixture components 1 and 2.

which is a polynomial of fourth degree in time. The diagram confirms that the district-level variances of the second component are higher, except for CV of NZ$250 000 at the end of the third year, shortly before the next valuation (compare curves C1 and C2). Although by necessity the two panels are on different scales, it is obvious that the standard deviations are of greater order of magnitude than the differences between the pairs of expectations. The within-district standard deviations (0.24 and 0.30) are much greater still. In conclusion, the two groups are distinguished more by their patterns of variation than by their expectations. The three-component solution has similar features; it 'distils' the two categories and collects the remainder in a 'compromise' third category.

Suggested Reading

Two established textbooks on longitudinal analysis are [37] and [192]. Alternative terms used for longitudinal data or substantially overlapping with it are repeated measures [30] and [104] and growth curves [186] and [85]. Longitudinal studies are often considered as an application of random coefficient models [97]. Further analytical challenges are presented by nonnormality of the outcomes [101] and [188], nonlinearity [31], and nonresponse [172] and nonignorable drop-out in particular [111]. For normally distributed outcomes, [89] and [105] discuss details of model-fitting algorithms for a wide range of dependence structures. The method of generalised estimating equations [198] was an important breakthrough in the analysis of nonnormally distributed outcomes in the late 1980s, but it has largely been superseded by computationally intensive methods.

A very good introduction to time-series analysis, with many examples, is [17]; [68] is a textbook suitable for the more advanced student. A monograph on the theory and applications of functional data analysis is [152]. An example of multivariate mixture models for longitudinal data is given in [127].

Problems and Exercises

11.1. Plot the trajectories for simulated normally distributed longitudinal datasets observed completely at three time points on $n = 50$ subjects. Choose a range of patterns for the vector of expectations μ (increasing, decreasing, increasing first and then decreasing, and the like) and for the variance matrices Σ, including some that are close to singularity.
Hint: Compose a variance matrix from its eigenvalue decomposition.

Compare the diagrams and the patterns of expectations and variation for the data on the original scale and after some common transformations, such as exponentiation and square, and square root if all the values are positive.

11.2. The triplet of outcomes for a subject can be summarised by the angle of the trajectory at the second time point; see Figure 11.10 for an illustration. (This angle depends on the scales used for the two axes.) Plot these angles and relate their distribution to the vector of expectations μ and variance matrix Σ. Supplement it with another summary that would provide more information about μ and Σ.

11.3. For a dataset used (or generated) in Exercise 11.1, predict the outcomes at the third time point based on the previous two outcomes or only the outcomes at point 2. Assess the result by the absolute difference $|\hat{y}_{3j} - y_{3j}|$ for the two predictors of y_{3j}. Relate the relative success of the simpler predictor to the (1,3) element of the concentration matrix and to the relative sizes of the two conditional variances.
Repeat this exercise after a transformation of the outcomes so that they are not normally distributed but use the predictors that assume normality. Assess to what extent the prediction is now deficient.

11.4. Check that the sequence of partial totals of a sequence of independent variables has the Markov property. That is, let $X_1, X_2, \ldots$ be independent variables; then the sequence $X_1, X_1 + X_2, \ldots, X_1 + X_2 + \cdots + X_m, \ldots$ has the Markov property. Note that the variables $X_1, X_2, \ldots$ can have arbitrary and unrelated distributions.

11.5. Construct an example that shows that a submatrix of a concentration matrix can differ substantially from the inverse of the corresponding

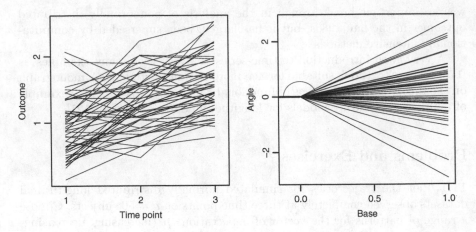

Fig. 11.10. The trajectories and angles for a longitudinal dataset with three time points. The angles are distorted because the horizontal and vertical axes have different scales.

submatrix of the variance matrix. That is, using the standard notation, $C_{ss} \neq (V_{ss})^{-1}$, where s denotes a set of indices. Explain why this happens.

11.6. Verify the formula for the inverse of a partitioned matrix in (11.3). Derive an expression for the determinant of this matrix in terms of its blocks.

11.7. Derive the maximum likelihood estimator of the parameters β_0 and β_1 of an AR(1) sequence.
Hints: Use the parameterisation in terms of the concentration matrix. Derive the determinant of the concentration matrix by induction, using the identity $E_{k+2} = a_1 E_{k+1} - a_{12}^2 E_k$ for the determinants E_k of a sequence of symmetric tridiagonal matrices $\mathbf{E}_k$, $k = 1, 2, \ldots$, with diagonal elements a_h and off-diagonal elements $a_{h,h+1} = a_{h+1,h}$; $\mathbf{E}_k$ is the submatrix of $\mathbf{E}_{k+1}$ formed by deleting its first row and column.

Derive a predictor of the next outcome. Explain why outcomes from the past beyond the immediate are useful for prediction.

11.8. On the web site of the Labour Force Survey in the UK or your country, find the details of the sampling design, as well as the information about the imperfect conduct, nonresponse in particular. If a rotating panel design is used, find out how it was started (full sample size in the first quarter, early retirements from the panel, or a combination). Find out how nonresponse is handled.

11.9. Draw a graphical summary of the dates (days) in the dataset `EXLb.dat` obtainable from `www.sntl.co.uk/BookA/Data`. The outcomes in the data are the measurements of the concentration of the human placental lactogen (log-transformed) on 69 healthy women during their (normal) pregnancies; the measurements are made irregularly. The stature (height) of the women is also given (in meters). Classify the women into a small number of categories according to how regularly they attended the clinic for the measurement and compare these groups on summaries of the outcomes (by numbers or graphs). Redraw the diagram so that these categories can be easily distinguished and explore ways of indicating the women's heights, suitably coarsened if necessary.

11.10. Fit a random coefficient model to the data in EXLb.dat with a polynomial average regression on gestational age and parallel regressions. Assess whether the assumption of parallelness is appropriate by simulations from the fitted model. If your conclusion is negative fit a more complex model (e.g., with linear variation of the women's regressions) and describe the pattern of patient-level variation.

11.11. Suppose a vector of K outcomes is recorded for each subject in a study at time points $k = 1, \ldots, K$. Suppose the vectors have a multivariate normal distribution. Show that the general model $\mathbf{X} \sim \mathcal{N}(\boldsymbol{\mu}, \boldsymbol{\Sigma})$ with no constraints on $\boldsymbol{\mu}$ or $\boldsymbol{\Sigma}$ is equivalent to the random coefficient model with a polynomial of degree $K-1$ on time and unrestricted subject-level variation. Explain why the scale used for the time $(1, 2, \ldots, K)$ is immaterial. That is, if a different scale is used, such as $(1, 2, 4, 7, \ldots)$, the population can be described by the same random coefficient model, although with different values of the parameters.

11.12. Fit a mixture of two random coefficient models, both with parallel regressions, to the dataset in EXLb.dat and describe the features in which the two mixture components differ most radically. How much certainty is there in the assignment of the women to the components? Can the assignment be guessed from their trajectories?

11.13. Generate a dataset from a mixture of two multivariate normal distributions, one with small variances and high correlations and the other with large variances and small correlations. Fit a mixture of two multivariate normals and check how well it identifies each subject's category. Explore how this depends on the sample size, number of observations per subject, and the difference between the two distributions.

11.14. Discuss how one might deal with nonresponse or erratic attendance in the study of pregnant women and human placental lactogen (dataset EXLb.dat in Exercise 11.10) and what difference it could make to the results. How should dropping in (first measurement at a later gestational age than planned) and dropping out (due to delivery in some cases) be treated?

11.15. Discuss how house-price inflation is assessed (informally) in the districts of your region or country and what its deficiencies are with regard to the causal interpretation of the inflation rate. Give reasons why the inflation may be uneven, for example, as properties of certain kinds and in certain price ranges become more sought after. How could this be reflected in a more complex description of the inflation?

11.16. *Semicontinuous outcomes.* A variable is said to be semicontinuous if it is a mixture of a constant (a degenerate variable) and a continuous variable. A common example of a semicontinuous outcome variable is the amount consumed or usage of a particular product, commodity or service, such as alcohol, bread, petrol (or miles travelled by car), and air travel. In the subpopulation of users (consumers), the distribution of the usage is continuous, but the nonconsumers contribute with identical zeros. In a longitudinal study with such an outcome variable, there are persistent and intermittent consumers and nonconsumers; persistent consumers may tend to consume less in periods when they do consume. Discuss how the data from such a study would be analysed. How could the consumption of a subject be predicted for the next time point? How could the amount consumed (which may be equal to zero) be related to a background variable?

Hint: For a nonconsumer, consider a negative 'hypothetical' consumption which is never observed because it is truncated at zero (left-censored). For each positive consumption, the value of the hypothetical consumption is the same. Regard the hypothetical consumption as having missing values whenever the observed consumption is equal to zero. Propose methods for missing data in this setting.

11.17. Devise a method for dealing with missing data that is suitable for the following setting. A longitudinal study inquires bi-monthly over a period of one year (seven time points) about subjects' attitudes toward their local authority. Nonresponse arises mainly because subjects are not at home during the week designated for the contact. Among those with complete records, there is a fair amount of consistency—the responses of a large proportion of subjects are the same on every occasion, and for most of the rest they differ by at most one point on an ordinal scale of seven points. The target of the analysis is the transition matrix, that is, the matrix of conditional probabilities

$$P(X_{k+1} = h_1 \mid X_k = h_0)$$

for $1 < h_0, h_1 \leq 7$, or the average of these probabilities over the six occasions, $k = 1, \ldots, 6$.

12
Meta-Analysis and Estimating Many Quantities

Meta-analysis is a term used for summarising a collection of studies that have the same or closely related targets. Each study may contain only modest information about the target, and meta-analysis seeks to synthesise this information and conclude with a single inferential statement. The main challenges in meta-analysis are related to the incompleteness of the studies: some are not reported at all, others are reported in a format that does not contain the items required for the meta-analysis, and, arguably, some studies that should have been were not conducted. Each study has its own context, such as the country or region in which it is conducted, time period (year), recruitment process, measurement and data-recording procedures, and other details of the design and protocol, which exert an influence on the targets of the studies and make the meta-analysis more complex.

Section 12.8 deals with a more general problem, that of estimating a large number of related quantities. If the quantities are similar all the observations can contribute to the estimation of each of them.

12.1 Introduction

In meta-analysis, we consider D studies, each of them yielding an estimator $\hat{\theta}_d$ and an estimator of its sampling variance $v_d = \mathrm{var}(\hat{\theta}_d)$. Each study has its target θ_d, $d = 1, \ldots, D$, such as the average effect of a new treatment over its established alternative in a particular population. It is usually reasonable to assume that such targets differ very little from one another, and that sometimes they even coincide. Why should the mean treatment effect in one country be different from that in another country? Why should it differ across time (years) or subpopulations? We do not seek any answers to these questions or any explanations; rather, we take such differences for granted, although we assume that they are not very large. Apart from the geographical domain (country) and time, the recruitment, administration, and data-recording processes exert an influence on the expectation $\mathrm{E}(\hat{\theta}_d \,|\, d)$ which is regarded as the target in study d. We refer collectively to the domain, time, and the processes involved in a study as the *context*. The context of a study comprises *elements*, such as the domain (country) and the data-management procedures, which may include the protocol for dealing with nonresponse and outlying (exceptional) values.

Meta-analysis seeks to estimate the parameter θ that is devoid of any context or that would be realised by a study in which each element of the context would be represented. This definition entails several difficulties. Good representation, if its meaning were well defined, would entail control over the context in which studies are conducted. This is impossible to arrange because a list of all possible contexts cannot be compiled, studies in the past were conducted without any regard for meta-analyses that might be carried out in the future, and the teams planning their studies may have preferences regarding some elements of the context that are not in accord with the requirements of a future meta-analysis. Some elements can be used only in conjunction with others. For instance, some countries have comprehensive medical registers, from which suitable patients can be drawn by specified sampling designs, and the records of the subjects used, with appropriate confidentiality safeguards. Elsewhere a study has to rely on recruitment of subjects.

The first step in a meta-analysis is to identify the rules for studies that will be included in it and the sources in which information about such studies will be searched. For example, of interest may be all the studies in which a specific treatment was used as the test treatment in comparison with an established alternative. The sources may be a list of medical journals and their volumes since 1975 or another year. The protocol for meta-analysis may include rules for following up on information with the authors of the identified journal articles or with their institutions. On no account would any subjects of the past studies be contacted; their identities are in any case hardly ever disclosed. The process of the search for studies, delineating them by a comprehensive definition, listing the sources to be searched (journals, agencies, and the like), keywords to be searched in them, and specifying the information to be extracted, is referred to as *systematic review*.

In most settings, the datasets or databases of the identified studies are not available. We assume that for each study we have an estimate $\hat{\theta}_d$ and an estimate of the associated sampling variance, $\hat{v}_d = \widehat{\mathrm{var}}(\hat{\theta}_d)$. Further, we assume that $\hat{\theta}_d$ is unbiased for its target θ_d, and $\hat{v}_d$ is unbiased for its target $v_d = \mathrm{var}(\hat{\theta}_d)$. These assumptions are not very restrictive. Covariates may be defined for the studies; the year of the study and its domain (country or region and its subpopulation) are obvious choices, and other covariates may be based on the details of the protocols of the studies. Throughout we assume that the studies are mutually independent. Cases when this assumption is not satisfied are rare. For example, some dependence arises when one study recruits from the participants of another.

Figure 12.1 gives an example of a set of $D = 28$ studies. Each study d is represented by a horizontal segment centred around the estimate $\hat{\theta}_d$, marked

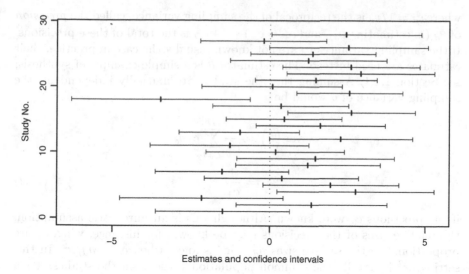

Fig. 12.1. Graphical summary of a set of 28 studies in a meta-analysis. Each study $d = 1, \ldots, D = 28$, is represented by a horizontal segment delimited by $\hat{\theta}_d \pm 2\sqrt{\hat{v}_d}$, with its centre $\hat{\theta}_d$ marked by a tick.

by a tick, and delimited by $\hat{\theta}_d - 2\sqrt{\hat{v}_d}$ and $\hat{\theta}_d + 2\sqrt{\hat{v}_d}$. Instead of $c = 2$, another factor could be used for the limits $\hat{\theta}_d \pm c\sqrt{\hat{v}_d}$. Such limits could be interpreted as confidence limits, but they are now redundant because they refer to a single study. It is not meaningful to count the numbers of studies that would yield a nominally significant result (indicating evidence that θ_d differs from zero), because the hypothesis tests involved are associated with errors of both types and the powers of these tests are unequal. By analysing all the studies together, we are bound to estimate with greater precision both a summary of the quantities θ_d and each value θ_d.

12.2 Studies with Identical Targets

The target of a meta-analysis, denoted by θ, is obvious only when the targets of the individual studies coincide; $\theta_1 = \ldots = \theta_D = \theta$. In this case, the context of the study is immaterial, or the studies have identical contexts. We consider this case first and then explore how its assumption may be contradicted by the data.

The D estimators $\hat{\theta}_d$ are unbiased for the common target θ, so their linear combination that is most efficient for θ is

$$\tilde{\theta} = \sum_{d=1}^{D} \frac{c_d}{c_+} \hat{\theta}_d , \qquad (12.1)$$

where $c_d = 1/v_d$ is the reciprocal of the sampling variance, called the *precision* of $\hat{\theta}_d$ (in estimating θ_d), and $c_+ = c_1 + \cdots + c_D$ is the total of these precisions. If the sampling variances v_d are not known, usually the case in practice, their estimates are used instead. The estimator $\tilde{\theta}$ is a simple example of synthesis; see Section 1.1.1. Assuming that the studies are mutually independent, the sampling variance of $\tilde{\theta}$ would be

$$\mathrm{var}\left(\tilde{\theta}\right) = \frac{1}{c_+^2} \sum_{d=1}^{D} c_d^2 v_d$$

$$= \frac{1}{c_+}, \tag{12.2}$$

if the precisions c_d were known. Although this is an unrealistic assumption, the relative sizes of the precisions may be known, for instance, when c_d are proportional to the sample sizes n_d, for instance, when $c_d = n_d/\sigma^2$. In this setting, σ^2 is usually the common population variance in the studies. Then the coefficients c_d/c_+ are proportional to the sample sizes of the studies, $c_d = c_+ n_d/(n_1 + \cdots + n_D)$. The sampling variance of $\tilde{\theta}$ is not known in this case but is a known multiple of the factor σ^2:

$$\mathrm{var}\left(\tilde{\theta}\right) = \frac{\sigma^2}{n_1 + \cdots + n_D}.$$

Note that we have made no reference to normality in the derivation of $\tilde{\theta}$.

Being common to the D studies, the variance σ^2 can be estimated by pooling its within-study estimates $\hat{\sigma}_d^2$. We can reuse the general idea of synthesis for this purpose, but this can no longer be done without a distributional assumption. If $\hat{\sigma}_d^2$ are distributed according to the scaled χ^2 distributions with $n_d^* = n_d - p_d$ degrees of freedom, then they are unbiased for their respective targets σ_d^2, and their respective sampling variances are $2\sigma^4/n_d^*$. Here p_d is the number of degrees of freedom lost due to estimation of model parameters in study d, typically by using ordinary regression. When $\hat{\theta}_d$ are sample means, $p_d = 1$. In complete analogy with (12.1) and (12.2), we obtain the combination

$$\tilde{\sigma}^2 = \sum_{d=1}^{D} \frac{n_d^*}{n_+^*} \hat{\sigma}_d^2 \tag{12.3}$$

$(n_+^* = n_1^* + \cdots + n_D^*)$ and

$$\mathrm{var}\left(\tilde{\sigma}^2\right) = \frac{2\sigma^4}{n_+^*}.$$

Of course, studies with $n_d^* < 1$ are of no use for estimating $\tilde{\sigma}^2$, because they contain no information about σ^2.

The assumptions of equal treatment effect, $\theta_1 = \ldots = \theta_D$, and proportional sampling variance, $v_d = \sigma^2/n_d^*$, represent the setting most congenial for analysis. When the variances v_d are known or estimated with high precision, the estimates $\hat{\theta}_d$ are unlikely to be identical, even when their targets θ_d are. Their expected dispersion is related to the variances v_d:

$$\mathrm{E}\left\{\frac{1}{D-1}\sum_{d=1}^{D}\left(\hat{\theta}_d - \bar{\theta}\right)^2\right\} = \frac{1}{D-1}\sum_{d=1}^{D}\mathrm{E}\left\{\left(\hat{\theta}_d - \bar{\theta}\right)^2\right\}$$

$$= \frac{1}{D-1}\sum_{d=1}^{D}\left\{\frac{(D-1)^2}{D^2}v_d + \frac{1}{D^2}\sum_{d'\neq d}v_{d'}\right\}$$

$$= \frac{1}{D^2(D-1)}\sum_{d=1}^{D}\left\{(D-1)^2 + (D-1)\right\}v_d$$

$$= \frac{1}{D}\sum_{d=1}^{D}v_d,$$

where $\bar{\theta} = (\hat{\theta}_1 + \cdots + \hat{\theta}_D)/D$ is the average of the study-level estimates. Therefore, when the sample variance of the estimates $\hat{\theta}_d$ is way in excess of the average sampling variance of the estimators $\hat{\theta}_d$, we have evidence that the targets of these estimators, θ_d, are not identical. The distribution of the sample variance, which would aid us in judging what amounts to being in excess, is not straightforward to derive. It is more practical to generate it empirically, by drawing random vectors from the distribution $\mathcal{N}(\mathbf{0}, \mathbf{V})$, where $\mathbf{V} = \mathrm{diag}_d(v_d)$. An example based on the setting of Figure 12.1 is given in Figure 12.2. The histogram summarises 25 000 replicate values of the sample variance of the set of 28 estimates $\hat{\theta}_d$ with the variances v_d equal to their estimates $\hat{v}_d$. The vertical dashes mark the 0.025 and 0.975 quantiles, equal to 0.70 and 2.09, respectively; the expectation of the distribution is equal to 1.29 and median to 1.26. For the realised dataset, the sample variance is 2.86, equal to the percentile 99.3 of the empirical distribution. That is ample evidence that the targets of the studies are not identical. The distribution of the sample variance is close to normal, but it is closer to a scaled χ^2 distribution with degrees of freedom close to $D - 1 = 27$. In fact, it would be 27 if each study had the same variance v_d.

12.3 Study-Specific Targets

If the subjects' records for all the studies in a meta-analysis were available, we would consider a two-level (regression) model with subjects within studies, allowing for differences among the within-study regressions in their intercepts and possibly also in the slopes on some of the covariates. In such a model, the

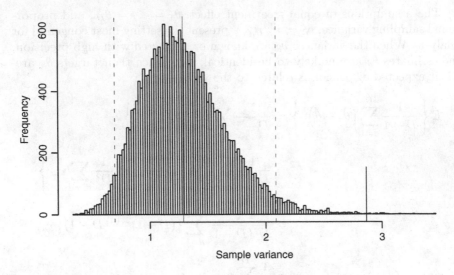

Fig. 12.2. Empirical distribution of the average dispersion of a set of studies that are assumed to have a common target; based on the setting of Figure 12.1. The vertical line marks the empirical mean and the vertical dashes the 2.5th and 97.5th percentiles. The realised value of the dispersion is marked by the short solid vertical segment.

average regression describes the associations in an average context and the study-level variance (matrix) the extent and pattern of variation among the study-specific regressions. Usually the subject-level records are not available for all the studies, and the sufficient statistics for the two-level model, which include the totals of crossproducts of the outcome variable with the covariates, cannot be recovered from the available information. Therefore this avenue cannot be pursued.

When only the D pairs of the sample quantities $(\hat{\theta}_d, \hat{v}_d)$ are available we consider the model

$$\hat{\theta}_d = \theta + \delta_d + \varepsilon_d, \tag{12.4}$$

where δ_d, $d = 1, \ldots, D$, are the deviations of the study-specific effects θ_d from their (superpopulation) average θ and ε_d are the errors in estimating the study-specific effects $\hat{\theta}_d$. The deviations are assumed to be a random sample from a centred normal distribution with unknown variance σ_{B}^2. We refer to σ_{B}^2 as the *context-level variance*. The estimation errors are mutually independent and are independent also from the deviations δ_d, both within and across studies. Even though the model contains two random terms for studies, it is well identified because the variance of one of them is assumed to be known. In fact, only $\hat{v}_d = \widehat{\mathrm{var}}(\varepsilon_d)$ are available, but we regard the confusion of the estimate $\hat{v}_d$ with its target v_d as a minor transgression.

The pair of parameters θ and σ_B^2 may seem to be an attractive and compact summary of the D studies; θ is the expected effect in an average context and σ_B^2 describes the variation of the within-context expected effects. The variance σ_B^2 can also be motivated as the variation of the D estimates that is in excess of what one might expect if the studies had a common target:

$$\text{var}_D(\theta_\bullet) = \text{E}_D(v_\bullet) + \sigma_B^2,$$

where the subscript D indicates averaging over the studies. For example, the studies summarised in Figure 12.1 have sample variance 2.86 and the average sampling variance is 1.29, yielding the estimate $\hat{\sigma}_B^2 = 1.57$. In the next section, we derive an alternative estimator.

Provisionally, we adopt the average of the study-level estimates $\hat{\theta}_d$, equal to 0.81, as an estimate of θ. If it were equal to θ, and σ_B were equal to $\hat{\sigma}_B = 1.25$, we would conclude that the average expected treatment effect is positive but the expected effect in some studies (contexts) is negative. Such a conclusion implies a reference to a population of contexts, and hence their representation among the studies that were conducted and were identified for the meta-analysis. Usually each study responds to a specific need and is funded after approval of a carefully formulated proposal. The proposal may review and draw on the experiences of other studies conducted in the past that have similar inferential agendas, but an appeal to good geographical or temporal representation rarely carries much weight. Other elements of the context, definitions of the outcomes and measurement and recording procedures in particular, could, with good reason, be proposed only as pursuing the practice believed to be the best at the time and best suited for the current circumstances. Therefore, good representation of these elements of the context is not feasible, but neither can the meaning of 'good representation' be defined without ambiguity and temporal dependence.

In brief, for a straightforward interpretation of the parameters θ and σ_B^2 we would require a *meta-design* which controls the representation of the contexts in the collection of studies to be conducted. This is not feasible. However, even setting this problem aside, θ may not be a meaningful or useful quantity. For example, if the most important element of the context is the country in which the study is conducted, the average of these elements is not well defined. For example, suppose studies of methods for encouraging cessation of smoking have been conducted mainly in the United States, Canada, some western European countries, and Japan. The average of the treatment effects is not a useful quantity because we cannot identify a (human) population that would correspond to the 'average' context (country). Similarly, for time (year) as the element of the context, we are interested in the present and near future, and the main purpose of the studies conducted in the past is to contribute to such inference, not to make θ refer to the average or median year of the studies.

Time is an example of an element of the context that is ordered, and so, at least in principle, we can consider the inference about present or near future as a slight extrapolation. This can be incorporated in the model in (12.4) by a regression on time. Most other contexts are categorical, such as the method of measurement. The mean or average for such a categorical variable is not defined and, in fact, one of the categories, such as the practice established as present, may be the most appropriate context for inference.

12.4 Maximum Likelihood Estimation

We describe the Fisher scoring algorithm for fitting the model in (12.4) to which we add regression,

$$\hat{\theta}_d = \mathbf{x}_d \boldsymbol{\beta} + \delta_d + \varepsilon_d , \tag{12.5}$$

with the assumptions of independence and normality of δ_d and ε_d; $\mathbf{x}_d$ is the vector of covariates for study d; its first element is the intercept 1. The log-likelihood associated with this model is

$$l = -\frac{1}{2} \left\{ D \log(2\pi) + \sum_{d=1}^{D} \log \left(\sigma_{\mathrm{B}}^2 + v_d \right) + \sum_{d=1}^{D} \frac{e_d^2}{\sigma_{\mathrm{B}}^2 + v_d} \right\} ,$$

where $e_d = \hat{\theta}_d - \mathbf{x}_d \boldsymbol{\beta}$. Differentiation of l with respect to $\boldsymbol{\beta}$ yields

$$\frac{\partial l}{\partial \boldsymbol{\beta}} = \sum_{d=1}^{D} \frac{e_d \, \mathbf{x}_d}{\sigma_{\mathrm{B}}^2 + v_d} ,$$

which can be expressed in matrix notation as

$$\frac{\partial l}{\partial \boldsymbol{\beta}} = \mathbf{X}^{\top} \mathbf{V}^{-1} \mathbf{e} , \tag{12.6}$$

where $\mathbf{X}$ is the matrix constructed by vertically stacking the rows $\mathbf{x}_d$, $\mathbf{e} = (e_1, \ldots, e_D)^{\top}$ is the vector of residuals, also expressible as $\mathbf{e} = \hat{\boldsymbol{\theta}} - \mathbf{X} \boldsymbol{\beta}$ with $\hat{\boldsymbol{\theta}} = (\hat{\theta}_1, \ldots, \hat{\theta}_D)^{\top}$, and $\mathbf{V}$ is the diagonal matrix with the variances $\sigma_{\mathrm{B}}^2 + v_d$ on its diagonal. Equation (12.6) has the solution

$$\hat{\boldsymbol{\beta}} = \left(\mathbf{X}^{\top} \hat{\mathbf{V}}^{-1} \mathbf{X} \right)^{-1} \mathbf{X}^{\top} \hat{\mathbf{V}}^{-1} \hat{\boldsymbol{\theta}} , \tag{12.7}$$

which depends on $\hat{\sigma}_{\mathrm{B}}^2$ through an estimate $\hat{\mathbf{V}}$ of $\mathbf{V}$. If σ_{B}^2 were known, the sampling variance of $\hat{\boldsymbol{\beta}}$ would be $\mathrm{var}(\hat{\boldsymbol{\beta}} \mid \sigma_{\mathrm{B}}^2) = (\mathbf{X}^{\top} \mathbf{V}^{-1} \mathbf{X})^{-1}$. The estimator in (12.7), similar to (9.9), is a weighted least squares estimator. Each study contributes to the quadratic forms $\mathbf{X}^{\top} \mathbf{V}^{-1} \mathbf{X}$ and $\mathbf{X}^{\top} \mathbf{V}^{-1} \hat{\boldsymbol{\theta}}$ with weights $1/(\sigma_{\mathrm{B}}^2 + v_d)$; smaller sampling variance v_d results in greater weight, but the disparities in the contributions are moderated by σ_{B}^2 or its estimate.

The study-level variance σ_B^2 is estimated from its score and expected information. The score is

$$s = \frac{\partial l}{\partial \sigma^2} = -\frac{1}{2}\sum_{d=1}^{D}\frac{1}{\sigma_B^2 + v_d} + \frac{1}{2}\sum_{d=1}^{D}\frac{e_d^2}{(\sigma_B^2 + v_d)^2},$$

and the expected information is

$$\mathcal{I} = -E\left\{\frac{\partial^2 l}{\partial(\sigma^2)^2}\right\} = -\frac{1}{2}\sum_{d=1}^{D}\frac{1}{(\sigma_B^2 + v_d)^2} + \sum_{d=1}^{D}\frac{E\left(e_d^2\right)}{(\sigma_B^2 + v_d)^3}$$

$$= \frac{1}{2}\sum_{d=1}^{D}\frac{1}{(\sigma_B^2 + v_d)^2}.$$

Hence the iterative updating formula

$$\hat{\sigma}_{\text{new}}^2 = \hat{\sigma}_{\text{old}}^2 + \frac{s_{\text{old}}}{\mathcal{I}_{\text{old}}},$$

using the same notational conventions as in Section 9.3.

For the example in Figure 12.1, we obtain $\hat{\theta} = 0.851$, with estimated standard error 0.297, and estimated study-level variance $\hat{\sigma}_B^2 = 1.207$, with estimated standard error 0.654. The latter estimator has the same problem as discussed in Section 9.5, that the estimator and the estimator of its standard error are highly correlated. The likelihood ratio test statistic, which compares the deviances of the model fits with σ_B^2 estimated on the one hand and set to zero on the other, provides a more suitable assessment of the evidence against the hypothesis that $\sigma_B^2 = 0$. The value of this test statistic is 7.87, and it should be compared with a high quantile of the χ_1^2 distribution. For example, the 95th percentile is 3.84 and the 99.5th percentile is 7.88. Thus we have ample evidence that the studies do not have a common target. This is in accord with the conclusion based on Figure 12.2.

The studies were conducted over a period of 25 years, between 1970 and 1995, and most of them took more than a year to complete. With an element of arbitrariness, we classify the studies into five ordinal categories according to the year in which they commenced. The first five studies in ascending order in Figure 12.1, started in 1970–1974, are in the first category, the next four (1975–1979) in the second, then seven in the third, nine in the fourth, and the top three (1990–1995) in the fifth category. We regard this categorical variable as ordinal, so that by including it in the regression model in (12.5) we introduce only one new parameter. The regression fit with this covariate t is $0.003 + 0.277t$; the deviance is reduced by only 1.39 vis-à-vis the model without the covariate. Therefore we have no evidence of any trend over the period covered by the studies. The estimate of the between-study variance $\hat{\sigma}_B^2$ is reduced to 1.064 (from 1.207). The date of the study does not contribute substantially to the between-study variation.

The analysis presented here is tainted with the problem of improper use of the regression. The year of the study, or the related category, cannot be assigned (manipulated) for a study, and so the regression parameter as a target cannot be regarded as an effect of time. Related to this is the problem that the studies have subjects drawn from different populations, with differences that may have substantial systematic components over time. For example, the success rates of an emergency operation cannot be compared straightforwardly over a long period of time if the subjects (patients) in the different periods have very different medical histories. One reason for such differences is that certain operations that were experimental many years ago have become routine since, so that many of the subjects in recent years would not have survived had they been treated for their illnesses and conditions earlier in their lives by methods current at that time. At an extreme, the success rate may be dropping over the years because more and more acute cases are presented that in the past would not have been considered for surgery at all. The comparison of the success rates would not be appropriate for assessing the effectiveness of the surgeons and their teams, or of a health care system as a whole.

In brief, infeasibility of a meta-design is an obstacle to making inferences about effects. We cannot assign subjects to studies (e.g., by randomisation), nor can we assign at will values of covariates to studies as assumed by the regression models that are applied.

12.5 Publication Bias

The results of studies that have large sample sizes and are conducted over a long period of time or in several countries are usually published and discussed extensively in the literature. Being expensive, such a study may have a range of inferential goals. The team of researchers working on the study may publish details of its design, some results based on intermediate outcomes, results of some preliminary analyses, and results of analyses on peripheral issues in addition to those responding to the main inferential agenda. In contrast, small studies are less likely to be published. The team may find the results of little importance, for example, because no evidence of a treatment effect was found. (Setting aside numerous other factors, no evidence is a more likely outcome in small studies than in large ones.) Journal editors may reject a submitted manuscript for the same reason, or simply because of the small sample size of the study, or because submissions about other more prominent studies are regarded as more important and a better 'value' for the limited space in their journals. Also, larger studies tend to be conducted by bigger and more competent teams, with greater experience in all aspects of research, including the publication process.

Attainment of a significant outcome of a key hypothesis test is often regarded as a kudos by the authors and as a positive point by manuscript reviewers. This is inappropriate; if such practice were pursued consistently, we would not be able to assess the extent of false positive indications of significance. Another undesirable consequence of such practice is that studies are published selectively. Studies should be published as documents of their good conduct and analysis, and the statistical significance is not directly related to these. Of course, the design of a study may influence the likelihood of a significant outcome, but this should not be confused with the actual realisation (result) of the planned hypothesis test.

We are unable to estimate θ without bias because, in essence, some studies that should have been conducted, to arrange good representation of the contexts, were not carried out. It may still be meaningful to consider what the outcome of a meta-analysis would be if the results of all the studies were available. For this goal, it is appropriate to refer to the missing-data framework. In it we regard the corresponding data as the complete dataset and the available results as the incomplete dataset (see Chapter 5 for the terminology used). Such an analysis is concerned principally with the bias in estimating the average effect θ relatively to the complete-data analysis. The issue is referred to as *publication bias*. We could similarly refer to the uneven representation of the contexts among the studies as *conduct bias*.

Apart from the failure to publish the results of a study, we include under the heading of publication bias all other reasons for not having the results of some of the studies. These include publication in journals not included in the search, in languages other than English (and some other western European languages), and the failure to identify all the appropriate articles and their details in the searched literature. Including a study in the meta-analysis inappropriately or more than once are other possible sources of error, but they are easy to avoid when the meta-analysis comprises only a moderate number of studies, as is often the case.

12.5.1 Funnel Plot

The fundamental difficulty in constructing a plausible complete dataset is that we do not know how many studies, if any, are missing from our list and can merely hypothesise about the reasons for not publishing a study, or failing to find any publications about it.

If all studies were published, without any prejudice, studies with large sample sizes n_d and small sampling variances v_d would tend to have estimates $\hat{\theta}_d$ in a narrow range and studies with small sample sizes in a wider range. Both would be approximately symmetrically distributed around the estimate $\hat{\theta}$. Therefore, a plot of the estimates $\hat{\theta}_d$ against the (estimated) sampling variances $\hat{v}_d$, or their transformation, would have a funnel shape for the complete data. Departure from this shape would indicate that some studies are omitted from the analysis. The plot of $\hat{\theta}_d$ against $f(\hat{v}_d)$ for a suitable monotone function f is called the *funnel plot*. An example is presented in Figure 12.3 for a set of 75 studies. The estimated sampling variation of the studies is drawn

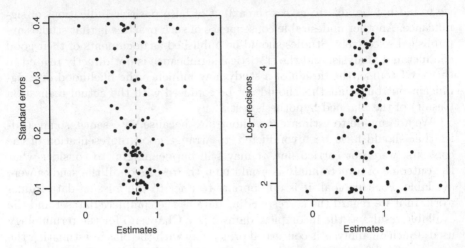

Fig. 12.3. Example of funnel plots for a collection of 75 studies. The median of the study-specific estimates $\hat{\theta}_d$ is marked by vertical dashes.

on two scales, as standard deviations, $\sqrt{\hat{v}_d}$, in the left-hand panel, and log-precisions, $-\log(\hat{v}_d)$, in the right-hand panel. Although some asymmetry can be discerned in both panels, completing either plot to make it symmetric is a nontrivial task. Moreover, we cannot expect a perfectly symmetric diagram even with a complete set of studies because of sampling variation within each study and a relatively small number of studies within any narrow range of estimated standard errors $\sqrt{\hat{v}_d}$. This is easy to illustrate by simulations.

We borrow the context of Figure 12.3, that is, the number of studies $D = 75$ and their (estimated) mean 0.73 and the standard errors, and generate sets of D estimates $\hat{\theta}_d$ according to the model in (12.4), with $\theta = 0.73$, $\delta_d \sim \mathcal{N}(0, 0.01)$, and $\varepsilon_d \sim \mathcal{N}(0, \hat{v}_d)$. We define a measure of asymmetry, evaluate it on every replicate collection of the D studies, and compare the distribution of these simulated features with its realised version. The purpose of this is to assess how much asymmetry is generated by a complete-data (symmetric) model. First we define a measure of asymmetry of a $K \times 1$ vector $\mathbf{u}$ with respect to a constant c as

$$S(\mathbf{u}, c) = \max \left| \tfrac{1}{2}(\mathbf{u}_A + \mathbf{u}_D) - c \right|,$$

where $\mathbf{u}_A$ and $\mathbf{u}_D$ are the versions of vector $\mathbf{u}$ obtained by sorting it in ascending and descending order, respectively. This is the largest of the (absolute) deviations of the means of the kth and $(K + 1 - k)$th largest values, $k = 1, \ldots, [K/2]$, from the 'centre' c.

We define the measure of asymmetry for a collection of studies as follows. We sort the realised studies according to their estimated sampling variances $\hat{v}_d$. We take segments of $K = 10$ studies, and for each segment evaluate their measure of asymmetry around the estimated mean $\hat{\theta}$. Let $\hat{\boldsymbol{\theta}}^{(A)}$ be the permutation of $\hat{\boldsymbol{\theta}}$ into ascending order according to the estimated variances. The first segment, composed of $(\hat{\theta}_1^{(A)}, \ldots, \hat{\theta}_K^{(A)})$, yields the value S_1, the next, $(\hat{\theta}_2^{(A)}, \ldots, \hat{\theta}_{K+1}^{(A)})$, yields S_2, and the last, $(\hat{\theta}_{D-K+1}^{(A)}, \ldots, \hat{\theta}_D^{(A)})$, yields S_{D-K+1}. Denote $\mathbf{S} = (S_1, \ldots, S_{D-K+1})$.

We repeat this exercise, but this time exclude from each segment the study with the smallest value of the estimate $\hat{\theta}_d$, so that the measure of asymmetry is evaluated for only $K - 1$ studies in each instance. The resulting vector of measures is denoted by $\mathbf{S}^{(A)}$. Finally, we carry out the mirror image of this exercise and evaluate the measure of asymmetry after excluding from each segment the study with the largest value of $\hat{\theta}_d$. The result in denoted by $\mathbf{S}^{(D)}$.

If by excluding a study with $(\hat{\theta}_d, \hat{v}_d)$ we reduce the value of S substantially, the funnel plot could be made much more symmetric by adding a study near the mirror image of this study, that is, with $(2\hat{\theta}_d - \hat{\theta}, \hat{v}_d)$. From the vectors $\mathbf{S}$, $\mathbf{S}^{(A)}$, and $\mathbf{S}^{(D)}$ we can identify the study which, when excluded, would result in the greatest reduction of the measure of asymmetry. Thus, we identify the segments for which $\mathbf{S} - \mathbf{S}^{(A)}$ and $\mathbf{S} - \mathbf{S}^{(D)}$ attain their respective maxima s_A and s_D and take the segment with the greater of these two values. Let $s^* = \max(s_A, s_D)$. This is the maximum reduction of asymmetry by excluding a single study, and we denote it by MRA1. The maximum reduction of asymmetry by excluding $m > 1$ studies from the meta-analysis is defined similarly, and is denoted by MRAm. In the segment in which the value of s^* is realised, we identify the study that was excluded to attain s^*. This is the study with the smallest value of $\hat{\theta}_d$ in the segment if $s^* = s^{(A)}$ and the maximum occurs for $\mathbf{S}^{(A)}$, and the study with the largest value of $\hat{\theta}_d$ otherwise. If we could add the results of a single study to our collection, symmetry of the funnel plot would be improved most by adding a study with results equal to the mirror image of the results of this study.

We adopt MRA1, the value of s^*, as our feature. We fit the model in (12.4) and simulate from the fit 999 sets of estimates $\hat{\theta}_d$, $d = 1, \ldots, D$, with the same values of $\hat{v}_d$ as in the realised study. For each replicate dataset we evaluate the feature s^*. For the realised set of D studies, $s^* = 0.350$, and among the 1000 values it is the 917th largest. Therefore, we have very weak evidence of an omitted study. The study that brings about more asymmetry than any other has $\hat{\theta}_d = 1.801$, the largest of all of the estimates, with $\hat{v}_d = 0.143$, close to the largest value, which is 0.159.

The appropriate conclusion is that we have failed to find any evidence of a missing study. This we cannot interpret as certainty that all the relevant studies have been identified. We could add fictitious study results to the funnel plot without upsetting the symmetry and yet alter the estimates $\hat{\theta}$ and $\hat{\sigma}_B^2$ appreciably. Further, if we found evidence of a missing study and did identify a study d^*, the results of which upset the symmetry more than any other study, the missing study need not have results in the vicinity of $(2\hat{\theta}_{d^*} - \hat{\theta}, \hat{v}_{d^*})$, because symmetry of the funnel plot could be promoted by adding (imputing) one or several study results elsewhere. Attaching any importance to study d^* or to the mirror image of its results would amount to personalisation (Section 9.7).

The procedure described finds or fails to find evidence of a single missing study. If some evidence is found, the procedure can be repeated as many times as necessary, with the studies that upset the symmetry most in each of the earlier applications removed, until no evidence is found. By each removal, the funnel plot becomes more symmetric, so it is unlikely that evidence could be found of more than a handful of studies missing. After each removal, the estimate $\hat{\theta}$ can be updated.

Although the problem of missing studies (publication bias) can be formulated as a problem of missing data, addressing it with integrity, for example, by multiple imputation (Section 5.5), is difficult because we have uncertainty about both the number of missing studies and their results. In the described procedure, the width of the segment, $K = 10$, is chosen partly by convention. On the one hand, the studies in each segment should have a narrow range of variances $\hat{v}_d$. On the other hand, K should not be too small, otherwise substantial departures from symmetry can be expected in many segments even when the funnel plot is symmetric. The procedure can be used in another mode. By simulating measures of asymmetry for a range of scenarios (number of studies D, sampling variances v_d, and study-level variance σ_B^2), we can get a feel for how much asymmetry can be expected in the funnel plot when no studies are missing.

In conclusion we note that large-scale studies are unlikely to be missing, so the impact of the studies that might be hypothesised to be missing would be overstated by their number. However, missing studies are only one element of uncertainty about the ideal target θ associated with the average (or no) context. For example, when no studies with the relevant agenda were conducted in a particular period or a particular geographical region, we could not draw a conclusion to the contrary, that some studies must have been conducted, but we may consider what the results of the meta-analysis would be if such studies were conducted and these and other elements of the context were represented in the meta-analysis more evenly.

12.6 Inference for a Particular Context

We return to the setting in which we assume that all the relevant studies have been identified and the contexts are represented among these studies evenly. A weakness of the target θ, and consequently of its estimator $\hat{\theta}$, is that it refers to an unrealisable context. For example, the 'average' of a collection of countries does not have a meaningful definition. For inferences about θ applicable to the present or the recent past, studies conducted decades ago should be less relevant than more recent studies. In brief, it is more meaningful to make inferences for a given context, instead of the ambiguously defined and often nonexistent 'average' or a typical context. Extrapolation to the near future and a country not represented among the studies would be even more useful, but it is a more difficult problem.

We consider first estimation of θ for one of the realised contexts, say, d^*, so that our target is θ_{d^*}. We derive an estimator of θ_{d^*} that draws on the information in all the studies. This is the estimator of the conditional expectation of θ_{d^*} given $\hat{\theta}_{d^*}$. When both θ_{d^*} and $\hat{\theta}_{d^*}$ are regarded as random variables their joint distribution is

$$
\begin{pmatrix} \theta_{d^*} \\ \hat{\theta}_{d^*} \end{pmatrix} \sim \mathcal{N} \left\{ \begin{pmatrix} \theta \\ \theta \end{pmatrix}, \begin{pmatrix} \sigma_B^2 & \sigma_B^2 \\ \sigma_B^2 & v_{d^*} + \sigma_B^2 \end{pmatrix} \right\}.
$$

Hence,

$$
\left(\theta_{d^*} \mid \hat{\theta}_{d^*} \right) \sim \mathcal{N} \left\{ \theta + \frac{\sigma_B^2}{v_{d^*} + \sigma_B^2} \left(\hat{\theta}_{d^*} - \theta \right), \sigma_B^2 - \frac{\sigma_B^4}{v_{d^*} + \sigma_B^2} \right\},
$$

which motivates the estimator

$$
\tilde{\theta}_{d^*} = \hat{\theta} + \frac{\hat{\sigma}_B^2}{\hat{v}_{d^*} + \hat{\sigma}_B^2} \left(\hat{\theta}_{d^*} - \hat{\theta} \right). \tag{12.8}
$$

This is a shrinkage estimator, pulling the unbiased estimator $\hat{\theta}_{d^*}$ toward the average estimator $\hat{\theta}$. The amount of shrinkage, or pull, depends on the relative sizes of the sampling and between-study variances. For instance, if σ_B^2 were very small, $\hat{\theta}_{d^*}$ could be improved a great deal, because all D studies would contribute substantially to $\tilde{\theta}_{d^*}$. In contrast, when σ_B^2 is large, the studies have very different targets, and one study contributes very little to the shrinkage estimation of the other. We can describe $\tilde{\theta}_{d^*}$ as exploiting the similarity of the studies; see Section 3.8 for a similar application to small-area estimation.

The estimator $\tilde{\theta}_{d^*}$ can also be derived by synthesis. The unbiased $\hat{\theta}_{d^*}$ and small-variance $\hat{\theta}$ are alternative estimators of θ_{d^*}. Instead of choosing one of them, we combine them with the coefficient for which the combination has the smallest MSE. For simplicity, we ignore the uncertainty about $\hat{\theta}$, that is, assume that $\theta = \hat{\theta}$. Then

$$
\mathrm{MSE} \left\{ (1 - b)\hat{\theta}_{d^*} + b\hat{\theta}; \theta_{d^*} \right\} \doteq (1 - b)^2 v_{d^*} + b^2 (\theta_{d^*} - \theta)^2, \tag{12.9}
$$

and the minimum of this quadratic function is attained for

$$
b_{d^*} = \frac{v_{d^*}}{v_{d^*} + (\theta_{d^*} - \theta)^2}.
$$

We estimate b_{d^*} by $\hat{b}_{d^*} = \hat{v}_{d^*} / (\hat{v}_{d^*} + \hat{\sigma}_B^2)$, replacing the squared deviation $(\theta_{d^*} - \theta)^2$ by its estimated expectation $\hat{\sigma}_B^2$. The estimator $(1 - \hat{b}_{d^*})\hat{\theta}_{d^*} + \hat{b}_{d^*}\hat{\theta}$ coincides with $\tilde{\theta}_{d^*}$ in (12.8).

The estimator $\tilde{\theta}_{d*}$ can be adapted for the regression model in (12.5) by replacing the estimated average effect $\hat{\theta}$ with its fit $\mathbf{x}_{d*}\hat{\boldsymbol{\beta}}$:

$$\tilde{\theta}_{d*} = \frac{\hat{\sigma}_{\mathrm{B}}^2}{\hat{v}_{d*} + \hat{\sigma}_{\mathrm{B}}^2}\hat{\theta}_{d*} + \frac{\hat{v}_{d*}}{\hat{v}_{d*} + \hat{\sigma}_{\mathrm{B}}^2}\mathbf{x}_{d*}\hat{\boldsymbol{\beta}}.$$

Note that σ_{B}^2 and its estimator in this expression refer to the study-level variance after adjusting for the covariates in $\mathbf{X}$.

The squared deviation $\Delta_{d*}^2 = (\theta_{d*} - \theta)^2$ might be estimated more efficiently by combining its alternative estimators, $(\hat{\theta}_{d*} - \hat{\theta})^2$ and $\hat{\sigma}_{\mathrm{B}}^2$. However, the relevant combination (coefficients) is easy to find only in some simple settings that are not realistic.

The uncertainty about $\hat{\theta}$ is easy to incorporate, although it makes very little difference to $\tilde{\theta}_d$. Assuming that σ_{B}^2 and v_d are known, the exact version of equation (12.9) is

$$\mathrm{MSE}\left\{(1-b)\hat{\theta}_{d*} + b\hat{\theta}; \theta_d\right\} = (1-b)^2 v_{d*} + b^2\left(v + \Delta_{d*}^2\right) - 2b(1-b)\,\mathrm{cov}\left(\hat{\theta}_{d*}, \hat{\theta}\right)$$

and

$$\mathrm{cov}\left(\hat{\theta}_{d*}, \hat{\theta}\right) = \frac{1}{c_+}\mathrm{cov}\left(\hat{\theta}_{d*}, \sum_{d=1}^{D} c_d\hat{\theta}_d\right)$$

$$= \frac{c_{d*}}{c_+}v_{d*},$$

where $v = \mathrm{var}(\hat{\theta})$, $c_d = 1/(v_d + \sigma_{\mathrm{B}}^2)$, and $c_+ = c_1 + \cdots + c_D$. Hence the MSE is

$$b^2\left\{v + v_{d*}\left(1 - 2\frac{c_{d*}}{c_+}\right) + \Delta_{d*}^2\right\} - 2bv_{d*}\left(1 - \frac{c_{d*}}{c_+}\right) + v_{d*},$$

and this quadratic function of b attains its minimum for

$$b_{d*} = \frac{v_{d*}\left(1 - c_{d*}/c_+\right)}{v + v_{d*}\left(1 - 2c_{d*}/c_+\right) + \Delta_{d*}^2}.$$

As earlier, we replace the squared deviation Δ_{d*}^2 by σ_{B}^2, its expectation over the studies, and the unknown quantities v_{d*}, θ, and σ_{B}^2 by their estimates. Usually, v_{d*} is much greater than v, so the impact of v on the coefficient b_{d*} is negligible. When σ_{B}^2 is small the fraction c_{d*}/c_+ is substantial for at most one or two studies that have variances v_{d*} much smaller than the other studies. For other studies the fraction c_{d*}/c_+ is small and can be ignored. Then we obtain the original shrinkage estimator in (12.8).

The estimator $\tilde{\theta}_{d*}$ can be improved by exploring alternatives to estimation of Δ_{d*}^2. A conservative strategy is to specify an upper bound for Δ_{d*}^2, and combine $\hat{\theta}_{d*}$ and $\hat{\theta}$ optimally, assuming that Δ_{d*}^2 attains this bound. It can be shown, as in Section 8.3.2, that this is a minimax estimator among the linear combinations of $\hat{\theta}_{d*}$ and $\hat{\theta}$ for feasible deviations Δ_{d*}. In most contexts, an upper bound for Δ_{d*}^2 would be set to a multiple of $\hat{\sigma}_B^2$, such as $4\hat{\sigma}_B^2$. Information specific to study d^* may be available, and that might enable one to set the bound much lower, although only for study d^*.

12.6.1 Prediction for an Unrealised Context

We turn next to estimating θ for a context not realised by any of the studies; we refer to this as the *target context*. Prediction of θ for the near future in a given population is a realistic example. If the context can be represented in a regression model, this is a standard prediction problem. However, we should be wary of any extrapolation, especially when the values of $\mathbf{x}$ have not been set by design. As the number of studies is never very large, we cannot rely on any asymptotic results or properties, and the procedures based on search for a parsimonious valid model are not very effective. Every degree of freedom expended by defining a more complex regression model inflates the sampling variance of the prediction a lot, so a covariate is useful only when it reduces the bias of the prediction substantially. In practice, clear cut associations are difficult to identify because each study result is subject to considerable uncertainty. Therefore we may have no useful model on which to base our prediction, other than the model in (12.4), or (12.5) with one or a few covariates.

If we regard all the realised or plausible contexts as an unstructured collection, our best prediction for a specific context is $\hat{\theta}$, with MSE equal to $\sigma_B^2 + \mathrm{var}(\hat{\theta})$. This may be unsatisfactory when some information, originating from another data source or from expert opinion, suggests that certain studies have contexts that are closer to the target context. When the target context is estimated by $\hat{\theta}$, the realised studies contribute to the prediction with weights $w_d = v_d/(v_d + \sigma_B^2)$. We can alter these weights to $w_d' = w_d u_d/u_+$, where $u_+ = (u_1 + \cdots + u_D)/D$. The adjustment factors u_d are set subjectively, reflecting expert opinion. Their purpose is to alter the influence each study exerts on the prediction; for those with contexts closer to the target, u_d is set greater than for those with more distant contexts. The concerns about the ambiguity of how u_d are set can be allayed by a sensitivity study, considering several plausible sets of factors u_d. The favourable outcome of such a study is that the predictions based on these sets differ insubstantially. Otherwise it is difficult to draw a firm conclusion.

12.7 Multivariate Meta-Analysis

Meta-analysis is usually concerned with estimating a single target or one target per study. Examples where two or more targets are estimated for the typical or a specific context are rare because, within a relevant theme, many studies that do not record all the relevant outcomes would have to be excluded.

We nevertheless study this setting and explore how one outcome variable can contribute to estimating a summary of another.

Suppose studies $d = 1, \ldots, D$ concluded with K-variate vectors of estimates $\hat{\boldsymbol{\theta}}_d$ and estimated sampling variance matrices $\hat{\mathbf{V}}_d$. We assume that the estimators $\hat{\boldsymbol{\theta}}_d$ are unbiased for their respective targets $\boldsymbol{\theta}_d$ and $\hat{\mathbf{V}}_d$ are unbiased for the sampling variances $\mathbf{V}_d = \mathrm{var}(\hat{\boldsymbol{\theta}}_d)$. We can estimate the vector $\boldsymbol{\theta}$ for the average context componentwise, but a more elegant approach is by direct maximum likelihood. The model considered is

$$\hat{\boldsymbol{\theta}}_d = \boldsymbol{\theta} + \boldsymbol{\delta}_d + \boldsymbol{\varepsilon}_d,$$

where $\boldsymbol{\delta}_d$ is a random sample from $\mathcal{N}_K(\mathbf{0}, \boldsymbol{\Sigma}_\mathrm{B})$ and $\boldsymbol{\varepsilon}_d$ is a random draw from $\mathcal{N}_K(\mathbf{0}, \mathbf{V}_d)$; we ignore the uncertainty about $\mathbf{V}_d$. The constant vector $\boldsymbol{\theta}$ can be replaced by multivariate regression $\mathbf{X}_d \boldsymbol{\beta}$ with a matrix of regressors for $\hat{\boldsymbol{\theta}}$. We impose no constraints on $\boldsymbol{\Sigma}_\mathrm{B}$; in particular, the components of $\boldsymbol{\delta}_d$ (or of $\boldsymbol{\theta}_d = \boldsymbol{\theta} + \boldsymbol{\delta}_d$) may be highly correlated. Maximum likelihood estimators of $\boldsymbol{\theta}$ and $\boldsymbol{\Sigma}_\mathrm{B}$ are derived by Fisher scoring, yielding equations similar to their counterparts for the univariate case:

$$\hat{\boldsymbol{\beta}} = \left(\sum_{d=1}^{D} \mathbf{X}_d^\top \hat{\mathbf{W}}_d \mathbf{X} \right)^{-1} \sum_{d=1}^{D} \mathbf{X}_d^\top \hat{\mathbf{W}}_d \hat{\boldsymbol{\theta}},$$

$$\hat{\boldsymbol{\Sigma}}_\mathrm{B,new} = \hat{\boldsymbol{\Sigma}}_\mathrm{B,old} + \left(\sum_{d=1}^{D} \hat{\mathbf{W}}_d^{(2)} \right)^{-1} \sum_{d=1}^{D} \left\{ -\hat{\mathbf{W}}_d + \left(\mathbf{e}_{d,\mathrm{W}}\, \mathbf{e}_{d,\mathrm{W}}^\top \right) \right\}, \quad (12.10)$$

where $\mathbf{W}_d = (\mathbf{V}_d + \boldsymbol{\Sigma}_\mathrm{B})^{-1}$, $\mathbf{W}_d^{(2)}$ is the matrix formed by elementwise squaring of $\mathbf{W}_d$, and $\mathbf{e}_{d,\mathrm{W}} = \hat{\mathbf{W}}_d^{-1} \hat{\mathbf{e}}_d$. As an alternative, $\boldsymbol{\Sigma}_\mathrm{B}$ may be estimated by moment matching as the matrix difference between the sample variance matrix of the estimates $\hat{\boldsymbol{\theta}}_d$ and the average of the estimated sampling variances $\mathbf{V}_d$. Weights can be used in this averaging, and the weights can be iterative, adjusted after each updating of $\boldsymbol{\Sigma}_\mathrm{B}$.

The vectors $\boldsymbol{\theta}_d$ are estimated by shrinkage as their estimated conditional expectations given the model fit:

$$\tilde{\boldsymbol{\theta}}_d = \hat{\boldsymbol{\theta}} + \boldsymbol{\Sigma}_\mathrm{B} \left(\boldsymbol{\Sigma}_\mathrm{B} + \mathbf{V}_d \right)^{-1} \left(\hat{\boldsymbol{\theta}}_d - \hat{\boldsymbol{\theta}} \right).$$

Like its univariate version, this estimator can be interpreted as exploiting the similarity of the context-specific values $\boldsymbol{\theta}_d$. When $\boldsymbol{\Sigma}_\mathrm{B}$ involves high correlations, components k of $\tilde{\boldsymbol{\theta}}_d$, $d \neq d^*$, contribute to component k of $\tilde{\boldsymbol{\theta}}_d$. However, the other components of $\hat{\boldsymbol{\theta}}_d$ also contribute to component k of $\tilde{\boldsymbol{\theta}}_d$. This is obvious as the weight matrix $\boldsymbol{\Sigma}_\mathrm{B} \left(\boldsymbol{\Sigma}_\mathrm{B} + \mathbf{V}_d \right)^{-1}$ is not diagonal. Thus, similarity is exploited not merely across the studies but also across the components of the outcome vector.

12.8 Estimating Many Quantities

Inference about a specific context is an example of estimating one (or several) of a large number of related quantities. In this section, we study a more general setting in which there are D independent estimators $\hat{\theta}_d$, each based on a separate dataset (study), with target θ_d. Suppose each estimator $\hat{\theta}_d$ is unbiased for its target θ_d and has sampling variance $v_d = f(n_d)g(\theta_d)$, where f and g are known functions. An example is provided by the setting $f(n) = 1/n$ and $g(\theta) = \theta$, which may be suitable for the means of Poisson-distributed samples. For estimating the within-sample variances of homoscedastic normally distributed samples, $f(n) = 1/(n-1)$ and $g(\theta) = 2\theta^2$. Note that there is some indeterminacy in the product $f(n)g(\theta)$; a constant factor can be extracted from one function and included in the other.

Let θ be the mean of the D quantities θ_d, and $\sigma_\theta^2 = \sum_d (\theta_d - \theta)^2/D$ their variance. As an alternative to $\hat{\theta}_d$, we might consider an (unbiased) estimator of θ, such as the mean of the estimators, $\hat{\theta} = (\hat{\theta}_1 + \cdots + \hat{\theta}_D)/D$, or their weighted version

$$\hat{\theta} = \left(\sum_{d=1}^{D} \frac{1}{v_d} \right)^{-1} \sum_{d=1}^{D} \frac{\hat{\theta}_d}{v_d}. \tag{12.11}$$

Denote the sampling variance of $\hat{\theta}$ by v.

Instead of choosing either $\hat{\theta}_d$ or $\hat{\theta}$ to estimate θ_d, we combine them as

$$\tilde{\theta}_d = (1 - b_d)\hat{\theta}_d + b_d\hat{\theta}, \tag{12.12}$$

with the coefficient b_d for which $\mathrm{MSE}(\tilde{\theta}_d; \theta_d)$ is minimised. This coefficient depends on some unknown quantities, so we use its estimator instead. The MSE of the composition $\tilde{\theta}_d$ is

$$\mathrm{MSE}\left(\tilde{\theta}_d; \theta_d\right) = (1 - b_d)^2 v_d + b_d^2 v + 2b_d(1 - b_d)\frac{c_d}{c_+}v_d + b_d^2(\theta_d - \theta)^2,$$

where $c_d = 1/v_d$ are the coefficients in the estimator $\hat{\theta}$ in (12.11) and c_+ is their total. We ignore the bias of $\hat{\theta}$ in estimating θ, but not its bias in estimating θ_d. The MSE attains its minimum for

$$b_d^* = \frac{v_d\left(1 - \dfrac{c_d}{c_+}\right)}{v_d\left(1 - \dfrac{2c_d}{c_+}\right) + v + (\theta_d - \theta)^2}. \tag{12.13}$$

Since θ_d is the target, we replace the squared deviation $(\theta_d - \theta)^2$ in b_d^* by its mean σ_B^2. When there are many studies this variance is estimated with much greater precision than the squared deviation it replaces. For example, based on the statistic $S = \sum_{d=1}^{D}(\hat{\theta}_d - \hat{\theta})^2$, the estimator

$$\hat{\sigma}_B^2 = \frac{1}{D}\left\{S - \left(1 - \frac{2}{D}\right)\sum_{d=1}^{D} v_d\right\} - v,$$

derived by moment matching, is approximately unbiased for $\hat{\sigma}_B^2$. In this approach, the variance σ_B^2 or its estimator has a pivotal role, as we rely on an assessment of how similar the targets θ_d are. As an alternative to estimating $(\theta_d - \theta)^2$ by $\hat{\sigma}_B^2$, we may adhere to the form of b_d^* in (12.13) but explore the consequences of substituting an incorrect value for θ_d or $\theta_d - \theta$ and attempt to ameliorate the error.

By way of an illustration, we explore estimation of within-group variances in an ANOVA setting with heteroscedasticity. There are D groups, with normally distributed outcomes y_{jd}, $j = 1, \ldots, n_d$, $d = 1, \ldots, D$, and within-group variances σ_d^2, $d = 1, \ldots, D$. The pooled variance is

$$\sigma^2 = \frac{1}{n - D}\sum_{d=1}^{D}(n_d - 1)\sigma_d^2,$$

where $n = n_1 + \cdots + n_D$ is the overall sample size. We assume that $n_d \ll n$ for all groups for which we are interested in improving on the obvious unbiased estimator of σ_d^2,

$$\hat{\sigma}_d^2 = \frac{1}{n_d - 1}\sum_{j=1}^{n_d}(y_{jd} - \bar{y}_d)^2,$$

where $\bar{y}_d$ is the sample mean in group d. We consider the synthetic estimator

$$\tilde{\sigma}_d^2 = (1 - b_d)\hat{\sigma}_d^2 + b_d\hat{\sigma}^2,$$

where

$$\hat{\sigma}^2 = \frac{1}{n - D}\sum_{d=1}^{D}(n_d - 1)\hat{\sigma}_d^2$$

is the pooled (unbiased) estimator of σ^2. The MSE of $\tilde{\sigma}_d^2$ is

$$\frac{2(1 - b_d)^2\sigma_d^4}{n_d - 1} + \frac{2b_d^2\sigma^4}{n - D} + 4b_d(1 - b_d)\frac{\sigma_d^4}{n - D} + b_d^2(\sigma_d^2 - \sigma^2)^2$$

$$= \sigma^4 b_d^2\left\{2r_d^2\left(\frac{1}{n_d - 1} - \frac{2}{n - D}\right) + \frac{2}{n - D} + (r_d - 1)^2\right\}$$

$$- 4\sigma^4 b_d r_d^2\left(\frac{1}{n_d - 1} - \frac{1}{n - D}\right) + \frac{2r_d^2\sigma^4}{n_d - 1}, \tag{12.14}$$

where $r_d = \sigma_d^2/\sigma^2$ is the ratio of the group-specific and pooled variances. If all the quantities involved in this quadratic function of b_d were known, its minimum would be attained for

$$b_d^* = \frac{2r_d^2 \left(\dfrac{1}{n_d - 1} - \dfrac{1}{n - D} \right)}{2r_d^2 \left(\dfrac{1}{n_d - 1} - \dfrac{2}{n - D} \right) + \dfrac{2}{n - D} + (r_d - 1)^2}$$

$$\doteq \frac{2r_d^2}{2r_d^2 + (n_d - 1)(r_d - 1)^2} \, ,$$

after dropping all fractions with the denominator $n - D$. This function of r_d increases from zero to unity for $0 \le r_d \le 1$ and decreases from unity to $2/(n_d + 1)$ for $1 \le r_d < +\infty$. The minimum MSE that would be attained with b_d^* is

$$\text{MSE}\{\tilde{\sigma}_d^2(b_d^*); \sigma_d^2\} \doteq \sigma^4 \left\{ \frac{2r_d^2}{n_d - 1} - \frac{2r_d^2}{2r_d^2 + (n_d - 1)(r_d - 1)^2} \frac{2r_d^2}{n_d - 1} \right\}$$

$$= \sigma^4 \frac{2r_d^2 (r_d - 1)^2}{2r_d^2 + (n_d - 1)(r_d - 1)^2}$$

$$= \frac{2\sigma_d^4}{n_d - 1 + \dfrac{2r_d^2}{(r_d - 1)^2}} \, .$$

This is the (unattainable) lower bound for the MSE of $\tilde{\sigma}_d^2$ when an estimated or guessed value of b_d^* is used. We have a great potential for improvement when $r_d \doteq 1$ because the pooled variance σ^2 is estimated with high precision. For a given value of r_d, the potential for improvement is greater for smaller n_d.

Suppose we do not have any prior information about the variance ratio r_d. What value of b_d should $\tilde{\sigma}_d^2$ be based on? Let u_d be our estimate, or guess, of r_d, and c_d the corresponding coefficient:

$$c_d = \frac{2u_d^2}{2u_d^2 + (n_d - 1)(u_d - 1)^2} \, .$$

Then the MSE of $\tilde{\sigma}_d^2(c_d)$ is equal to

$$\sigma^4 \left[\frac{2r_d^2}{n_d - 1} + \left\{ \frac{2r_d^2}{n_d - 1} + (r_d - 1)^2 \right\} c_d(c_d - 2b_d) \right] \, .$$

Therefore we should strive to make $c_d(c_d - 2b_d) = (c_d - b_d)^2 - b_d^2$ as small as possible. If we prefer a conservative strategy we should base c_d on a value of r_d as far from zero and infinity as possible, while being confident that $c_d < b_d$. In this way, we avoid the largest possible deviations $|c_d - b_d|$. If we can rule out neither that $r_d < 1$ nor that $r_d > 1$, it is better to err on the side of overstating r_d, that is, choosing u_d as the largest plausible value of r_d, because b_d has a higher limit and the MSE a lower limit as r_d diverges to $+\infty$.

Suggested Reading

Analyses that can be regarded as meta-analyses have been conducted for a long time without recognising their special nature. A milestone paper that is generally agreed to have set off the modern meta-analysis is [59], and [72] is the first systematic treatment of the topic. For a review of later developments, see [140]. Research synthesis and synthesis of evidence are two commonly used synonyms for meta-analysis. The term *systematic review* is used for protocol-based search for studies in the literature and the subsequent analysis. It implies a codification of the process for literature search and extraction of information. See www.cochrane.org/resources/handbook for guidelines for meta-analysis in medical research and information about the Cochrane Collaboration, a library of systematic reviews. The principal areas in which meta-analysis is conducted are clinical trials [36], epidemiology [64], and educational research [106] and [155]. The book [187] deals with methods for and applications of meta-analysis in medical research (clinical and epidemiology). Ever since [40], the topic has been of keen interest to Bayesians. Key references to publication bias are [41] and [24]; the latter emphasises sensitivity analysis as a way of addressing the uncertainties not accounted for by the analysis directly.

Problems and Exercises

12.1. Recall the definitions of the terms *standard deviation* and *standard error*. Relate them to the terms *concentration* and *precision*.

12.2. Figure 12.1 can be redrawn with the studies ordered according to their values of $\hat{\theta}_d$. Such diagrams, and the identification of pairs of studies for which there is evidence that their targets θ_d differ, is described in [61]. Study this paper and discuss its relevance to meta-analysis. Verify the conclusions of the paper by simulations using a setting similar to that of Figure 12.1.

12.3. For a set of $D = 12$ studies with identically normally distributed estimators $\hat{\theta}_d$ with sampling variances $v_d = v_1$, $d = 1, \ldots, D$, study by simulations the error involved in the identity in (12.3) arising from substituting the estimator $\hat{v}_d$ for v_d. For simplicity, assume that the variance estimators also have the same scaled χ^2 distribution. Relate the scaling σ^2 and the common number of degrees of freedom to the bias of the estimator of $\mathrm{var}(\tilde{\sigma}^2)$. Repeat this exercise for a similar setting with studies that have distinct targets.

12.4. Describe how the hypothesis that the context-level variance σ_B^2 vanishes could be tested and describe the rationale for testing the hypothesis that $\sigma_B^2 < \Delta$ for a suitably selected value Δ. Relate this problem to the hypothesis test of small treatment effect in (individual) bioequivalence in Section 8.5.

12.5. Consider a meta-analysis of the average grades in a standardised examination in an academic subject, such as the A-levels in the UK or the Placement Test in the United States. Suppose a comparison of the average grades between two types of schools is of interest. Compile a list of causes that confound the straightforward interpretation of (substantial) differences of the sample means as the effect of the school type. Discuss how the difference in the coming year could be predicted. Compile another list of reasons why the changes in the differences over time cannot be interpreted as changes in the quality of the education/instruction provided by the schools.

12.6. Implement the Fisher scoring algorithm described in Section 12.4. (To simplify the task, suppose there are no covariates.) Construct a moment-matching estimator of the context-level variance σ_B^2 and compare it with the maximum likelihood estimator on real or artificially generated examples.

12.7. Translate the arguments for restricted maximum likelihood (REML) (see Section 9.3.1) to the setting of meta-analysis and devise an adaptation of the maximum likelihood that takes into account the lost degree of freedom. Compare REML and ML estimates on a few examples from the previous exercise.

12.8. Revisit the example in Section 7.5.1 about RAAA. Several studies have been conducted (in the UK) since the 1950s (and register information may be available from more recent years). Discuss what results one might expect from a meta-analyis of these studies. How should time (e.g., the year of the study) be treated in a meta-analysis? How could the results be interpreted? Compare your conclusions with those of [86].

12.9. Construct funnel plots for the datasets you used in Exercise 12.6 and, ignoring all the theory in Section 12.5, make a judgment about the symmetry of each of them. Construct a dataset comprising (θ_d, v_d), $d = 1, \ldots, D$, where θ_d is the target and v_d the sampling variance of its unbiased estimator, in such a way that the funnel plot of your choice, with θ_d instead of $\hat{\theta}_d$, is perfectly symmetric. Generate replicates of $(\hat{\theta}_d, \hat{v}_d)$ and assess the symmetry of the plots for these datasets.

12.10. Implement the measure of asymmetry MRA1 or a similar measure that you design yourself or find in the literature and assess its performance on the replicates generated in the previous exercise or Exercise 12.6. As an alternative, delete a study from a dataset and explore whether MRA1 indicates that such a study (with similar values of $\hat{\theta}_d$ and $\hat{v}_d$) is missing. Construct scenarios in which the task of detection might be easier.

12.11. Implement the shrinkage estimator $\tilde{\theta}_{d*}$ given by (12.8). Assess the loss of efficiency due to estimating (not knowing) the values of θ, σ_B^2, and v_{d*}. That is, on a set of replications, compare the MSEs of $\tilde{\theta}_{d*}$ based on estimates $\hat{\theta}$, $\hat{\sigma}_B^2$, and $\hat{v}_{d*}$ on the one hand and $\tilde{\theta}_{d*}$ based on the values of θ, σ_B^2, and v_{d*}

on the other.

Consider an alternative way of assessing these estimators. For each replication, count the number of studies for which the estimate based on the values of the parameters is closer to the target θ_d than the estimate based on estimated values of the parameters. Discuss the merits of the two assessments.

12.12. Explore how the minimax estimator based on an upper bound for the plausible value of the context-level variance σ_B^2 could be implemented and whether it would have properties similar to those of the estimator derived in Section 1.1.1 or Section 8.3.2.

12.13. Discuss how a meta-analysis could take advantage of a register (census or some other form of enumeration) in the following scenario. Each study included in the meta-analysis is associated with a domain (region or country) and time period (year), and the estimate $\hat{\theta}_d$ of its target θ_d can be augmented by a similar quantity derived from the register. The register-based quantity is biased for θ_d because the relevant variable is defined (slightly) differently from the outcome variable in the studies included in the meta-analysis, but its sampling variance is effectively zero. The study-based estimators are unbiased, but their sampling variances are large. Relate this problem to its counterpart in small-area estimation in which districts are in the role of studies.

12.14. Summarise the information lost because the subject-level records from the studies included in a meta-analysis are not available.

Hint: Consider the set of sufficient statistics that are used by meta-analysis and the set of sufficient statistics that you would prefer to use, e.g., for fitting a random coefficient model to the subject-level data. Discuss how the results of a study commonly reported at present (consult the relevant literature for examples) could be augmented to facilitate a more efficient meta-analysis in the future.

12.15. Derive an estimator of the squared deviation $(\theta_{d^*} - \theta)^2$ that combines the naive estimator $(\hat{\theta}_{d^*} - \hat{\theta})^2$ and the context-level variance σ_B^2 (or its approximately unbiased estimator).

Hint: See [124] for the solution of a related problem in small-area estimation.

12.16. Consider the problem of estimating many quantities in Section 12.8 for a set of concentrations (reciprocals of variances). Work out all the details and compare the conclusions with those for estimating the variances.

Appendix. A Refresher

This appendix gives a condensed summary of the basic terminology used throughout the book. To the extent possible it is organised in the order of the chapters, indicating how they are connected. Not all the terms are standard or used in the same way as in the statistical literature. The appendix can be used as a glossary, although the principal definitions are accompanied by motivating examples.

A.1 Populations and Variables

We define *statistics* as the study of the values of variables on the members of populations. Any collection of units can be regarded as a population. Formally, a *population* is defined by a rule that arbitrates without any ambiguity, about any entity, as to whether it does or does not belong to (is a member of) the population. For instance, the population of the residents of a country is defined by a qualification stipulated by the relevant laws of the country. Such a population has to be associated with a date, to resolve the membership of those who were born or died, emigrated, immigrated, or qualified for residence by some other means around the designated date. The rule may be revised from time to time. A population need not comprise human subjects or other living organisms. Moments in time, repeated operations (e.g., in a production process), locations, or computer records may form a population, as can organisations defined by human subjects, such as companies, households, schools, and (local) administrative authorities.

A *variable* is defined on a population by its value for each member. Instead of these values, the variable may be defined by a procedure that establishes its value for each member. For instance, the income of a resident of a country is defined as the sum of all the payments received by the member in a given period of time. More details may be given to classify the payments into categories, such as income from employment, investments, pension, rents, sale of property, winnings in games of chance, and the like. The details of a definition of a population or a variable that are essential to remove any ambiguity but are not listed every time we refer to the population or the variable are called the *small print*.

The *support* of a variable is defined as the set of all values that occur for the variable. The values of a variable may be counts (integers), numbers, categories, lists, or (unordered) sets of objects. They define the *type* of the variable. A variable is said to be *categorical* if its support comprises a finite number of values. These values may be associated with ordering, such as for the integers from one to six. Such a variable is called *ordered categorical*; its support consists of ordered categories. An unordered categorical variable is also called a *factor*. A variable is said to be *discrete* if its support comprises isolated values; around any value x in the support there is a neighbourhood that contains no value other than x. A variable is said to be *continuous* if its support contains no isolated values; any neighbourhood of any value x in the support contains at least one other value that belongs to the support. This definition is revised in Section A.3.

These definitions imply that the support is a subset of a space in which certain structures and operations are defined. For example, ordering is an operation; it assigns to each pair of values their comparison (the same, greater than, or smaller than). Whether two values are the same or not can also be regarded as a (trivial) operation. Neighbourhoods of points define a structure. Neighbourhoods are commonly defined by a *metric*. A metric is an operation that assigns to each pair of values (points) in the space their distance. The distance is nonnegative; $d(x_1, x_2) \geq 0$ for any pair of points x_1 and x_2 in the space. The only point in the distance of zero from any given point is the point itself; $d(x_1, x_2) = 0$ only when $x_1 = x_2$. The distance is symmetric, $d(x_1, x_2) = d(x_2, x_1)$, and satisfies the triangular inequality:

$$d(x_1, x_3) \leq d(x_1, x_2) + d(x_2, x_3)$$

for any three points x_1, x_2, and x_3. We can define the size of a value by its distance from a common reference point, called the *origin* and denoted by 0; that is, $s(x) = d(x, 0)$. The origin (its existence and location) is an element of the structure. A space is said to be *bounded* if there is a positive number M such that the distance between any two points in the space is shorter than M. The triangular inequality implies that a space is bounded only when there is an upper bound on the size of the values. If there is no such bound the space is said to be *unbounded*. Bounded and unbounded support are defined similarly.

Usually several variables are defined in a population. From one or several such variables, new variables can be defined by transformations, using operations that are well defined in the supports of the variables concerned. For instance, when the values of a variable are real numbers new variables can be defined by the usual arithmetic operations.

Clustering is a commonly occurring structure in populations of human subjects. For example, the members of a family, each of them also a member of the population, form a cluster. Clusters may be nested, such as families (households) within streets, towns or villages, and districts, or cross-classified, such as families and birthplaces. Other structures can be defined by the values of one or several variables. For instance, the geographical location of a member of the population can be indicated by a categorical variable (place name) or even by its coordinates (latitude and longitude, both continuous variables).

Variables are defined because their values provide useful descriptions of the members of the population. For large populations, containing tens of thousands or even millions of members, a list of the values of a variable is not very useful for learning about the population; the values require some processing and summarising. This often takes the form of calculating certain *summaries* of the values. Examples of such summaries are the mean (average), range (the difference between the maximum and minimum value), the fraction of the members whose value exceeds a given threshold, and the proportion of the members who have a particular value. Such summaries are popularly referred to as *information*. A summary need not be a single number; it may comprise several numbers, although not many, because a summary is intended as an easy-to-digest, even if not comprehensive, description of the population.

Although it is usually derived from a single variable, a summary may involve several variables. For example, the proportion of members whose value of one variable exceeds the value of another variable is derived from two variables. However, this proportion depends only on the difference of the two variables. By defining this difference as another variable, the summary depends only on this new (constructed) variable.

An elementary task in statistics is associated with establishing the value of a population summary of a variable. This value could be determined by *enumeration*—by establishing the value of the variable on each member of the population and then evaluating the summary. We regard the task of evaluating a summary as elementary, requiring only minimum effort and expertise, *if* all the values are available. The principal difficulty is that enumeration requires resources, such as labour, equipment, services (including transport and telecommunications), and time, and therefore funding, and these are usually insufficient for an enumeration. Cooperation of the studied population, their goodwill, is another important resource.

Collecting information from every member of a large population is often a singularly unreasonable proposition, from the perspectives of both the member of the population (*respondent*) and the *consumer* of the information. The consumer associates the required information with a financial, ethical, professional, or some other benefit (value). They would be willing to finance, and assist by other means, the effort of collecting the information if the investment (expenditure) they make was recovered by the outcome—by valuable information that would facilitate the conduct of their business, such as governing the country (by adjusting policies and incentives), production and distribution for the retail trade, and location of service outlets. Instead of enumeration, the values of the variable of interest could be collected on only a subset of the population. Such a subset is called a *sample*. The members of the population who belong to the sample are called *subjects*. The number of subjects in the sample is called the *sample size*. The value of the summary of interest, called the *target*, could not be established with precision but, hopefully, a summary of the sample would not be far off. Thus, the expense is reduced, but precision is sacrificed in the process.

The cost can be further reduced by establishing the value of the variable not precisely but subject to some approximation. For instance, instead of asking for a complete list of food and drink consumed in a given period of time (say, in a week), a questionnaire would inquire merely about the frequencies of eating certain kinds of food and consuming beverages in a short list of categories (types of food and drink). In this way, less detail is collected, but the exercise of eliciting information from the subjects is made easier and less intrusive.

In this description, we can readily identify two activities: selecting a sample (*sampling*) and eliciting the value (*measurement*). They are referred to as *processes*, because they are defined not by the selected sample and the recorded values, respectively, but by how they would be applied (methods) in any conceivable instance. Examples of these processes are all the adult human passengers on a selected list of rail services (date and number of the service) who are not employees of the railways, and requesting the subjects to complete a particular questionnaire that inquires about their experiences as railway passengers in the last few months. With this sampling process, members of the population who use rail services infrequently are less likely to be included in the sample than those who travel by rail frequently.

Ideally, we would like to draw (select) a sample in which the country's regions, age groups, occupational categories, and other attributes of the members of the studied population are represented in proportions that resemble their composition in the country. Similarly, a more elaborate process of measurement, with more detailed and clearly formulated questions, may be more useful than the responses to a single ambiguous question for which there is a limited set of response options, such as, at the extreme, only 'Agree' and 'Disagree'. More detailed questioning takes longer and detains the respondent for longer; it requires more preparation, instruction, and training of the interviewers and, as a result, a sample with fewer subjects (a smaller sample) can be afforded for the fixed resources available. Thus, higher quality of the measurement process may not serve well the primary purpose of the survey.

From the values of a variable recorded, possibly not precisely, on a sample of subjects, we cannot establish the value of the target; we can merely make a guess based on the available values and informed by the details of the sampling and measurement processes. Such a guess is called an *estimate*, and the process of deriving it is referred to as drawing (making) an *inference*. The process may be described by a mathematical formula, a verbal description, such as 'the proportion of subjects who responded with "Yes"', or it may be implemented in a computer program. The process (or procedure) by which the estimate is evaluated (calculated) is called an *estimator*. A typical estimator is intended for a specific target. A desirable property of an estimator is that it is close to the target. The difference between estimates (numbers) and estimators (procedures) will become clearer in Section A.2.

Among the values and summaries defined so far, we can distinguish between population and sample quantities. A summary and a target are examples of population quantities; they can be established only when the values of the relevant variable are available for every member of the population. An estimate and the sample size are examples of sample quantities; they can be established from the values of the variable on the sample, after one application, or *realisation*, of the sampling and measurement processes.

With the terms defined so far, we can specify the role of statistics as making inferences about population quantities related to variables, when the resources available for these activities are limited. This entails specifying the processes of sampling, measurement, and estimation that yield the best inference that can be afforded with the available resources. To solve this problem, we have to agree first on what to regard as 'best' inference. Next, we require formulae for the cost of executing any considered sampling and measurement processes. The estimation process can also be associated with a cost, although it is usually fixed and trivial in comparison with the expenditure on the sampling and measurement processes.

A.2 Replications and Randomness

Replication is a key device for comparing alternative sampling, measurement, and estimation processes (*schemes*). Replication is the act of repeating (repeatedly applying) a set of processes, doing so each time without being affected in any way by the previous applications. Replications are *independent* applications of the same scheme. The outcome of a replication is called a *replicate*. Thus, we talk about replicate samples, replicate measurements, and replicate values of an estimator.

We assume that the estimator is perfectly replicable. That is, its application on the values of a variable for a given (*fixed*) set of subjects always yields the same estimate. In general, replicate estimates are not constant (are dispersed) because replications of the sampling process yield different sets of subjects, and they have different values of the observed variable. The replications of the measurement process might yield different values of the variable even if the same sample were drawn in the replications, or the measurement process were replicated on the entire population. The sampling and measurement processes involve randomness; we say that they are *stochastic*. Note that the sampling process cannot be replicated in practice; resources are usually available only for one application. Nevertheless, in some circumstances at least, we can discuss what results would be obtained in a long sequence of replications. In Section A.8.1, we discuss a general method for generating replications on the computer.

Replicate measurements on the same subject are not constant because the measurement process is affected by the idiosyncrasies of the measurement instruments or agents (interviewers), momentary distractions influencing the respondents (subjects), and imperfect communication between the respondent and the interviewer. In some settings, measurements can be replicated (on the same set of subjects), especially when they leave no trace on the subject, are not costly to conduct, and have no ethical consequences. Such replications enable us to learn about the quality of the measurement.

Measurements are difficult to replicate when the subject or the interviewer can recall, even if only partially, the previous measurement. For instance, a school examination would be very difficult to replicate, especially if the same questions were presented in the second version of the exam. Nevertheless, we can speculate how different the results would be if a replication took place, with students unaffected by the experience of having taken the same exam in the past. We say that such a replication is *hypothetical*. When the idiosyncrasy of the measurement process is mainly due to the interviewer, his or her *assessment*, independence of the measurements can be ensured by engaging different interviewers who are not informed about each other's assessments or workloads (which subjects they assessed).

A.2.1 Efficiency

An estimator in a particular scheme is said to be *efficient* if its values obtained by replications (replicate estimates) are tightly concentrated around the target. To assess how close an estimate is to the target, we need a measure of its distance, the *deviation* of the estimate from the target. The difference of the estimate from the target is the obvious choice, although the sign of the difference is immaterial for the assessment of the size of the deviation. For an estimator in a scheme, represented by its replicate values, it is necessary to summarise its deviations from the target. Two important summaries, capturing two aspects of the deviations are *bias* and *dispersion*.

The bias is defined as the average deviation, with the sign of the deviation not ignored. The dispersion of an estimator is defined as the spread of its values around its mean. No bias, or being *unbiased*, and having small dispersion are desirable properties of an estimator. However, small bias is of little value if it is accompanied by large dispersion, and small dispersion is not useful if the bias is very large. Figure A.1 illustrates this with four examples of combinations of small and large bias with small and large dispersion. In each panel, the diagram, called a *histogram*, comprises bars. The height of each bar is proportional to the number of replicate estimates that fall into the (horizontal) range covered by the bar. Each histogram is based on 10 000 replications. The target is marked by a vertical line. The four panels have the same horizontal and vertical scales.

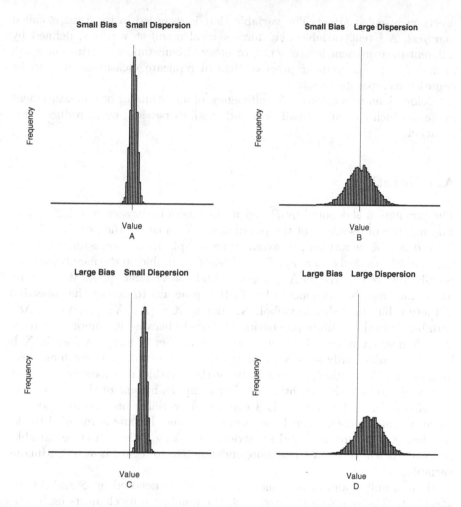

Fig. A.1. Histograms of replicate estimates for estimators with small and large biases and dispersions. The target is marked by a thin vertical line in each panel. The horizontal axes of the four histograms have the same scale.

The measurement process can be considered similarly, with the genuine value of the variable for a subject regarded as the target. The ideal measurement process recovers the target value in each replication. Otherwise, replicate measurements concentrated more tightly around the target are preferred. Note that the value of the variable for each member of the population is a potential target, and so the properties of the measurement process have to be considered for all members. The replicate measurements may be constant for some or all members of the population, and they may agree with the target for some members. The variable for which the value cannot be recovered with precision is called *latent*. The variable that is recorded in its stead is called *manifest*. A latent variable may have several manifest versions, defined by different measurement instruments, or other circumstances (settings or small print) of the measurement process. Sets of replicate measurements can be regarded as separate variables.

Before defining a criterion for efficiency, of an estimator or a measurement process, which combines small bias and small dispersion, we introduce some notation.

A.3 Notation

The population is denoted by $\mathcal{P}$ and its members by integers $i = 1, 2, \ldots, N$. The number of members of the population, N, is called the *population size*. It need not be known but, to avoid some complications, we assume it to be finite, until specified otherwise. The values of a variable on the members of the population are denoted as $X_1, \ldots, X_N$, and the variable, or its value on an unspecified member, is denoted by X. It is practical to denote the collection of these values by a single symbol, $\mathbf{X}$; that is, $\mathbf{X} = (X_1, X_2, \ldots, X_N)^\top$. Any variable defined in a finite population is discrete because it cannot have more than N distinct values. However, when the number of unique values in $\mathbf{X}$ is large (then necessarily so is N), and any point on a continuum, such as a real interval, could, in principle, be a value of the variable, it is more appropriate to regard the variable as continuous. For example, income of the members of the labour force of a country is a continuous variable because any positive value, within a range, could be someone's income. Income is rounded to the smallest unit of currency, and so, strictly speaking, it is a discrete variable. However, it will turn out to be more constructive to regard it as a continuous variable.

The sampling and measurement processes are denoted by $\mathcal{S}$ and $\mathcal{M}$, respectively. The sample is denoted by $\mathbf{s}$, the number of its elements (subjects) by n, the subjects by $j = 1, \ldots, n$, and the values of the variable on the subjects by $x_1, \ldots, x_n$, or as $\mathbf{x}$. Note that (sample) subject $j = 1$ is distinct from (population) member $i = 1$, and their respective values x_1 and X_1 are not related in any way other than both being one of the N values in $\mathbf{X}$.

A population quantity, such as a target, is denoted by θ. For instance, θ may stand for the mean of a variable in a population. As the mean can be calculated for any numerical variable, a more complete notation includes the variable involved: $\theta(\mathbf{X})$. The 'same' variable may be defined in another population, and so the population may be added as another argument of θ, in addition to $\mathbf{X}$; $\theta(\mathbf{X}; \mathcal{P})$. As in most cases we work with a single population, this is not necessary. We regard two variables as different if they are defined in different populations, even if their descriptions are the same. In other words, the population is part of the small print in the definition of a variable.

An estimator of θ is denoted by $\hat{\theta}$ or $\hat{\theta}(\mathbf{x})$, although a more rigorous notation would include the sampling and measurement processes as arguments. The measurement process may be subsumed in the definition of the variable X. Then the values of one variable (on a sample of subjects) are used for making inferences about the summary of another variable. The sampling and measurement processes cannot be recognised from the sample values $\mathbf{x}$. That is, a particular sample $\mathbf{x}$, a set of n values, could be realised by several distinct pairs of sampling and measurement processes.

The replicate samples are denoted by $\mathbf{x}^{(1)}, \ldots, \mathbf{x}^{(H)}$, where H is the number of replicates. Each of these samples is associated with an estimate, and these are denoted by $\hat{\theta}^{(1)}, \ldots, \hat{\theta}^{(H)}$, or, more completely, as $\hat{\theta}^{(1)} = \hat{\theta}\left(\mathbf{x}^{(1)}\right), \ldots, \hat{\theta}^{(H)} = \hat{\theta}\left(\mathbf{x}^{(H)}\right)$, emphasising that we use the same estimator $\hat{\theta}$. The *expectation* of an estimator $\hat{\theta}$ is defined as the mean of the estimates in a large number of replications, that is, as

$$\frac{1}{H}\left(\hat{\theta}^{(1)} + \cdots + \hat{\theta}^{(H)}\right)$$

or, more precisely, as the limit of this expression with H diverging to infinity $(H \rightarrow +\infty)$. The expectation of $\hat{\theta}$ is denoted as $\mathrm{E}(\hat{\theta})$. The expectation depends on the sampling process. We add the sampling process $\mathcal{S}$ to the notation, as $\mathrm{E}(\hat{\theta}; \mathcal{S})$ or $\mathrm{E}_{\mathcal{S}}(\hat{\theta})$, for emphasis or when we operate with several sampling processes.

The bias of $\hat{\theta}$ is denoted by $\mathrm{B}(\hat{\theta}; \theta)$:

$$\mathrm{B}\left(\hat{\theta}; \theta\right) = \mathrm{E}\left(\hat{\theta} - \theta\right).$$

It is essential to retain the target θ as an argument of B because an estimator may be used for more than one target; it may be unbiased for one target, and biased for another.

An obvious candidate for the estimator of a population quantity $\theta = \theta(\mathbf{X})$ is the same function of the sample values: $\hat{\theta} = \theta(\mathbf{x})$. For instance, the population mean may be estimated by the sample mean. Such estimators are called *naive*. (The term is not intended to be derogatory.) Note that θ has to be well defined for both N values in the population quantity $\theta(\mathbf{X})$ and n values in the estimator (sample quantity) $\theta(\mathbf{x})$. In fact, many estimators have to be similarly flexible, because the (replicate) samples need not have constant size n.

The *sampling variance* of an estimator $\hat{\theta}$ is defined as the expectation of the squared deviation of $\hat{\theta}$ from its expectation $\mathrm{E}(\hat{\theta})$:

$$\mathrm{var}\left(\hat{\theta}\right) = \mathrm{E}\left[\left\{\hat{\theta} - \mathrm{E}\left(\hat{\theta}\right)\right\}^2\right].$$

The mean squared error (MSE) of an estimator $\hat{\theta}$ is defined as the expectation of its squared deviation from the target θ:

$$\text{MSE}(\hat{\theta};\,\theta) = \text{E}\left\{\left(\hat{\theta} - \theta\right)^2\right\}.$$

The sampling variance and MSE depend on the sampling and measurement processes, and the MSE depends also on the target. The MSE, sampling variance, and bias are connected by the identity

$$\text{MSE}\left(\hat{\theta};\,\theta\right) = \text{var}\left(\hat{\theta}\right) + \left\{\text{B}\left(\hat{\theta};\,\theta\right)\right\}^2. \tag{A.1}$$

Thus the sampling variance and the squared bias are two contributors to the MSE. An estimator with small MSE cannot have a large bias or a large sampling variance. We adopt the MSE as a measure of efficiency. Suppose $\hat{\theta}_A$ and $\hat{\theta}_B$ are estimators intended for the same target θ. Then $\hat{\theta}_A$ is said to be more efficient than $\hat{\theta}_B$ for θ if $\text{MSE}(\hat{\theta}_A;\,\theta) < \text{MSE}(\hat{\theta}_B;\,\theta)$.

The MSE is an example of a *sampling-process quantity*. It characterises the sampling and estimation processes engaged. Except for some simple cases, it can be established only by replicating the sampling process many times. Usually, the MSE (of an estimator $\hat{\theta}$ for a target θ) depends on some population quantities, often the target itself, and so the MSE can itself be regarded as a target and estimated. As the MSE depends on some unknown (population) quantities, we may consider properties of the estimator $\hat{\theta}$ assuming specific values of these population quantities. One estimator of θ is said to be *uniformly more efficient* than another estimator of the same target if it is more efficient for any configuration of the population quantities on which their MSEs depend.

Estimators of a target may have strengths and weaknesses; they may be more efficient than their competitors for some configurations of population quantities and less efficient for others. When striving to choose an efficient estimator, information, however incomplete, about the relevant population quantities is sometimes invaluable; it can assist in discarding estimators that are inefficient for the particular setting.

A.4 Distributions

When studying the values of a variable in a population, we are usually not interested in the identities of the members; we say that the members are *anonymous*. Each member has a unique identifier. It is useful for tracing the various steps in the construction of the dataset and for connecting the values of two (or more) variables of a member. Given the values of all the defined variables for a member, the member's identifier has no information content and we treat it as a mere label.

We often wish to summarise a variable by how frequently certain values, and their ranges, arise. Examples of such summaries are:

- What proportion of the households in a country have income below a certain level?
- How many households comprise a single person each?
- How many students fail a particular examination?

To address the first of the listed questions, we define a new variable, U, equal to unity (or 'Yes') for members whose answer to the question

Is your household's income below £...?

is affirmative, and equal to zero (or 'No') if the answer is negative. The summary of interest, the proportion of 'Yes', is equal to the mean of the variable U. Such a *population proportion* is called a probability. We write $P(U = 1)$ for this probability, but also as $P(X < c^*)$, where X is income and c^* the value of the threshold income in the question.

The *distribution* of a variable X with real values is defined as any collection of probabilities from which the probability $P(X < c)$ could be recovered for any real value c. Of course, such a collection is not unique. For instance, $P(X < c)$ for every value c that occurs in the population is a distribution, but so is $P(X > c)$ for every such c, or indeed $P(X = c)$, so long as the number of distinct values c of X is finite. As every population we consider has a finite population size, the number of distinct values of the variable in the population is finite. By definition, it can be established whether two collections of probabilities correspond to the same set of probabilities $P(X = c)$ for values c in their supports. If they do, it is practical to regard them as identical distributions. With this convention, the distribution is uniquely defined, and any conceivable probability involving X, such as $P(X = c_1$ or $X = c_2$ or $\ldots$ or $X = c_K)$ can be derived by adding up the relevant probabilities $P(X = c_k)$, $k = 1, 2, \ldots, K$, so long as the values $c_1, \ldots, c_K$ are distinct.

The distribution of a variable often comprises many probabilities, so it cannot be effectively presented in any tabular form. The distribution of a variable can be presented graphically by a *histogram*. An example is presented in Figure A.2 for a variable with 400 distinct values in a population of size 25 000. The vertical segments represent the distinct values and the height of each segment is equal to the *frequency*—how many times the value occurs in the population. Note the similarity in the layout with the histograms in Figure A.1. Part of the distribution is presented in tabular form in Table A.1, giving the frequencies of the 15 smallest values of the variable.

Some of the detail in Figure A.2 is unnecessary. The segments that are very close to one another could be represented by a single segment, or a bar, as in Figure A.1. Two examples of this are given in Figure A.3. Either histogram conveys much better that the most frequent values are around zero, all the values are nonnegative, very few values exceed 7.0, there are fewer values in the neighbourhood of 3.0 than elsewhere in the support, and so on. The vertical axis in Figure A.1 is in fractions (probabilities), whereas in Figure A.2 it is in counts (numbers of members). This has no impact on what we can

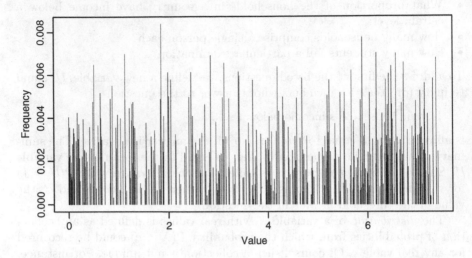

Fig. A.2. Histogram—graphical representation of the distribution of a variable.

Table A.1. The distribution of the variable in Figure A.2 (an extract).

Value	Frequency	Value	Frequency	Value	Frequency
0.0004	15	0.0035	52	0.0128	71
0.0008	52	0.0042	52	0.0160	155
0.0009	87	0.0048	43	0.0165	134
0.0022	62	0.0059	80	0.0231	23
0.0025	250	0.0115	18	0.0242	73

learn about the distribution; that is, the same information could be extracted from the diagrams with either layout.

The histogram in panel A is more detailed and the histogram in panel B somewhat coarser. The coarseness is given by the width of the bars or by the number of bars that cover the entire range of the values, in this example, from zero to 7.41. The more detailed histogram in panel A has 50 bars and the histogram in panel B 20 bars. Each histogram is associated with a table that lists the range of each bar with the corresponding frequency. Table A.2 presents such a table for the histogram in panel B.

A.4.1 Describing Distributions

Although we can reconstruct from the distribution most of the important facts about a variable, we do not always need to convey all the details of

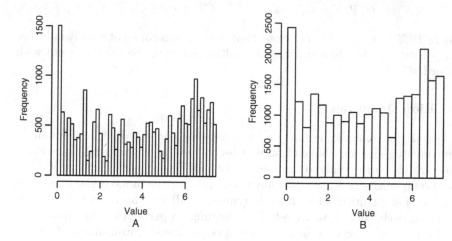

Fig. A.3. Coarse histograms of the variable in Figure A.2.

Table A.2. The ranges and frequencies associated with the histogram in panel B of Figure A.3.

Range	Frequency	Range	Frequency	Range	Frequency
0.000–0.370	3819	2.594–2.964	566	5.187–5.558	1218
0.370–0.741	811	2.964–3.334	914	5.558–5.928	1506
0.741–1.111	1412	3.334–3.705	1341	5.928–6.298	1503
1.111–1.482	616	3.705–4.075	709	6.298–6.669	1202
1.482–1.852	1046	4.075–4.446	1112	6.669–7.040	1478
1.852–2.223	345	4.446–4.816	1638	7.040–7.410	2066
2.223–2.594	721	4.816–5.187	977		

the distribution. Coarse histograms and the associated tables of frequencies condense the information about the distribution and present it in a form that is easy to digest. Often it useful to have a single-number or a succinct verbal description of a particular feature of the distribution. In this section, we define a few such features.

Any summary of the values of a variable that can be derived directly from the distribution is also a summary, or feature, of the distribution. For instance, the population mean of a variable can be expressed as

$$E(X) = \frac{1}{N}\left(M_1 C_1 + M_2 C_2 + \cdots + M_K C_K\right),$$

where $M_1, \ldots, M_K$ are the frequencies (*multiplicities*) of the respective (unique) values $C_1, \ldots, C_K$ of X in the population, or as

$$E(X) = C_1 P(X = C_1) + C_2 P(X = C_2) + \cdots + C_K P(X = C_K),$$

where $P(X = C_k) = M_k/N$. Note that a more rigorous notation would use M_{C_k} instead of M_k, to associate the multiplicity with the value C_k, not with its order k.

Location Quantities

A population quantity is said to be a *location quantity* if it is a summary that involves one variable and adding a constant to or changing the scale of the variable corresponds to the same change of the quantity. That is, if d is a location quantity of X, then, for any given values (constants) a and b, $ad+b$ is the location quantity of the (linearly transformed) variable $aX + b$, formed by changing each value X_i to aX_i+b. This defining property of location quantities is also referred to as *invariance* with respect to linear transformations. Apart from the mean, the minimum and maximum are obvious location quantities.

The (population) *median* of a variable, or of a distribution, is defined as the value that is exceeded by exactly half the members of the population. For example, in a population that comprises $N = 41$ members, the median is equal to the 21st highest value of the variable. When the population size N is even, the median is not always unique. For example, any value between the 20th and 21st highest value is a median in a population of 40 members. If these two values coincide, then the median is unique. Otherwise, we may choose as the median the mean of these two values. If either of these values occurs more than once the weighted mean of the values may be used, with weights equal to the frequencies. The median of the distribution in Figure A.2 is 4.200; in this case it is a value that occurs in the population, for 131 members, so the median is unique, even though the population size N is even.

The upper quartile of a variable or distribution is defined as a value that is exceeded by exactly 25% of the values, and the lower quartile as a value exceeded by exactly 75% of the values. For the distribution in Figure A.2, these quartiles are 1.218 and 5.915. Both values occur in the population multiply, so both quartiles are unique.

More generally, for any number q between zero and unity, the q-quantile is defined as a value R_q for which $P(X < R_q) = q$. In a more complete notation, we would write $R_q(X)$ instead of R_q, because the quantile depends on the values of the variable. We drop the argument X only when there is no ambiguity about the variable on which the quantile is evaluated. The p-percentile is defined as the $p/100$-quantile. For example, an upper quartile is a 0.75-quantile and a 75th percentile of the distribution. A particular quantile may not be unique. When it is not, any point in the interval between two consecutive values of the variable is this quantile, or a convention for averaging or weighting of the adjacent values may be adopted. With any convention that makes the quantiles unique we can refer to any particular quantile as *the* quantile. The quantiles and percentiles are location quantities. They have a general invariance property that for any increasing function g, $R_q\{g(X)\} = g\{R_q(X)\}$; swapping the operations 'quantile' and 'function' does not alter the result.

A compact, though incomplete, description of a distribution is by the values of the minimum, lower quartile, median, upper quartile, and the maximum, possibly supplemented by the mean. For example, these values for the distribution in Figure A.2 are

$$(0.000,\ 1.218,\ 4.200,\ 5.915,\ 7.408)$$

and the mean is $E(X) = 3.753$. The minimum can be regarded as the 0-quantile and the maximum as the 1-quantile of the distribution.

Dispersion Quantities

A population quantity, defined for a variable or a distribution, is called a *dispersion quantity* if it is unchanged when a constant is added to each value of the variable and is multiplied by $|b|$ when each value is multiplied by a constant b. The difference of any two quantiles (higher quantile – lower quantile) is a dispersion quantity, as is the *range*, the difference between the maximum and minimum. The difference between the two quartiles, $R_{0.75}(X) - R_{0.25}(X)$, is called the *interquantile range*.

The population variance is defined as the mean squared distance of the values from their mean:

$$\text{var}(X) = E\left[\{X - E(X)\}^2\right] ;$$

compare this with the definition of the sampling variance in Section A.3. When the context is insufficient to distinguish between the two kinds of variance the notation can be supplemented by subscripts to indicate whether a variance is over sampling or population, var_S and var_P, respectively. The square root of the population variance, $\sqrt{\text{var}_P(X)}$, is called the *standard deviation*. The standard deviation is a dispersion quantity.

Symmetry and Unimodality

A distribution is said to be *symmetric* if it coincides with its reflection across the (suitably defined) median, that is, when the distributions of X and $2R_{0.50}(X) - X$ coincide. An example of a symmetric distribution is given in Figure A.4.

The mean and median of a symmetric distribution coincide; $E(X) = R_{0.50}(X)$. Further, for any $0 \le q \le 1$, the q- and $(1-q)$-quantiles are equidistant from the median:

$$R_q(X) - R_{0.50}(X) = R_{0.50}(X) - R_{1-q}(X).$$

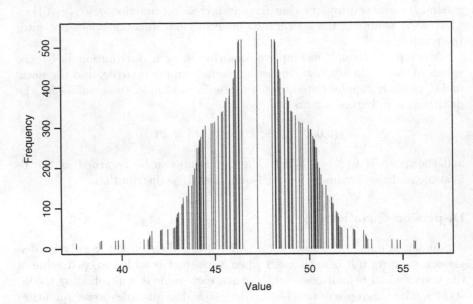

Fig. A.4. Example of a symmetric distribution.

A distribution is said to have a *mode* at a value X^* if both the nearest value smaller than X^* and the nearest value greater than X^* have smaller frequencies. Every distribution has a mode, but some distributions have several modes. For example, the distribution in Figure A.4 has one mode, at its median, but the distribution in Figure A.2 has numerous modes. The modes of a symmetric distribution are located symmetrically around the median. If X^* is a mode, then so is $2R_{0.50}(X) - X^*$. A distribution with a single mode is called *unimodal*, with two modes *bimodal* and, generally, with more than one mode as *multimodal*.

A.4.2 Approximating the Distribution by a Histogram

The graphs of the distributions in Figures A.2 and A.4 are rather unwieldy and contain too much detail that may not be relevant and would be better omitted from a compact summary. One way of achieving this is by *rounding* the values of the variable. The resulting variable can be regarded as a manifest, or *coarsened* version of the original variable. The distribution of the coarse variable is simpler because the variable has fewer possible values and these (the support) are located regularly.

In general, a coarsening is defined by a set of cut points $c_0 < c_1 < \ldots < c_K$ and values $d_1, \ldots, d_K$, such that $c_{k-1} \leq d_k \leq c_k$, $k = 1, \ldots, K$. If the original value of X is in the range $(c_{k-1}, c_k]$ the value of the coarse variable is set to d_k. Instead of the coarse variable we can define a variable $X^\dagger$ with values equal to the category k into which the original value falls: if $c_{k-1} < X \leq c_k$, then $X^\dagger = k$. When the original variable is equal to one of the cut points c_k, coarsening can allocate it either to d_k (category k) or to d_{k+1} (category $k+1$). A coarsening with cut points $c_0 < c_1 < \ldots < c_K$ is said to be coarser than with cut points $c'_0 < c'_1 < \ldots < c'_{K'}$ if the set of values $(c_0, c_1, \ldots, c_K)$ is a subset of the set $(c'_0, c'_1, \ldots, c'_{K'})$. Necessarily, $K < K'$. A coarsening can be refined by introducing new cut points (and defining appropriate new values d_k), and made coarser by discarding one or several cut points c_k (and defining new values d_k in the affected intervals).

For a given variable, such as the annual income of a household, we may consider a few alternative ways of coarsening that are ordered according to their coarseness. For example, the income could be rounded to units, tens, hundreds, or thousands of £UK. The choice of the coarseness should be guided by the purpose of the analysis (summary) to which the variable (income) is to be subjected. For example, if the difference of several hundreds of £UK is not important, rounding to thousands is appropriate. By a coarser rounding we obtain a variable that is easier to handle, because is has fewer possible values, but we may lose some detail in the process. In contrast, less coarse (finer) rounding yields values that are closer to (or the same distance from) the original values but may contain too much detail for an effective presentation and study.

A (coarse) histogram of a variable can be identified with the distribution of a coarsened version of the variable. The cut points of the coarsening applied coincide with the limits of the bars. Figure A.3 gave an example of the impact on coarsening of a continuous variable.

A.5 Sampling Design

When we cannot afford to enumerate the population, we establish the values of the target variable only for a sample of subjects. Such an exercise is called a *survey*. Every survey involves a sampling process by which subjects are selected. Substantial advantages accrue when we can select the sampling process purposefully. Such a sampling process is said to be *controlled* or planned and is referred to as a *sampling design*.

A sampling design can be defined by its (unambiguous) description, such as

1. Select a member completely at random.
2. Select one member completely at random from those not yet selected.
3. Repeat step 2 until the specified number of subjects has been selected.

More formally, a sampling design is defined as a way of assigning to every subset of the population the probability that it would form the sample. That is, the collection of all subsets of the population's members, denoted by $\exp(\mathcal{P})$, is regarded as a new population, and a probability in this population is interpreted by a reference to replications. This definition does not seem to be constructive, because most populations have very many subsets, equal to 2^N, where N is the population size. In a typical sampling design, most subsets have zero probability of forming a sample. For instance, when the sample size is set (prescribed or fixed) to be n the number of possible samples is $\binom{N}{n} = N! / \{n!(N-n)!\}$. The controlled nature of a sampling design rests not on which member is selected into the sample but on how the selection is conducted.

Sampling designs in which each member has the same probability p of being included in the sample, each pair of members has the same probability $p^{(2)}$, and so on, are called *simple random*. Of course, $p \neq p^{(2)}$. A member can be included in the sample several times. Sampling designs in which this is possible are called designs *with replacement*, and designs in which this is ruled out are called *without replacement*. The term *replacement* refers to the description of the sampling design by a mechanism of drawing subjects into the sample one by one. In designs with replacement, after being selected, a subject is retained in the pool of candidates for being selected in subsequent draws. Thus, in simple random sampling design with replacement, each member has the same probability of being drawn as the first subject, equal to $1/N$, but, irrespective of who was drawn first, the probability of being drawn as the second subject is also equal to $1/N$ for every member of the population. The number of times a member of the population is included in the sample is referred to as its *multiplicity*.

A sample is most conveniently specified as a list of its subjects. The order of the subjects in such a list is immaterial; (i_1, i_2, i_3, i_4) and (i_1, i_4, i_3, i_2) are identical samples, even when $i_2 \neq i_4$. However, multiplicity is an important feature; when $i_2 \neq i_3$, (i_1, i_2, i_3, i_3), (i_1, i_2, i_3, i_2), and $(i_1, i_2, i_2, i_3, i_2)$ are different samples, even though each of them comprises the same set of subjects, i_1, i_2, and i_3.

From the sampling design, we can derive the probability that a given member is included in the sample by adding up the probabilities of all the subsets that contain the member:

$$p_i = \sum_{\mathbf{s} \in \exp(\mathcal{P})} I(i \in \mathbf{s}) P(\mathbf{s}; \mathcal{D}),$$

where P denotes the probability as a function of the set $\mathbf{s}$ and design $\mathcal{D}$ and I is the indicator function, equal to unity when its argument is true and to zero otherwise. A sampling design $\mathcal{D}$ is called *proper* if each member has a positive probability of being included in the sample. Members who have zero probability of being included in the sample are, in effect, excluded from the population that is studied because they are not considered in the sampling process.

A.5.1 Complex Sampling Designs

Stratification and clustering are two ways of defining a wide range of sampling designs. For stratification, the population is divided into subpopulations (groups) called *strata*, and a different sampling design is applied in each stratum. The sampling processes in the strata are independent; the *subsample* drawn in one stratum has no impact on the subsample drawn in another. Stratification has two important advantages. First, the unwieldy task of drawing a sample from one large population is simplified to a number of simpler tasks of drawing a sample from each of several smaller subpopulations, and second, the design can exercise tighter control over the within-stratum subsamples. For example, the within-stratum sampling designs may sample much more densely (with relatively greater subsample sizes) in some strata, at the expense of sparser sampling in other strata.

In most large populations of practical importance, the members are related; such populations are said to be *structured*. The most common element of the structure is clustering—members form small groups (such as families or households), the groups are further clustered (say, to clusters at level 2, such as neighbourhoods or classrooms), and these groups may be further clustered (clusters at level 3, such as districts or schools). In a *clustered sampling design*, a sampling design is applied to the clusters (at a particular level), and independent sampling designs are then applied in each selected cluster. The design applied in a cluster may itself be clustered. Such designs are called *multistage clustered*. The clusters involved in the first round of clustering (say, districts) are called *primary sampling units*, clusters in the next round (say, neighbourhoods) *secondary* sampling units, and so on. Subjects are the *elementary-level* sampling units (elements), unless all members of the selected clusters at level 2 (or at another level) are included in the sample.

An advantage of clustered sampling design is that it is focussed; the sampling in some (randomly selected) clusters is dense, at the expense of no sampling in some other clusters. Dense sampling may provide more information about the associations within the clusters, such as similarity of the members' values of the observed variables. In a clustered sampling design, we have a cluster-level design for each level of clustering and within-cluster designs. Clustered designs are in general easier to organise and manage. When the cost of accessing a cluster is substantial it is more economic to collect data in fewer clusters, but to do so from more (or all) subjects in the selected clusters.

A.5.2 Sampling Frame

A sampling design can be constructed with purpose and implemented effectively only when some basic information about the population is available. The *sampling frame* is a list of all the members of the population. In ideal circumstances, a sampling frame is *complete*, containing all members of the population (without any omissions); *exclusive*, containing no objects that do not belong to the population; and *nonredundant*, containing no duplicates. A sampling frame that satisfies these three conditions is said to be perfect. For stratification and clustering, it would also identify the relevant strata and clusters into which the members belong.

Construction of a perfect sampling frame for a large population is rarely feasible. Commonly, a sampling frame of clusters is used, with some information about the composition of each cluster. For instance, a sampling frame may comprise the country's districts, or smaller administrative units, and the population size of each cluster may be available, usually subject to some approximation, for instance, because is it based on a population register that is a few months out of date. When a clustered sampling design is planned, construction of the sampling frame may be reduced to the selected clusters. For example, clustering by schools is a practical proposition in a survey of students. The school enrollments (sizes) may be available from a previous year, informing the sampling design for the schools as clusters, and within-school subsampling frames are obtained only from the schools that have been selected into the sample.

A.5.3 The Planned and Realised Sampling Processes

The sampling design reduces the study of a population to operations applied to a sample—eliciting information from the subjects and processing their responses (or information recorded about them) to make inferences about the population. A sampling design is essential to ensure good *representation* (representativeness) of the population by the sample. Good representation means that, in replications of the designed sampling process, samples would tend to have features similar to the population and, as a consequence, efficient inferences could be made about the population quantities related to the observed variables. The requirement of good representation has to be qualified by the targets—the population quantities for which inferences are sought.

Without a sampling design, the sampling process may conspire to yield samples that present a distorted image of the population. The image would be distorted in many replications. The image (a feature) may be distorted even in a sample drawn by a well-chosen sampling design because a distortion cannot be ruled out. As an example, consider a population that comprises $N = 100$ members and a binary variable, with values of zero and unity for 50 members each. A simple random sampling design without replacement and with fixed sample size $n = 10$ may yield a sample in which each subject's value of the variable is equal to zero. The probability of this event is $\binom{50}{40} / \binom{100}{90} = (50 \times \ldots \times 41)/(100 \times \ldots \times 91) \doteq 0.0006$. Thus, even an extreme distortion is possible, but its probability is very small; it would be present in only a small fraction of replicate samples.

Without a sampling design, such a 'protection' would not be available. Some distortion in the sample may be introduced by the sampling design.

For instance, by using a stratified sampling design, the smallest regions of the country may be overrepresented in the sample. If these regions tend to have high values of the observed variable the sample will tend to contain more high values than what might be regarded as an appropriate representation of the country. However, such a 'misrepresentation' can be taken into account when the sampling process is known. Without a sampling design we do not know how the sample is likely to have been distorted.

Suppose $\theta(\mathbf{X})$ is a population quantity of interest (a target). Here, θ can be interpreted as a mathematical formula or a computer program. Good representation can be interpreted that θ applied on the sample $\mathbf{x}$, $\theta(\mathbf{x})$, would be close to $\theta(\mathbf{X})$. Of course, an adjustment is necessary when θ is a total, but this can be 'built in' to the definition of θ. At the outset, when the sampling design is specified, the sample is not yet available; only the process by which it is formed is specified. We say that at that point the sample is *random*. Any sample quantity is also random at that point; its value is not known, but its distribution could, in principle, be established, by replications. In particular, it is meaningful to discuss how a population quantity would be estimated.

As a result of applying the sampling design, a sample is drawn. It is referred to as the *realised* sample. With it or, more precisely, with the values of the relevant variable on the subjects, the selected estimator can be evaluated and an estimate obtained. If the sampling design is implemented as prescribed the survey is concluded by reporting the estimate. In practice, the analysis (calculations made on the realised sample) is more extensive—several estimators are evaluated and each estimator is associated with its estimated MSE. Other forms of inference may be conducted, such as evaluating confidence intervals; these are dealt with in Section A.20.

The good properties of an estimator are usually contingent on the sampling design. In large populations, most sampling designs are impossible to implement exactly as planned. The sampling frame is usually imperfect and some of the selected subjects may not be available for an interview or may exercise their right not to cooperate with the survey. As a result, the probabilities of the samples that could be realised are altered. The sampling design as a process is contaminated by an *imperfection* process. This 'contaminated' version of the sampling design is called the *realised* sampling process. We cannot refer to it as a sampling design because it is not under our control. Without a detailed description of the imperfection process, the probabilities of the possible samples for a realised sampling process are not known.

The estimator selected at the planning stage may be efficient when the planned and realised sampling processes coincide, but with the imperfections its properties may have been altered somewhat. The estimator does not have the properties it would have had had the planned sampling design been implemented perfectly. When the realised process deviates from the plan only slightly we can expect the 'realised' properties of the estimators to deviate from the 'planned' properties also only slightly. Hence the strong incentive to reduce the difference between the planned and realised processes, even if it cannot be eliminated altogether.

A.6 Measurement Processes

This section deals with describing measurement processes. In general, we intend to make inferences about a variable X, but we can obtain or record (measure, elicit, or the like) only the values of a related variable Y. The measurement process can be motivated as the way in which a particular value of the latent (underlying) variable X is 'converted' (distorted) to the value of the manifest (observed or recorded) variable Y. The measurement process can either be described by the mechanism that distorts the value of X in the process of its measurement, or by the distribution of the differences $Y - X$. Instead of these differences, the ratios Y/X, their logarithms, $\log(Y/X)$, or the differences after some other monotone transformation, $f(Y) - f(X)$, may be considered. As an alternative, the distributions of Y may be described in each of the subpopulations defined by the unique values of X. Of course, this is not practical when X is continuous, unless these distributions have some features in common.

When X is a categorical variable and Y is an attempt to recover the value of X, we refer to a *misclassification* process. Such a process can be described by the table of the probabilities $P(X = x, Y = y)$ for each pair of possible values x and y. A desirable property of a misclassification process is that the probability of agreement, $P(X = Y)$, equal to the total of the probabilities $P(X = x, Y = x)$ over the possible values x, is close to unity. When X is an ordinal categorical variable another desirable property is that when disagreement occurs, $X \neq Y$, it is frequently by only one point on the scale. For instance, when the possible values of X are $1, 2, \ldots, K$, we prefer a manifest variable Y for which $P(|X - Y| \geq 2)$ is small.

Apart from the latent value X_i, the manifest value Y_i may depend on the values of some other variables. For instance, if the task of measurement is assigned to several judges, the identity of the judge assigned to assess a particular subject is a relevant (categorical) variable. The manifest value Y_i may be influenced even by the values of some variables, including X, for other subjects. For instance, a judge's assessment may be influenced by the other assessments made (recently) by the same judge, or by instructions received (or made aware of) halfway through the assessment process. Of course, it is wise to avoid such influences (by training and appropriately instructing the judges), but the process of measurement is not always under our control and training and instruction entail costs drawn from the same budget as the other survey tasks.

If the value of X can be established we can learn about the distortion $Y - X$ directly, by applying the measurement process on a sample of subjects. Otherwise, when the act of measurement alters the state of the subject at most temporarily (in particular, it does not destroy it) and is not costly, we can learn about the measurement process by replicating it on subjects. Thus, we observe two (or more) versions of the variable Y, $Y^{(1)}$ and $Y^{(2)}$; the pairs may be observed on the entire sample of subjects, a subsample of the subjects, or an entirely different sample drawn from the same population. These two variables have identical distributions. Observations from other populations have to be considered with care because the properties of the measurement process may be specific to the population. By the same token, if repeated observations are made on a subsample of subjects, this subsample (just like the sample) should be representative of the population.

The variables $Y^{(1)}$ and $Y^{(2)}$ differ because they are affected by different settings, such as the assigned judge, observed circumstances that are beyond our control, such as the temperature and the environment in which the interview is conducted, and other inexplicable influences (circumstances) that defy our understanding. We may consider versions of Y associated with each conceivable set of circumstances (moments or *contexts*). These contexts can themselves be regarded as a population. Unlike populations considered so far, they may be *infinite*. To draw a clearer distinction, we refer to the population that is the original target of our inferences, as the *target population*, and to the contexts as an *incidental* or *nuisance* population. This qualifier reflects our position—if the context had no impact on the measurement, or indeed, if Y coincided with X, our task of making inferences about X would be simpler.

The properties of a measurement process are described by the distribution of the measurements on a member of the target population. The measurements are taken in the population of contexts. For each member i of the target population, we denote by $Y_i^{(m)}$ the variable defined as the manifest value in the population of contexts. The bias of the measurement $B_i^{(m)}$ is defined as the expectation of the measurement deviations,

$$B_i^{(m)} = E\left(Y_i^{(m)} \mid i\right) - X_i,$$

taken over the population of contexts. We write i behind the bar $|$ to indicate that the expectation is taken with the member i fixed; the expectation is *conditional* on and relates solely to member i. The expression for bias requires a definition of the expectation, because E has so far been defined only for finite populations. The expectation for an infinite population is defined as the limit over sequences of increasing subpopulations, such that each member is eventually included in a subpopulation. The details are postponed to Section A.7. We considered similar limits in the context of replications of a sampling process in Section A.3.

The measurement variance and mean squared error (MSE) are defined similarly to the expectation:

$$\text{var}\left(Y_i^{(m)} \mid i\right) = E\left[\left\{Y_i^{(m)} - E\left(Y_i^{(m)}\right)\right\}^2 \mid i\right],$$

$$\mathrm{MSE}\left(Y_i^{(\mathrm{m})};\, X_i\,\middle|\, i\right) = \mathrm{E}\left\{\left(Y_i^{(\mathrm{m})} - X_i\right)^2\,\middle|\, i\right\};$$

they coincide for unbiased measurement processes, when $\mathrm{B}_i^{(\mathrm{m})} = 0$ for each member i.

Conditioning on member i in these equations is essential. Without it the measurement process would be replicated on a different member each time and $\mathrm{var}(Y_i^{(1)})$ would depend also on the dispersion of the values of X and on the process used for selecting the member to be observed.

Just like the expectation, variance, and MSE, other features and properties defined for a (finite) target population can be defined also for a population of measurements. These features include symmetry, the median, and quantiles (percentiles), except for minimum and maximum (the zero- and unity-quantiles) that need not exist. The definition of the mode is also problematic.

Every feature defined for one subject or member of the population has an obvious equivalent for every other member; after all, the ordering (labelling) of the members of the population is immaterial. Description of the measurement process by one or a few quantities for each member is impractical for a population of moderate or large size. The ultimate simplification is attained when the measurement process has the same properties for every member. Of course, this is a very special case. For example, suppose X has possible values 0, 1, 2, ..., 10, and its manifest version Y deviates by at most one unit in either direction, with probability 0.1:

$$\mathrm{P}(Y = X - 1 \mid 1 < X < 10) = \mathrm{P}(Y = X + 1 \mid 1 < X < 10) = 0.1\,,$$

unless $X = 0$ or $X = 10$. When $X = 0$ or $X = 10$, only one kind of deviation is possible: observing $Y = 1$ instead of $X = 0$ and observing $Y = 9$ instead of $X = 10$. This measurement process is symmetric and unbiased, so long as $X \neq 0$ and $X \neq 10$.

We prefer measurement processes that have smaller MSEs, and among those with identical MSEs, those with smaller absolute bias $|\mathrm{B}|$. Of course, it may be difficult to compare measurement processes when their properties are specific to the members of the population. The distribution of the deviations $Y - X$ may be the same within each subpopulation defined by a categorical variable (such as men and women, or occupational categories in human populations), or by the value of X itself.

An appealing property of a measurement process is that its distribution depends on the observed subject only through the values of a limited set of variables, and the identity of the observed member is irrelevant otherwise. A measurement process is said to be *impartial* if the distribution of Y depends only on the value of X. A measurement process is said to be *additive* if the deviations $Y - X$ have the same distribution for every member of the population. Such a process can be described as

$$Y = X + \varepsilon\,,$$

where the distribution of ε is independent of the observed members' values of X. Additive processes for which ε is independent of the background variables are impartial. Section 6.2 contains more details on impartiality and additivity.

Properties of a measurement process can be changed dramatically by a transformation. By way of an example, suppose X is a monetary value, such as the total value of a company's liabilities. For many companies, their total liabilities are not defined with precision because guesses have to be made about some of its elements, and other elements may depend on the prices in the near future. A plausible model for a particular measurement (assessment or audit) process is that

$$Y_i = X_i \delta_i,$$

where the distribution of δ_i does not depend on the company (i). Such a measurement process is called *multiplicative*. The logarithms of the assessed and 'true' liabilities satisfy an additive measurement model. For instance, suppose a typical deviation from X is by 1%, and deviations in access of 2.5% are very rare. A deviation of 1% corresponds to £10 000 for a large company with liabilities of £1 million, but only £100 for a small company with liabilities of £10 000. After taking logarithms, such deviations correspond to log-deviations of $\log(0.01) = 0.0095$, irrespective of the underlying value of the liabilities.

A.7 Infinite Populations

The distribution of a variable in an infinite population cannot be established by counting the number of members with each specific value because these counts may be infinite for some or all of the possible values. Even when the counts are infinite it is meaningful to consider how much more frequently one value occurs than another. For example, the distribution of the outcomes of the single toss of a fair coin is given by the probabilities:

$$P(Y = \text{head}) = P(Y = \text{tail}) = \tfrac{1}{2}.$$

We could verify this by replicating the toss many times and observing that about half the outcomes are heads. (The number of replications has to be large and specified up front.)

The distribution of a general variable in an infinite population is defined similarly. The distributions are considered for a sequence of samples s_h, $h = 1, 2, \ldots$, such that each sample is a subsample of the following sample, that is, $s_h \subset s_{h+1}$, and the union of all the samples coincides with the population; every member i belongs to all samples s_h for $h \geq h_i$; the index h_i is specific to member i. The distribution of the variable is defined as the limiting distribution as h increases above all bounds.

This definition requires two qualifications: how a limiting distribution is defined and by what process the sequence of samples is constructed. For simplicity, we consider first variables that have only a finite number of possible

Table A.3. The observed counts of the outcomes in replicate draws from the distribution with probabilities 0.08, 0.15, 0.27, 0.32, and 0.18 of the respective categories 1–5. The corresponding frequencies are plotted in Figure A.5.

	Outcome				
Replications	1	2	3	4	5
100	10	10	25	38	17
1000	79	155	250	334	182
10 000	798	1489	2694	3184	1837
100 000	7835	15 058	27 005	32 295	17 807

values. With the increasing sample size, the segments or bars of the histogram become taller, even if their relative sizes are not changed radically. The effect of the sample size can be removed by plotting the proportions of subjects in each value category, while keeping the total length of the segments constant, equal to unity. With such a *standardisation*, the limiting distribution is defined by the limits of the proportions for each category.

An example of convergence in distribution is given in Figure A.5. The numbers of replicates (sample sizes) on which the plotted distributions are based are 100, 1000, 10 000 and 100 000, given in the subtitle of each panel. The probabilities, 0.08, 0.15, 0.27, 0.32, and 0.18, of the respective categories 1–5 are marked in each panel by thin horizontal bars. On the scale used for plotting, the five deviations of the sample proportions from the corresponding probabilities are substantial for $n = 100$ in panel A and minute for $n = 100\,000$ in panel D. Table A.3 gives the four distributions in tabular form, expressed as counts for each category. In contrast to the proportions, the counts tend to differ from their expectations by wider margins with more replications; for instance, in 100 replications, outcome 1 was observed ten times, in two more cases than expected, whereas in 100 000 replications, outcome 1 was observed 165 fewer times than the expected count of 8000. Convergence occurs for the proportions, not for the counts.

Control over the sampling process is essential to avoid distortions such as overrepresentation of a category. To simplify matters, we define simple random sampling from an infinite population by a sequence of replications of drawing a single subject without any prejudice for or against any of the members' attributes. This sounds like a circular definition, but we cannot define a sampling process by probabilities because the probability of any one member being drawn is equal to zero.

The distributions drawn in Figure A.5 are called *sampling distributions* because they depend on the sample (of occasions) drawn. Their limit is called the *population distribution*. The adjectives *sampling* and *population* are used

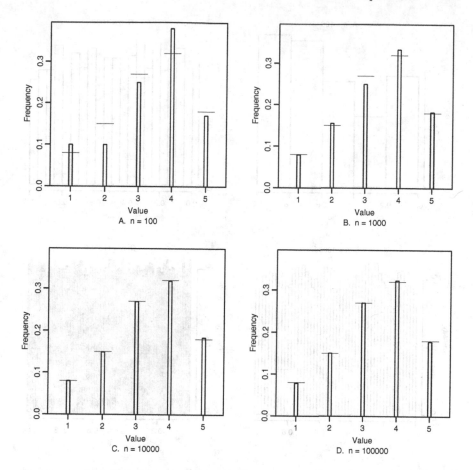

Fig. A.5. Illustration of convergence in distribution. The sample size for each distribution is given in the subtitle of each panel. The limiting frequencies are marked by horizontal bars.

in the same way as for quantities or sets of quantities derived from them. A distribution can be regarded as a collection of quantities.

A.7.1 Continuous Distributions

The possible values of some variables cover the entire continuum or an interval of real numbers, and so, without rounding, each value may be unique. The distribution of such a variable cannot be described as a limit of sampling distributions, because each (finite) sampling distribution is full of spikes corresponding to the values of the individual subjects. Yet the density of the spikes informs us about the ranges in which values are more or less frequent. Such features are more succinctly depicted by a coarsened histogram. It is practical

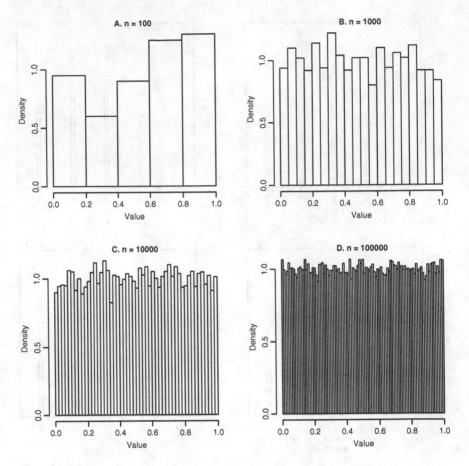

Fig. A.6. Illustration of the convergence in distribution for a continuous variable. The sample size for each distribution is given in the title of each panel.

to plot the standardised histogram, in which the area covered by the bars is equal to a set value, such as unity. The distribution of a continuous variable in an infinite population is defined as the limit of the standardised histograms for random samples with sample sizes increasing beyond all bounds, while the bars of the histograms get narrower (the coarsening is refined) as the sample size increases.

An illustration paralleling Figure A.5 is given in Figure A.6. In the limiting distribution, each bar has the same (unit) height. For the sample size $n = 100$, this could not be anticipated, but for $n = 100\,000$ it is obvious, although one may argue that the limit could still have an irregular pattern. The limiting histogram, with the bar widths converging to zero, is called the *density* of the distribution, if the limit is well defined. A distribution that has a density is called *absolutely continuous*. We drop the qualifier 'absolutely' because we very rarely come across variables or distributions that are continuous but not absolutely continuous.

A distribution with a constant density on its support is called *uniform*. The *standard uniform* distribution is the uniform distribution with the support on $(0, 1)$. Its density is $f(x) = 1$ for $x \in (0, 1)$ and $f(x) = 0$ otherwise. The limiting distribution in Figure A.6 is standard uniform.

For any continuous distribution, the area under the density is equal to unity:

$$\int_{-\infty}^{+\infty} f(x)\, dx = 1\,.$$

A density defines a unique distribution by the identity

$$P(c < X < d) = \int_{c}^{d} f(x)\, dx$$

for any pair of real numbers $c < d$.

For a variable X or its distribution, the distribution function is defined as

$$F(x) = P(X \le x)\,,$$

a function in $(-\infty, +\infty)$. It is nondecreasing, with limits of zero and unity at $-\infty$ and $+\infty$, respectively. The distribution function and the density of a continuous distribution are related by the identity

$$f(x) = F'(x)$$

(the derivative of F at x). Therefore, the distribution function of a continuous distribution is differentiable.

Strictly speaking, it cannot be proven that the limiting distribution in Figure A.6 is the uniform or any other distribution. To justify the uniform as the limit, we have to supplement the evidence based from sampling with the conjecture, or appeal to 'good reason', that the density is smooth. In the case of Figure A.6, it may be difficult to argue why the density should deviate from a constant (unity) according to no apparent pattern. In practice, it is often much more difficult to integrate the information extracted from the data and obtained from other sources, such as descriptions of the studied setting and relevant findings made by other parties, and conclude with a simple description of the sought distribution and its properties.

A.7.2 Superpopulations: Models

Although finite, many human populations are large, with several million members, and the distributions of variables defined for them are often very close to continuous distributions with densities that contain no sharp edges or sudden changes. Such densities are called *smooth*. Formally, a density $f(x)$ is said to be smooth in an interval if it is differentiable at each point of the interval and its derivative, denoted by $f'(x)$, is a continuous function. Note that a smooth density f corresponds to an 'even smoother' distribution function F; since $f(x) = F'(x)$, F is twice continuously differentiable.

Using a continuous distribution has several advantages; continuous distributions tend to be easier to describe, by a mathematical formula or graph, and various operations with them are easier to execute. The use of such a distribution may be justified by a reference to an infinite-size *superpopulation*. This is a hypothetical (nonexistent) population from which the studied population is assumed to have been drawn as a random sample. For instance, in a different context, such as the same survey conducted at a different time point and using slightly different questions, the survey would be conducted on a different population, but the population would have been realised by the same sampling process applied to the same superpopulation. We may even make inferences about the superpopulation, regarding its features as more stable (less transient) than the features of the population. After all, the population, regarded as a simple random sample, is, by definition, a faithful miniature of the superpopulation.

Superpopulation and its description (by a distribution) are an example of a *model*, an analyst's construct. A model is a stylised (simplified) description of a studied population using one or several variables defined on it. For instance, a model may provide a description of how the values of several variables are related in a population. The price of the simplification is a loss of precision and detail, but it may well be worth it if the result is greater insight and better understanding of the studied population.

A.8 Distributions

Any sequence of values $v_1, v_2, \ldots$, of finite or infinite length, and a corresponding sequence of positive numbers $p_1, p_2, \ldots$ that add up to unity, forms a discrete distribution, by prescribing for a random variable X that

$$P(X = v_k) = p_k.$$

Any nonnegative function $f^\dagger$ that has a finite area underneath it,

$$\int f^\dagger(u)\,du < +\infty,$$

defines a continuous distribution by the density obtained by standardising $f^\dagger$, that is, by defining

$$f(x) = \frac{f^\dagger(x)}{\int f^\dagger(u)\,du}.$$

For example, the exponential distribution is defined by the density

$$f(x) = \theta \exp(-\theta x), \tag{A.2}$$

for $x > 0$ and $f(x) = 0$ otherwise; θ is a positive constant. The distribution function is obtained from the density by integration:

$$F(x) = \int_{-\infty}^{x} f(x) \, dx,$$

and the density is obtained from the distribution by differentiation: $f(x) = F'(x)$. The distribution function of the exponential distribution given by (A.2) is

$$F(x) = P(X \le x) = 1 - \exp(-\theta x),$$

for $x > 0$. We use the singular *distribution* for the density $f(x)$ in (A.2) with a specific *parameter* θ, and the plural *distributions* for the collection of distributions, for θ in the entire range $(0, +\infty)$ or its subset.

The exponential distributions are a special case of the gamma distributions given by the densities

$$f(x) = \frac{1}{\Gamma(b)} \theta^b x^{b-1} \exp(-\theta x),$$

for $x > 0$ and $f(x) = 0$ otherwise; b and θ are positive constants and Γ is the gamma function; see Section A.12 for more details.

An important role in statistics is played by the *normal* distributions. They are defined by the densities

$$f(x) = \frac{1}{\sqrt{2\pi\sigma^2}} \exp\left\{ -\frac{(x - \mu)^2}{2\sigma^2} \right\}, \tag{A.3}$$

where μ is a real and σ^2 a positive constant. We denote this distribution by $\mathcal{N}(\mu, \sigma^2)$. The normal distribution with $\mu = 0$ and $\sigma^2 = 1$ is called the *standard normal* distribution.

For continuous distributions, we can define various features similarly to their counterparts for discrete distributions, with probabilities $P(X = x_k)$ replaced by the values of the density $f(x)$. A continuous distribution is said to be symmetric around a value c if $f(c - \Delta) = f(c + \Delta)$ for every constant Δ. For example, the normal distribution $\mathcal{N}(\mu, \sigma^2)$ is symmetric around μ. A continuous distribution is said to have a mode at value c if its density has a local maximum at c. The distribution is said to be unimodal (bimodal, trimodal, and so on), if it has one (two, three, or more) modes.

The expectation of a continuous distribution with density $f(x)$ is defined as

$$E(X) = \int_{-\infty}^{+\infty} x f(x) \, dx,$$

if the integral is well defined. Equivalently, the expectation can be defined as the limit of the expectations of a sequence of discrete distributions that converge to the distribution with density f, so long as the limit exists and the integral is well defined. The variance of a continuous distribution with density $f(x)$ is defined as

$$\text{var}(X) = \text{E}\left[\{X - \text{E}(X)\}^2\right]$$

if the integrals involved are well defined. Equivalently, we have

$$\text{var}(X) = \text{E}\left(X^2\right) - \{\text{E}(X)\}^2,$$

so long as $\text{E}\left(X^2\right)$ is well defined. If it is, then so is $\text{E}(X)$. For example, the mean of the normal distribution $\mathcal{N}(\mu, \sigma^2)$ is μ, and its variance is equal to σ^2.

The q-quantile of a continuous distribution with density $f(x)$ is the value u for which

$$P(X < u) = \int_{-\infty}^{u} f(x)\,dx = q. \tag{A.4}$$

This probability, the distribution function, in fact, is a continuous nondecreasing function of u, and so the equation in (A.4) always has a solution, for every $q \in (0, 1)$; the solution either is unique or is any point in an interval. In the latter case, a sensible convention is to declare the centre of the interval as the quantile.

Earlier we defined sampling processes for finite populations. Sampling from a continuous distribution or a related superpopulation requires a new definition, because the probability of any particular real value is equal to zero. We define a random draw from the standard uniform distribution by the process of drawing a single value in the range $(0, 1)$ without any prejudice. A practical implementation of this can rely on a sequence of independent draws from the discrete uniform distribution on $(0, 1, \ldots, 9)$. Let these draws be $(l_1, l_2, \ldots)$. Then the draw from the standard uniform distribution is

$$\sum_{h=1}^{\infty} 10^{-h} l_h,$$

that is, l_h is the digit in the decimal place h. A random draw from a continuous distribution is defined as the q-quantile of this distribution, where q is a random draw from the standard uniform distribution. A random sample of size n is defined as a sequence of n replicate (independent) random draws from a distribution. Note that this definition confers a pivotal role on the standard uniform distribution. From a random sample $\mathbf{X} = (X_1, X_2, \ldots, X_n)$ from the standard uniform distribution we obtain a random sample from a continuous distribution with distribution function F by the elementwise quantile transformation

$$F^{-1}(\mathbf{X}) = \left\{ F^{-1}(X_1), F^{-1}(X_2), \ldots, F^{-1}(X_n) \right\}.$$

A distribution is given by a set of probabilities, a density, a distribution function, or the like. Frequently we consider a *class of distributions*; they are a finite or infinite set of distributions that have a common (or similar) functional form and are distinguished by the values of one or several parameters.

For example, the set of all exponential distributions, given by the density $f(x) = \theta \exp(-\theta x)$, where θ is in the range $(0, +\infty)$, is a class of distributions. The distributions in this class are characterised by the value of one parameter, θ. Such a class is said to be single-parameter. The class of all the normal distributions $\mathcal{N}(\mu, \sigma^2)$, where $\mu \in (-\infty, +\infty)$ and $\sigma^2 \in (0, +\infty)$, is a two-parameter class of distributions. In principle, any collection of distributions can be regarded as a class, and they need not have a description in terms of one or a few parameters.

A.8.1 Simulations

With a considerable simplification, a typical problem in statistics can be described as follows. The values of a variable are available for a random sample drawn from an infinite population, and the population distribution of the variable is known to belong to a given class of distributions. The task is to estimate this distribution or its summary. Ideally, we would like to identify it, but that is rarely possible. For a one-parameter class, the quantity of interest may be the value of the characterising parameter, such as θ for the exponential distributions given by (A.2). The key assumption made is that the process that generates the values of the studied variable is well described by one of the distributions in the posited class. We can *simulate* (mimic) the process of generating a random sample from an infinite population (distribution) on the computer.

Figure A.7 displays the histogram of a computer-generated random sample of size 50 000 drawn from the standard normal distribution. The density of the normal distribution, suitably scaled, is superimposed. The distribution of the computer-generated values is called *empirical*. Any summary of the empirical distribution, such as its mean and variance and, in relation to an estimator, bias and MSE, are also called empirical.

The histogram shows that with a large sample size the empirical and population distributions differ only slightly and have essentially the same features, except for a modicum of roughness of the empirical distribution. For instance, unlike the population distribution, the empirical distribution may have more than one mode. The symmetry is not reproduced, but the empirical distribution is very close to symmetry.

The term (computer) *simulation* refers to replications of the assumed data-generating process (on a computer). In principle, any device could be used for simulation, but the modern computer has no practical competitor, especially when a large number of replicates and a nontrivial amount of computing are required. By simulation, we can generate replicates fast and at a fraction of the cost of replicates generated by the studied processes ('real life') and can assess the properties and, more generally, learn about the posited distributions. To this process, we can attach estimation, using several (candidate) estimators,

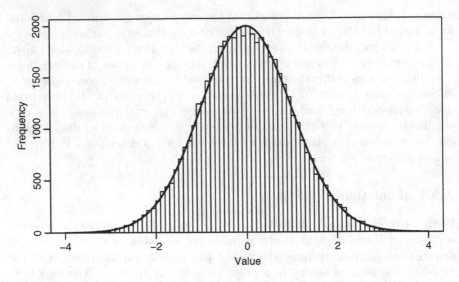

Fig. A.7. Histogram of a computer-generated random sample of size 50 000 from the standard normal distribution, with the density of $\mathcal{N}(0,1)$ superimposed.

and compare their properties, efficiency in particular. In this way, we can engage in an informed planning of a study in which observations are expensive (as regards finance, labour, ethics or any form of undesirable destruction), and decide how to strike a balance between the conflicting goals of high precision in estimating a target and low expenditure.

A.9 Classes of Distributions and Models

Simulations can use the computing power as a replacement for the analytical ability to derive properties of estimators. Sampling and measurement processes can be explored similarly. In practice, we face a task much more difficult than simulation because only one replication of a process, governed by a distribution that is not known to us, is available. When we know, or assume, that the sought distribution belongs to a particular class, we might look for the member of the class that resembles the observed values more closely than any other. For this, we have to define a metric for 'resemblance' but also develop approaches to identifying suitable classes of distributions based on the information about the studied processes.

If we had a perfect understanding of how a particular process operates, we could anticipate what kind of values it would produce. In a typical setting, our understanding is far from complete but is not totally hollow. We study a process to enhance or supplement our partial understanding of it. We can entice the process to run its course and yield values of one or several key variables on a sample of subjects or occasions (observational units). From this output, commonly referred to as *data*, we want to estimate certain population quantities related to the process. We can interpret this problem as an *inverse* task to simulations. While in simulations we can implement a process and obtain output (data), the task in practice is to infer from the data obtained some properties (details) of the underlying process.

A powerful general approach to addressing this problem is by specifying a model for the studied (target) process. This model is a collection of processes, and we assume that one of them is the studied process. For instance, if we believe that the process generates values drawn at random from one of a class of distributions, then this class forms the model. Suppose the class comprises all the normal distributions, $\mathcal{N}(\mu, \sigma^2)$, with unknown values of μ and σ^2, and it would be valuable to know the values of these *parameters*, μ and σ^2. The target process may be more complex than one of the model distributions, but the simplicity in the model specification may be rewarded by a better choice of an estimator or, more importantly, a better understanding of the studied process.

For models or classes of distributions in general, we can define a partial ordering. Model A is said to be narrower than model B if every distribution in model A is also contained in model B. A model with a narrower class of distributions has the advantage that we have fewer candidates for the target process, so the search among them is, in principle, easier. On the other hand, if we choose a wider class of distributions we do not reduce the possibility that this class contains the target distribution or contains a distribution that is close to the target distribution. This balancing act between *specificity* (narrowness) and *validity* (containing the 'true' distribution) is one of the principal unresolved problems in statistics. A model that contains the target distribution is called *valid*. In later chapters we will also find that estimation based on narrower models is more efficient, *if* the model is valid.

A.10 Normal Distributions

The class of normal distributions appears in many theoretical derivations as well as in practical applications. It has some very useful properties which make it a popular choice for a model. From its density given by (A.3), we can easily deduce that the normal distribution $\mathcal{N}(\mu, \sigma^2)$ is symmetric and has a single mode at μ. These properties imply that its mean, if it exists, is equal to μ. This can be verified by evaluating the integral

$$E(X) = \int_{-\infty}^{+\infty} \frac{x}{\sqrt{2\pi\sigma^2}} \exp\left\{-\frac{(x-\mu)^2}{2\sigma^2}\right\} dx$$

$$= \mu \int_{-\infty}^{+\infty} \frac{1}{\sqrt{2\pi}} \exp\left(-\frac{y^2}{2}\right) dy + \frac{1}{\sqrt{2\pi}} \int_{-\infty}^{+\infty} y \exp\left(-\frac{y^2}{2}\right) dy = \mu,$$

after the transformation $y = (x - \mu)/\sigma$, and realising that the first integrand in the second line is the density of the standard normal distribution. The second integrand is symmetric and has the primitive function $-\exp(-y^2/2)$, so its integrals over $(-\infty, 0)$ and $(0, +\infty)$ are well defined and add up to zero. Similarly, it can be shown that the variance of the normal distribution $\mathcal{N}(\mu, \sigma^2)$ is equal to σ^2. A more elegant proof of this is provided after deriving another property of the class of normal distributions.

If X has the distribution $\mathcal{N}(\mu, \sigma^2)$, then $Y = (X - \mu)/\sigma$ has the standard normal distribution $\mathcal{N}(0, 1)$. This can be derived by expressing the distribution of Y by the probabilities

$$P(Y < c) = P(X < \mu + c\sigma),$$

and expressing this as

$$P(X < \mu + c\sigma) = \frac{1}{\sqrt{2\pi\sigma^2}} \int_{-\infty}^{\mu + c\sigma} \exp\left\{-\frac{(x - \mu)^2}{2\sigma^2}\right\} \, \mathrm{d}x$$

$$= \frac{1}{\sqrt{2\pi}} \int_{-\infty}^{c} \exp\left(-\tfrac{1}{2}y^2\right) \, \mathrm{d}y,$$

which is the distribution function of the standard normal distribution. The variance of the standard normal distribution is equal to

$$\frac{1}{\sqrt{2\pi}} \int_{-\infty}^{\infty} y^2 \exp\left(-\tfrac{1}{2}y^2\right) \, \mathrm{d}y = 1,$$

derived by integrating by parts, using the primitive function $-\exp(-y^2/2)$ for $y \exp(-y^2/2)$. As the standard deviation is a dispersion quantity, the standard deviation of $\mathcal{N}(\mu, \sigma^2)$ is equal to σ and the variance to σ^2.

We can declare each constant μ the (degenerate) normal distribution $\mathcal{N}(\mu, 0)$. With this convention, any linear transformation of a normally distributed variable is normally distributed. We say that the normal distributions are closed with respect to linear transformations. Any normal distribution can be formed by a linear transformation of the standard normal distribution, and any normal distribution $\mathcal{N}(\mu, \sigma^2)$ with positive variance σ^2 can be transformed linearly, as from X to $(X - \mu)/\sigma$, to become the standard normal. The application of this transformation, $g(X) = (X - \mu)/\sigma$, is referred to as *standardisation*.

Owing to the closure of the normal distribution with respect to linear transformations, an arbitrary quantile of any normal distribution can be derived straightforwardly from the corresponding quantile of the standard normal distribution. Denote by Φ the distribution function of $\mathcal{N}(0, 1)$, so that its inverse $\Phi^{-1}(q)$ is the quantile as a function of the probability q. As every quantile is a location quantity, the q-quantile of $\mathcal{N}(\mu, \sigma^2)$ is equal to $\mu + \sigma\Phi^{-1}(q)$. Many estimators encountered in practice are approximately normally distributed with the approximation being very close when the sample size is large.

A.10.1 Log-Normal Distributions

Many variables are expressed in physical units, such as degrees Fahrenheit, miles, or degrees of latitude, which have alternatives, such as degrees Celsius, kilometres, and radians, respectively. A class of distributions would have a strong appeal if, among other conditions, it would be equally well suited for either of the scales defined by the alternative units. When the units are linearly related, as in the listed examples, the normal distribution has the obvious advantage because it is closed with respect to linear transformations.

In practice, we often encounter variables for which classes that are closed with respect to multiplication would be suitable. For example, a natural operation for values defined in monetary units is multiplication, often expressed in terms of percentages. By taking logarithms, multiplication converts to addition, a linear transformation. Some laws of physics involve multiplication (or division) and units that imply multiplication. Area and volume are cases in point, and speed and shape involve division. By taking logarithms, length, area, and volume are expressed in identical units, such as 'log-meter'.

These examples motivate the *log-normal* distribution. A variable X is said to have a log-normal distribution if its logarithm has a normal distribution. If a variable X is distributed according to $\mathcal{N}(\mu, \sigma^2)$, then its exponential (the inverse of logarithm) has mean $\exp(\mu + \frac{1}{2}\sigma^2)$ and variance $\exp(2\mu)\exp(\sigma^2)\{\exp(\sigma^2) - 1\}$. To prove this, we evaluate $E\{\exp(kX)\}$ for $k = 1$ and $k = 2$. By reorganising the terms in the arguments of the exponentials we obtain

$$
\begin{aligned}
E\{\exp(kX)\} &= \frac{1}{\sqrt{2\pi\sigma^2}} \int_{-\infty}^{+\infty} \exp(kx) \exp\left\{-\frac{(x-\mu)^2}{2\sigma^2}\right\} \\
&= \frac{1}{\sqrt{2\pi\sigma^2}} \exp\left\{-\frac{\mu^2}{2\sigma^2} + \frac{(\mu + k\sigma^2)^2}{2\sigma^2}\right\} \int_{-\infty}^{+\infty} \exp\left[-\frac{\{x - (\mu + k\sigma^2)\}^2}{2\sigma^2}\right] \\
&= \exp\left(k\mu + \tfrac{1}{2}k^2\sigma^2\right),
\end{aligned}
$$

exploiting the fact that the density of $\mathcal{N}(\mu + k^2\sigma^2, \sigma^2)$ integrates to unity. The expression for the mean follows directly ($k = 1$), and the variance is derived from the identity

$$
\text{var}\{\exp(X)\} = E\{\exp(2X)\} - [E\{\exp(X)\}]^2.
$$

The normal and log-normal distributions provide an effective illustration that nonlinear transformations and expectation E do not commute. We have

$$
E\{\exp(X)\} \geq \exp\{E(X)\},
$$

with equality only when $\sigma^2 = 0$. The finite-sample version of this inequality is equivalent to the statement that the geometric mean of a set of positive numbers never exceeds the arithmetic mean:

$$\sqrt[n]{\prod_{i=1}^{n} x_i} \leq \frac{1}{n} \sum_{i=1}^{n} x_i \,,$$

with equality only when all n values x_i coincide.

A.11 Uniform Distributions

The uniform distribution was introduced in Section A.7.1. In this section, we explore it in greater detail. The class of continuous uniform distributions is given by the densities $f(x) = 1/(\theta_2 - \theta_1)$ for $x \in (\theta_1, \theta_2)$ and $f(x) = 0$ elsewhere; $\theta_1 < \theta_2$ are the two parameters that define a distribution. We denote the uniform distribution on (θ_1, θ_2) by $\mathcal{U}(\theta_1, \theta_2)$. Although θ_1 has to be smaller than θ_2, it is expedient to regard the constant θ as the (degenerate) uniform distribution $\mathcal{U}(\theta, \theta)$. For $\theta_1 < \theta_2$, the distribution function of $\mathcal{U}(\theta_1, \theta_2)$ is piecewise linear: $F(x) = 0$ for $x < \theta_1$, $F(x) = (x - \theta_1)/(\theta_2 - \theta_1)$ for $x \in [\theta_1, \theta_2]$ and $F(x) = 1$ for $x > \theta_2$.

Similarly to the standard normal distribution, the standard uniform distribution is obtained from an arbitrary nondegenerate distribution $\mathcal{U}(\theta_1, \theta_2)$, with $\theta_1 < \theta_2$, by the linear transformation $g(X) = (X - \theta_1)/(\theta_2 - \theta_1)$. Conversely, any uniform distribution is obtained from the standard uniform by the transformation $\theta_1 + (\theta_2 - \theta_1)X$. The class of uniform distributions is closed with respect to linear transformations.

The distribution $\mathcal{U}(\theta_1, \theta_2)$ is symmetric, with mean $(\theta_1 - \theta_2)/2$ and variance $(\theta_1 - \theta_2)^2/12$. The latter expression is obtained by integration (for the standard uniform distribution),

$$\int_0^1 \left(x - \tfrac{1}{2}\right)^2 \, \mathrm{d}x = \tfrac{1}{12} \,,$$

and using the fact that the standard deviation is a dispersion quantity. The class of uniform distributions defines a model for randomness in a variety of settings. By a number randomly drawn from a given range, such as $(0, 100)$, we mean a random draw from the distribution $\mathcal{U}(0, 100)$. The condition of 'no prejudice' for or against any particular value in the support is interpreted as a constant density of the distribution from which a draw (selection) is to be made. It implies that the probability of a draw falling to any particular interval depends solely on the length of the interval; $\mathrm{P}(a < X < b) = (b - a)/(\theta_2 - \theta_1)$, so long as $\theta_1 \leq a \leq b \leq \theta_2$.

The standard uniform distribution has the role of a pivot among all the continuous distributions. Suppose variable X has a continuous distribution with distribution function $F(x)$, strictly increasing throughout its support (ξ_1, ξ_2); either bound ξ_1 or ξ_2 may be infinite. Then $F(X)$, the distribution function applied as a transformation, has the standard uniform distribution. This follows immediately from the identity

$$P\{F(X) < u\} = u$$

for $u = F(x) = P(X < x)$.

Suppose continuous variable X has distribution function $F(x)$ and $G(x)$ is another distribution function with a density. Then the variable $G^{-1}\{F(X)\}$ has the distribution function $G(x)$. Thus, a continuous variable can be transformed to have any other continuous distribution. In particular, we can construct (by simulations) a variable with any conceivable continuous distribution.

Polynomial and Other Distributions Derived from Uniform

A polynomial distribution is derived by taking a power of a variable with uniform distribution. We focus here on polynomial distributions with support on $(0,1)$; distributions with supports on other intervals are derived straightforwardly. Suppose variable X has uniform distribution on $(0,1)$, $X \sim \mathcal{U}(0,1)$, so that $P(X < x) = x$ for any $x \in (0,1)$. Then the variable $Y = X^k$ has the distribution function $P(Y < x) = \sqrt[k]{x}$, density $k^{-1}x^{1/k-1}$, expectation $1/(k+1)$ and standard deviation $k/(k+1)/\sqrt{2k+1}$.

The exponential distribution is obtained as the negative logarithm of the uniform distribution. If $X \sim \mathcal{U}(0,1)$, then the distribution function of $-\log(X)$ is $P\{-\log(X) < x\} = P\{X > \exp(-x)\} = 1 - \exp(-x)$. Note that while $E(X) = \frac{1}{2}$, $E\{-\log(X)\} = 1$, different from $\exp(\frac{1}{2})$; exponentiation and expectation cannot be exchanged. An arbitrary exponential distribution is obtained by the transformation $-\theta^{-1}\log(X)$ from $X \sim \mathcal{U}(0,1)$ for a positive θ.

A.12 Beta and Gamma Distributions

The class of beta distributions is defined by the densities

$$f(x) = \frac{\Gamma(a+b)}{\Gamma(a)\Gamma(b)}x^{a-1}(1-x)^{b-1} \tag{A.5}$$

for $x \in (0,1)$ and positive constants a and b. The gamma function $\Gamma(a)$ is defined for positive arguments a as

$$\Gamma(a) = \int_0^{+\infty} x^{a-1}e^{-x}\,dx.$$

For integers a, $\Gamma(a) = (a-1)! = 2 \times 3 \times \ldots \times (a-1)$. The beta density with parameters a and b is denoted as $B(a,b)$. Its expectation is $a/(a+b)$ and its variance is $ab/\{(a+b)^2(a+b+1)\}$. The expectations of the beta distributions are in the entire range $(0,1)$ and their variances in the range

$\{0, \mu(1 - \mu)\}$ where μ is the expectation. Beta distributions with mean equal to $\frac{1}{2}$, when $a = b$, are symmetric.

The gamma distributions are defined by the densities

$$f(x) = \frac{1}{\Gamma(\alpha)} \theta^\alpha x^{\alpha-1} \exp(-\theta x),$$

where α and θ are arbitrary positive constants and $x > 0$. The mean and variance of a gamma distribution are α/θ and α/θ^2, respectively. The parameter α is referred to as the shape and θ as the scale. Exponential distributions are a special case (a *subclass*) of gamma, with shape $\alpha = 1$. A gamma distribution with shape parameter equal to integer α can be derived as the distribution of the sum of α independent variables each with the exponential distribution with the same parameter θ; see Section 2.2.

A.13 Classes of Discrete Distributions

The simplest nontrivial discrete distribution is the binary distribution, also known as the Bernoulli distribution. It has probabilities $1-p$ and p, $0 < p < 1$, on the two points of its support, 0 and 1, respectively. Its expectation is p and variance $p(1 - p)$, obtained directly from the corresponding definitions for a general discrete distribution.

A *binomial distribution* is defined as the number of successes in a sequence of n independent trials, each of which has the same probability p of yielding a successful outcome. Thus, it is a sum of n independent and identically distributed binary variables. Its distribution is given by the probabilities

$$P(X = k) = \binom{n}{k} p^k (1 - p)^{n-k}. \tag{A.6}$$

Its expectation and variance are np and $np(1-p)$, respectively. They are both n-multiples of the Bernoulli distribution from which the binomial is generated. This is not a coincidence; see Section A.17. Every binomial distribution is either unimodal or its highest probability is attained at two consecutive points. The latter is the case when $k = p(n + 1)$ is an integer, and then the highest probabilities are attained at $k - 1$ and k. Otherwise it is unimodal, with mode either at the integer part of $p(n + 1) - 1$, denoted by $[p(n + 1) - 1]$, or at the following integer, $[p(n + 1)]$. Every binomial distribution with $p = \frac{1}{2}$ is symmetric, but no other binomials are, unless we define the degenerate binomial distributions with $p = 0$ and $p = 1$.

A *Poisson distribution* can be derived as the limit of binomial distributions as the probability p converges to zero and the number of trials diverges to infinity at such a speed that np converges to a finite constant λ. The Poisson distributions are given by the probabilities

$$P(X = k) = \frac{e^{-\lambda}\lambda^k}{k!},$$

for $k = 0, 1, \ldots$ and parameter $\lambda > 0$. The expectation and variance of this distribution are both equal to λ. Every Poisson distribution is either unimodal, with mode at one of the integers next to λ, or, when λ is an integer, the highest probability is shared by the points $\lambda - 1$ and λ.

A geometric distribution is derived as the number of failures prior to the first success in a sequence of independent binary trials. Let $q = 1 - p$ be the probability of failure; $q \in (0, 1)$. Then

$$P(X = k) = pq^k,$$

for a geometrically distributed variable X. The expectation of this variable is q/p and variance q/p^2. To prove this, we differentiate both sides of the identity

$$\sum_{k=0}^{\infty} p(1 - p)^k = 1;$$

$$\sum_{k=0}^{\infty} (1 - p)^k - \sum_{k=1}^{\infty} kp(1 - p)^{k-1} = 0. \tag{A.7}$$

The first summation, the total of a geometric sequence, is equal to $1/p$ and second to the $1/q$-multiple of the expectation; hence $E(X) = q/p$. Another differentiation of (A.7) yields the identity

$$-2 \sum_{k=1}^{\infty} k(1 - p)^{k-1} + \sum_{k=2}^{\infty} k(k - 1)p(1 - p)^{k-2} = 0,$$

and by relating the two summations to $E(X)$ and $E\{X(X - 1)\}$, respectively, we obtain the identity

$$E\{X(X - 1)\} = \frac{2q^2}{p^2},$$

from which the result for $\text{var}(X) = E\{X(X - 1)\} + E(X) - \{E(X)\}^2$ follows immediately.

A.13.1 Discrete Uniform Distributions

The class of discrete uniform distributions is defined by equal probabilities on each possible outcome. For example, the toss of a fair coin is represented by the uniform distribution on the set (H,T), head and tail of the coin. Casting a die corresponds to the uniform distribution on its six faces, or on the digits $1, \ldots, 6$. Similarly, by drawing a random digit, we mean drawing one member from the population $(0, 1, \ldots, 9)$ with probability equal to 0.1 for each digit. Lottery and games of chance provide further examples (and applications) of discrete uniform distributions.

The distributions supported on a finite number of values are called *multinomial*. The discrete uniform and binomial are their subclasses. A discrete distribution that is supported on infinitely many values can be approximated with arbitrary precision by a distribution that has the same probabilities on a suitably selected finite subset of the support, and the remaining probability is gathered in a single point. This sequence of subsets can be set to the n values that have the highest probabilities, with an arbitrary way of resolving ties, and letting n diverge to infinity.

A.14 Discrete Bivariate Distributions

So far, we have considered in detail only distributions defined on the real numbers, $(-\infty, +\infty)$, or its subsets, such as finite-length intervals and integers. We refer to such distributions as *univariate*. However, distributions can be defined in any space. In this section, we consider distributions on $\mathcal{I}^2 = \mathcal{I} \times \mathcal{I}$, where $\mathcal{I}$ is the set of integers $0, 1, \ldots$. They are essential for dealing with pairs of univariate variables and for studying how they are associated.

A discrete bivariate distribution is derived from a pair of random variables, X_1 and X_2; it is given by the probabilities

$$P(X_1 = x_1 \text{ and } X_2 = x_2),$$

for all integers x_1 and x_2. The two variables are said to be *independent* if

$$P(X_1 = x_1 \text{ and } X_2 = x_2) = P(X_1 = x_1) P(X_2 = x_2) \tag{A.8}$$

for all x_1 and x_2. Independence is a special case of association. A trivial case of dependence (the negation of independence) is the association of the variable with itself; the identity

$$P(X = x) = \{P(X = x)\}^2,$$

required for independence, holds only when $P(X = x)$ is equal to zero or unity, so a variable is independent with itself only when it is degenerate (supported by a single value x). As a nontrivial example of dependence, consider a single cast of a die and denote by X_1 and X_2 the dichotomous variables that indicate whether the outcome is even (2, 4 or 6), and whether it exceeds 3. Both variables have binary distributions on (Yes, No), with identical distributions given by $P(X_1 = \text{Yes}) = P(X_2 = \text{Yes}) = \frac{1}{2}$. However,

$$P(X_1 = \text{Yes and } X_2 = \text{Yes}) = \frac{1}{3},$$

different from $P(X_1 = \text{Yes}) \times P(X_2 = \text{Yes}) = \frac{1}{4}$.

A probability that involves both variables X_1 and X_2 is called *joint*, and a probability that involves only one of them is called *marginal*. These terms are motivated by the table of the (joint) probabilities in Table A.4.

In general, we have the identity

Table A.4. Joint and marginal probabilities (an example).

	X_2		
X_1	Yes	No	*Margin*
Yes	$\frac{1}{3}$	$\frac{1}{6}$	$\frac{1}{2}$
No	$\frac{1}{6}$	$\frac{1}{3}$	$\frac{1}{2}$
Margin	$\frac{1}{2}$	$\frac{1}{2}$	

$$P(X_1 = x_1) = \sum_x P(X_1 = x_1 \text{ and } X_2 = x),$$

where the summation is over the support of X_2. From the joint distribution (probabilities) we can derive the marginal distributions, but these are not sufficient for recovering the joint distribution of a pair of variables. If we know that X_1 and X_2 are independent, then their joint distribution is easily reconstructed from the marginal distributions according to (A.8).

A.14.1 Conditional Distributions

A conditional distribution is defined for a variable and a condition. A simple example is drawn from Table A.4. The conditional distribution of X_1, given that the outcome of casting a die exceeds 3 (X_2 is equal to 'Yes'), is defined by

$$P(X_1 = \text{Yes} \,|\, X_2 = \text{Yes}) = \tfrac{2}{3}.$$

This is derived by reducing our attention to the outcomes that satisfy the condition stated behind the vertical bar $|$. The probability is derived from the first column of the table as $\frac{1}{3} / \left(\frac{1}{3} + \frac{1}{6}\right)$ or, in general, as

$$P(X_1 = x_1 \,|\, X_2 = x_2) = \frac{P(X_1 = x_1 \text{ and } X_2 = x_2)}{P(X_2 = x_2)}.$$

This may be easier to motivate by replacing the probabilities in the table by counts. It corresponds to multiplying each entry in the table by a large number, but it has no impact on the ratio.

The roles of the two variables in the probability $P(X_1 = x_1 \,|\, X_2 = x_2)$ differ substantially. In general,

$$P(X_1 = x_1 \,|\, X_2 = x_2) \neq P(X_2 = x_2 \,|\, X_1 = x_1)$$

even though $P(X_1 = \text{Yes} \,|\, X_2 = \text{Yes}) = P(X_2 = \text{Yes} \,|\, X_1 = \text{Yes}) = \tfrac{2}{3}$ in Table A.4. The following example confirms this rule. Let X_1 be the higher outcome of the two casts of a die and X_2 the sum of the two outcomes. The conditional probability that $X_1 = 6$, given that the total is $X_2 = 8$, is $P(X_1 = 6 \mid X_2 = 8) = \frac{2}{5}$, whereas the conditional probability that $X_2 = 8$ given that six has come up at least once is $P(X_2 = 8 \mid X_1 = 6) = \frac{2}{11}$. A conditional probability is well defined only when the condition itself has a positive probability.

The two sets of probabilities are connected by the identity

$$P(X_1 = x_1 \mid X_2 = x_2) = \frac{P(X_2 = x_2 \mid X_1 = x_1)\, P(X_1 = x_1)}{P(X_2 = x_2)} \qquad (A.9)$$

(assuming that $P(X_2 = x_2)$ and $P(X_1 = x_1)$ are both positive), called the *Bayes theorem*. Further, the denominator in (A.9) can be expressed as

$$P(X_2 = x_2) = \sum_x P(X_2 = x_2 \mid X_1 = x)\, P(X_1 = x),$$

where the summation is over the (finite) support of X_1.

Let $p_{kh} = P(X_1 = k \text{ and } X_2 = h)$, $k = 1, \ldots, K$ and $h = 1, \ldots, H$, be the two-way table of the joint probabilities (rows k and columns h) associated with discrete variables X_1 and X_2. Then the conditional distribution of X_1 given $X_2 = h$ is derived by standardising column h of the table, that is, dividing its entries by the column total (so that they add up to unity):

$$P(X_1 = k \mid X_2 = h) = \frac{p_{kh}}{p_{1h} + p_{2h} + \cdots + p_{Kh}}.$$

It is useful to introduce the notation p_{k+} and p_{+h} for the marginal probabilities, as they are derived by summing up over the index that is replaced by the summation sign '+'. The conditional distribution of X_2 given $X_1 = k$ is derived by interchanging the roles of the rows and columns:

$$P(X_2 = h \mid X_1 = k) = \frac{p_{kh}}{p_{k+}}.$$

Of course, we assume that none of the margins (row or column totals) vanish; otherwise the row or the column concerned could be deleted.

Variables X_1 and X_2 are independent when none of the conditional probabilities $P(X_1 = k \mid X_2 = h)$ depend on the condition and all are equal to $P(X_1 = k)$. This follows immediately from the definition of independence. When the conditional probabilities $P(X_1 = k \mid X_2 = h)$ do not depend on h for any h in the support of X_2, the conditional probabilities $P(X_2 = h \mid X_1 = k)$ do not depend on the condition either. Independence is a symmetric property, but conditional probabilities are not symmetric.

A.15 Bivariate Continuous Distributions

Most of the definitions and theory of bivariate discrete distributions carry directly over to bivariate continuous distributions, with the various probabilities replaced by densities. A pair of continuous random variables X_1 and X_2 is said to have a continuous joint distribution when the limit

$$\lim_{\delta \to 0+} \frac{P(|X_1 - x_1| < \delta \text{ and } |X_2 - x_2| < \delta)}{\delta^2} \tag{A.10}$$

exists for every x_1 and x_2 in the respective supports of X_1 and X_2. The limit is called their *joint density* and is denoted by $f(x_1, x_2)$. When any ambiguity might arise, we indicate the variables as subscripts of the density function, such as f_{X_1, X_2} for the density of (X_1, X_2).

Even though every (univariate) continuous distribution has a density, not every pair of continuous distributions has a (bivariate) joint density. As an example, suppose X_1 has the standard uniform distribution and let $X_2 = 1 - X_1$. It is easy to show that the limit in (A.10) is either equal to zero (when $x_1 + x_2 \neq 1$) or diverges to $+\infty$. Therefore the joint distribution of the pair (X_1, X_2) is not continuous.

Two continuous distributions are independent when they have a joint density $f(x_1, x_2)$ and it is equal to the product of the (marginal) densities of the (univariate) component variables: $f(x_1, x_2) = f_{X_1}(x_1) f_{X_2}(x_2)$. This definition is equivalent to the natural definition of independence, requiring that

$$P(X_1 \in U_1 \text{ and } X_2 \in U_2) = P(X_1 \in U_1)\, P(X_2 \in U_2)$$

for any pair of intervals U_1 and U_2.

The marginal densities are obtained from the joint density of a pair of variables by integration:

$$f_{X_1}(x_1) = \int_{-\infty}^{+\infty} f(x_1, x)\, dx$$

and similarly for X_2.

The conditional density of X_1, given a value of X_2, is defined as

$$f_{X_1}(x_1 \mid X_2 = x_2) = \frac{f(x_1, x_2)}{f_{X_2}(x_2)},$$

so long as the denominator is positive. In parallel with conditional probabilities, in general, $f_{X_1}(x_1 \mid X_2 = x_2) \neq f_{X_2}(x_2 \mid X_1 = x_1)$. The two sets of conditional distributions are connected by the Bayes theorem for conditional densities,

$$f_{X_1}(x_1 \mid X_2 = x_2) = \frac{f_{X_2}(x_2 \mid X_1 = x_1)\, f_{X_1}(x_1)}{f_{X_2}(x_2)},$$

and $f_{X_2}(x_2) = \int f_{X_2}(x_2 \mid X_1 = x)\, f_{X_1}(x)\, dx$; compare with (A.9).

Two continuous random variables are independent when the conditional distribution of one, given a value of the other, does not depend on the value, that is, when $f_{X_1}(x_1 \mid X_2 = x_2) = f_{X_1}(x_1)$ for all x_1 and x_2 in the respective supports of X_1 and X_2.

A bivariate distribution is defined for *any* two random variables, and these may be of different types, such as one continuous and one discrete. A practical way of defining their joint distribution is by the set of (continuous) conditional distributions $f_{X_1}(x_1 \mid X_2 = x_2)$ given category x_2 of the discrete variable X_2. The marginal density of X_1 is

$$f_{X_1}(x_1) = \sum_x f_{X_1}(x_1 \mid X_2 = x)\, P(X_2 = x),$$

where the summation is over the (discrete) support of X_2. The distribution of X_1 is called a *discrete mixture* (of the conditional distributions given the categories of X_2). When X_2 is supported by a finite set of values, the mixture is said to be finite. A natural mechanism (process) for generating a draw from such a distribution is by drawing first a value of X_2, which determines the distribution from which X_1 is to be drawn next. A finite mixture of variables can be expressed as

$$X = I_1 X_1 + I_2 X_2 + \cdots + I_K X_K,$$

where I_k is the *indicator* of category k: $I_k = 1$ if category k is realised and variable X_k used, so that $X = X_k$, and $I_k = 0$ otherwise. It is assumed that $I_1, \ldots, I_K$ are independent of all the *constituent* variables $X_1, \ldots, X_K$. However, they are correlated among themselves, as $I_1 + \cdots + I_K = 1$.

A.16 Operating with Bivariate Distributions

The expectations, medians, quantiles, variances, and the like, are defined for bivariate distributions componentwise, that is, separately for each variable (component), so they entail no new definitions. An important quantity that describes the association of two variables X_1 and X_2 is the *covariance*, denoted by $\mathrm{cov}(X_1, X_2)$. It is defined as

$$\mathrm{cov}(X_1, X_2) = \mathrm{E}\left[\{X_1 - \mathrm{E}(X_1)\}\{X_2 - \mathrm{E}(X_2)\}\right]$$

so long as all three expectations (including those of X_1 and X_2) are well defined. Simple operations yield the identity

$$\mathrm{cov}(X_1, X_2) = \mathrm{E}(X_1 X_2) - \mathrm{E}(X_1)\mathrm{E}(X_2), \qquad (A.11)$$

if the expectations are well defined. Variance is a special case of covariance—it is the covariance of a variable with itself: $\mathrm{var}(X) = \mathrm{cov}(X, X)$.

It is expedient to use a single symbol for the pair of variables; $\mathbf{X} = (X_1, X_2)^\top$, so that $\mathbf{X}$ is a 2×1 column vector. A clash with the notation introduced in the context of sample surveys in Section A.3 is unavoidable. Later we will use boldface symbols for vectors of arbitrary (unspecified) finite length. We write $E(\mathbf{X}) = \{E(X_1), E(X_2)\}^\top$, and define the variance matrix $\mathrm{var}(\mathbf{X})$ as the matrix

$$\mathrm{var}(\mathbf{X}) = \begin{pmatrix} \mathrm{var}(X_1) & \mathrm{cov}(X_1, X_2) \\ \mathrm{cov}(X_1, X_2) & \mathrm{var}(X_2) \end{pmatrix}.$$

For an arbitrary 2×1 vector $\mathbf{a}$, $E(\mathbf{a}^\top \mathbf{X}) = \mathbf{a}^\top E(\mathbf{X})$ and $\mathrm{var}(\mathbf{a}^\top \mathbf{X}) = \mathbf{a}^\top \mathrm{var}(\mathbf{X})\mathbf{a}$, so long as each element of $E(\mathbf{X})$ and $\mathrm{var}(\mathbf{X})$ is well defined. The latter identity implies that $\mathrm{var}(\mathbf{X})$ is a nonnegative definite matrix, and hence

$$\{\mathrm{cov}(X_1, X_2)\}^2 \le \mathrm{var}(X_1)\,\mathrm{var}(X_2), \tag{A.12}$$

with equality only when X_1 and X_2 are linearly dependent (and when $\mathbf{a}^\top \mathbf{X}$ is equal to a constant for a nonzero vector $\mathbf{a}$).

The *correlation* of two variables X_1 and X_2 that have well-defined (finite) positive variances is defined as

$$\mathrm{cor}(X_1, X_2) = \frac{\mathrm{cov}(X_1, X_2)}{\sqrt{\mathrm{var}(X_1)}\,\sqrt{\mathrm{var}(X_2)}}.$$

The inequality in (A.12) implies that $-1 \le \mathrm{cor}(X_1, X_2) \le 1$. Further, $\mathrm{cor}(X_1, X_2) = \pm 1$ only when X_1 and X_2 are linearly dependent. In such a case, X_1 and X_2 are said to be *perfectly correlated*; $\mathrm{cor}(X_1, X_2) = 1$ when $X_1 - cX_2$ is constant for a positive constant c, and $\mathrm{cor}(X_1, X_2) = -1$ when $X_1 - cX_2$ is constant for a negative constant c.

Variables X_1 and X_2 are said to be uncorrelated when $\mathrm{cov}(X_1, X_2) = 0$. When X_1 and X_2 are independent they are also uncorrelated. To prove this, we evaluate first $E(X_1 X_2)$. The distribution of the product $Y = X_1 X_2$ is in general given by the density

$$f_Y(y) = \int f_{X_1}\left(\frac{y}{x_2}\,\middle|\, X_2 = x_2\right) f_{X_2}(x_2)\,\mathrm{d}x_2,$$

obtained by conditioning on X_2. Hence, discarding the condition (owing to independence),

$$E(X_1 X_2) = \int y \int f_{X_1}\left(\frac{y}{x_2}\right) f_{X_2}(x_2)\,\mathrm{d}x_2\,\mathrm{d}y,$$

and the change of variables $x_1 = y/x_2$ yields the identity

$$E(X_1 X_2) = \int x_1 f(x_1)\,\mathrm{d}x_1 \int x_2 f(x_2)\,\mathrm{d}x_2,$$

that is, $E(X_1)\,E(X_2)$. Now, $\mathrm{cov}(X_1, X_2) = 0$, according to (A.11), and so also $\mathrm{cor}(X_1, X_2) = 0$. The proof carries over to discrete variables, by replacing each integral with the corresponding summation.

Table A.5. Example of a pair of variables that are uncorrelated but dependent.

X_2	-2	-1	1	2
		X_1		
1	0	$\frac{1}{4}$	$\frac{1}{4}$	0
2	$\frac{1}{4}$	0	0	$\frac{1}{4}$

Note however, that absence of correlation does not imply independence. The following is a simple example of two dependent uncorrelated discrete variables. Variable X_1 is uniformly distributed on $(-2, -1, 1, 2)$, that is, each value in its support has probability $\frac{1}{4}$. Variable X_2 is equal to the absolute value of X_1, so it is uniformly distributed on $(1, 2)$; see Table A.5. The two variables are dependent because $P(X_1 = 1 \text{ and } X_2 = 2) = 0$ whereas $P(X_1 = 1) = \frac{1}{4}$ and $P(X_2 = 2) = \frac{1}{2}$, yet they are uncorrelated because $E(X_1 X_2) = E(X_1) = 0$.

Independence is maintained by transformations. If X_1 and X_2 are independent variables, then so are their transformations $g_1(X_1)$ and $g_2(X_2)$. Of course, the transformed variables $g_1(X_1)$ and $g_2(X_2)$ may be independent when the original variables X_1 and X_2 are not. Further, if X_1 and X_2 are both independent of X_3, then any function of X_1 and X_2 is also independent of X_3.

The covariance has the following 'quadratic' property. If $\text{cov}(X_1, X_2)$ is well defined for a pair of variables X_1 and X_2, then

$$\text{cov}(a_1 X_1 + c_1, a_2 X_2 + c_2) = a_1 a_2 \, \text{cov}(X_1, X_2)$$

for arbitrary constants a_1, a_2, c_1, and c_2. Hence

$$\text{cor}(a_1 X_1 + c_1, a_2 X_2 + c_2) = \text{sign}(a_1 a_2) \, \text{cor}(X_1, X_2),$$

where sign is the function equal to $+1$ for positive, -1 for negative arguments, and $\text{sign}(0) = 0$; the absolute value of the correlation is unaffected by (nontrivial) linear transformations. Recall that $\text{var}(aX + b) = a^2 \text{var}(X)$, since standard deviation is a dispersion quantity.

For any two variables with finite variances,

$$\text{var}(X_1 + X_2) = \text{var}(X_1) + \text{var}(X_2) + 2\text{cov}(X_1, X_2);$$

the covariance is well defined, so long as any two variances in this expression are. For independent variables X_1 and X_2

$$\text{var}(X_1 + X_2) = \text{var}(X_1) + \text{var}(X_2). \tag{A.13}$$

This is a key identity for working with random samples, sequences of independent and identically distributed random variables.

For expectations, we have an identity similar to (A.13), except that it holds even when X_1 and X_2 are correlated;

$$E(X_1 + X_2) = E(X_1) + E(X_2),\qquad\qquad (A.14)$$

so long as two of the expectations are well defined. This result is derived similarly to its counterpart for the product of two independent variables:

$$E(X_1 + X_2) = \int \int y f_{X_1}(y - x_2 \mid X_2 = x_2)\, f_{X_2}(x_2)\, dx_2\, dy$$
$$= \int x f_{X_1}(x)\, dx + \int x_2 f_{X_2}(x_2)\, dx_2$$
$$= E(X_1) + E(X_2),$$

after the change of variables $x = y - x_2$.

A.17 Random Samples

A single observation of a process, yielding a random draw from a distribution, is rarely of much use because it conveys little information. Much more commonly we work with a sequence of independent realisations of the studied process and the resulting random sample from a distribution. This section summarises the properties of random samples.

Suppose $X_1, X_2, \ldots, X_n$ is a random sample from a distribution with finite mean μ and finite variance σ^2. Then the mean of the sample, $\bar{X} = (X_1 + \cdots + X_n)/n$ has the expectation μ and variance σ^2/n. This result, derived from (A.14), supports the estimation of the (finite) expectation of a distribution. It can be rephrased as follows: if the population mean μ is finite, then the sample mean of a random sample is an unbiased estimator of μ and, if the population variance is finite, its sampling variance converges to zero as the sample size increases above all bounds. That is, greater sample size is rewarded by greater precision, confirming the intuition that more data amounts to more information and yields better inference (about μ).

The sample mean is unbiased for the population mean even when the observations are correlated. However, independence is essential for the result about the variance, $\mathrm{var}(\bar{X}) = \sigma^2/n$. In fact, absence of any correlation among X_j would suffice, but the additional generality is of little practical importance. When any pair of observations X_j have the same positive correlation ρ, then

$$\mathrm{var}(\bar{X}) = \frac{\sigma^2}{n}\left(1 + \frac{n-1}{n}\rho\right),$$

so inferences are profoundly handicapped vis-à-vis independent observations with the same sample size.

It might seem that the variance σ^2 would also be estimated without bias naively, as

$$\hat{\sigma}_{\dagger}^2 = \frac{1}{n}\sum_{j=1}^{n}\left(X_j - \bar{X}\right)^2 .$$

That is not the case;

$$\mathrm{E}\left(\hat{\sigma}_{\dagger}^2\right) = \frac{1}{n}\sum_{j=1}^{n}\mathrm{E}\left\{(X_j - \mu)^2\right\} - \mathrm{E}\left\{(\bar{X} - \mu)^2\right\}$$

$$= \sigma^2 - \mathrm{var}\left(\bar{X}\right) = \frac{n-1}{n}\sigma^2 ,$$

and so

$$\hat{\sigma}^2 = \frac{1}{n-1}\sum_{j=1}^{n}\left(X_j - \bar{X}\right)^2$$

is unbiased for σ^2. The unity subtracted from the divisor for $\hat{\sigma}^2$ is interpreted as a *degree of freedom* lost due to estimating a parameter, in this case μ. Indeed, if μ were known, the estimator

$$\hat{\sigma}^2 = \frac{1}{n}\sum_{j=1}^{n}(X_j - \mu)^2$$

would be unbiased.

In many settings, the sample mean $\bar{X}$ is efficient, or nearly so, but that is not always the case. For example, for a uniform distribution $\mathcal{U}(\theta_1 , \theta_2)$, the sample mean is a very inefficient estimator of the population mean $\frac{1}{2}(\theta_1 + \theta_2)$; the average of the extremes, $\frac{1}{2}(\max x_j + \min x_j)$, is much more efficient. In contrast, the sample mean of a normally distributed random sample is efficient for the population mean, and the average of its extremes is very inefficient.

A.18 Regression

Regression of one variable, Y, on another, X, is the term used for the conditional expectation of Y given a value of X, $\mathrm{E}(Y \mid X = x)$, treated as a function of the value x. It provides a description, alternative or additional to covariance and correlation, for the association of the two variables. For example, when X and Y are independent, $\mathrm{E}(Y \mid X = x) = \mathrm{E}(Y)$, and regression of Y on X is constant. The conditional variance $\mathrm{var}(Y \mid X = x)$, as a function of x, is called the *residual variance*.

The regression can be interpreted as the contribution made by X to the information about Y. When we know the distribution of Y but we do not observe Y, its expectation $\mathrm{E}(Y)$ is a reasonable estimate (prediction) of the value of Y that would or might be observed in the future, especially when the distribution of Y is symmetric. By definition, $E(Y)$ is unbiased for the realisation of Y, and its variance is $\text{var}(Y)$. If we know the value of X that accompanies Y, we should be able to predict the value of Y more efficiently (with smaller MSE)—the additional information, in the form of the value of X, should not be detrimental to our efforts at predicting the value of Y. The logic of this statement does not hold up all the time, certainly not when the expectation or the variance of Y is not defined, but a weaker result is obtained from the identity

$$\text{var}(Y) = E_X \{\text{var}(Y \mid X = x)\} + \text{var}_X \{E(Y \mid X = x)\} ,$$

in which the 'outer' expectation and variance, with the subscript X, are over the distribution of X, that is, over all possible conditions $X = x$. This identity implies that $\text{var}(Y) \geq E_X \{\text{var}(Y \mid X = x)\}$, and equality occurs only when the regression $E(Y \mid X = x)$ is constant, that is, when X and Y are uncorrelated. Therefore, by using the regression X helps us in predicting Y *on average*.

A.19 Multivariate Distributions

For a vector of more than two variables, some but not all of the definitions for bivariate distributions are extended straightforwardly. Let $\mathbf{X} = (X_1, \ldots, X_K)^\top$ be a vector of K variables. Its expectation is defined componentwise,

$$E(\mathbf{X}) = \{E(X_1), \ldots, E(X_K)\}^\top ,$$

and its variance matrix is defined as the matrix of the variances and covariances of its components,

$$\text{var}(\mathbf{X}) = \begin{pmatrix} \text{var}(X_1) & \text{cov}(X_1, X_2) & \cdots & \text{cov}(X_1, X_K) \\ \text{cov}(X_2, X_1) & \text{var}(X_2) & \cdots & \text{cov}(X_2, X_K) \\ \vdots & \vdots & \ddots & \vdots \\ \text{cov}(X_K, X_1) & \text{cov}(X_K, X_2) & \cdots & \text{var}(X_K) \end{pmatrix} .$$

Commonly, the following notation is used: $\boldsymbol{\Sigma} = \text{var}(\mathbf{X})$, with diagonal elements $\sigma_k^2 = \text{var}(X_k)$, and $\sigma_{kh} = \text{cov}(X_k, X_h)$, with the convention that $\sigma_{kk} = \sigma_k^2$.

The correlation matrix of $\mathbf{X}$ is defined as the matrix of the pairwise correlations $\text{cor}(X_k, X_h)$, with unities on the diagonal. Let $\boldsymbol{\sigma} = \text{diag}_{(k)}(\sigma_k)$ be the diagonal matrix with the standard deviations of $\mathbf{X}$ on its diagonal; then $\text{cor}(\mathbf{X}) = \boldsymbol{\sigma}^{-1}\boldsymbol{\Sigma}\boldsymbol{\sigma}^{-1}$. The variables in $\mathbf{X}$ are said to be uncorrelated if they are pairwise uncorrelated, so that the correlation and variance matrices of $\mathbf{X}$ are diagonal. Recall that the correlation of two variables is not defined if one of them has zero variance or its variance is not defined.

The variables in $\mathbf{X}$ are said to be *mutually independent* if each variable X_k is independent of any transformation $g\left(\mathbf{X}_{-k}\right)$ that involves the variables in $\mathbf{X}$ except for X_k. Mutual independence is a stricter condition than pairwise independence.

A multivariate distribution, say of a vector $\mathbf{X}$, has univariate marginals, the distributions of X_1, X_2, ..., X_K, bivariate marginals, the joint distributions of any pair of components X_k and X_h of $\mathbf{X}$ ($k \neq h$), and so on, $(K-1)$-variate marginals, the distributions of $\mathbf{X}_{-k}$, $k = 1, \ldots, K$, obtained by dropping one of the components of $\mathbf{X}$.

A.19.1 Multivariate Normal Distributions

A random vector $\mathbf{X}$ is said to have multivariate normal distribution if any linear combination of its components, $\mathbf{a}^\top \mathbf{X}$, has a univariate normal distribution. This definition may appear a bit awkward, but a vector comprising normally distributed variables as its components may not satisfy this definition, and it is desirable to exclude such (joint) distributions. The joint density of the multivariate normal distribution is

$$ f(\mathbf{x}) = \frac{1}{\left(\sqrt{2\pi}\right)^K} \det(\mathbf{\Sigma})^{-\frac{1}{2}} \exp\left\{ -\frac{1}{2}(\mathbf{x} - \boldsymbol{\mu})^\top \mathbf{\Sigma}^{-1}(\mathbf{x} - \boldsymbol{\mu}) \right\}, $$

where $\boldsymbol{\mu}$ and $\mathbf{\Sigma}$ are a vector of length K and a $K \times K$ symmetric positive definite matrix, respectively. It turns out that $\mathrm{E}(\mathbf{X}) = \boldsymbol{\mu}$ and $\mathrm{var}(\mathbf{X}) = \mathbf{\Sigma}$; this can be verified directly by integration. We denote a K-variate normal distribution by $\mathcal{N}_K(\boldsymbol{\mu}, \mathbf{\Sigma})$; the subscript K will be dropped whenever the dimension K is immaterial or is obvious from the context (e.g., when the length of $\boldsymbol{\mu}$ is specified).

Any marginal distribution of $\mathcal{N}(\boldsymbol{\mu}, \mathbf{\Sigma})$ is also (multi- or univariate) normal with its mean vector and variance matrix obtained as the corresponding subvector of $\boldsymbol{\mu}$ and submatrix of $\mathbf{\Sigma}$. The proof of this is immediate from the definition of $\mathcal{N}(\boldsymbol{\mu}; \mathbf{\Sigma})$, since any linear combination of a subvector is also a linear combination of the original vector. More generally, let $\mathbf{A}$ be a $H \times K$ matrix of constants of full rank H ($H \leq K$). Then $\mathbf{X} \sim \mathcal{N}(\boldsymbol{\mu}, \mathbf{\Sigma})$ implies that $\mathbf{AX} \sim \mathcal{N}\left(\mathbf{A}\boldsymbol{\mu}, \mathbf{A}\mathbf{\Sigma}\mathbf{A}^\top\right)$. For a choice of $\mathbf{A}$ such that $\mathbf{A}\mathbf{A}^\top = \mathbf{\Sigma}^{-1}$, $\mathbf{A}(\mathbf{X} - \boldsymbol{\mu}) \sim \mathcal{N}(\mathbf{0}, \mathbf{I})$, where $\mathbf{0}$ is the vector of zeros (of length K) and $\mathbf{I}$ the $K \times K$ identity matrix. A vector with the distribution $\mathcal{N}_K(\mathbf{0}, \mathbf{I})$ can be constructed from K independent standard normal variates, variables distributed identically according to $\mathcal{N}(0, 1)$.

The class of multivariate normal distributions is complete in the sense that a distribution can be constructed for any vector of means $\boldsymbol{\mu}$ and any positive definite matrix $\mathbf{\Sigma}$ of compatible dimensions. The class of multivariate normal distributions can be extended by attaching to a vector $\mathbf{X} \sim \mathcal{N}(\boldsymbol{\mu}, \mathbf{\Sigma})$ linear combinations of the components of $\mathbf{X}$, and permuting the resulting vector. The variance matrix of this vector is not positive definite, but it has no negative eigenvalues—it is nonnegative definite.

The class of multivariate log-normal distributions is formed by component-wise log-transformations of vectors with multivariate normal distributions. Other classes of distributions, with prescribed univariate marginals can be formed by componentwise transformations, using the standardized uniform distribution as a pivot.

A.19.2 Regression with Normally Distributed Variables

A common task in statistics is concerned with the (joint) distribution of a vector or variable constructed by mathematical operations. In most cases, the solution involves expressions that are not analytic and can at best be evaluated only approximately. Some exceptions from this 'rule' involve the class of normal distributions.

Suppose (X, Y) have bivariate normal distribution with the vector of expectations (μ_X, μ_Y), variances σ_X^2 and σ_Y^2 and covariance σ_{XY}. We derive the regression of Y on X. First, we require the conditional distribution of Y given X, which we denote by $(Y \mid X)$. Its density is given by the ratio $f(x, y)/f_X(x)$, and this is equal to

$$\frac{\sigma_X}{\sqrt{2\pi \det(\Sigma)}} \exp\left\{-\frac{1}{2}\begin{pmatrix} x - \mu_X \\ y - \mu_Y \end{pmatrix}^\top \Sigma^{-1} \begin{pmatrix} x - \mu_X \\ y - \mu_Y \end{pmatrix} + \frac{(x - \mu_X)^2}{2\sigma_X^2}\right\},$$

where Σ is the variance matrix of (X, Y). Its inverse is

$$\Sigma^{-1} = \frac{1}{\sigma_X^2 \sigma_Y^2 - \sigma_{XY}^2} \begin{pmatrix} \sigma_Y^2 & -\sigma_{XY} \\ -\sigma_{XY} & \sigma_Y^2 \end{pmatrix}.$$

Hence, after simplifying the argument of the exponential, we obtain

$$(Y \mid X = x) \sim \mathcal{N}\left\{\mu_Y + \frac{\sigma_{XY}}{\sigma_X^2}(x - \mu_X), \sigma_Y^2 - \frac{\sigma_{XY}^2}{\sigma_X^2}\right\}.$$

Several aspects of this result are remarkable. First, the normal distribution is 'closed' with respect to conditioning; if (X, Y) is (bivariate) normally distributed, then $(Y \mid X = x)$ is also normally distributed. Next, the regression of Y on X is linear, with slope equal to σ_{XY}/σ_X^2. And finally, the residual variance is constant, not depending on the value of X in the condition. The ratio σ_{XY}^2/σ_X^2 is the reduction of the variance due to knowing the value of X. The squared correlation

$$\rho^2 = \frac{\sigma_{XY}^2}{\sigma_X^2 \sigma_Y^2}, \tag{A.15}$$

is the fraction of the variance of Y by which the variance of the prediction of the value of Y is reduced when we know the value of X. Prediction with smaller MSE and, when the prediction is unbiased, with smaller variance is preferred, so variables X for which ρ^2 is high are particularly valuable,

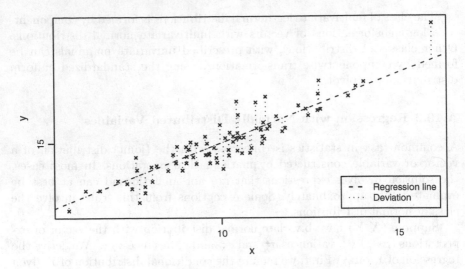

Fig. A.8. Example of ordinary regression.

especially when their observation is easy and inexpensive. When X and Y are strongly associated and observing X is much cheaper than observing Y, we may observe only X and pay a small 'penalty' of uncertainty due to the positive residual variance.

The regression of Y on X can be obtained also as the linear transformation $a + bX$ that differs from Y least, that is, by minimising $E\left\{(Y - a - bX)^2\right\}$. This expectation is equal to

$$\text{var}(Y - bX) + \{E(Y - a - bX)\}^2 = \sigma_Y^2 - 2b\sigma_{XY} + b^2\sigma_X^2 + (\mu_Y - a - b\mu_X)^2,$$

a quadratic function of a and b. Its minimum is attained when $a = \mu_Y + b\mu_X$ and $b\sigma_X^2 - \sigma_{XY} = 0$. Hence $b = \sigma_{XY}/\sigma_X^2$.

A geometric interpretation of regression of Y on X is that in the plot of the values of X against Y, the points are scattered around the straight (regression) line with intercept $a = \mu_Y + b\mu_X$ and slope σ_{XY}/σ_X^2; hence the terms *regression slope* for $b = \sigma_{XY}/\sigma_X^2$ and regression line for $a + bx$. The dispersion of the points around the regression line, measured vertically, is equal to the residual variance. See Figure A.8 for an illustration.

A.20 Formulating Inferences

The starting point of a statistical analysis is to specify the target—the population quantity that we would like, in ideal circumstances, to determine. This goal is reduced to estimation, based on the values of the key (and maybe some other) variables on a sample of subjects. The outcome of the analysis is an estimate of the target. It is an established practice in statistics to indicate the precision of the estimator that was applied, to inform how much faith can be placed in the estimate. The MSE is commonly adopted as a measure of the precision. It is equal to the sampling variance when the estimator is unbiased. Usually the MSE cannot be determined and has to be estimated. Thus, the estimation task comprises two parts:

- estimation of the target θ, by evaluating an estimator $\hat{\theta}$;
- estimation of $\mathrm{MSE}(\hat{\theta}; \theta)$, by evaluating an estimator $\widehat{\mathrm{MSE}}\left(\hat{\theta}; \theta\right)$.

Since efficient estimation is valued, the analyst's reward should be inversely proportional to $\mathrm{MSE}(\hat{\theta}; \theta)$ and the analyst has an obvious incentive to present the estimate in as good a light as possible. One unfair means of doing this is by estimating $\mathrm{MSE}(\hat{\theta}; \theta)$ with a negative bias (underestimating the MSE). In contrast, overestimating the MSE is comparable to underselling the product of the analyst's effort—understating the quality of the analysis.

Commonly, the term *estimation* is used for generating a statement of the form $\{\hat{\theta}, \widehat{\mathrm{MSE}}(\hat{\theta}; \theta)\}$ for a target θ. We say that such an estimation is *dishonest* if the MSE is underestimated. Note that underestimation does not mean that $\widehat{\mathrm{MSE}}(\hat{\theta}; \theta) < \mathrm{MSE}(\hat{\theta}; \theta)$, because the realised value of $\widehat{\mathrm{MSE}}$ may exceed the MSE even when it does not do so in expectation (on average in replications). A more appropriate, although rather cumbersome, term for underestimation might be 'dishonest in the long run', standing for $\mathrm{E}\{\widehat{\mathrm{MSE}}(\hat{\theta}; \theta)\} \leq \mathrm{MSE}(\hat{\theta}; \theta)$.

A.20.1 Confidence Intervals

The 'honestly' estimated root-MSE indicates how far we can expect the estimate to be from the target on average, if we replicated the sampling and estimation processes many times. An alternative formulation of the inference is by a *confidence interval*. The confidence interval is defined as an interval $(C_\mathrm{L}, C_\mathrm{H})$ delimited by sample quantities C_L and C_H that satisfy the inequality

$$P(C_\mathrm{L} < \theta \text{ and } C_\mathrm{H} > \theta) \geq \alpha, \tag{A.16}$$

where α, called the *level of confidence*, is a prescribed (a priori set) value in the range $(0, 1)$. Practical choices for α are values close to unity, so that the interval with the data-dependent (random) bounds C_L and C_H is very likely to contain the target, an unknown constant. As a convention, $\alpha = 0.95$ and $\alpha = 0.99$ are often used, allowing an error rate (probability of not covering the target by the confidence interval) of not more than 5% and 1%, respectively. We may set out to obtain a confidence interval with a particular level of confidence, but as a result of errors, incorrect assumptions, or approximations, we end up with a level of confidence that does not satisfy the condition in (A.16). The probability on the left-hand side of (A.16) is called the *coverage rate*. It may depend on some parameters, even on the target itself.

In analogy with honest estimation, we say that a confidence interval is honest if condition (A.16) is satisfied; that is, if the coverage rate does not fall short of the (intended) level of confidence. For the confidence intervals for a specified target and level of confidence, we can define a partial ordering. Confidence interval A is said to be narrower than confidence interval B, if A is a subset of B. Note that both A and B are data-dependent, so the lengths of A and B, as random variables, may overlap even when A is narrower than B.

For a given target and confidence level, there may be several alternative confidence intervals. We should discard all dishonest intervals and compare the honest ones by their length or expected length. Shorter (narrower) confidence intervals are preferred because they narrow down the range of plausible values of the target. Suppose confidence interval A has coverage rate 95%, equal to the level of confidence, and has constant length 2.7. Suppose another confidence interval, B, has coverage rate 96.5% and length constant 2.5. Confidence interval B is preferred because it is shorter. The fact that it could, in principle, be improved by reducing it so that its coverage rate would match the level of confidence is beside the point; there may be a confidence interval better than B, but it is not A. The length of a confidence interval is a sample quantity, so it may be random. This makes the comparison of confidence intervals more difficult than this example may suggest. Comparison of the realisations of the two confidence intervals is not sufficient, although it may happen that one confidence interval is longer than another for every replication (with probability equal to one).

In some settings, only confidence intervals of the form $(-\infty, C_H)$ are of interest. Such intervals, as well as intervals of the form $(C_L, +\infty)$ are called *one-sided*. We can adopt any function of the pair (C_L, C_H) as the criterion for what we regard an optimal confidence interval among the intervals with the prescribed level of confidence. However, only three criteria are of any practical relevance: minimum width of the interval, preferring intervals that are symmetric around the estimate ($C_L = \hat{\theta} - \xi$ and $C_C = \hat{\theta} + \xi$ for a suitably defined sample quantity ξ), and using only one-sided intervals (either $C_L = -\infty$ and preferring small C_H or $C_H = +\infty$ and preferring large C_L). And finally, instead of confidence intervals, we may consider confidence *regions*, which may be any subsets of real numbers. We need to do this very rarely, most often to consider a pair of intervals symmetric around zero, such as $(-a, -b) \cup (a, b)$ for some positive numbers $a < b$, when (a^2, b^2) would be a confidence interval for the square of the parameter.

A confidence interval (or region) is interpreted as *a* range of plausible values of a parameter. Naturally, it is often corrupted to *the* range of possible values. We should bear in mind that the confidence limits are sample quantities and a 'surprise', in the form of $\theta \notin (C_L, C_H)$, has a positive probability. When several confidence intervals are considered, the probability of such a surprise in connection with at least one of the intervals may be much greater than the error rate associated with a single interval.

Problems and Exercises

A.1. Formulate for your country the current definitions of

(a) the citizen;
(b) the resident.

Consult the appropriate sources for the legal definitions. Discuss elements or clauses in these definitions that might be ambiguous or contentious.

A.2. Describe the population of all applications to study at a university in your country in a recent year. Relate it to the population of all applicants in the year, to all functioning universities and their departments, and to the population of all eligible persons. Define some variables and structures (divisions into clusters) for these populations. Describe the variables by type and specify their supports.

A.3. On the web site of a national statistical institute, such as the Office for National Statistics (ONS, www.ons.gov.uk) or the Catalan Statistical Institute (IDESCAT, www.idescat.es), find summaries of basic socio-demographic and economic indicators for a recent year and determine which of them were established by enumeration and which by a survey. Identify some consumers of such information and how they would draw benefit from them. For any sample quantity you come across, identify its target and look for any information about its precision. Are these sample quantities estimates or estimators? What about their precision?

A.4. In the training of assessors (graders) of essays in a particular academic subject, the trainees are presented essays as typical examples that should be marked with a particular score. The trainees are not informed about these scores. In one such exercise, copies of an essay that is supposed to be marked 75 are distributed and the twelve trainees mark it, without conferring, as 72, 70, 83, 79, 76, 76, 75, 69, 73, 80, 70, and 75. In another scheme, the trainees discuss an essay that is supposed to be marked 62 and collectively come to the conclusion that it should be marked 65. In a third scheme, the trainees are presented an essay that is supposed to be marked 95, are informed about this score, and are asked to agree or raise objections to the score. Discuss the merits and drawbacks of each scheme for essay marking and for assessment of the accuracy of the marking in the case when each essay is marked only by one person assigned at random from the pool of qualified assessors.

A.5. In a particular context, the sampling variance of an estimator is 2.6 and its bias for a given target θ is 1.2. An alternative estimator of the same target θ is unbiased, with the sampling variance 3.5. Which estimator of θ is more efficient? Could your choice, when applied to a dataset, be more distant from the target than the other estimate?

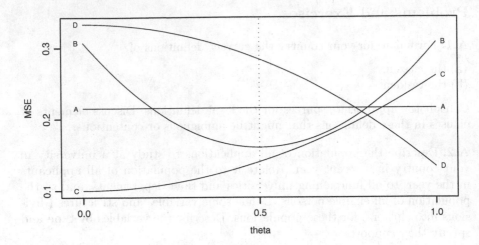

Fig. A.9. Plot of the MSEs of four estimators of θ as functions of θ. For Exercise A.9.

A.6. In a population of households in a region, the percentage of those with per capita income below a certain level is of interest. A simple random sample of households is selected and their size (number of members of the household) and income in the last year, rounded to hundreds of $US, are established. Define the naive estimator of the sought percentage. Consider how different it would be if the income were established with greater or smaller precision.

A.7. Derive the identity in (A.1)

(a) from the definitions of expectation and variance;
(b) from the definition of replications.

Suppose the square root of the MSE (root-MSE) is equal to the bias. What can be said about the sampling variance?

A.8. Calculate the mean and variance of the variable defined on a population of 22 members by their values:

$$3, 7, 11, 11, 13, \ 4, 7, 8, 11, 12, \ 2, 7, 9, 15, 18, \ 6, 6, 9, 12, 12, \ 10, 15 \,.$$

Find the interquantile range of this variable. Present these values in a way that is more informative about the distribution of the variable.

A.9. Figure A.9 is a plot of the MSEs of four estimators of the same target θ as functions of the parameter θ in the interval $(0, 1)$. Is any of the estimators uniformly more efficient than one of the others? Describe the strengths and weaknesses of the four estimators. Suppose we can reduce our attention to θ in the interval $\left(0, \frac{1}{2}\right)$. Would your answer be different?

A.10. Which of the following summaries of a variable X are location quantities?

median; $\max_i X_i$; the standard deviation of X; the value for member 1, X_1; the interquantile range; sum of squares of the values of X; the number of positive values of X; the distribution of X.

Which are dispersion quantities?

A.11. What is the mode of a distribution with support on the digits $0, 1, \ldots, 9$, if the value 0 is attained for more than 60% of the population? Is there a distribution with the same support that has mode at 5 and the frequency of this value is 15%? Give an example of a symmetric trimodal distribution with this support.

A.12. Construct a without-replacement sampling design that is different from the simple random sampling design and in which every member has the same probability of being included in the sample. On a population of small size, say, $N = 4$, construct a sampling design in which each pair has the same probability of being included in the sample but each member has a different probability.

A.13. Summarise the advantages of designs with stratification and clustering in a national survey of individuals or households. Find in the literature or on the Web an example of a national survey with a stratified clustered sampling design and discuss its details and what information about the design is not given.

A.14. A market research company engages interviewers who are assigned to be at particular locations in the centres of some cities and large shopping areas of the UK or United States at selected times of the day (lunchtime, the afternoon rush hour, Saturday morning, and the like). They collect responses to a questionnaire about a car brand from a given number (quota) of adult English-speaking passersby. Comment on the difficulties in making population inferences based on the collected data.

A.15. Construct a small population with the values of one variable and design a sampling scheme for this population. Replicate the sampling design in this population and record the values of an estimator based on the sample drawn. Compare the replicate values of the estimator with the target and estimate the bias and MSE of the estimator.

This exercise can be conducted on paper, with a device for random selection, e.g., based on a table of random numbers, but it is much more effective when executed on a computer using a more extensive population.

A.16. Generate at least 100 values of the discrete manifest variable Y for a latent variable X according to the matrix of probabilities $P(Y = k, X = h)$ for $k = 1, 2, 3, 4$ (rows) and $h = 1, 2, 3, 4$ (columns)

$$\begin{pmatrix} \frac{1}{10} & \frac{1}{25} & \frac{1}{100} & 0 \\ \frac{1}{20} & \frac{1}{5} & \frac{1}{20} & \frac{1}{100} \\ \frac{1}{100} & \frac{1}{10} & \frac{1}{5} & \frac{1}{20} \\ \frac{1}{50} & \frac{1}{50} & \frac{1}{25} & \frac{1}{10} \end{pmatrix}.$$

Find the marginal distributions of X and Y from this matrix and estimate the latter from the generated values of Y.

For each value $k = 1, 2, 3$, and 4 of X, find the bias, measurement variance, and MSE of the misclassification process given by this matrix. How can it be verified using computer-generated values of X and Y?

A.17. Relate what is commonly understood by the term 'impartial jury' in the criminal justice system, 'impartial assessment' in educational testing, and 'impartial referee' in a sport event to the definition of impartiality in Section A.6. How is impartiality related to the frequency of incorrect decisions in these examples?

A.18. Replicate the example in Figure A.5 and Table A.3 in your own computational environment with probabilities and numbers of replications of your choice.

A.19. Revise the rules for integration of continuous functions on finite intervals and how integration and differentiation are associated. When can the order of integration and differentiation be exchanged, that is,

$$\frac{\partial}{\partial x} \int_0^1 f(u, x)\, du = \int_0^1 \frac{\partial f(u, x)}{\partial x}\, du\,?$$

Under what conditions do we have the identity

$$\frac{\partial}{\partial x} \int_0^x f(u)\, du = f(x)$$

for a continuous function f?

A.20. Find the distribution function $F(x) = P(X < x)$ of a continuous variable with support on $(-1, 1)$ and density $f(x) = C(x+1)(x+2)$ for a suitable constant C. Sketch the density and describe the properties of this distribution. What is the probability of a positive value of X?

A.21. For a random sample from the uniform distribution on (θ_1, θ_2), consider the following estimators of the population mean:

(a) the sample mean;
(b) the sample median;
(c) the average of the first and third sample quartiles;
(d) the average of the maximum and minimum of the sample.

Compare these estimators by simulation. That is, set a sample size n (say, $n = 150$) and the limits $\theta_1 < \theta_2$, and replicate many (say, $K = 1000$) times the following steps:

(A) draw a random sample of size n from $\mathcal{U}(\theta_1, \theta_2)$;
(B) evaluate the estimators a,–d, on this sample.

Finally, calculate the empirical biases, variances, and MSEs of these estimators. Explain why the study can focus on the standard uniform distribution, setting $\theta_1 = 0$ and $\theta_2 = 1$, so that the target is $\frac{1}{2}$.

If you have difficulties with this question, repeat the study for several settings of θ_1 and θ_2 and compare the results. As an alternative, you could conduct the separate studies within a single simulation study by linearly transforming each sample from $\mathcal{U}(0, 1)$ to be a sample from $\mathcal{U}(\theta_1, \theta_2)$.

A.22. Repeat the study in the previous exercise, with the normal distribution in place of the uniform. Explain why this study can focus on the standard normal distribution.

A.23. For revision. How is the integral of a function over an infinite interval defined? Revise the calculus of infinite sequences and sums, in particular the principal results about their convergence.

Let $p_k = 1/k - 1/(k+1)$ for $k = 1, 2, \ldots$. Do these values define a distribution on the integers? If not, do Cp_k for a positive constant C?

A.24. Show that when the expectation of the square of a distribution, $\mathrm{E}\left(X^2\right)$, is well defined, then so is the expectation $\mathrm{E}(X)$. Find a distribution for which $\mathrm{E}(X)$ is well defined, but $\mathrm{var}(X)$ is not.
Hint: Consider the functions $f(x) = x^{-k}$ on $(0, 1)$ and $(1, +\infty)$ for $k > 0$.

A.25. Show that when a discrete distribution on the integers $0, 1, \ldots$ has an expectation, then the summation $\sum_{k=1}^{\infty} F_k$, where $F_k = p_0 + \cdots + p_k$, converges and its limit is equal to the expectation.

A.26. Generate the empirical distribution of the continuous uniform distribution on $(0, 1)$ and the negative logarithm, $-\log(X)$, of the values. Compare the latter with the empirical distribution of the exponential distribution with parameter $\theta = 1$.

A.27. Carry out a simulation study to compare estimators of your choice for the expectation of the distribution with density $f(x) = 2x$ for $x \in (0, 1)$. Include the trimmed mean among the estimators. The $p\%$-trimmed mean is defined as the mean of the subsample formed by discarding $\frac{1}{2}p\%$ of the smallest and $\frac{1}{2}p\%$ of the largest observations.

A.28. Derive $\mathrm{E}\left(X^k\right)$ for a centred normally distributed random variable X and integer k. Derive $\mathrm{var}\{(X - \mu)^2\}$ for an arbitrary distribution $\mathcal{N}(\mu, \sigma^2)$.
Hint: Apply integration by parts.

A.29. *Asymptotic normality.* For an estimator of your choice, show empirically that its distribution approaches normality as the sample size increases. Hint: Conduct separate simulations of the estimator for samples of sizes 10, 30, 100, 300, 1000, or similar, and draw the empirical distributions. Each simulation should be based on the same number of replications.

A.30. Derive the moments $\mathrm{E}\left(X^k\right)$ for X with distribution $\mathcal{U}(0,1)$. Confirm that

$$-\log\left\{\mathrm{E}(X^k)\right\} < \mathrm{E}\left\{-\log(X^k)\right\}$$

both analytically and by simulations. Check that

$$\mathrm{var}\left(X^k\right) = \frac{k^2}{(k+1)^2(2k+1)}.$$

Derive an expression for $\mathrm{E}\{X^k - 1/(k+1)\}^3$.

A.31. Check the expressions for the expectations and variances of the beta and gamma distributions given in Section A.12. Prove the identity

$$\mathrm{E}\left\{(X-\mu)^3\right\} = \mathrm{E}\left(X^3\right) - 3\mu\,\mathrm{var}(X) - \mu^3$$

for any distribution with expectation μ and finite third moment $\mathrm{E}(X^3)$.

A.32. Derive the probability in (A.6) and prove the statements about the modes of binomial distributions made in Section A.13.
Hint: Consider the ratios of $\mathrm{P}(X = k)/\mathrm{P}(X = k+1)$ for integers k and variable X with binomial distribution.

A.33. Prove that for every fixed integer k the probability $\mathrm{P}(X = k\,;\,n,p)$ for a binomial variable $\mathcal{B}(n,p)$ converges to the probability $\mathrm{P}(Y = k;\lambda)$ for a Poisson-distributed variable when n and p are such that $np_n \to \lambda$ as $n \to \infty$.

A.34. Devise a way of drawing a random sample from a binomial distribution using a source of independent draws from a uniform distribution.

Describe how a random sample from a discrete uniform distribution could be generated using a source of independent draws from the standard uniform distribution. How about a random sample from a multinomial distribution?

A.35. Show that for an exponentially distributed variable X, its conditional distribution given that $X > t$ is also exponential for every real constant t. Show that no binomial distribution $\mathcal{B}(n,p)$ with $n > 2$ has this property for any $k < n$. What about the geometric distributions?

A.36. Table A.6 gives the conditional probabilities $\mathrm{P}(X_1 = k\,|\,X_2 = h)$ for $h = 0,1,\ldots,9$. Marginally, X_2 has the binomial distribution $\mathcal{B}(9,0.4)$. Find the marginal distribution of X_1. Construct the table of conditional probabilities $\mathrm{P}(X_2 = h\,|\,X_1 = k)$.
Note: This exercise is intended not for pencil and paper but for computer programming.

Table A.6. The conditional distributions of X_1 given values of X_2. The entries of the table are $P(X_1 = k \mid X_2 = h)$, $h = 0, 1, \ldots, 9$ and $k = 0, 1, 2$.

					X_2					
X_1	0	1	2	3	4	5	6	7	8	9
0	0.70	0.60	0.55	0.50	0.40	0.40	0.35	0.30	0.25	0.15
1	0.20	0.20	0.20	0.20	0.25	0.30	0.35	0.40	0.40	0.45
2	0.10	0.20	0.25	0.30	0.35	0.30	0.30	0.30	0.35	0.40

A.37. Show that independence is maintained by transformations. That is, if X_1 and X_2 are independent, then so are $g_1(X_1)$ and $g_2(X_2)$ for any two functions g_1 and g_2. Show by example that the converse does not apply. That is, find transformations g_1 and g_2 and variables X_1 and X_2 such that X_1 and X_2 are not independent, but $g_1(X_1)$ are $g_2(X_2)$ are.
Hint: Focus on discrete variables with few categories.

A.38. Explore the variety of distributions that can be generated as mixtures of two or three univariate normal distributions. Write a programme for plotting the densities of such distributions and execute it for a range of trinomial probabilities (p_1, p_2, p_3), expectations (μ_1, μ_2, μ_3), and variances $(\sigma_1^2, \sigma_2^2, \sigma_3^2)$. Explain why no generality is lost by setting $\mu_1 = 0$ and $\sigma_1^2 = 1$. Present the conditional and the mixture densities in a suitable graph.

A.39. For a discrete mixture of a set of continuous distributions with densities $f_1, f_2, \ldots, f_K$, derive the conditional distribution of the category given the realised value of the mixture.

A.40. Find a class of distributions that are closed with respect to mixing. That is, if K distributions belong to this class, then so does their finite mixture with any multinomial distribution.

A.41. Revise the following topics: matrix calculus, including inverse and determinant; properties of (symmetric) positive and nonnegative definite matrices; and eigenvalue and other decompositions.

A.42. Show that if variable X is a mixture of variables $X_1, \ldots, X_K$, each of them with finite variance, then

$$E(X) = \sum_{k=1}^{K} p_k \, E(X_k) \, ,$$

$$\text{cov}(X, X_k) = p_k \, \text{var}(X_k) \, ,$$

$$\text{var}(X) = \sum_{k=1}^{K} p_k \left[\text{var}(X_k) + \{E(X_k)\}^2 \right] - \{E(X)\}^2,$$

where p_k is the probability of category k.

A.43. Derive the covariance and correlation of a pair of indicators I_k and I_h in a multinomial distribution. The indicator for category k is defined as $I_k = 1$ if component k is realised and $I_k = 0$ otherwise.

A.44. Derive the distributions of the sum and product of two independent uniformly distributed variables. Check your results by simulations.

A.45. Suppose a set of identically distributed variables $X_1, X_2, \ldots, X_K$ is such that each pair of them has the same correlation $\rho = \text{cor}(X_{k_1}, X_{k_2})$. Find the highest lower bound for ρ.
Hint: Consider the variance of the sample mean.
Relate this result to the correlation of the K-nomial distribution with equal probabilities $1/K$.

A.46. Construct a symmetric matrix with unities on its diagonal and all other entries in the range $(-1, 1)$ that is not a correlation matrix. Interpret this matrix as an example that its symmetry and all correlations in the range $[-1, 1]$ are not sufficient for it to be a variance matrix.

A.47. Compare the regressions $\text{E}(X \mid Y)$ and $\text{E}(Y \mid X)$ for a vector (X, Y) with bivariate normal distribution and relate them to the correlation $\text{cor}(X, Y)$. Explain why the product of the regression slopes is not equal to unity when the two variables are not perfectly correlated.

A.48. Explore how the regression $\text{E}(Y \mid X)$ for a vector (X, Y) with bivariate normal distribution is altered when Y is replaced by $Y + \xi$, where $\xi \sim \mathcal{N}(0, \sigma^2)$ is independent of of both X and Y. What change is brought about by replacing X with $X + \xi$?

A.49. Suppose (C_L, C_H) is an honest confidence interval for a population quantity μ. Find honest confidence intervals for $\exp(\mu)$ and μ^2. Discuss the advantages and drawbacks of constructing confidence intervals for σ^2, $\log(\sigma)$, and $\sqrt{\sigma}$ for a population variance σ^2.

References

1. Aitkin, M., Anderson, D. A., Hinde, J. P., and Francis, B. J.: *Statistical Modelling in GLIM*, 2nd ed. Oxford University Press, Oxford (2003)
2. Aitkin, M., and Longford, N. T.: Statistical modelling issues in school effectiveness studies. *Journal of the Royal Statistical Society* Series A **149**, 1–43 (1986)
3. Akaike, H.: A new look at statistical model identification. *IEEE Transactions on Automatic Control* AU–**19**, 716–722 (1974)
4. Armitage, P.: *Statistical Methods in Medical Research*. Blackwell, Oxford (1971)
5. Bayes, T.: An essay towards solving a problem in the doctrine of chances. *Philosophical Transactions of the Royal Society*, 330–418 (1763)
6. Benjamini, Y., and Hochberg, Y.: Controlling the false discovery rate: a practical and powerful approach to multiple testing. *Journal of the Royal Statistical Society* Series B **57**, 289–300 (1995)
7. Berger, J. O.: *Statistical Decision Theory and Bayesian Analysis*, 2nd ed. Springer-Verlag, New York (1985)
8. Bernardo, J. M., and Smith, A. F. M.: *Bayesian Theory*. Wiley, New York (1994)
9. Bird, S. M. (Chair of the Working Party), Cox, D. R., Farewell, V. T., Goldstein, H., Holt, D., Smith, P. C.: Performance indicators: good, bad, and ugly. *Journal of the Royal Statistical Society* Series A **168**, 1–27 (2005)
10. Box, G. E. P., and Tiao, G. C.: *Bayesian Inference in Statistical Analysis*. Wiley, New York (1973)
11. Breslow, N.: Extra-Poisson variation in log-linear models. *Applied Statistics* **33**, 38–44 (1984)
12. Breslow, N., and Clayton, D. G.: Approximate inference in generalized linear models. *Journal of the American Statistical Association* **88**, 9–25 (1993)
13. Bryk, A. S., and Raudenbush, S. W.: *Hierarchical Linear Models: Applications and Data Analysis Methods*. Sage, Newbury Park, CA (1992)
14. van Buuren, S., Boshuizen, H. C., and Knook, D. L.: Multiple imputation of missing blood pressure covariates in survival analysis. *Statistics in Medicine* **18**, 681–694 (1999)
15. Carroll, R. J., Ruppert, D., and Stefanski, L. A.: *Measurement Error in Nonlinear Models*. Chapman and Hall, London (1995)

16. Cassella, G., and George, E. I.: Explaining the Gibbs sampler. *The American Statistician* **46**, 167–174 (1992)
17. Chatfield, C.: *The Analysis of Time Series: An Introduction*, 6th ed. Chapman and Hall/CRC, Boca Raton (2004)
18. Chow, S. C., and Liu, J. P.: *Design and Analysis of Bioequivalence and Bioavailability Studies*. Marcel Dekker, New York (1992)
19. Cochran, W. G.: The planning of observational studies of human populations. *Journal of the Royal Statistical Society* Series A **128**, 134–155 (1965)
20. Cochran, W. G.: *Sampling Techniques*, 3rd ed. Wiley, New York (1977)
21. Cochran, W. G., and Cox, G.: *Experimental Designs*. Wiley, New York (1957)
22. Cochran, W. G., and Rubin, D. B.: Controlling bias in observational studies: a review. *Sankya* A **35**, 417–446 (1973)
23. Cook, J. R., and Stefanski, L. A.: A simulation extrapolation method for parametric measurement error models. *Journal of the American Statistical Association* **89**, 1314–1328 (1995)
24. Copas, J. B., and Shi, J. Q.: A sensitivity analysis for publication bias in systematic reviews. *Statistical Methods in Medical Research* **10**, 1–15 (2001)
25. Cox, D. R.: *Planning of Experiments*. Wiley, New York (1958)
26. Cox, D. R.: Regression models and life tables. *Journal of the Royal Statistical Society* Series B **34**, 187–220 (1972)
27. Cox, D. R., and Hinkley, D. V.: *Theoretical Statistics*. Chapman and Hall, London (1974)
28. Cox, D. R., and Oakes, D.: *Analysis of Survival Data*. Chapman and Hall, London (1984)
29. Cronbach, L. J., Gleser, G. C., Nanda, H., and Rajaratnam, N.: *Dependability of Behavioral Measurements: Theory of Generalizability of Scores and Profiles*. Wiley, New York (1972)
30. Crowder, M. J., and Hand, D. J.: *Analysis of Repeated Measures*. Chapman and Hall, London (1990)
31. Davidian, M., and Giltinan, D. M.: *Nonlinear Models for Repeated Measurement Data*. Chapman and Hall, London (1995)
32. DeGroot, M. H.: *Optimal Statistical Decisions*. McGraw-Hill, New York (1970)
33. Dempster, A. P., Laird, N. M., and Rubin, D. B.: Maximum likelihood for incomplete data via the EM algorithm. *Journal of the Royal Statistical Society* Series B **39**, 1–38 (1977)
34. Dempster, A. P., Rubin, D. B., and Tsutakawa, R. K.: Estimation in covariance component models. *Journal of the American Statistical Association* **76**, 341–353 (1981)
35. Dennis, J. E. Jr., and Schnabel, R. B.: *Numerical Methods for Unconstrained Optimization and Nonlinear Equations*. Prentice-Hall, Englewood Cliffs, NJ (1983)
36. DerSimonian, R., and Laird, N. M.: Meta-analysis in clinical trials. *Controlled Clinical Trials* **7**, 177–188 (1986)
37. Diggle, P. J., Heagerty, P., Liang, K.-Y., and Zeger, S. L.: *Analysis of Longitudinal Data*, 2nd ed. Oxford University Press, Oxford (2002)
38. Dobson, A.: *An Introduction to Generalized Linear Models*, 2nd ed. Chapman and Hall/CRC, London (2001)

39. Draper, D., and Gittoes, M.: Statistical analysis of performance indicators in UK higher education. *Journal of the Royal Statistical Society* Series A **167**, 449–474 (2004)

40. DuMouchel, W. H., and Harris, J. E.: Bayes methods for combining results of cancer studies in humans and other species. *Journal of the American Statistical Association* **78**, 293–315 (1983)

41. Duval, S., and Tweedie, R.: Trim and fill: a simple funnel-plot-based method of testing and adjusting for publication bias in meta-analysis. *Biometrics* **56**, 455–463 (2000)

42. Efron, B., and Morris, C.: Limiting the risk of Bayes and empirical Bayes estimators—part I: the Bayes case. *Journal of the American Statistical Association* **66**, 807–815 (1971)

43. Efron, B., and Morris, C.: Limiting the risk of Bayes and empirical Bayes estimators—part II: the empirical Bayes case. *Journal of the American Statistical Association* **67**, 130–139 (1972)

44. Efron, B., and Morris, C.: Stein's estimation rule and its competitors—an empirical Bayes approach. *Journal of the American Statistical Association* **68**, 117–130 (1973)

45. Efron, B., and Morris, C.: Data analysis using Stein's estimator and its generalizations. *Journal of the American Statistical Association* **70**, 311–319 (1975)

46. Efron, B., and Tibshirani, R.: *An Introduction to the Bootstrap*. Chapman and Hall, London (1993)

47. Eisenhart, C.: Effect of rounding or grouping data. In: Eisenhart, C., Hastay, M. W., and Wallis, W. A. (eds.) *Selected Techniques of Statistical Analysis*. McGraw-Hill, New York (1947)

48. Fay, R. A., and Herriot, R. E.: Estimates of income for small places: an application of James-Stein procedures to census data. *Journal of the American Statistical Association* **74**, 269–277 (1979)

49. Firth, D., and Harris, I. R.: Quasi-likelihood for multiplicative random effects. *Biometrika* **78**, 545–555 (1991)

50. Fisher, R. A.: *The Design of Experiments*, 2nd ed. Oliver and Boyd, London (1949)

51. Fleiss, J. L.: *The Design and Analysis of Clinical Experiments*. Wiley, New York (1986)

52. Frangakis, C., and Rubin, D. B.: Principal stratification in causal inference. *Biometrics* **58**, 21–29 (2002)

53. Freeman, P. R.: The performance of the two-stage analysis of two-treatment cross-over designs. *Statistics in Medicine* **8**, 1421–1432 (1989)

54. Fuller, W. A.: *Measurement Error Models*. Wiley, New York (1987)

55. Gelfand, A. E., and Smith, A. F. M.: Sampling-based approaches to calculating marginal densities. *Journal of the American Statistical Association* **85**, 398–409 (1990)

56. Gelman, A., Carlin, J. B., Stern, H., and Rubin, D. B.: *Bayesian Data Analysis*, 2nd ed. Chapman and Hall/CRC, New York (2003)

57. Gilks, W. R., Richardson, S., and Spiegelhalter, D. (eds.): *Practical Markov Chain Monte Carlo*. Chapman and Hall, New York (1996)

58. Gill, P. E., Murray, W., and Wright, M. H.: *Practical Optimization*. Academic Press, New York (1981)

59. Glass, G.: Primary, secondary, and meta-analysis of research. *Educational Researcher* **5**, 3–8 (1976)

462   References

60. Goldstein, H.: *Multilevel Statistical Models*, 3rd ed. Edward Arnold, London (2003)
61. Goldstein, H., and Healy, M. J. R.: The graphical presentation of a collection of means. *Journal of the Royal Statistical Society* Series A **158**, 175–177 (1995)
62. Goldstein, H., and Spiegelhalter, D. J.: League tables and their limitations: statistical issues in comparisons of institutional performance. *Journal of the Royal Statistical Society* Series A **159**, 385–443 (1996)
63. Good, I. J.: *The Estimation of Probabilities: An Essay on Modern Bayesian Methods*. MIT Press, Cambridge, MA (1965)
64. Greenland, S.: Invited commentary: a critical look at some popular meta-analytic methods. *American Journal of Epidemiology* **135**, 1301–1309 (1994)
65. Greenland, S.: Multiple-bias modelling for analysis of observational data. *Journal of the Royal Statistical Society* Series A **168**, 267–306 (2005)
66. Hartigan, J. A.: *Bayes Theory*. Springer-Verlag, New York (1983)
67. Hartley, H. O., and Rao, J. N. K.: Maximum likelihood estimation for the mixed analysis of variance model. *Biometrika* **54**, 93–108 (1967)
68. Harvey, A. C.: *Time Series Models*, 2nd ed. Harvester Wheatsheaf, London (1993)
69. Harville, D. A.: Bayesian inference for variance components using only error contrasts. *Journal of the American Statistical Association* **69**, 383–385 (1974)
70. Harville, D. A.: *Matrix Algebra from a Statistician's Perspective*. Springer-Verlag, New York (1997)
71. Healy, M. J., and Westmacott, M.: Missing values in experiments analyzed on automatic computers. *Applied Statistics* **5**, 203–206 (1956)
72. Hedges, L. V., and Olkin, I.: *Statistical Methods for Meta-Analysis*. Academic Press, Orlando (1985)
73. Heitjan, D. F.: Inference from grouped continuous data: a review. *Statistical Science* **4**, 164–183 (1989)
74. Heitjan, D. F., and Little, R. J. A.: Multiple imputation for the Fatal Accident Reporting System. *Applied Statistics* **40**, 13–29 (1991)
75. Heitjan, D. F., and Rubin, D. B.: Inference from coarse data via multiple imputation with application to age heaping. *Journal of the American Statistical Association* **85**, 304–314 (1990)
76. Henderson, C. R.: Estimation of variance and covariance components. *Biometrics* **9**, 226–252 (1953)
77. Henderson, C. R.: *Applications of Linear Models in Animal Breeding*. University of Guelph, Canada (1984)
78. Hochberg, Y., and Tamhane, A.: *Multiple Comparison Procedures*. Wiley, New York (1987)
79. Hoeting, J., Madigan, D., Raftery, A. E., and Volinsky, C. T.: Bayesian model averaging: a tutorial. *Statistical Science* **14**, 381–417 (1998)
80. Holt, D., and Smith, T. F. M.: Post-stratification. *Journal of the Royal Statistical Society* Series A **142**, 33–46 (1979)
81. Holland, P. W.: Statistics and causal inference. *Journal of the American Statistical Association* **81**, 945–970 (1986)
82. Horton, N. J., and Kleinman, K. P.: Much ado about nothing: a comparison of missing data methods and software to fit incomplete data regression models. *The American Statistician* **61** 79–90 (2007)

83. Horvitz, D. G., and Thompson, D. J. A generalization of sampling without replacement from a finite universe. *Journal of the American Statistical Association* **47**, 663–685 (1952)

84. Hosmer, D. W., and Lemeshow, S.: *Applied Logistic Regression.* Wiley, New York (1989)

85. Huggins, R. M., and Loesch, D. Z.: On the analysis of mixed longitudinal growth data. *Biometrics* **54**, 583–595 (1998)

86. Jackson, D., Copas, J., and Sutton, A. J.: Modelling reporting bias: the operative mortality rate for ruptured abdominal aortic aneurysm repair. *Journal of the Royal Statistical Society* Series A **168**, 737–752 (2005)

87. Jamshidian, M., and Jennrich, R. I.: Acceleration of the EM algorithm by using quasi-Newton methods. *Journal of the Royal Statistical Society* Series B **59**, 569–587 (1997)

88. Jeffreys, H.: *Theory of Probability*, 3rd ed. Oxford University Press, New York (1961)

89. Jennrich, R. I., and Schluchter, M. D.: Unbalanced repeated measures models with structured covariance matrices. *Biometrics* **42**, 805–820 (1986)

90. Jones, B., and Kenward, M. G.: *Design and Analysis of Cross-over Trials.* Chapman and Hall, London (1989)

91. Kalbfleisch, J. D., and Prentice, R. L.: *The Statistical Analysis of Failure Time Data.* Wiley, New York (1980)

92. Kass, R. E., and Raftery, A. E.: Bayes factors and model uncertainty. *Journal of the American Statistical Association* **90**, 773–795 (1995)

93. Kass, R. E., and Steffey, D.: Approximate Bayesian inference in conditionally independent hierarchical models (parametric empirical Bayes models). *Journal of the American Statistical Association* **84**, 717–726 (1989)

94. Kennedy, W. J. Jr., and Gentle, J. E.: *Statistical Computing.* Marcel Dekker, New York (1980)

95. Kish, L.: *Survey Sampling.* Wiley, New York (1965)

96. Kish, L.: *Statistical Design for Research.* Wiley, New York (1987)

97. Laird, N. M., and Ware, J. H.: Random-effects models for longitudinal data. *Biometrics* **38**, 963–974 (1982)

98. Lange, K.: *Numerical Analysis for Statisticians.* Springer-Verlag, New York (1999)

99. Lee, Y., and Nelder, J. A.: Hierarchical generalized linear models. *Journal of the Royal Statistical Society* Series B **58**, 619–678 (1996)

100. Lee, Y., and Nelder, J. A.: Hierarchical generalized linear models: a synthesis of generalized linear models, random-effect models and structured dispersions. *Biometrika* **88**, 987–1006 (2001)

101. Liang, K.-Y., and Zeger, S. L.: Longitudinal data analysis using generalized linear models. *Biometrika* **73**, 13–22 (1986)

102. Lindley, D. V.: *Introduction to Probability and Statistics from a Bayesian Viewpoint*, two volumes. Cambridge University Press, New York (1965)

103. Lindley, D. V.: Decision analysis and bioequivalence trials. *Statistical Science* **13**, 136–141 (1998)

104. Lindsey, J. K.: *Models for Repeated Measurements.* Oxford University Press, Oxford (1993)

105. Lindstrom, M. J., and Bates, D. M.: Nonlinear mixed effects models for repeated measures data. *Biometrics* **46**, 673–687 (1988)

106. Linn, R. L., and Hastings, C. N.: A meta-analysis of the validity of predictors of performance in law school. *Journal of Educational Measurement* **21**, 245–259 (1984)

107. Little, R. J. A.: Regression with missing X's: a review. *Journal of the American Statistical Association* **87**, 1227–1237 (1992)

108. Little, R. J. A.: Pattern-mixture models for multivariate incomplete data. *Journal of the American Statistical Association* **88**, 125–134 (1993)

109. Little, R. J. A.: Modelling the drop-out mechanism in repeated-measures studies. *Journal of the American Statistical Association* **90**, 1112–1121 (1995)

110. Little, R. J. A., and Rubin, D. B.: *Statistical Analysis with Missing Data*, 2nd ed. Wiley, New York (2002)

111. Little, R. J. A., and Yau, L.: Intent-to-treat analysis for longitudinal studies with drop-outs. *Biometrics* **52**, 1324–1333 (1996)

112. Longford, N. T.: A fast scoring algorithm for maximum likelihood estimation in unbalanced mixed models with nested random effects. *Biometrika* **74**, 817–827 (1987)

113. Longford, N. T.: *Random Coefficient Models*. Oxford University Press, Oxford (1993)

114. Longford, N. T.: Logistic regression with random coefficients. *Computational Statistics and Data Analysis* **17**, 1–15 (1994)

115. Longford, N. T.: *Models for Uncertainty in Educational Testing*. Springer-Verlag, New York (1995)

116. Longford, N. T.: Multivariate shrinkage estimation of small area means and proportions. *Journal of the Royal Statistical Society* Series A **162**, 227–245 (1999)

117. Longford, N. T.: Selection bias and treatment heterogeneity in clinical trials. *Statistics in Medicine* **18**, 1467–1474 (1999)

118. Longford, N. T.: An alternative definition of individual bioequivalence. *Statistica Neerlandica* **54**, 14–36 (2000)

119. Longford, N. T.: Synthetic estimators with moderating influence: carryover in crossover trials revisited. *Statistics in Medicine* **20**, 3189–3203 (2001)

120. Longford, N. T.: An alternative to model selection in ordinary regression. *Statistics and Computing* **13**, 67–80 (2003)

121. Longford, N. T.: Editorial: Model selection and efficiency: is 'Which model ...?' the right question? *Journal of the Royal Statistical Society* Series A **168**, 469–472 (2005)

122. Longford, N. T.: *Missing Data and Small-Area Estimation: Modern Analytical Equipment for the Survey Statistician*. Springer-Verlag, New York (2005)

123. Longford, N. T.: Correspondence: a comment on Jackson, Copas and Sutton (2005). *Journal of the Royal Statistical Society* Series A **169**, 647–648 (2006)

124. Longford, N. T.: On standard errors of model-based small-area estimators. *Survey Methodology* **33**, 69–79 (2007)

125. Longford, N. T., Ely, M., Hardy, R., and Wadsworth, M. E. J.: Handling missing data in diaries of alcohol consumption. *Journal of the Royal Statistical Society* Series A **163**, 381–402 (2000)

126. Longford, N. T., McCarthy, I., and Dowse, G.: Patterns of house price inflation in New Zealand. In: van Montfort, K., Oud, J., and Satorra, A.: *Longitudinal Models in the Behavioral and Related Sciences*, chapter 17, pp. 403–433. L. Erlbaum Associates, Mahwah, NJ (2007)

127. Longford, N. T., and Pittau, M. G.: Stability of household income in European countries in the 1990's. *Computational Statistics and Data Analysis* **51**, 1364–1383 (2006)

128. Longford, N. T., and Rubin, D. B.: Performance assessment and league tables: comparing like with like. Working paper No. 994, Department of Economics and Business Studies, University Pompeu Fabra, Barcelona, Spain (2006)

129. Longford, N. T., Tyrer, P., Nur, U. A. M., and Seivewright, H.: Analysis of a long-term study of neurotic disorder, with insight into the process of non-response. *Journal of the Royal Statistical Society* Series A **169**, 507–523 (2006)

130. Lord, F. M., and Novick, M.: *Statistical Theories of Mental Test Scores*. Addison-Wesley, Reading, MA (1968)

131. Louis, T. A.: Finding the observed information matrix when using the EM algorithm. *Journal of the Royal Statistical Society* Series B **44**, 226–233 (1982)

132. McCullagh, P., and Nelder, J. A.: *Generalized Linear Models*, 2nd ed. Chapman and Hall, London (1989)

133. McCulloch, C. E.: Maximum likelihood algorithms for generalized linear mixed models. *Journal of the American Statistical Association* **92**, 162–170 (1997)

134. McLachlan, G. J., and Krishnan, T.: *The EM Algorithm and Extensions*. Wiley, New York (1997)

135. Meijlijson, I.: A fast improvement to the EM algorithm on its own terms. *Journal of the Royal Statistical Society* Series B **51**, 127–138 (1989)

136. Meng, X.-L., and van Dyk, D.: The EM algorithm—an old folk-song sung to a fast new tune. *Journal of the Royal Statistical Society* Series B **59**, 511–567 (1997)

137. Nelder, J. A., and Pregibon, D.: An extended quasi-likelihood function. *Biometrika* **74**, 221–232 (1987)

138. Nelder, J. A., and Wedderburn, R. W. M.: Generalized linear models. *Journal of the Royal Statistical Society* Series A **135**, 370–384 (1972)

139. O'Hagan, A: Fractional Bayes factors and model comparison. *Journal of the Royal Statistical Society* Series B **57**, 99–138 (1995)

140. Olkin, I.: Meta-analysis: current issues in research synthesis. *Statistics in Medicine* **15**, 1253–1257 (1996)

141. Orchard, T., and Woodbury, M. A.: A missing information principle: theory and applications. In: *Proceedings of the 6th Berkeley Symposium on Mathematical Statistics and Probability*, Vol. 1., pp. 697–715. University of California, Berkeley (1972)

142. Patterson, H. D., and Thompson, R.: Recovery of inter-block information when block sizes are unequal. *Biometrika* **58**, 545–554 (1971)

143. Pawitan, Y.: *In All Likelihood: Statistical Modelling and Inference Using Likelihood*. Oxford University Press, Oxford (2001)

144. Pearl, J.: *Causality*. Cambridge University Press, New York (2000)

145. Piantadosi, S.: *Clinical Trials: A Methodological Perspective*. Wiley, New York (1997)

146. Pinheiro, J. C., and Bates, D. M.: *Mixed-Effects Models in* S *and* Splus. Springer-Verlag, New York (2000)

147. Pocock, S. J.: *Clinical Trials: A Practical Approach*. Wiley, Chichester, UK (1983)

148. Potthoff, R. F., Woodbury, M. A., and Manton, K. G.: 'Equivalent sample size' and 'equivalent degrees of freedom' refinements for inference using survey weights under superpopulation models. *Journal of the American Statistical Association* **87**, 383–396 (1992)

149. Prentice, R. L.: Surrogate end points in clinical trials: definitions and operational criteria. *Statistics in Medicine* **8**, 431–440 (1989)

150. Press, S. J.: *Subjective and Objective Bayesian Statistics: Principles, Models, and Applications*, 2nd ed. Wiley, New York (2003)

151. R Development Core Team: R: *A Language and Environment for Statistical Computing.* R Foundation for Statistical Computing, Vienna, Austria, 2006

152. Ramsay, J. O., and Silverman, B. W.: *Functional Data Analysis.* Springer-Verlag, New York (1997)

153. Rao, C. R.: *Linear Statistical Inference and Its Applications.* Wiley, New York (1973)

154. Rao, J. N. K.: *Small Area Estimation.* Wiley, New York (2003)

155. Raudenbush, S. W., and Bryk, A. S.: Empirical Bayes meta-analysis. *Journal of Educational Statistics* **10**, 75–98 (1985)

156. Rosenbaum, P. R.: *Observational Studies*, 2nd ed. Springer-Verlag, New York (2002)

157. Rubin, D. B.: Estimation of causal effects of treatments in randomized and nonrandomized studies. *Journal of Educational Psychology* **66**, 688–701 (1974)

158. Rubin, D. B.: Inference and missing data. *Biometrika* **63**, 581–592 (1976)

159. Rubin, D. B.: Using empirical Bayes techniques in the law school validity studies. *Journal of the American Statistical Association* **75**, 373–380 (1980)

160. Rubin, D. B.: Bayesianly justifiable and relevant frequency calculations for the applied statistician. *Annals of Statistics* **12**, 1151–1172 (1984)

161. Rubin, D. B.: Neyman (1923) and causal inference in experiments and observational studies. *Statistical Science* **5**, 472–480 (1990)

162. Rubin, D. B.: EM and beyond. *Psychometrika* **56**, 241–254 (1991)

163. Rubin, D. B.: Practical implications of modes of statistical inference for causal effects and the critical role of the assignment mechanism. *Biometrics* **46**, 1213–1234 (1991)

164. Rubin, D. B.: Multiple imputation after 18+ years. *Journal of the American Statistical Association* **91**, 473–489 (1996)

165. Rubin, D. B.: *Multiple Imputation for Nonresponse in Surveys*, 2nd ed. Wiley, New York (2002)

166. Rubin, D. B.: Causal inference using potential outcomes: design, modelling, decisions. 2004 Fisher Lecture. *Journal of the American Statistical Association* **100**, 322–331 (2005)

167. Rubin, D. B., and Schenker, N.: Multiple imputation in health-care databases: an overview and some applications. *Statistics in Medicine* **10**, 585–598 (1991)

168. Särndal, C.-E., Swensson, B., and Wretman, J.: *Model Assisted Survey Sampling.* Springer-Verlag, New York (1992)

169. Schafer, J. L.: *Analysis of Incomplete Multivariate Data.* Chapman and Hall, London (1996)

170. Schafer, J. L.: Multiple imputation: a primer. *Statistical Methods in Medical Research* **8**, 3–15 (1999)

171. Schall, R., and Luus, H. G.: On population and individual bioequivalence. *Statistics in Medicine* **12**, 1109–1124 (1993)

172. Scharfstein, D. O., Rotnitzky, A., and Robins, J. M.: Adjusting for nonignorable drop-out using semiparametric nonresponse models. *Journal of the American Statistical Association* **94**, 1096–1146 (1999)

173. Schenker, N., Treiman, D. J., and Weidmann, L.: Analyses of public use Decennial Census data with multiply imputed industry and occupation codes. *Applied Statistics* **42**, 545–556 (1990)

174. Schuirmann, D., J.: A comparison of two one-sided tests procedure and the power approach for assessing the equivalence of average bioavailability. *Journal of Pharmacokinetics and Biopharmaceutics* **15**, 657–680 (1987)

175. Schwartz, G.: Estimating the dimension of a model. *Annals of Statistics* **6**, 461–464 (1978)

176. Searle, S. R.: *Linear Models for Unbalanced Data.* Wiley, New York (1987)

177. Searle, S. R., Cassella, G., and McCulloch, C. E.: *Variance Components.* Wiley, New York (1992)

178. Seber, G. A. F.: *Linear Regression Analysis.* Wiley, New York (1977)

179. Senn, S. J.: *Cross-over Trials in Clinical Research.* Wiley, Chichester, UK (1993)

180. Senn, S. J.: *Statistical Issues in Drug Development.* Wiley, Chichester, UK (1997)

181. Sheiner, L. B.: Bioequivalence revisited. *Statistics in Medicine* **11**, 1777–1788 (1992)

182. Sheppard, W. F.: On the calculation of the most probable values of frequency constants for data arranged according to equidistant divisions of a scale. *Proceedings of the London Mathematical Society* **29**, 353–380 (1898)

183. Smith, A. F. M., and Roberts, G. O.: Bayesian computation via the Gibbs sampler and related Markov chain Monte Carlo methods. *Journal of the Royal Statistical Society* Series B **55**, 3–102 (1993)

184. Spiegelhalter, D. J.: Surgical audit: statistical lessons from Nightingale and Codman. *Journal of the Royal Statistical Society* Series A **162**, 45–58 (1999)

185. Spiegelhalter, D. J., Aylin, P., Best, N. G., Evans, S. J. W., and Murray, G. D.: Commissioned analysis of surgical performance by using routine data: lessons from the Bristol inquiry. *Journal of the Royal Statistical Society* Series A **165**, 1–31 (2002)

186. Strenio, J. F., Weisberg, H. I., and Bryk, A. S.: Empirical Bayes estimation of individual growth-curve parameters and their relationship to covariates. *Biometrics* **39**, 71–86 (1983)

187. Sutton, A. J., Abrams, K. R., Jones, D. R., and Sheldon, T. A.: *Methods for Meta-Analysis in Medical Research.* Wiley, Chichester, UK (2000)

188. Thall, P. F., and Vail, S. C.: Some covariance models for longitudinal count data with overdispersion. *Biometrics* **46**, 657–671 (1990)

189. Tanner, M. A.: *Tools for Statistical Inference: Methods for the Exploration of Posterior Distributions and Likelihood Functions*, 2nd ed. Springer-Verlag, New York (1993)

190. Tanner, M. A., and Wong, W. H.: The calculation of posterior distribution by data augmentation. *Journal of the American Statistical Association* **82**, 528–550 (1987)

191. Venables, W. N., and Ripley, B. D.: *Modern Applied Statistics with S-plus*, 4th ed. Springer-Verlag, New York, 2002

192. Verbeke, G., and Molenberghs, G.: *Linear Mixed Models for Longitudinal Data.* Springer-Verlag, New York (2000)

193. Wedderburn, R. W. M.: Quasi-likelihood functions, generalized linear models and the Gauss-Newton method. *Biometrika* **61**, 439–447 (1974)

194. Whitehead, J.: *The Design and Analysis of Sequential Clinical Trials*, 2nd ed. Wiley, Chichester, UK (1997)

195. Williams, D. A.: Extra-binomial variation in logistic linear models. *Applied Statistics* **31**, 144–148 (1982)

196. Wolter, K. M.: *Introduction to Variance Estimation.* Springer-Verlag, New York (1985)

197. Wu, C. F. J.: On convergence properties of the EM algorithm. *Annals of Statistics* **11**, 95–103 (1983)

198. Zeger, S. L., Liang, K.-Y., and Albert, P.: Models for longitudinal data: a generalized estimating equation approach. *Biometrics* **44**, 1049–1060 (1988)

Index

Springer Texts in Statistics

(continued from p. ii)

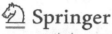
springer.com

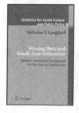

Missing Data and Small-Area Estimation

Nicholas T. Longford

This book develops methods for two key problems in the analysis of large-scale surveys: dealing with incomplete data and making inferences about sparsely represented subdomains. The presentation is committed to two particular methods, multiple imputation for missing data and multivariate composition for small-area estimation. The methods are presented as developments of established approaches by attending to their deficiencies. The general tone of the book is not "from theory to practice," but "from current practice to better practice."

2005. 360 pp. (Statistics for Social and Behavioral Sciences) Hardcover
ISBN 978-1-85233-760-5

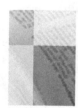

Correlated Data Analysis

Peter X-K. Song

This book presents some recent developments in correlated data analysis. It utilizes the class of dispersion models as marginal components in the formulation of joint models for correlated data. This enables the book to handle a broader range of data types than those analyzed by traditional generalized linear models. One example is correlated angular data. Various real-world data examples, numerical illustrations and software usage tips are presented throughout the book.

2007. 365 pp. (Springer Series in Statistics) Hardcover
ISBN 978-0-387-71392-2

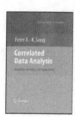

Introduction to Applied Bayesian Statistics and Estimation for Social Scientists

Scott M. Lynch

Introduction to Applied Bayesian Statistics and Estimation for Social Scientists covers the complete process of Bayesian statistical analysis in great detail from the development of a model through the process of making statistical inference. The key feature of this book is that it covers models that are most commonly used in social science research including the linear re gression model, generalized linear models, hierarchical models, and multivariate regression models and it thoroughl y develops each real-data example in painstaking detail.

2007. 400 pp. (Statistics for Social and Behavioral Sciences) Hardcover
ISBN 978-0-387-71264-2

Easy Ways to Order ▶ Call: Toll-Free 1-800-SPRINGER • E-mail: orders-ny@springer.com • Write: Springer, Dept. S8113, PO Box 2485, Secaucus, NJ 07096-2485 • Visit: Your local scientific bookstore or urge your librarian to order.